HAMILTON AND HARDY'S
INDUSTRIAL TOXICOLOGY

FOURTH EDITION

HAMILTON AND HARDY'S
INDUSTRIAL TOXICOLOGY

FOURTH EDITION

Revised by
Asher J. Finkel

John Wright • PSG Inc
Boston   Bristol   London
1983

Library of Congress Cataloging in Publication Data
Main entry under title:

Hamilton and Hardy's industrial toxicology.

Hamilton, Alice, 1869–1970.
Hamilton and Hardy's industrial toxicology.

    Rev. ed. of: Industrial toxicology. 2nd ed.,
rev. and enl. [1949]
    Bibliography: p.
    Includes index.
    1. Industrial toxicology. I. Hardy, Harriet Louise,
1906–   II. Finkel, Asher Joseph, 1915–
III. Title. IV. Title: Industrial toxicology.
[DNLM: 1. Occupational medicine. 2. Poisons. WA 465
H217h]
RA1229.H35 1982   615.9′02   82-8613
ISBN 0-7236-7027-7   AACR2

Published by:
John Wright • PSG Inc, 545 Great Road, Littleton,
Massachusetts 01460, U.S.A.
John Wright & Sons Ltd, 823–825 Bath Road,
Bristol BS4 5NU, England

Printed in the United States of America.

International Standard Book Number: 0-7236-7027-7

Library of Congress Catalog Card Number: 82-8613

ABOUT THE AUTHORS

Asher J. Finkel, M.D., Ph.D., F.A.C.P., FA.A.O.M.

Former Director, Health Division, Argonne National
Laboratory, Argonne, Illinois
Former Group Vice-President for Scientific Affairs,
American Medical Association, Chicago, Illinois

Alice Hamilton, M.D.

Late Assistant Professor Emerita of Industrial Medicine,
Harvard School of Public Health, Boston, Massachusetts

Harriet L. Hardy, M.D., F.A.C.P., F.A.A.O.M.

Clinical Professor of Occupational Medicine Emerita,
Department of Preventive Medicine, Harvard Medical
School, Boston, Massachusetts
Honorary Consultant, Massachusetts General Hospital,
Boston, Massachusetts
Assistant Medical Director, Occupational Medical Service
(Retired), Massachusetts Institute of Technology,
Cambridge, Massachusetts

TABLE OF CONTENTS

FOREWORD

This fourth edition of *Hamilton and Hardy's Industrial Toxicology,* prepared as were the earlier editions to alert and excite students of medicine to the harmful effects of industrialization in the United States, has a history.

In the early years of the United States, after the signing of the Declaration of Independence, this vast continent was used chiefly for agriculture, while lands settled earlier in Europe and Asia had years before begun and developed a wide variety of trades and arts. When America proved to have land with mineral ores and coal, men with ambition from here and abroad moved to develop these resources. Likewise our countrymen, seeking riches and also the cultural and trade advantages of the Old World, traveled abroad. And so manufacturing and trades of all kinds, together with flourishing of the arts, took root. The great wars of the French and American Revolution and the Civil War of the mid-19th century had finally burned out, allowing a burst of industrial activity in the United States.

Dr. Alice Hamilton in her autobiography describes the state of industry in America in the late 19th and early 20th centuries as applied to the health of the worker.* Most laborers were immigrants, largely of peasant stock, who were used to feudalism as a way of life. Since, at the date she began her work (1910), there was no recognizable field of industrial medicine except that of necessary traumatic surgery for the many accidents in mine and mill, the physician of the period lacked any knowledge of the harmful effects of industrial poisons. A gentle, highly educated upbringing gave Dr. Alice the vision and courage to combine her medical training with her own charity. Thus she plunged single-handed into the first Illinois Lead Survey. After 30-odd years of field work, advising, writing, and teaching of occupational medicine at Harvard, in industry, and to labor and its lawyers, Dr. Alice had accomplished much for the prevention of workers' injury and illness and for their freedom to organize, and had brought a sense of responsibility to plant managers.

*Hamilton, A: *Exploring the Dangerous Trades.* Boston, Little, Brown, 1943.

In 1946, at the time of my identification of beryllium as the most likely cause of the epidemic of illness in the fluorescent lighting industry, Dr. Hamilton asked me to serve as junior author in producing a second edition of her text, *Industrial Toxicology,* originally published in 1929. I accepted this invitation with much advantage to myself by study in the Boston Medical Library and by spending weekends at Dr. Hamilton's home in Connecticut. Here she lived with her sister, Miss Margaret, exheadmistress of an excellent girls' school, and Miss Clara, a friend who had traveled far and wide. As my own travel and writing developed, the four of us became a small, exciting teaching and learning seminar. It was only the deaths of Miss Clara at the age of 92, Miss Margaret at 98, and Dr. Alice at 103 that halted this seminar in 1970.

The present edition is the fourth; the third, appearing in 1974, I wrote with the aid of an engineer, a chemist, and a radiation physicist who were colleagues experienced in the field now called occupational or environmental hygiene or medicine.

What is the status of occupational medicine in 1982 as compared to what my senior wrote 40 years ago of her experience in the field of worker illness? My years of work in occupational medicine (1945–1972) have been as clinical as I could make them and still be able to boast that my working philosophy was basically prevention of job-related disease. Thus Dr. Hamilton and I held similar views and methods of work in this field new to the medical profession.

I found many workers educated and devoted to liberal, or even radical, ideas for the labor movement. Most wanted country-wide unionization with the right to strike. One segment of labor wanted to become politically active, running for office as union members. Some union officials in this period were corrupt; some, perhaps most, unions were vigorously anticommunist. Perhaps the managerial establishment in America set the pace and example for the organized worker in the mid-20th century. These statements about union members I have found true also of executives of our industries. Both were free in the American sense, and both wanted all the good things of life—which they thought could be achieved by hard work and hard bargaining.

And what of the physicians and nurses in industry since Dr. Hamilton first worked in the field of identifying and controlling work-related disease and injury? The report is a mixture of good, less good, and some evil. Since United States' industry is so vast and so varied in size and character of work, the patterns of health services are numerous. First, the "bad." The profit motive dominates too many decisions, and often the medical budget is handled by the same officials responsible for workmen's compensation and, in large companies, legal support. Great secrecy because of trade competition may be required of the medical team. I have known plant doctors who have testified in a compensation court against worker-patients whom they had treated. A disturbing, growing practice is that of appointing or hiring physicians as corporate—not patient—doctors who claim publicly that their loyalty is to the company, not to the worker. Some unions have their own physicians for advice in combating this practice.

Less good service is provided by plant workers who have had first aid courses, nurses who often have had no training in industrial illness, and part-time doctors, many with specialties in other fields, such as dermatology or obstetrics.

There are, indeed, in some United States' industries well-trained occupational health teams provided with appropriate support for the physician and nurse, such as engineer, chemist, biologist, and radiation health officer as required.

Government has done much in this field, beginning with a small branch of the United States Public Health Service in the First World War, expanded greatly in the Second World War, followed by the large, federally funded Occupational Safety and Health Administration under the Department of Labor for enforcement and the National Institute of Occupational Safety and Health to identify and study industrial disease.

Finally, there are in my judgment two serious gaps in current study and control of man-made disease. Conclusions and decisions used by government and industry are based on small animal study. No one can dispute the value of understanding metabolic pathways and basic mechanisms of the way mammals handle foreign materials. However, decisions about human illness based only on dosages and experiments in animals are not necessarily valid ones. The second, quite tragic fact is that undergraduate medical colleges or teaching hospitals with rare exception fail to include occupational medicine in the curriculum.

This fourth edition of *Hamilton and Hardy's Industrial Toxicology,* revised and updated by Dr. Asher J. Finkel, is intended to help close the gap. Dr. Finkel is unusually well equipped for this assignment because of his active participation in occupational medicine, research with small animals, and an unusual facility in writing.

Harriet L. Hardy, M.D.
Concord, Massachusetts
January 1982

PREFACE

The preface, wrote Alfred J. Lotka in his *Elements of Physical Biology* (1925), is written last, placed first, and read least. Nevertheless, I feel that I must make a brief statement describing my purposes and intentions in preparing this volume. It was a great honor indeed when Dr. Harriet L. Hardy invited me to prepare a new edition of the well-known Hamilton/Hardy *Industrial Toxicology*, a task that has occupied most of my free time since 1977. In now presenting this new edition to the public, I should explain that in the face of an enormous world literature there was no intention of making the work encyclopedic in scope and that consequently there are many untouched subjects as well as uncited papers. As with the previous editions, the emphasis continues to be mainly clinical. I did want to make the book something of an introduction both to the older medical literature as well as to the more recent publications. To this end I have not restricted the cited references to those in English, although these predominate. Nor have I written an entirely new book. Perceptive and knowledgeable readers will readily note the extent to which I have used and built upon the previous edition. For the opportunity to do this I am most grateful since in utilizing the earlier work of Drs. Hamilton and Hardy, and of their colleagues, I have truly stood on the shoulders of some very accomplished persons.

I want to express my gratitude to the reference librarians of the Archives-Library of the American Medical Association, in particular to Miss Mary Jo Dwyer, for their superb help in unraveling knotty bibliographic problems. Mrs. Rebecca Smith of the Biology Library, Argonne National Laboratory, was always most gracious and helpful. My profound thanks go to Dr. Frank N. Paparello, of John Wright • PSG Inc, for his encouragement and, above all, for his patience in the face of a tardy performance on my part in delivering a completed typescript.

I will be delighted and appreciative to hear from readers who will undoubtedly catch errors of fact, interpretation, or citation. I do hope that the present edition will be sufficiently worthy to stand alongside its predecessors.

My efforts in preparing this edition are dedicated to the memory of my parents, Morris Finkel, M.D., and Henrietta Israelson Finkel.

A.J.F.
Chicago
January 1982

From the Previous Edition

It was the privilege of HLH to serve as junior in the preparation of Dr. Alice Hamilton's volume, *Industrial Toxicology,* for its second edition in 1949. The intention of this third volume is to help practitioners and to attract medical students and physicians in the field of occupational disease by combining Dr. Hamilton's pioneer wisdom with current industrial hygiene practice and the authors' clinical experience as internists especially interested in industrial illness. To include every reported occupational insult and the reaction to it would make this book unwieldy. This volume does not attempt to include a description of every industrial operation and of each use of a potentially hazardous material. Aside from the problem of size of such an undertaking, it is a fact that, during the period this book is being printed, technical innovations will be introduced that may result in new hazards to workers. The plan, therefore, has been that this edition serve both as a ready reference and a point of view toward job-related disease as etiology, an often neglected possibility. Attention is drawn to Section One, designed to be of practical value in guiding the clinician to the criteria needed for a correct diagnosis of occupational disease.

The updating of certain sections of the 1949 edition of *Industrial Toxicology* has required considerable reworking. Updating and revision with needed additions have been developed by me and

xi

my colleagues, Drs. Asher Finkel, Clarence Maloof, John Stoeckle, and Lloyd Tepper. This edition has been enlarged by new sections dealing with potential risks from exposure to plastics and pesticides, occupational causes of pulmonary disease, and biologic hazards to workers of importance to the physician. The section on radiant energy includes the great advances in knowledge since 1949 with emphasis on facts of importance to physicians. Edwin D. Flack prepared the chapter on lasers and microwave radiation and updated those on ultraviolet and infrared radiations.

H.L.H.
Lincoln, Massachusetts
December 1973

INTRODUCTION

1 • *The Diagnosis of Occupational Disease*

In the 17th century, Ramazzini, the first great student of industrial disease, laid down a rule for the diagnosis of such illness. He bade the physicians of Italy, when they had a case of illness in a working man, to ask the patient not only about his symptoms but to go carefully into all the details of his occupation for, without this knowledge, a correct diagnosis could not be made. Ramazzini's advice is still needed, at least by medical students and hospital house staffs, for most medical schools still leave occupational medicine out of the curriculum, and students graduate with more information about endocrine diseases than about lead poisoning. And, as anyone who has had to go through hospital records will agree, many a physician has little intelligent interest in the history of a patient's work. Often he is content with the word "laborer," or perhaps he goes so far as to write "lead worker," but that tells us far too little. We do not know how great the lead exposure may have been or how long it lasted, and these factors have an important bearing on the diagnosis. Mixing white lead paint in an open chaser may bring on a form of plumbism that could never occur in a man who handled freshly made lead grids for storage batteries. The slow accumulation of metallic lead dust in the body gives rise to one clinical picture; the sudden flooding of the body with soluble lead, to quite a different one.

The diagnosis of occupational disease is important, not only for the care of the patient, but also because accurate diagnosis makes it possible to seek control of job hazards and so to prevent disease. A diagnosis depends upon the traditional steps of the clinical method—history, physical examination, laboratory tests, and x-ray examinations—but, in particular, an occupational history. Symptoms such as cough and dyspnea and signs such as opacities on a chest x-ray are by themselves not specific for the diagnosis of a single disorder. But a history of work experience is critical for diagnosis. It may provide the information that relates the patient's symptoms and signs with exposure to a specific, toxic job hazard.

Technique of Occupational History Taking

Four components in taking an occupational history can be identified: 1) the patient's symptoms and their relation to his work, past or present; 2) the character of the hazardous exposure; 3) the quantity and duration of these hazards; and 4) the presence of similar illness in co-workers with similar jobs.

Such a history is often complicated and difficult to elicit. It is not sufficient simply to make a note of present occupation; a history of past potential exposures must also be obtained. But the worker may have forgotten dates of employment and dates of short, but critical, work periods. His own beliefs about the causes of his disease may even make him forget to mention a crucial work experience or deny its importance. Through ignorance, fear of losing a job, advice from fellow workers, family or a lawyer, a patient may be reluctant to reveal work exposures. Although often a false lead, a patient's story of fellow workers suffering similar illness should be investigated. The physician who first interviews a patient with occupational disease has the best opportunity to get an accurate account of what the patient knows about his work exposure and how he views his illness.

Since patients often have had several jobs, a chronological lifetime work history, not just a current job description, must be obtained. Particularly in the United States, workers often move from place to place and job to job, with few political or economic restraints, so that many workers hold several jobs in a lifetime. Hazardous exposures occurring early in a worker's life may have a long latent period before their effects produce symptoms or the worker seeks medical help. Certain occupationally induced malignancies, for example, may not be clinically detectable for as long as 30 to 40 years after the last exposure to the etiologic agent. A chronological job and medical history should include smoking habits, residence, and chronic infections, since it is likely that more than one environmental insult is responsible for the disease. For example, tuberculous infection combined with exposure to silica dust produces more severe disease than infection by tubercle bacilli alone. Similarly, smoking is thought to contribute to the development of carcinoma of the lung in patients with asbestosis.

The occupational history supplied by the patient can provide some but not all the information needed as to the *quality* of exposure. The patient may know only the trade name of the material with which he has worked, yet it is necessary to learn not only what metal or chemical compound may have been involved, but also its physical state and concentration. For example, at high temperatures the chlorinated hydrocarbon, trichloroethylene, widely used as an industrial solvent, produces phosgene, which is capable of causing pulmonary edema. Similarly, freshly generated cadmium oxide fumes can result in an acute chemical pneumonitis, whereas "old" cadmium compounds have no such effect. Although the materials in use may be similar in chemical structure, they may differ completely in toxic effect. An important example is the hazard associated with exposure to benzene (C_6H_6), which is well known to cause bone marrow damage. In contrast, toluene ($C_6H_5CH_3$) has no harmful effect on blood-forming tissue. Yet both benzene and toluene are excellent organic solvents.

Besides the character of an exposure, history-taking must not neglect the *quantity*. Factors governing the total dose of an occupational exposure are many. Duration of work is of obvious first importance. Whether or not the job was done with protection or in close proximity to the worker's breathing zone is also important. Whether the exposures were intermittent or steady, the levels high or low, are the next questions. Conditions of work are also significant. If the work took place in a hot climate with great physical effort, the increased respiratory demands could have resulted in a greater dose of inhaled material. If drilling work was done in a wet atmosphere, airborne dust would have been less than if, for example, dry drilling or surface grind-ing had been done. When industrial hygiene data are available, the task of acquiring a quantitative exposure history is obviously facilitated (see next chapter). More often, however, information must be ferreted out by the interrogating physician.

Standards of Safe Work

Terms such as safe dose, threshold limit value, maximum allowable concentration, or maximum permissible limit are used to express the concept that there is a level below which no exposed worker will become ill. *Maximum allowable concentration* (MAC) has been in use the longest time but has been supplanted in recent years by the term, *threshold limit value* (TLV). Such levels of environmental contamination usually refer to exposures during a 40-hour workweek over a working lifetime, except in a few instances where exposure restrictions are specified. An extreme position against the TLV concept is taken by some who believe that no amount of evidence can assure that any exposure will be harmless for all workers.

The physician seeing cases of possible occupational disease or trying to evaluate the potential harm of neighborhood industrial exposures needs to know the current MAC or TLV. The latter are developed, revised and published each year by the American Conference of Governmental Industrial Hygienists (ACGIH) in Cincinnati. This group was organized in 1938 and its members are professional personnel in government agencies or educational institutions who are engaged in occupational health and safety programs. Maximum permissible limits for a large number of hazardous substances have been promulgated in the United States by the Occupational Safety and Health Administration (OSHA), and in some cases revisions have been recommended by the National Institute for Occupational Safety and Health (NIOSH), for which see the list of "Criteria Documents" in the Appendix. Individual states also publish such lists, which often tend to differ. The United Kingdom and European countries have also set standards although, not surprisingly, there is frequently no real agreement.

What is the evidence that forms the basis for the MACs that are in use? A number of safe dose levels are based on experience with death and impairment of exposed workers. The MAC value for benzene (C_6H_6) has such a history. Benzene has been a widely used solvent and was important in explosives manufacturing in World War I. Unprotected workers exposed to as much as 1000 parts per million (ppm) or more died of its narcotic effect. At lower levels of exposure, the unique action of benzene on the hematopoietic system caused fatal aplastic anemias. A number of workers exposed to benzene escaped these outcomes, but at a later date developed leukemias. As this experience with benzene toxicity was collected and publicized, the safe dose level was reduced to 25 ppm, and is now 1 ppm. This experience with benzene illustrates an important point in understanding other man-made diseases. Toluene and xylene, which are related to benzene chemically, do not elicit the same toxic response except for narcosis at high levels. In general, a toxic effect to an unknown chemical cannot always be predicted from its chemical likeness to a compound of known toxicity.

While accidental or unanticipated human exposures provide toxicity information, a systematic study of toxicity may require studies with animals. One approach, a "range-finding toxicity study," may be of use by determining the median lethal dose of a substance in several species of animals to help establish a safe upper upper limit for man. Whether a material is inert or harmful may be assessed by experimental animal studies. However, there are difficulties in studying low-level long-term effects, and the variation, in response from species to species provide additional obstacles in extrapolating from animal exposure to man. Some of the problems are illustrated by animal studies of beryllium toxicity. In spite of experience with chronic illness in 800 beryllium workers, some authorities believed that failure to reproduce the disease in animals ruled out beryllium as a cause. Rabbits exposed to beryllium compounds develop osteogenic sarcomas, while pulmonary tumors are produced experimentally in rats, a difference illustrating the difficulty in predicting a response from one species to another.

Further Sources of Information

Because the patient can rarely supply accurate and complete information about his job, other sources must be used to supply additional facts or to confirm reported knowledge about his work and exposures. Trade secrecy, fear of litigation, and union interference are serious deterrents to easy discovery of the precise facts of a sick worker's exposure.

The physician may get help from: 1) the patient's foreman, employer, or the plant physician; 2) the state agency responsible for monitoring and preventing occupational disease; 3) a university laboratory interested in occupational disease; 4) the insurance company carrying the workmen's compensation coverage of the employer; 5) occupational physicians and industrial hygienists on the staff of large companies or in independent consulting firms; and 6) reference texts that identify ingredients in materials that are known only by trade names (e.g., Gosselin et al., 1976).

Role of Host and Other Factors

While the occupational history focuses on the knowledge about hazardous agents that is needed to make an etiologic diagnosis, other factors may be important in understanding the development of such disease.

A crucial factor in the development of disease due to toxic substances is the *mode of entry* of harmful materials into the body. Far and away the most important route is by inhalation. Some organic compounds penetrate the unbroken skin, but the amount of inorganic material reaching the blood stream through the intact skin is of little importance.

Economic and social factors may also affect an individual case or help to account for illness differences in a group of similarly exposed workers. Low income workers may have poor diets and less resistance to infections and toxins. Because of economic pressures, some workers, such as disabled coal miners, continue on the job in spite of suffering from active respiratory tract disease. Lack of education can also be a problem. An example was provided during World War II by the behavior of poorly educated American Indians and Spanish Americans employed in some laboratories for atomic energy development in the southwestern United States. Because they were either unreasonably frightened or utterly careless of precautions, control of their radiation exposures was difficult. Important economic factors in the development of disease are the fast production demanded by piece-work remuneration and the extra work undertaken by employees concerned about debts at home, both of which may lead workers to avoid using protective devices in order to maintain production output. Still additional economic pressure results from the attitude of some trade unions. Not until relatively recently have unions been concerned enough about the health of workers in dangerous trades to take an interest in removing hazards through negotiated labor contracts. Instead, job hazards have been viewed as a means of getting extra pay, understandably in periods of economic depression.

The pollution of urban air with oxides of nitrogen from motor vehicle exhausts and nearby industrial plants may be a residential factor in the development of obstructive lung disease and one that may act together with occupational agents. Individuals exposed to long-term low doses of toxic agents in soil, water, and food present a special problem. For example, leaded gasoline has been a continuing source of small but definite amounts of lead in the bodies of most city dwellers. Exposure to lead in the atmosphere presents a problem of interpretation when it is found in urine or tissue of a worker known to be exposed to toxic lead compounds at his job. The body burden of such a toxic agent is additional to that from the occupational exposure and may be critical in the development of disease. While the general significance of low concentrations of metals in the environment is still largely unknown, they may be important cofactors in the development of occupational disease.

A wise physician will be alert to the possibility that *psychological factors* such as the patient's attitude toward life, his temperament, or his problems at home can favorably limit or enhance his reaction to a hazardous exposure. The discouraged, depressed worker may have less chance of acquiring a disease-producing exposure at his job since, being less productive, he inhales less workroom air in a day. The worker from an unhappy home, the one with a seriously ill wife or child, the chronic alcoholic, the person with a strenuous second job—all of these come to a potential occupational risk with problems that may influence the dose, total exposure, or response. Heavy cigarette smokers are in greater jeopardy of developing lung cancer when exposed to relatively low doses of a known occupational carcinogen such as asbestos. An emotionally ill worker with both lead poisoning and anxiety may respond to lead colic with such severe pain and tenderness that the surgeon is induced to operate in the belief that he is dealing with an acute abdomen.

Why do workers apparently exposed to the same hazard, at the same exposure level, and for the same duration vary in their response? Some

of this variation may be due to differing *immunologic responses*. Environmental and job-related insults are thought by some observers to be sensitizing agents acting as antigens, with the disease a result of antigen-antibody complexes that produce tissue injury. Without sufficient evidence to confirm this hypothesis in many disorders, a limited conclusion seems to be that in some cases inherited or acquired immune responses are indeed responsible for occupational disease such as the pulmonary hypersensitivities to organic dusts. Despite this explanation, the increase in case incidence as the amount of exposure increases suggests that dose level of the toxic agent remains of basic importance.

Another factor in this immunologic situation may be the effect of tobacco smoking. Zetterström et al. (1981) found mean serum IgE concentrations to be higher in smokers than in nonsmokers. They also produced evidence that sensitization against occupational allergens, such as those found in laxative manufacture from *Plantago* seeds and in coffee roasting, was more common in workers who smoked.

The study of inborn errors of metabolism is yielding to special techniques. Two examples illustrate the importance of *genetic influence* in the diagnosis of occupational disease. Workers with Mediterranean or with sickle-cell anemia who are exposed to toxic lead compounds develop far more serious effects because lead destroys the more vulnerable red cells in such patients. Persons with hereditary asthma and eczema may be more easily sensitized to environmental irritants, in particular to certain vegetable dusts (Stokinger and Scheel, 1963).

It is useful to know that persons who serve as foremen, production engineers, research chemists, secretaries, and maintenance men may be exposed to higher doses of a harmful material than are the regular workers because of the needs of their jobs, chance failure of ventilation, or failure to utilize proper protection.

There has been considerable attention to so-called *neighborhood poisoning* in recent years. This phenomenon is due in part to publicity and in part to increasing concern over industrial air pollution. In the 18th century it was common experience that a boy sharing a bed with his father, a mercury miner, developed mercury poisoning; and infants in families where lead was used in pottery manufacture, a cottage industry, suffered central nervous system damage. From Japan in the past two decades have come reports of disease caused by industrial methyl mercury pollution of fish used for food, called Minamata disease after the bay into which the waste was dumped (Matsumoto et al., 1965). Recently, a painful bone disease in rice field workers in Japan, named Itai-itai disease, resulted from cadmium pollution by nearby mines producing zinc and lead as well (Kobayashi, 1971).

In the United States a dramatic example of neighborhood disease was provided by 60 cases of chronic beryllium poisoning suffered by women, children, and a few men, none of whom had entered a beryllium-using plant (Hardy et al., 1967). Beryllium in nearby community air from factory stacks was one source; clothes brought from the workplace into the home proved to be a more serious source; and recent study makes it likely that soil heavily contaminated with beryllium may prove to be the most important cause of long-delayed cases of chronic toxicity. Another startling example of neighborhood disease is provided by the accumulating reports of the hazards of asbestos exposure. Wagner et al. (1960) published their finding of 32 cases of malignant mesothelioma correlated with neighborhood asbestos exposure. Native women and

children, living in South African villages close to plants refining asbestos from nearby mines, were the chief victims. Newhouse and Thompson (1965) reported a series of fatal cases of mesothelioma among residents of a dwelling adjacent to a London asbestos factory. As in the United States experience in the beryllium industry, both close proximity and contaminated work clothes were etiologic factors in these cases. Kiviluoto (1960) found x-ray evidence of pleural calcification in a significant number of inhabitants of a geographically limited area in Finland, with no other evidence of disease. Further study demonstrated that dust from a neighboring asbestos plant was responsible for the x-ray findings.

It cannot be overemphasized that correct diagnosis, rational treatment, and prognosis of occupational disease rests chiefly on knowledge of harmful work or incidental exposure. Assay of blood, urine, or tissue may in some cases lead to a diagnosis of industrial illness; in other cases it may serve to create confusion because the findings reflect only exposure or levels also found in nonindustrially exposed individuals.

References

ACGIH: *Documentation of the Threshold Limit Values,* ed 4. American Conference of Governmental Industrial Hygienists, Cincinnati OH, 1980.

Gosselin RE, Hodge HC, Smith RP, et al: *Clinical Toxicology of Commercial Products: Acute Poisoning,* ed 4. Williams & Wilkins, Baltimore, 1976.

Hardy HL, Rabe EW, Lorch S: United States Beryllium Case Registry (1952–1966): Review of its methods and utility. *J Occup Med* 1967;9: 271–276.

Kiviluoto R: Pleural calcification as a roentgenologic sign of nonoccupational endemic anthophyllite asbestosis. *Acta Radiol* 1960;194 (suppl 1):1–67.

Kobayashi J: Relation between the "Itai-Itai" disease and the pollution of river water by cadmium from a mine. *Proc 5th Intern Water Pollution Res Conf* 1971;I-25:1–7.

Matsumoto H, Koya G, Takeuchi T: Fatal Minamata disease: A neuropathological study of two cases of intrauterine intoxication by a methyl

mercury compound. *J Neuropathol Exp Neurol* 1965;24:563–574.

Newhouse ML, Thompson H: Mesothelioma of pleura and peritoneum following exposure to asbestos in the London area. *Br J Ind Med* 1965;22:261–269.

NIOSH/OSHA: *Pocket Guide to Chemical Hazards.* Washington, DC, National Institute for Occupational Safety and Health; Occupational Safety and Health Administration, (NIOSH 78-210), 1978.

Stokinger HE, Scheel LD: Hypersusceptibility and genetic problems in occupational medicine—a consensus report. *J Occup Med* 1973;15:564–573.

Wagner JC, Sleggs CA, Marchand P: Diffuse pleural mesothelioma and asbestos exposure in the North Western Cape Province. *Br J Ind Med* 1960;17:260–271.

Zetterström O, Osterman K, Machado L, et al: Another smoking hazard: Raised serum IgE concentration and increased risk of occupational allergy. *Br Med J* 1981;283:1215–1217.

2 • *Methods of Control of Occupational Disease*

There are five ways to correct a recognized industrial hazard. The ideal method is to discover a harmless replacement for the toxic material. This approach was successfully used in 1949 in the United States fluorescent lamp industry because of the serious epidemic of worker illness caused by beryllium-containing phosphors. If this ideal cannot be achieved, a second choice is to isolate the dangerous operation as is done, for example, in nuclear power plant construction and operations, where glove boxes are used or where manipulations with highly radioactive materials are carried out behind shielding by means of master slave manipulators. The third method is engineering appropriate ventilation to carry harmful vapors, fumes, and dusts away from the worker's breathing zone. A fourth, and least desirable, method is to fit the exposed worker with a respirator. However, it is difficult to provide a respirator mask that fits a worker's face well enough to afford real protection. Special knowledge of the protection requirements is needed to provide the proper filtering device within the mask. Not surprisingly, experience shows that workers do not wear respiratory protection except for short periods, for the equipment places a physiological load on the user (Johnson, 1976; Raven et al., 1979). If the job entails physical effort, the respirator interferes with breathing. If the work is done at great height, as in bridge repair, interference with vision by the mask creates a risk of falling. For such reasons, individual masks are a poor substitute for proper ventilation and should be used for short-term, hazardous jobs only after expert guidance as to the kind of equipment required by a particular operation. Finally, some extremely hazardous operations require special protective clothing and supplied air systems. This fifth method obviously applies to highly special situations and cannot be used for routine work.

Professional Personnel for Control of Industrial Hazards

Control of occupational hazards as developed in the United States and other highly industrialized countries follows from the point of view that illness arises from old and new man-made inventions and technology. Its focus is not the patient *per se,* as has been the tradition in clinical medicine, but the interaction of the worker and his workplace environment. The word "occupational" is preferred to the often used term "industrial medicine" because it broadens the definition of the field to include scientists, laboratory technicians, farmers, executives, and office workers.

Charged with monitoring hazardous occupations, those working in this field describe their technical preventive activity as occupational or industrial hygiene; physicians refer to their work as occupational medicine. It is useful to realize that a great variety of methods of using such manpower exists in different countries dependent upon industrial development. To describe the various technical skills that may be involved, the following list is offered:

1. *Industrial or occupational hygiene chemist.* Tasks include sampling workroom air, assaying biological samples from exposed workers, identifying materials thought to be harmful. When newly introduced substances are thought to be hazardous, assay methods need to be developed. Chemical engineering or chemistry are the usual professional fields of training although a few institutions offer specific training in industrial hygiene.

2. *Industrial or occupational hygiene engineer.* Identification and measurement of size and amounts of dust; design of proper ventilation; control of excessive noise levels; decision as to

correct respirator. Chemical engineering may be the prior field of training.

3. *Radiation protection officer, health physicist.* This profession was developed in World War II to serve the needs of atomic energy development. This field, which has become highly specialized throughout the world, requires a background in physics or electrical engineering. Work involves radiation monitoring, development of instrumentation, assay of biological samples for radioactivity, planning for response to radiation accidents, decontamination.

4. *Industrial or occupational safety engineer.* Serves to prevent accidents, explosions, fires, and supplies protective devices such as safety glasses. In small plants the person who fills this post may also carry out duties of those listed above. Technical or academic training for this job is the exception rather than the rule, and often the plant safety officer is an ex-worker.

5. *Other professions* engaged in the prevention of occupational disease include physicians, nurses, dentists, dieticians, psychologists, and health educators, who may be employed full- or part-time, depending on the size of the company and the interest of executives.

Control of Industrial Hazards

Until very recently in the United States, the federal government has acted to control worker illness and injury only when asked to do so by industry or state authorities. State legislatures have traditionally passed regulations governing, and created agencies to investigate, industrial hazards. In only a few states have county authorities or local health departments legally forced compliance by industry. Because of variation from state to state, a physician seeking information about industrial hazards must discover the local or regional agencies that are responsible for investigation and control.

Two recent exceptions enlarging federal control in the United States are the Federal Coal Mine Health and Safety Act of 1969 (P.L. 91-173) and the Occupational Safety and Health Act of 1970 (P.L. 91-596). The first gave components of the federal government expanded powers not only to set standards for dust control along with enforcement authority to insure compliance, but also to set standards for work conditions that may affect the health of miners, particularly accidents, noise control, and sanitation. The Occupational Safety

and Health Act does the same for many other industries where toxic exposures may occur. In addition, the Act created the National Institute for Occupational Safety and Health (NIOSH) that is responsible for research into the detection, cause, control, and treatment of occupational disorders. While the intent of P.L. 91-596 was excellent, there have been problems in its implementation because enforcement is in one federal agency, the Occupational Safety and Health Administration (OSHA), while recommendations on safe levels, the character of new hazards, and research are the responsibility of another (NIOSH).

Both the older industrialized countries and the developing nations have adopted the use of the factory inspectorate system with authority from the central government to carry out inspections and enforcement of regulations, with more or less right of appeal by industry. Benefits to disabled workers and their families are a part of social insurance and are awarded without the need for court action, with support derived from general governmental funds rather than the practice in the United States where such payments come from profit-making free enterprise insurance carriers.

In the United States only a few states require physicians to report cases of occupational disease. Knowledge about the prevalence of cases may come only from compensation awards, a registry that is incomplete and inaccurate for several reasons. Many workers may never claim compensation, and so their diseases go unrecorded. Since diagnostic standards are variable, the compensation list is intrinsically inaccurate. For example, if compensation claims are settled only on the basis of x-ray changes, as they often are, then other respiratory disease of occupational origin will not be identified. In some states, patients with known occupational disease are not eligible for compensation simply because their disease has not been recognized within a prescribed time limit. Also, some states, by limiting compensation to disorders on approved lists, ignore occupational illnesses that result from newly introduced harmful materials.

International Agencies

Important international organizations in the field of occupational disease and its control are the International Labour Office and the World Health Organization. The International Labour Office (ILO) is the older of the two, and is the remaining unit of the post-World War I League of Nations, founded in 1919. The ILO is made up of government delegates plus one employer and one union representative from each member country. It promotes continuing interest in labor problems with a permanent safety and health section publishing details of good practices in such subjects as lead poisoning, maternity protection, and medical examination of young workers. Similarly, the World Health Organization (WHO), the more recently established health agency of the United Nations, has become active in the field of occupational hazards. One branch of WHO is devoted to the study of hazards arising from the use of nuclear energy, a topic on which it collaborates with the International Atomic Energy Agency (IAEA) in Vienna, Austria. Another component of WHO is the International Agency for Research on Cancer (IARC), with headquarters and laboratories in Lyon, France, much of whose effort is directed to the study of occupational malignancy.

References

Johnson AT: The energetics of mask wear. *Am Ind Hyg Assoc J* 1976;37:479–488.

Raven PB, Dodson AT, Davis TO: The physiological consequences of wearing industrial respirators. A review. *Am Ind Hyg Assoc J* 1979; 40:517–534.

SECTION TWO
METALS AND METALLOIDS

1 • *Aluminum*

Industrial Uses

Aluminum, for more than 100 years, has found wide application in industry, more recently in atomic energy development and aircraft manufacture. It is widely distributed in nature as bauxite, cryolite, corundum, and combinations of aluminum with a variety of constituents — chiefly, fluorine, silicon, oxygen. Electrolytic reduction of bauxite was developed in 1886 by Hall in the United States and Héroult in France. Aluminum is used alone and alloyed with copper, zinc, magnesium, manganese, and silicon in building construction materials, insulated cables and wiring, household utensils and laboratory equipment, all kinds of packaging material, and reflectors. Important, less well-known uses for aluminum and its compounds are in the paper industry, printing inks, the glass industry, water purification, and waterproofing in the textile industry. Various aluminum oxides are used as abrasives and refractories in many different industrial operations.

Harmful Effects in Industry

The major health hazards associated with the electrolytic reduction of Al_2O_3 result from the use of ground coke and coal-tar pitch applied to the anode, and from the addition of CaF_2 (fluorspar) to lower the melting point of the mixture and of AlF_3 to increase current efficiency (Taylor, 1978). Consequently, there has been concern for possible toxic effects from pitch (skin, lung, hematopoietic malignancies) and from fluorides (occupational fluorosis). Lung cancer mortality has been correlated with tar-years of exposure in aluminum reduction plant workers (Gibbs and Horowitz, 1979). Another study confirmed an excess of lung cancer deaths as well as pancreatic, lymphatic,

and hematopoietic cancers, fatal benign tumors of the brain, and pulmonary emphysema among workers in an aluminum reduction plant (Milham, 1979). Fluoride metabolism and prevention of bone fluorosis in aluminum smelter workers have been studied extensively and will be discussed in the chapter on fluorine compounds.

When cooking utensils made of aluminum were first introduced, it was thought that they caused aluminum poisoning. This has proved not to be so. Aluminum is absorbed poorly, if at all, from the gastrointestinal tract. The combination of aluminum with available phosphate makes an insoluble compound, a fact utilized in preparing drugs used in peptic ulcer therapy.

In contrast, a number of older reports describe harm to industrial workers after inhalation of aluminum or one of its compounds as a dust. The literature is by no means clear as to the character of exposure causing lung damage. A review of these reports of toxic effect provides a background for judging the hazard due to inhalation of finely divided aluminum and its compounds. The German literature during World War II is discussed in Hamilton and Hardy (1949, pp. 199–202). Cases were reported of x-ray changes "similar to silicosis" in workers exposed to inhalation of aluminum dust who complained of dyspnea and developed spontaneous pneumothorax. Another paper reported a case with a strikingly rapid course of the disease and absence of hypertrophy of the right side of the heart in spite of the extensive induration and shrinking of the lung tissue. Regional lymph glands contained little aluminum dust, a finding suggesting that aluminum remains in the lung.

Yet another paper reported an autopsy on a 35-year-old man who had worked four years in an atmosphere of finely divided pure aluminum dust. Extensive, bilateral, chronic interstitial pneumonia with right-sided cardiac hypertrophy was

9

found. Stress was placed on the short exposure and rapid course of the disease. The interstitial tissue of the lung was thickened with narrowing of the alveolar spaces and with little compensatory emphysema. Koelsch, an investigator commissioned by the German government to examine the situation in German aluminum works, found descriptions of 181 cases of aluminum lung. The victims were young and the period of dust exposure was brief. A high level of exposure was attributed to wartime conditions of blackout and poor ventilation. Koelsch believed that there is no specific character of aluminum pneumoconiosis and that the picture is similar to that caused by excessive inhalation of a variety of relatively inert silica-free dusts. The pneumothorax that also occurs in connection with these dusts is thought to be due to rupture of an emphysematous patch or the tearing of a pleural adhesion by excessive coughing.

An important report is that of Shaver and Riddell (1947) who described a series of 23 cases of pulmonary disease in a group of 344 furnace workers processing bauxite. There were seven deaths. Bauxite, which is aluminum oxide ($Al_2O_3 \cdot 2H_2O$), is used in the manufacture of artificial abrasives. In the process, bauxite, plus small quantities of iron and coal, is heated to 2000°C. White fumes are evolved and on analysis these proved to consist of 60% alumina and 25% silica with 12% iron and magnesium oxides. Shaver's disease, as this occupational disease has been named, is clinically characterized by dyspnea, cough, substernal pain, weakness, and fatigue. The chest x-ray picture shows bilateral "lacelike shadowing," especially in the upper halves, more intense toward the lung roots. Emphysematous changes are seen at the periphery as well as varying degrees of pneumothorax. Dyspnea depends in severity on the degree of pneumothorax and is a distinctive and frequent finding. At autopsy, advanced emphysema and interstitial pulmonary fibrosis are outstanding features. The occupational histories showed that 21 of the sufferers from Shaver's disease were furnace feeders and two were crane operators. In view of the high silica content of the fumes to which these workers were exposed, Shaver's disease may prove to be a hitherto undescribed form of silicosis. An additional report of importance is that of Smith and Perina (1949) describing seven of 35 workers in abrasive wheel manufacture who showed striking abnormalities on chest x-ray. The importance of this report lies

in the extensive use of these materials in modern abrasive wheels.

Reports of so-called aluminosis from Sweden, dated between 1950 and 1960, have been summarized and discussed by Ahlmark et al. (1960). These occurred among workers in the manufacture of aluminum metal powders for pyrotechnic uses and for bronze paints. Extremely fine dust (1 μm or less) was evolved in the crushing mills so that for about six hours certain workers were exposed to very dusty air. This small group of workers (five to ten) deserves study since the crushed aluminum to which they were exposed contained 98% pure aluminum, 2% aluminum oxide, and less than a few tenths of 1% of iron, silica, copper, lead, zinc, and tin. Five cases of aluminum pneumoconiosis were diagnosed from this plant between 1946 and 1947. All had chest x-ray abnormalities — at first mild, but in two cases progressive. One man died of pulmonary disease; another became seriously disabled. A United States case recorded in detail by Mitchell (1959) described clinical, x-ray, and postmortem findings of a young man heavily exposed to aluminum dust for two and a half years who died after a nine months' illness of increasing dyspnea and weight loss. Fibrosis and emphysema of generalized and marked character were found and the amount of aluminum, judged to be Al_2O_3, was 640 ppm dry weight.

A chest x-ray, sent to HLH for an opinion, of a dental technician who used aluminum powder to clean dentures revealed bilateral opacities. Lung biopsy showed these to be large-sized non-caseating granulomata. Since the patient had no symptoms or signs of chest disease, the diagnosis was benign pneumoconiosis caused by aluminum.

Quite different are two reports of workers exposed to aluminum with no toxic effects. Crombie, Blaisdell, and McPherson (1944) reported x-ray observations on a group of 125 workers exposed to high concentrations of metallic aluminum powder for periods ranging from six to 23 years with an average of 12 years. They reported no abnormal x-ray changes in the group except those found in a few cases of healed pulmonary tuberculosis. Hunter et al. (1944) reported observations made on a group of 92 men working as grinders of duraluminum airplane propellers. This operation involved grinding and polishing the metallic alloy with aluminum and alumina. Abnormal shadows at the lung periphery were found in the chest x-rays of seven of the workers, but the rest of the group had no unusual findings. The authors considered that the abnormal shadows may have been due to deposits of aluminum dust and concluded that there is no evidence that the dust in the working environment of the grinders of duraluminum airplane propellers produces disease of the trachea, bronchi, or lungs.

On the other hand, two reports from England presenting evidence of pulmonary fibrosis, confirmed the fact that, depending on total dose inhaled, aluminum is damaging to the lung. Mitchell et al. (1961) found that of 27 workmen examined, six had pulmonary fibrosis after exposure to finely divided aluminum powder. Two cases were fatal after less than three years' exposure. McLaughlin et al. (1962) described a single case of a 49-year-old aluminum worker exposed for 13½ years who, in addition to pulmonary fibrosis, suffered symptoms of a severe encephalopathy. At autopsy, lungs and brain contained 20 times, and liver 122 times, more aluminum than normal. Although these authors found no other reports of encephalopathy associated with aluminum exposure, they quoted experimental studies with primates who developed an encephalopathy when certain aluminum compounds were applied to the surface of the brain.

Indeed, recent reports incriminate aluminum as a cause of neurofibrillary degeneration of rabbit brain after repeated subcutaneous administration of soluble aluminum salts (DeBoni et al., 1976). Crapper and his colleagues (1976) emphasized the neurotoxic properties of aluminum as a result of finding elevated concentrations of Al in brains of patients with Alzheimer's disease, although whether the pathological changes in this disease are caused by Al has been questioned by McDermott et al. (1979). Aluminum intoxication has been suggested as a cause of renal dialysis encephalopathy syndrome as a result of the use of Al-containing phosphate-binding gels to control serum phosphorus levels in uremic patients on dialysis (Alfrey et al., 1976), or as a result of aluminum being added to city water used as a dialysate (Rozas and Port, 1979). However, dialysis dementia probably has multiple causation and is not the result of elevated brain Al alone (Arieff et al., 1979).

None of these neurotoxic effects is related to occupational exposure, but acroanesthesia, described as a congestive numbness of the fingers, is reported from cotton mills in operations where there is long contact with aluminum in wet bobbin winding.

Organometallic substances, alkylaluminum compounds are being used more and more as catalysts according to Stokinger (1963). They are extremely reactive; as a result, their use presents great danger of burns. Powdered aluminum ignites easily and has been responsible for fires and explosions in many instances.

Interpretation of Reports of Aluminum Illness

Conflicting reports of the risk involved in inhaling aluminum or its compounds can be only partially explained. Of first importance are the precise character and size of the dose of aluminum-containing dust that reaches the lower respiratory tract. Aluminum and aluminum oxide used in industry may also be inhaled together with other dusts of more or less hazard to the lung. The most striking example of this is in the case of Shaver's disease, where the dust contained at least 25% silica. A technical change of importance arose from the military requirement during World War II for aluminum free from stearine or paraffin previously used to coat the metal as a lubricant and that acted to prevent finely divided dust from reaching the alveoli. As in many industrial disease descriptions, aluminosis is thought by some to be a disease of hypersensitivity with great variation in individual idiosyncrasy. Since aluminum can combine with protein, it may behave as an antigen, although to date this has not been proved.

Clinical experience recorded in the literature varies from no illness, to slight and hard-to-assess chest x-ray changes, to a rapidly progressive, irreversible lung disease among workers exposed to aluminum or its compounds. Susceptibility to acid-fast infection is reported not to be a problem in aluminum exposures, but true bacterial infection causes progression of the lung disease. Dyspnea, spontaneous pneumothorax, weight loss, and cardiac failure mark the course of a severe case of aluminosis, shown at autopsy to be due to interstitial fibrosis and emphysema.

In the United States, aluminum is considered harmless. Aluminum oxide, Al_2O_3, is regulated as a nuisance dust, safe if exposure does not exceed 50 million parts per cubic foot (15 mg/m^3), where particles are small enough, 5 μm in diameter or less, to reach the lower respiratory tract. In view of the reports reviewed here, the United States concept may be in error. Inhalation studies with experimental alumina fibers with median diameters of 3.5 μm have shown only occasional aggregates of fiber-containing alveolar macrophages in rats and no indication of progressive fibrosis after two years (Piggott and Ishmael, 1979). The use of aluminum as a preventive and as therapy for silicosis was popular in the United States and Canada for a short time but has now been abandoned almost entirely.

Much of the animal experimental work has been done because of the suggested use of aluminum for therapy and prevention of silicosis. Some has been done to evaluate the toxicity and mechanism of aluminum-containing antiperspirants. Irritation of human and laboratory animal skin depends on the acidity of the compound and its affinity for epidermal keratin. The antiperspirant effect appears to result from plug formation at the openings of the sweat ducts (Lansdown, 1974). Many experiments with a variety of aluminum preparations have failed to produce pulmonary lesions in animals. For a review of animal studies of aluminum toxicity, see Browning (1969, pp. 3–22).

References

Ahlmark A, Bruce T, Nyström A: *Silicosis and Other Pneumoconioses in Sweden.* Stockholm, Svenska Bokförlaget, 1960.

Alfrey AC, LeGendre MS, Kaehny WD: The dialysis encephalopathy syndrome. Possible aluminum intoxication. *N Engl J Med* 1976;294:183–188.

Arieff AI, Cooper JD, Armstrong A, et al: Dementia renal failure, and brain aluminum. *Ann Intern Med* 1979;90:741–747.

Browning E: *Toxicity of Industrial Metals,* ed 2. New York, Appleton-Century-Crofts, 1969, pp 3–22.

Crapper DR, Krishnan SS, Quittkat S: Aluminium, neurofibrillary degeneration and Alzheimer's disease. *Brain* 1976;99:67–80.

Crombie DW, Blaisdell JD, McPherson G: The treatment of silicosis by aluminum powder. *Can Med Assoc J* 1944;50:318–328.

DeBoni U, Otvos A, Scott JW, et al: Neurofibrillary degeneration induced by systemic aluminum. *Acta Neuropathol* (Berl) 1976;35:285–294.

Gibbs GW, Horowitz I: Lung cancer mortality in aluminum reduction plant workers. *J Occup Med* 1979;21:347–353.

Hamilton A, Hardy H: *Industrial Toxicology,* ed 2. New York, Paul B. Hoeber, 1949, pp 197–202.

Hunter D, Milton R, Perry KMA, et al: The effect of aluminium and alumina on the lungs in grinders of duraluminum aeroplane propellers. *Br J Ind Med* 1944;1:159–164.

Lansdown ABG: Aluminium compounds in the cosmetic industry. *Soap, Perfumery, and Cosmetics* 1974;47:209–212.

McDermott JR, Smith IA, Iqbal K, et al: Brain aluminum in aging and Alzheimer disease. *Neurology* 1979;29:809–814.

McLaughlin AIG, Kazantzis G, King E, et al: Pulmonary fibrosis and encephalopathy associated with the inhalation of aluminium dust. *Br J Ind Med* 1962;19:253–263.

Milham S Jr: Mortality in aluminum reduction plant workers. *J Occup Med* 1979;21:475–480.

Mitchell J: Pulmonary fibrosis in an aluminium worker. *Br J Ind Med* 1959;16:123–125.

Mitchell J, Manning GB, Molyneux M, et al: Pulmonary fibrosis in workers exposed to finely powdered aluminium. *Br J Ind Med* 1961;18:10–23.

Piggott GH, Ishmael J: Toxicological assessment of potential hazards from new inorganic fibres. *J Soc Occup Med* 1979;29:20–21.

Rozas VV, Port FK: Progressive dialysis encephalopathy. Prevention through control of aluminum levels in water. *Ann Neurol* 1979;6:88–89.

Shaver CG, Riddell AR: Lung changes associated with the manufacture of alumina abrasives. *J Ind Hyg Toxicol* 1947;29:145–157.

Smith AR, Perina AE: Pneumoconiosis among workers in plant engaged in grinding synthetic abrasive material. *New York Department of Labor Monthly Review* 1949;28:29–31.

Stokinger HE: The metals (excluding lead), in Patty FA (ed): *Industrial Hygiene and Toxicology,* ed 2. New York, John Wiley, 1963, vol 2.

Taylor W: Aluminium manufacture. *J Soc Occup Med* 1978;28:25–26.

2 • Antimony

Uses

Antimony has been used since ancient times, especially in the manufacture and plating of vases and domestic vessels. It occurs mainly as stibnite, Sb_2S_3, although other antimony-containing ores are known. It is widely used in industry as an alloy of tin, lead, and copper; in the compounding of rubber; in flameproofing of military textiles and in fire retardants; and has wide uses in dyes, paints, varnishes, glass and pottery, and pharmaceuticals such as tartar emetic (Browning, 1969). The most common industrial exposures occur during the mining, smelting and refining of ores in the course of which antimony dusts and fumes are produced.

Antimony is extensively used as a constituent of lead-antimony alloy, especially for printers' type, and as the "golden sulfide" in rubber compounding. Printers' type contains far more lead than antimony and it is difficult, if not impossible, to verify a case of antimony poisoning among printers because the symptoms of lead poisoning are so similar. It is only when symptoms include skin lesions that the possibility of antimony poisoning can be considered. The golden sulfides of the rubber industry are mixtures of trisulfide, pentasulfide, and oxysulfide, and are not very soluble in the human stomach, a factor that reduces the risk of toxic effect. Grids for electric storage battery plates, like printers' type, are made of an alloy of antimony and lead. No cases of antimony poisoning have ever been reported from this industry.

Industrial Illness Experience

Antimony resembles arsenic as well as lead in its action. Exposure to antimony can result in irritation of the skin and mucous membranes, eczema and other forms of dermatitis, and inflammation of the lining of mouth, nose, and throat. Like lead, antimony causes metallic taste, vomiting, colic, and diarrhea, if it is acute; if it is chronic, it causes indigestion, loss of appetite and weight, but diarrhea is more common than in lead poisoning. Sores in the mouth and sore throat help to distinguish antimony poisoning from that of lead. It must not be forgotten that practically all industrial antimony contains some arsenic. Because of this, Rambousek (1913, p. 146) doubted that industrial antimony poisoning existed; instead, he attributed any symptoms to the presence of arsenic occurring with the antimony.

A brief review of reports in the literature will summarize current knowledge of occupational antimony poisoning. Older authorities, especially among the Germans, who do draw a clear picture of antimony poisoning, described 200 cases of industrial dermatitis in men who used antimony salts as a mordant in dyeing cloth or who handled the dyed cloth. The lesions are described as a pustular necrotic dermatitis. Seitz (1925) reported that antimony dust in the foundry was an important cause of the gastrointestinal symptoms of exposed workers. German workmen became ill and were incapacitated for ten days, suffering from dyspnea, headache, vomiting, conjunctivitis, and bloody purulent discharge from the nose as a result of grinding metallic antimony.

Dernehl and his colleagues (1945) quoted Feil who, in 1939, found among workers in antimony smelters the following symptoms: conjunctivitis, tracheitis, pharyngitis, anemia, headache, anorexia, and vomiting. Feil ruled out arsenic as the cause since the ore contained less than 10 mg per kilogram. Taylor (1966) described acute intoxication from antimony trichloride fumes that caused gastrointestinal symptoms with persistent nausea and respiratory tract irritation. Urine antimony

14

concentrations were estimated to be in excess of 1.0 mg/L.

In 1953 Renes reported 69 cases of illness among workers in an antimony smelter where they were exposed to dust and fume at high levels (5 to 12 mg/m³) and where the particle sizes were less than 1 μm. Since the arsenic concentrations in these exposures were low, the toxic effect was attributed to antimony. Dermatitis in sweaty, hairy, friction areas and upper respiratory tract inflammation occurred most frequently, and in six cases an acute pneumonitis was demonstrated by chest x-ray and was completely reversed by penicillin and freedom from exposure. The skin lesions are well known in the industry as "antimony spots."

Antimony process workers exposed to very fine, white trioxide fumes, as well as those of antimony sulfide, have been found on occasion to have a simple benign pneumoconiosis resembling that seen in siderosis, stannosis, and baritosis (Cooper et al., 1968; McCallum, 1967). Clinical examinations and lung function tests have not shown any harmful effects of this deposition; histological sections of lung have shown an accumulation of dust particles and dust-laden macrophages in alveolar septa and in perivascular tissues without fibrosis or inflammatory reaction (McCallum, 1967). Similar findings have been reported for antimony workers in a Serbian smelter, but silicosis may have been a complicating factor here since the patients developed massive lesions that might have represented an antimony-silicosis (Karajovic et al., 1958).

Bulmer and Johnson (1948) described, in contrast, their practical experience with industrial antimony exposure. Over a period of years they never encountered an industrial exposure to antimony that caused ill health, not even after gross exposure to the trisulfide. They record concentrations of 42 to 52 mg/m³ of this compound without discernible effect on the men breathing it. This accords with the experience of Hamilton in the early years of the century when antimony sulfides were used in the coloring of rubber goods, and the men handling it were dyed with the color from head to foot. Yet no evidence of damage could be found. The low toxicity of antimony trisulfide and larger particle size of the dust may explain the discrepancy in the outcome.

A serious toxic effect of exposure to antimony as the compound Sb_2S_3 was reported by Brieger et al. in 1954. They studied 125 workers who had been employed in the abrasive industry for less than two years. Of these, six died suddenly of heart failure, and 37 of 75 examined showed abnormal electrocardiograms, chiefly T wave changes. The use of antimony had to be stopped since values of 3 to 5.5 mg/m³ of antimony were found in the air and up to 9.6 mg/L in urine, in spite of engineering control. This experience recalled the cardiac complications arising from the therapeutic use of antimony compounds as therapy for parasitic disease. Stokinger (1963) summarized the two following reports of toxic antimony effect. A 1955 report from Morocco antimony mines described chronic symptoms of headache, vertigo, anorexia, and muscle pains. The second report is of exposure to antimony pentasulfide in Italian glass manufacture. The workers complained of gastrointestinal irritation, and, as in other reports, there were unusual changes in the hemogram. As much as 1.3 to 2.1 mg/L of antimony was found in the urine. The discovery of Belyaeva (1967) that Russian women workers exposed to antimony suffer a significant increase in abortions is not reported anywhere else. Belyaeva found antimony in human milk and placental and amniotic fluid as well as in blood and urine of exposed workers.

More recently, Cordasco (1974) reported a case of severe pulmonary edema that followed inhalation exposure to antimony pentachloride that also produced severe burns of most of the body of a 39-year-old male. Immediate development of severe coughing, wheezing, dyspnea, and chest tightness was followed by pulmonary edema 12 hours later. Treatment required CPPB (constant positive pressure breathing), massive doses of corticosteroids, and eventually tracheostomy. Chest films at the height of respiratory distress revealed marked vascular congestion throughout both lungs. The patient gradually improved and was discharged 95 days after hospital admission.

Storage of food in containers glazed with an antimony compound has caused epidemics of sickness thought to result from the release of antimony when acid attacks the glass. Colic, nausea, vomiting, and, in severe cases, collapse are reported.

Stibine (SbH_3) is a colorless gas evolved when antimony is treated with acid, such as during the charging of electric batteries. Stibine resembles arsine in that both are extremely toxic gases, stibine having marked hemolytic properties with a history of a high death rate (Dernehl et al., 1944). While the threshold limit is set at 0.1 ppm, no chronic stibine poisoning has been reported for man (Browning, 1969).

Animal Studies

Fairhall and Hyslop (1947) believed that far too little attention has been paid to the toxicity of metallic antimony and certain of its salts. Tested on animals, metallic antimony dust appears to be much more toxic than the dust of insoluble antimony compounds used in industry and, when finely divided, remains suspended in the air much longer than would be expected of a heavy metal. The suggested order of descending toxicity is metallic antimony, the trisulfide, the pentasulfide, the trioxide, the pentoxide.

Most striking is the experimental finding by Bradley and Fredrick (1941) and by Brieger et al. (1954) that, as in human experience, antimony causes pathologic changes in the cardiac muscle of laboratory animals. Trivalent antimony compounds are more harmful in these studies than pentavalent. Interstitial pneumonitis, lipoid pneumonia, focal pulmonary hemorrhage, fatty degeneration of the liver, and a variety of changes in the peripheral blood picture are recorded by various authors in different species of animals as summarized by Browning (1969, pp. 28–31) and NIOSH (1978).

Therapy and Control

Antimony and arsenic are so alike both chemically and biologically that British antilewisite (BAL) is the treatment of choice in acute poisoning. Moeschlin (1965, p. 174) favors use of BAL by deep intramuscular injection for 10 days.

Urine assay for antimony is a satisfactory method of assessing clinical complaints. Elkins (1959, p. 256) suggests that a urinary level of 1.0 mg/L reflects a harmful antimony exposure. A level of 0.5 mg/m³ of antimony in air for steady work exposure (40 hours per week) is considered safe.

The *in vivo* measurement of antimony dust in human lungs by use of x-ray spectrophotometry has been reported by McCallum and his colleagues (1971).

The federal (OSHA) standard for antimony exposure is 0.5 mg/m³ determined as a time-weighted average (TWA) concentration limit, a value that agrees with the 1968 ACGIH TLV.

References

Belyaeva AP: The effect produced by antimony on the generative function. *Gig Truda Prof Zabol* 1967;11:32–37 (in Russian), abstracted, *Bull Hyg* 1967;42:615.

Bradley WR, Fredrick WG: Toxicity of antimony: Animal studies. *Ind Med* 1941;2:15–22.

Brieger H, Semisch CW, Stasney J, et al: Industrial antimony poisoning. *Ind Med Surg* 1954;23:521–523.

Browning E: *Toxicity of Industrial Metals,* ed 2. New York, Appleton-Century-Crofts, 1969, pp 23–38.

Bulmer FMR, Johnston JH: Antimony trisulfide. *J Ind Hyg Toxicol* 1948;30:26–28.

Cooper DA, Pendergrass EP, Vorwald AJ, et al: Pneumoconiosis among workers in an antimony industry. *Am J Roentgentol* 1968;103:495–508.

Cordasco EM: Newer concepts in the management of environmental pulmonary edema. *Angiology* 1974;25:590–601.

Dernehl CU, Stead FM, Nau CA: Arsine, stibine, and hydrogen sulfide: Accidental generation in a metal refinery. *Ind Med Surg* 1944;13:361–362.

Dernehl CU, Nau CA, Sweets HH: Animal studies on the toxicity of inhaled antimony trioxide. *J Ind Hyg Toxicol* 1945;27:256–262.

Elkins HB: *The Chemistry of Industrial Toxicology,* ed 2. New York, John Wiley, 1959, p 256.

Fairhall LT, Hyslop F: The toxicology of antimony. *Pub Health Rpts* (suppl 195) 1947.

Karajovic D: Pneumoconiosis in workers at an antimony smelting plant. *Proc 12th Intern Cong Occup Health* (in German). Helsinki, 1957, vol 3, pp 370–374.

McCallum RI: Detection of antimony in process workers' lungs by x-radiation. *Trans Soc Occup Med* 1967;17:134–138.

McCallum RI, Day MJ, Underhill J, et al: Measurement of antimony oxide dust in human lungs *in vivo* by x-ray spectrophotometry. *Inhaled Particles III,* 1971, pp 611–619.

Moeschlin S: *Poisoning: Diagnosis and Treatment.* New York, Grune & Stratton, 1965, p 174.

NIOSH: *Criteria for a Recommended Standard . . . . Occupational Exposure to Antimony.* Washington, DC, National Institute for Occupational Safety and Health (NIOSH 78-216), 1978.

Rambousek J: *Industrial Poisoning from Fumes, Gases and Poisons of Manufacturing Processes.* London, Longmans, 1913, p 146.

Renes LE: Antimony poisoning in industry. *Arch Ind Hyg Occup Med* 1953;7:99–108.

16

Seitz A: Hygiene in type-casting industry and experimental antimony poisoning. *Arch Hyg* 1924;94:284–297 (in German), abstracted, *J Ind Hyg Toxicol* 1925;7:188.

Stokinger HE: The metals (excluding lead), in Patty FA (ed): *Industrial Hygiene and Toxicology,* ed 2. New York, John Wiley, 1963, vol 2.

Taylor PJ: Acute intoxication from antimony trichloride. *Br J Ind Med* 1966;23:318–321.

3 • Arsenic

Solid Arsenic Compounds

White arsenic, the trioxide As_2O_3, is historically the most important of the poisons used for criminal purposes. It is profoundly irritating and corroding to tissues. It produces inflammation of the gastrointestinal tract, violent purging and vomiting, hemolytic jaundice, hematuria and anuria. A single dose of 0.12 g may be fatal. If death does not occur, changes in the peripheral sensory nerves cause pain, and paresthesias may follow. Later there may be motor paralysis, loss of hair, deformity of the nails, skin lesions, and symptoms of upper respiratory tract irritation. In cases that develop slowly, the same symptoms, although less severe, are noted.

The chief industrial uses of arsenic trioxide are in the manufacture of insecticides, weed killers, fungicides, and antifouling paints. Lesser amounts are used in the manufacture of special glass and enamels, and some arsenic is added to certain alloys (Browning, 1969). Arsenic was used for years as a drug, most widely in a tonic known as Fowler's solution, a preparation of 1% neutral arsenic trioxide. Sodium arsenite ($NaAsO_2$) is used as a solid sterilant. Arsenic pentoxide (As_2O_5) is used as a defoliant to prepare cotton for mechanical harvesting, as a wood preservative, and in the production of oxo-salts (AsO_4^{3-} arsenates). The trivalent compounds are much more toxic than the pentavalent arsenicals (Savory and Sedor, 1977). Because of the risk of poisoning, arsenical pigments are no longer used in domestic products such as ornaments, toys, carpets, and curtains. In the past there were reports of deaths and poisonings in homes caused by arsine and trimethyl arsine diffusing into the air from wallpaper as a result of decomposition by molds of Scheele's green, copper arsenite, which has since been abandoned as a paper pigment.

The principal occupational hazards of arsenic exposure are in the preparation of herbicides and pesticides, and in those industrial processes where arsenic trioxide is a by-product. Potential exposures derive from the presence of arsenic in coal and oil shales. Arsenic in copper and iron ores is oxidized to the trioxide in smelting operations. Exposure to the trivalent arsenites and the pentavalent arsenates may also occur by inhalation or skin contact. Unusual sources of arsenic poisoning occur in glass manufacture with the emptying of sacks of white arsenic and adding it to the glass mixture; in the stitching of window shades dyed with arsenic green; in the mixing of arsenic with enamel for iron bathtubs and shot-blasting such enamel from defective ware; and in the handling of hides and bird skins that have been treated with white arsenic.

Absorbed arsenic is deposited in skin, nails, and hair, and in liver and bone. Excretion is via the kidneys, and the rate of fall in urine arsenic values varies with the concentration of arsenic in the urine. Pinto et al. (1976) found a significant correlation between industrial exposure to airborne arsenic trioxide and urine arsenic values when the former did not exceed 300 $\mu g/m^3$ and the latter were below 500 $\mu g/L$. Background urine arsenic levels for adult males not exposed to arsenic trioxide in industry averaged 52.6 $\mu g/L$. Rate of decline of urine As levels after removal from exposure began at 9.5% per day for workers with urine As below 200 $\mu g/L$ and began at 21% per day for those whose levels exceeded 600 $\mu g/L$. These authors point out that trivalent inorganic arsenic may be slowly oxidized to the pentavalent form and then excreted. Since certain seafoods contain appreciable amounts of pentavalent arsenic, which is not known to be toxic in the amounts normally eaten, Pinto et al. (1976) recommended that evaluation of absorption of arsenic trioxide due to industrial exposure be based on urine samples collected at least two days after seafood has been eaten.

Systemic poisoning is rarely seen in industry,

17

and still more rarely is it severe in character. The usual effect is local, on skin and mucous membranes and conjunctiva, wherever the dust is deposited. Moist surfaces suffer most — the lips, nares, eyelids, pharynx, and scrotum. A hoarse voice is characteristic of an arsenic worker, and a perforated nasal septum is an occupational sign of the worker handling white arsenic. After short periods of exposure, the workers notice nasal obstruction with consequent mouth-breathing and usually some inflammation in pharynx and larynx, soreness of the tongue, and excessive salivation. Sloughing of the mucous membrane and necrosis of the nasal cartilage may follow. The bony septum is not involved. When exposure ceases, healing occurs without deformity.

The study of poisoning from arsenic trioxide and copper aceto-arsenite (Paris green) in industry is largely a study of skin lesions. Such lesions vary from local inflammation, with or without ulceration, to thickening and pigmentation, hyperkeratosis and slowly developing malignant transformation. Arsenic-induced skin cancer has a benign course and does not give rise to metastases. Opinions differ as to whether industrial exposures to arsenic compounds act only as irritants to the skin or whether they are sensitizing agents. Loss of hair and trophic changes in the nails are common. Such cases have been reported due to the handling of paper dyed with arsenic green (Ayres, 1920).

The picture of generalized, arsenical poisoning from solid arsenic as seen in exceptional cases in industry is rarely severe. Symmetrical peripheral neuropathy is a well-known complication of arsenic poisoning that begins 7 to 14 days after the acute intoxication episode, frequently after recovery from the gastrointestinal phase (Jenkins, 1966). Numbness and paresthesias (especially burning sensations of the soles) begin in the distal extremities, lower limbs before the upper, spread rapidly proximally, and increase in intensity. Motor weakness of the distal extremities may occur and the palsy is likely to affect the long extensors of fingers and toes, as does lead. It is distinguished from the latter by severe neuralgic pains. Neuropathy may develop whether the exposure is inhalation, ingestion, or cutaneous absorption. Garb and Hine (1977), in a discussion of their case of a worker who was splashed with arsenic acid, state that peripheral neuropathy from arsenic exposure is the same whatever the route of entry. Mayers (1954) reported a case of peripheral neuropathy in a worker exposed for 20 years to inhalation and skin absorption of Paris green. Heyman et al. (1956) reported arsenical neuropathy in seven farm workers exposed occupationally to arsenate sprays or dust. A rare form of industrial poisoning involving the optic nerve has been reported in a patient with skin lesions and bilateral optic atrophy who worked with arsenical insecticides (Moleen, 1913).

It is hard to explain the difference between industrial and nonindustrial arsenical poisoning, but such variation is recorded in all industrialized countries. The lack of serious symptoms in industrial arsenic poisoning is not to be explained on the ground of slight exposure, for in the great smelting works of western United States, the lead works in Colorado, and the copper works in Montana, the ores contain a high proportion of arsenic, which is volatilized in the furnaces and carried in the flues to be deposited in the baghouse and tunnels as white arsenic. Sometimes in Colorado smelting works, as much as 60% of the flue dust is arsenic trioxide. This dust must be shoveled into trucks and transported for a second sublimation, after which the product, almost pure, must be handled and packed; yet the men carrying on this work almost never show any but local effects on skin and upper respiratory tract (Pinto and McGill, 1953). Lundgren et al. (1951), studying 1500 Swedish smelter workers exposed both to arsenic trioxide and sulfur dioxide, described Rönnskär disease, a worker illness named for the location of the smelter. In contrast with 500 controls, the exposed men suffered chronic upper respiratory tract disease. Arsenic is given as the cause of a number of cases of poisoning among workers making or handling sheep dip. Ulceration of the nasal septum, irritation, dark pigmentation of exposed skin, especially around the neck and axillae, are reported. As in other arsenic exposures, a wide variety of skin reactions were found, including malignant changes.

It is impossible in many industries to protect nose and throat from arsenic without putting each worker into a protective mask, a procedure that is not practicable. The skin and eyes can be protected against the dust, and every effort should be made to do this to prevent painful ulceration, especially of the skin of the scrotum, the lips, and the nostrils. In industry this means a great deal of annoyance. Men will face poisoning of a dangerous character such as nitrous fumes, benzol, and take their chances without much fuss, but they will not endure an itching, burning eruption. Labor turnover is great in any plant where skin irritants are present.

Lead and Calcium Arsenate

A great deal of study has been devoted to the toxic action of the arsenates, lead and calcium, when present in minute quantities in food, because of wide use as insecticides, especially in fruit orchards (Calvery, 1938; Fairhall et al., 1943). Study of mortality data shows that, of compounds to which sprayers of orchards are exposed, calcium arsenate is most toxic; next is lead arsenate; and third is lead carbonate. A few cases of industrial poisoning from lead arsenate have been reported, all from its use as a spray in orchard or forestry work. The workers suffer signs and symptoms of lead rather than arsenic poisoning. A well-studied case showed that the worker suffered colic, then double wristdrop, after 27 years of exposure in spraying trees (Aub et al., 1925). Other reported cases have shown typical arsenical lesions after exposure to arsenic-containing insecticides (Hamilton and Hardy, 1949, p. 131). Unusual symptoms of arsenical poisoning have occurred in sprayers of grape vines. One worker suffered a generalized exfoliative dermatitis, severe conjunctivitis and keratitis, the result of direct toxic action of arsenic on the eye. Butzengeiger in 1949 (Buchanan, 1962, p. 17), studying wine growers exposed for long periods to arsenic-containing sprays, described abnormal electrocardiograms in 45% of several hundred men. These changes disappeared when arsenic was hard to get during World War II. Arsine (AsH_3) exposure has caused similar changes. Tarrant and Allard (1972) suggested that workers thinning forests who use arsenic compounds, so-called silvicides, chiefly cacodylic acid (dimethylarsinic acid) and monosodium methanearsonate (MSMA), are at risk of toxic effect if they are without complete protective clothes and gloves to prevent skin contact. HLH saw a forestry worker who had been injecting a silvicide into trees. The man complained of anorexia, nausea, and abdominal pain, and was found to have an elevated arsenic urine level. The worker's symptoms gradually subsided when he was free of exposure.

Toxic Effects of Arsenic Compounds

Knowledge of the biological behavior of arsenic and its compounds is relatively great because of their uses in drugs, and war gas, and as a homicidal and suicidal weapon. All arsenicals except arsine act by inhibiting sulfhydryl enzyme systems required for cell metabolism (Johnstone, 1963). The potency of action varies among arsenic compounds and depends on valency, trivalent compounds being most toxic. Arsine combines with hemoglobin to form a powerful hemolytic poison and does not act by sulfhydryl inhibition.

Although chronic arsenic ingestion has been reported to lead to cirrhosis of the liver and to noncirrhotic portal hypertension (Huet et al., 1975; Morris et al., 1974; Cowlishaw et al., 1979), there are a few documented cases of liver cirrhosis as a result of industrial exposure to arsenic. Jhaveri (1959) reported a case of primary liver carcinoma associated with liver cirrhosis in a man who had handled arsenious oxide and sodium arsenite for over 20 years in a chemical plant. Buchanan (1962) reviewed earlier work that had reported characteristic arsenic skin lesions and enlarged livers in 73 of 113 vineyard workers where the exposure may have been due to the practice of giving the workers a juice made of grapeskin, rich in arsenic, as a free drink. He also reviewed earlier reports of 23 similar cases of chronically ill Moselle vineyard workers suffering from cirrhosis, ascites, and peripheral neuritis. Because of exposure to both lead and arsenic in orchard workers, diagnosis of the causative agent requires careful analysis of urine for both of these substances.

Peripheral polyneuropathy in industrial occupational exposure to arsenic has already been discussed (see above). Electrophysiological studies in cases that followed a single exposure showed reduction of motor conduction velocity and marked abnormalities of sensory nerve action potentials, while sural nerve biopsies showed axonal degeneration (Le Quesne and McLeod, 1977). Recovery is slow, and sensory symptoms and abnormal signs may persist for several years.

The role of arsenic as an occupational carcinogen dates from the observations of Paris in 1820 on cancer of the scrotum in smeltery workers (Bishop and Kipling, 1978). Since that time a number of epidemiological studies have continued to implicate arsenic as an industrial carcinogen. Neubauer (1947) collected 24 cases of skin cancer among miners, smelters, sheep-dip workers, and agricultural laborers who had been exposed to arsenic. Hill and Faning (1948) found an increased incidence of cancers of the skin and respiratory tract in chemical process workers in a factory in Great Britain that prepared and packaged sodium arsenic powder. Lee and

Fraumeni (1969) reported an eightfold excess of respiratory tract malignancies in 8047 smeltery workers exposed to arsenic trioxide, although exposure to sulfur dioxide may also have been involved. Osburn (1969) noted a similar excess of carcinoma of the lung in South African gold miners who had worked in dusty mines with highly arsenical ores. Ott et al. (1974) found a significant increase in respiratory cancer among employees exposed primarily to arsenates of lead and calcium in the manufacture of insecticides.

While these and other epidemiological studies (Kuratsune et al., 1974; Axelson et al., 1978; Mabuchi et al., 1979) along with literature reviews (Sunderman, 1976; Pinto and Nelson, 1976) continue to point to arsenic as at least a low-grade carcinogen, there are dissenting views largely because arsenic carcinogenicity has not been demonstrated in experimental animals. Frost (1967), in addition to asserting that the observations of Paris are more appropriately ascribed to selenium toxicity, concluded from a critical review of the literature that arsenicals are "remarkably free from carcinogenicity" and that the natural association of arsenic with soot, tar, and fossil fuels has led to an indiscriminate acceptance of the concept of arsenical cancer. Similar skepticism regarding arsenic and cancer was voiced by Pelfrene (1976) in his evaluation of epidemiological reports and experimental studies with animals. This fascinating problem deserves further critical examination especially in view of recent reports of arsenic teratogenicity and mutagenicity (Pelfrene, 1976; Bencko, 1977; Beckman et al., 1977). The concomitant roles of sulfur dioxide and of tobacco smoke also need to be considered in evaluating industrial epidemiological studies.

Bioassay of Arsenic

The diagnosis of occupational arsenic poisoning is not easy in an individual case. Accurate work history with knowledge of the amount of arsenic and the compound to which the patient has been exposed are of first importance. An important clue may be illness in fellow workers. Absorbed arsenic is promptly distributed in various organs so that blood levels are of little value in measuring total body burden. Urine is the chief route of excretion; a small amount is lost in the feces.

Bioassay of nails, hair, and urine has been used

in studies of industrial arsenic intoxication and poisoning due to drugs as well as in forensic medicine. Urine arsenic values given in the literature for nonexposed persons range from 0.02 to 0.13 mg As/L (NIOSH, 1975). Elkins (1959) cited several series of industrially exposed arsenic workers in whom the urine arsenic level was 1.0 mg/L when the average air concentration in the workplace was 0.2 mg/m^3. Among 348 smeltery workers exposed to arsenic trioxide dust, the urine arsenic level averaged 0.82 mg/L (Pinto and McGill, 1953). While there were cases showing local irritation of skin and mucous membranes, no cases of systemic arsenic poisoning were seen, even though several workers had urine arsenic levels as high as 4 mg/L.

Various authors report that determinations of levels of arsenic in hair or nails are useful in diagnosis. Because of the affinity of arsenic for sulfhydryl groups, abundant in skin and its appendages, the amount of arsenic in hair or nails can be conveniently measured (Schroeder and Balassa, 1966). However, the values may be hard to interpret because of the amount of arsenic in certain foods, notably seafood, and drinking water in some areas. Values of arsenic given in the literature for normal nonexposed hair vary widely. Lenihan and Smith (1958) assayed 1000 hair samples, and Boylen and Hardy (1967) a small number (50); both studies agreed that the upper limit of normal is 1 ppm. Exposed workers are reported to have up to 100 ppm of arsenic in hair both with and without symptoms of poisoning. Chronic mild exposures, errors in assay, and the well-recognized acquired tolerance of the body for arsenic account for such a wide range of published values in reports of arsenic levels in biological material.

Arsine

Arsine (AsH_3), a highly toxic gas, is the most hemolytic poison encountered in industry. It is also known as arsenic hydride, arsenic trihydride, arsenous hydride, arseniuretted hydrogen, and hydrogen arsenide. It is produced when nascent (freshly formed) hydrogen is generated in the presence of arsenic or when water reacts with a metallic arsenide (Blackwell and Robbins, 1979). Colorless and nonirritating, it has a mild garlic odor that may be masked by other odors present at the same time.

Occupational arsine poisoning has occurred in

smelting and refining of metals, galvanizing, soldering, etching, lead plating, wetting of aluminum and phosphate dross, cleaning of furnaces and tanks, and mishandling of arsenical insecticides (Buchanan, 1962; Browning, 1969; Fowler and Weissberg, 1974). Less typical occurrences have been reported from the action of sewage fungi (Cox and Alexander, 1973) and from cleaning out of cattle dip vat (Rathus et al., 1979). Poisoning as a result of use of a galvanized pail in cleaning an acid vat and a clogged drain has been reported twice recently (Hocken and Bradshaw, 1970; Pinto, 1976). Arsine is used in the transistor industry to stabilize selenium, and leakage from a cylinder of this gas carried in the cargo hold of a freighter resulted in serious poisoning of four sailors (Wilkinson et al., 1975). Similar poisoning has been produced in the generation of hydrogen for filling balloons by the action of hydrochloric acid on zinc dust contaminated with arsenic. Most of the iron, lead, and antimony used in industry is likely to be contaminated with arsenic, as is also commercial sulfuric acid made by the ordinary chamber process and the hydrochloric acid that is made from it. In the production of aniline dyes and coal-tar drugs, one of the most important processes is reduction by nascent hydrogen, produced from iron or zinc dust and hydrochloric acid, and here there is always a risk that arsine may be formed.

A frequent cause of arsine poisoning is the cleaning out of tanks and tank cars that have contained either hydrochloric or sulfuric acid. Strong acid does not attack iron or steel tanks, but weak acid does. Consequently, there is no trouble while the tank is full but, when it is emptied and flushed out with water, weak acid is left in the residual sludge, and when the laborer or lead-burner goes in to dip out the sludge or make repairs, he is exposed to the risk of arsine rising from the action of the weak acid on the arsenic-contaminated iron. Three men in a plant in New Jersey were sent into an acid tank to make repairs after it had been supposedly well flushed out. There was about a bucketful of residue left at the bottom that contained enough arsine to affect the workers, two of whom died.

There is a general belief in industry that pickling metal (i.e., treating it in tanks of sulfuric or hydrochloric acid, hot or cold) is unhealthy work, and it seems that the small amounts of arsine formed from time to time in such tanks may be responsible for this view. In one serious shipyard incident, in which one man died after four days in

coma and another developed hemolytic anemia and nephritis, the acid in a pickling tank had been used over and over again so that the content of arsenic had increased from 0.005 to 0.05%. The same sort of accident is possible in the charging and forming departments in storage battery manufacture where the lead antimony grids are immersed in weak sulfuric acid. Epidemics of arsine poisoning have occurred in submarines where the acid in storage batteries had eaten into the lead antimony grids that had been contaminated, as is usually the case, with arsenic. In contrast, in the manufacture of batteries such cases are rare.

The principal effect of arsine poisoning is intravascular hemolysis. Varying periods of time elapse after the gas has been inhaled before the destruction of red cells shows its effect in clinical symptoms. Such intervals have been reported as ranging from six to 36 hours or more, depending on the severity and length of exposure. The initial symptoms of headache, malaise, weakness, dizziness and dyspnea are followed by abdominal pain, nausea and vomiting (Fowler and Weissberg, 1974). These acute symptoms are followed in four to six hours by the passage of dark or bloody urine, often the first symptom that alarms the victim. Jaundice appears later, after 24 to 48 hours, and the red cell count may fall below 2 million. The triad of abdominal pain, hemoglobinuria, and jaundice was pointed out by Jones (1907) as characteristic of arsine poisoning. Physical examination findings include fever, tachycardia, tachypnea, jaundice, abdominal tenderness, especially of the enlarged liver. Hemolytic anemia is evidenced by the low hemoglobin values, and the presence of reticulocytosis and red cell fragments and ghost cells. Toxic granules may be found in the leukocytes. Plasma hemoglobin may be present in concentrations as high as 2 mg/dL. Urinalysis will reveal the presence of hemoglobin as well as arsenic.

As the disease progresses, jaundice deepens and the urine grows scantier until in fatal cases there is complete suppression that results in death. Arsenic may continue to be excreted in nonfatal cases for many weeks after the acute symptoms have disappeared (Wignall, 1920; Kensler et al., 1946). The anemia is likely to persist even longer. In spite of modern therapy, the prognosis is grave.

Arsine intoxication is differentiated from acute poisoning with nitro and amido derivatives of benzene by the absence of methemoglobin formation and of cyanosis. Other conditions that need to be considered in the differential diagnosis include malaria, leptospirosis, paroxysmal nocturnal hemoglobinuria, and other forms of intravascular hemolysis, such as that produced by stibine, pyrogallic acid, or potassium chlorate (Fowler and Weissberg, 1974). A valuable observation confirming the direct toxic action of arsine on cardiac muscle has been provided by the reports of lowered or inversion of T waves on the electrocardiogram (Pinto et al., 1950; Weinberg, 1960). Such changes may persist for two months after apparent recovery.

Dimercaprol (British antilewisite, BAL) was developed for the specific need to treat cases of war gas poisoning caused by arsenicals. Its action is of greatest value when it is used promptly, and there are a number of recommended courses. Moeschlin (1965) suggested varying the dose depending on the severity of the case and recommended starting with 2.5 to 3 mg/kg every four to six hours and tapering to every six hours and then to every 12 hours between the fourth and 14th day. All injections should be given deep intramuscularly to prevent abscess formation. Fowler and Weissberg (1974), however, pointed out that BAL provides no protection against erythrocyte destruction and they stress that the treatment of choice for severe arsine poisoning is exchange transfusion and, if necessary in the face of renal failure, hemodialysis. The efficacy of renal dialysis has been supported by a number of reports, most recently by Pinto (1976). For less severe cases of arsine poisoning, BAL may be effective (Muehrcke and Pirani, 1968; Conrad et al., 1976). Since D-penicillamine has been used successfully in treating three cases of arsenic trioxide poisoning and one case of sodium arsenate ingestion (Peterson and Rumack, 1977), this chelating agent may also be useful in arsine poisoning.

Pulmonary edema secondary to the effect of arsine on cardiac muscle and dilatation of the heart due to the anoxemia resulting from hemolysis require heroic measures. Early death after acute arsine poisoning may be due to myocardial failure accompanied by massive pulmonary edema that precedes the onset of renal failure.

Chronic arsine poisoning has been reported in workers employed in the cyanide extraction of gold (Bulmer and Rothwell, 1940) and perhaps in workers in a zinc smeltery (Johnson, 1953). In the former situation, there was a progressive reduction in erythrocyte levels and hemoglobin values, marked basophilic stippling, and an elevation of urine arsenic. The workers had exertional dyspnea and the weakness typical of anemia.

Control

It has been estimated that in the United States 900,000 workers are occupationally exposed to sources of arsenic (Blackwell and Robbins, 1979). Arsine is the most toxic of the arsenic hazards in industry and the important weapon in its control is the anticipation that it will be generated. Equipment for complete respiratory protection and plans for emergency care by a physician who is informed about the toxic effects of arsine and appropriate therapy are required. So great is the risk associated with arsine exposure that in the United States the so-called safe level of exposure for all forms of arsenic is set at 0.05 ppm (0.2 mg/m³) as a TWA in any 8-hour work shift of a 40-hour workweek. However, NIOSH (1975) has recommended a more stringent standard of 0.002 mg/m³ determined by a 15-minute sample. The same exposure standard was proposed for all forms of inorganic arsenic as well as for arsine and other arsenical gases.

References

Aub JC, Fairhall LT, Minot AS, et al: Lead poisoning. *Medicine* 1925;4:1–250.

Axelson O, Dahlgren E, Jannson C-D, et al: Arsenic exposure and mortality: A case-referent study from a Swedish copper smelter. *Br J Ind Med* 1978;35:8–15.

Ayres S Jr: Scleroderma as a possible manifestation of chronic arsenic poisoning. *Arch Derm Syph* 1920;2:747–756.

Beckman G, Beckman L, Nordenson I: Chromosome aberrations in workers exposed to arsenic. *Environ Health Perspectives* 1977;19:145–146.

Bencko V: Carcinogenic, teratogenic, and mutagenic effects of arsenic. *Environ Health Perspectives* 1977;19:179–182.

Bishop C, Kipling MD: Dr. J. Ayrton Paris and cancer of the scrotum. *J Soc Occup Med* 1978;28:3–5.

Blackwell M, Robbins A: Arsine (arsenic hydride) poisoning in the workplace. NIOSH Current Intelligence Bulletin #32, August 3, 1979. Also published in *Am Ind Hyg Assoc J* 1979;40:A56–A61.

Boylen GW Jr, Hardy HL: Distribution of

arsenic in nonexposed persons (hair, liver, and wine). *Am Ind Hyg Assoc J* 1967;28:148–150.

Browning E: *Toxicity of Industrial Metals,* ed 2. New York, Appleton-Century-Crofts, 1969, pp 39–60.

Buchanan WD: *Toxicity of Arsenic Compounds.* New York, Elsevier, 1962, p 17.

Bulmer FMR, Rothwell HE: Chronic arsine poisoning among workers employed in the cyanide extraction of gold: A report of fourteen cases. *J Ind Hyg Toxicol* 1940;22:111–124.

Calvery HD: Chronic effects of ingested lead and arsenic. *J Am Med Assoc* 1938;111:1722–1728.

Conrad ME, Mazey RM, Reed JE: Industrial arsine poisoning: Report of three cases. *Ala J Med Sci* 1976;13:65–66.

Cowlishaw JL, Pollard EJ, Cowen AE, et al: Liver disease associated with chronic arsenic ingestion. *Aust NZ J Med* 1979;9:310–313.

Cox DP, Alexander M: Production of trimethylarsine gas from various arsenic compounds by three sewage fungi. *Bull Environ Contam Toxicol* 1973;9:84–88.

Elkins HB: *The Chemistry of Industrial Toxicology,* ed 2. New York, John Wiley, 1959.

Fairhall LT, Miller JW, Weaver FL: The effect of arsenates on the storage of lead. *Publ Health Rep* 1943;58:955–959.

Fowler BA, Weissberg JB: Arsine poisoning. *N Engl J Med* 1974;291:1171–1174.

Frost DV: Arsenicals in biology—retrospect and prospect. *Fed Proc* 1967;26:194–208.

Garb LG, Hine CH: Arsenical neuropathy: Residual effects following acute industrial exposure. *J Occup Med* 1977;19:567–568.

Hamilton A, Hardy HL: *Industrial Toxicology,* ed 2. New York, Hoeber, 1949, p 131.

Heyman A, Pfeiffer JB Jr, Willett RW, et al: Peripheral neuropathy caused by arsenical intoxication. *N Engl J Med* 1956;254:401–409.

Hill AB, Faning EL: Studies in the incidence of cancer in a factory handling inorganic compounds of arsenic: I. Mortality experience in the factory. *Br J Ind Med* 1948;5:1–6.

Hocken AG, Bradshaw G: Arsine poisoning. *Br J Ind Med* 1970;27:56–60.

Huet P-M, Guillaume E, Coté J, et al: Noncirrhotic presinusoidal portal hypertension associated with chronic arsenical intoxication. *Gastroenterol* 1975;68:1270–1277.

Jenkins RB: Inorganic arsenic and the nervous system. *Brain* 1966;89:479–498.

Jhaveri SS: A case of cirrhosis and primary carcinoma of the liver in chronic industrial arsenical intoxication. *Br J Ind Med* 1959;16:248–250.

Johnson GA: An arsine problem: Engineering notes. *Am Ind Hyg Assoc Q* 1953;14:188–190.

Johnstone RM: Sulfhydryl agents: Arsenicals, in Hochster RM, Quastel JH (eds): *Metabolic Inhibitors.* New York, Academic Press, 1963, vol 2, pp 99–118.

Jones NW: Arseniuretted hydrogen poisoning; with report of five cases. *J Am Med Assoc* 1907;48:1099–1105.

Kensler CJ, Abels JC, Rhoads CP: Arsine poisoning, mode of action and treatment. *J Pharmacol Exp Ther* 1946;88:99–108.

Kuratsune M, Tokudome S, Shirakusa T, et al: Occupational lung cancer among copper smelters. *Int J Cancer* 1974;13:552–558.

Lee AM, Fraumeni JF: Arsenic and respiratory cancer in man: An occupational study. *J Nat Cancer Inst* 1969;42:1045–1052.

Lenihan JMA, Smith H: Clinical applications of activation analysis. *Proceedings of the Second United Nations International Conference on the Peaceful Uses of Atomic Energy* 1958;26:238–241.

Le Quesne PM, McLeod JG: Peripheral neuropathy following a single exposure to arsenic. *J Neurological Sci* 1977;32:437–451.

Lundgren KD, Richtner NG, Sjöstrand T: Changes of respiratory tract in workers of Rönskär smelting works probably due to arsenic trioxide intoxication. *Nord Med* 1951;46:1556–1560.

Mabuchi K, Lilienfeld AM, Snell LM: Lung cancer among pesticide workers exposed to inorganic arsenicals. *Arch Environ Health* 1979;34:312–320.

Mayers MR: Occupational arsenic poisoning. *Arch Ind Hyg J Occup Med* 1954;9:384–388.

Moeschlin S: *Poisoning: Diagnosis and Treatment.* New York, Grune and Stratton, 1965.

Moleen GA: Metallic poisons and the nervous system. *Am J Med Sci* 1913;146:883–895.

Morris JS, Schmid M, Newman S, et al: Arsenic and noncirrhotic portal hypertension. *Gastroenterol* 1974;64:86–94.

Muehrcke RC, Pirani CL: Arsine-induced anuria. A correlative clinicopathological study with electron microscopic observations. *Ann Intern Med* 1968;68:853–866.

Neubauer O: Arsenical cancer: A review. *Br J Cancer* 1947;1:192–251.

NIOSH: *Criteria for a Recommended Standard . . . .Occupational Exposure to Inorganic Arsenic. New Criteria—1975.* Washington, DC, National

24

Institute for Occupational Safety and Health (NIOSH 75-149), 1975.

Osburn HS: Lung cancer in a mining district in Rhodesia. *South African Med J* 1969;43:1307–1312.

Ott MG, Holder BB, Gordon HL: Respiratory cancer and occupational exposure to arsenicals. *Arch Environ Health* 1974;29:250–255.

Pelfrene A: Arsenic and cancer: The still unanswered question. *J Toxicol Environ Health* 1976;1:1003–1016.

Peterson RG, Rumack BH: D-Penicillamine therapy of acute arsenic poisoning. *J Pediatr* 1977;91:661–666.

Pinto S: Arsine poisoning: Evaluation of the acute phase. *J Occup Med* 1976;18:633–635.

Pinto S, McGill CM: Arsenic trioxide exposure in industry. *Ind Med Surg* 1953;22:281–287.

Pinto S, Nelson KW: Arsenic toxicology and industrial exposure. *Ann Rev Pharmacol Toxicol* 1976;16:95–100.

Pinto S, Petronella SJ, Johns DR, et al: Arsine poisoning: A study of thirteen cases. *Arch Ind Hyg Occup Med* 1950;1:437–451.

Pinto S, Varner MO, Nelson KW, et al: Arsenic trioxide absorption and excretion in industry. *J Occup Med* 1976;18:677–680.

Rathus E, Stinton RG, Putman JL: Arsine poisoning, country style. *Med J Aust* 1979;1:163–166.

Savory J, Sedor FA: Arsenic poisoning, in Brown SS (ed): *Clinical Chemistry and Chemical Toxicology of Metals.* Amsterdam, Elsevier/North Holland, 1977, pp 271–286.

Schroeder HA, Balassa JJ: Abnormal trace metals in man: Arsenic. *J Chronic Dis* 1966;19:85–106.

Sunderman FW Jr: A review of the carcinogenicities of nickel, chromium and arsenic compounds in man and animals. *Prevent Med* 1976;5:279–294.

Tarrant RF, Allard J: Arsenic levels in urine of forest workers applying silvicides. *Arch Environ Health* 1972;24:277–280.

Weinberg SL: The electrocardiogram in acute arsenic poisoning. *Am Heart J* 1960;60:971–975.

Wignall TH: Poisoning by arseniuretted hydrogen. *Br Med J* 1920;1:826–827.

Wilkinson SP, McHugh P, Horsley S, et al: Arsine toxicity aboard the Asiafreighter. *Br Med J* 1975;2:559–563.

4 • Barium

Uses

Barium is found in two chief ores: barytes or barite ("heavy spar") ($BaSO_4$) and witherite ($BaCO_3$). It is used as a paint extender, principally in the manufacture of lithopone, a white pigment consisting of two thirds $BaSO_4$ and one-third ZnS. Barium is also used in metal alloys in automobile engine parts, as a filler for paper, textiles, leather, soap, rubber, and linoleum. It is used in salt-water resistant cement, in ceramic and glass industries, in insecticides and rodenticides, in dyestuffs, and pyrotechnics. Barium chloride is used to treat wool for stuffing mattresses to render it more elastic, whiter, and more moth resistant.

Industrial Toxicity

The soluble salts are highly toxic but they have not ordinarily been involved in industrial poisoning. Bertarelli (1931) found that prolonged contact with carded wool that had been treated with $BaCl_2$ never resulted in the inhalation of enough of this compound to cause a suspicion of toxic symptoms. Doig (1976) cites a fatal case of a worker exposed for several days in the mid-1920s to severe dust from barium peroxide crushing operations. The BaO, $BaCO_3$, and the peroxide were presumably converted to the soluble chloride in the stomach. Death on the third day was preceded by abdominal pain, vomiting, tachycardia, dyspnea, cyanosis, and right arm and leg paralysis. Nonoccupational poisonings have resulted from accidental ingestion from errors in food preparation (Browning, 1969).

Barium sulfate, on the other hand, is extremely insoluble, a property that makes it safe for use in contrast radiography.

Baritosis, a benign pneumoconiosis, has been reported in workers who have inhaled finely ground $BaSO_4$, in baryta (BaO) miners, and in lithopone workers (Arrigoni, 1933; Pendergrass

and Greening, 1953). There is no respiratory distress, but the chest radiographs show small, sharply circumscribed nodules evenly distributed throughout the lung fields. Some reports suggest that baritosis is accompanied by a significant increase in deaths due to pneumonia and tuberculosis. Closer study makes it likely that there has been exposure to the fibrogenic dust-free silica in such cases.

Doig (1976) has studied a group of workers in a barytes crushing factory over a span of years from 1947 to 1973. Baritosis was detected radiographically in some cases as early as 18 to 21 months after beginning of exposure. The chest radiographs were conspicuous for the "intense radioopacity of the discrete opacities" that were profuse and evenly disseminated and for the absence of any other abnormalities of the lungs. The radiographic opacities slowly disappeared after cessation of exposure. Pulmonary function tests were essentially normal and were in contrast to the severity of the appearance of the chest films. Doig comments that the chest radiographs of well-established baritosis are similar to those of stannosis while Pendergrass and Greening also caution that silicosis should be considered in the differential diagnosis.

References

Arrigoni A: Pneumoconiosi da bario. *Med lavoro* 1933;24:461–468.

Bertarelli E: Treatment of wool for mattresses with barium chloride from the hygienic aspect. Abstracted, *J Ind Hyg Toxicol* 1931;12:6.

Browning E: *Toxicity of Industrial Metals,* ed 2. New York. Appleton-Century-Crofts, 1969, pp 61–66.

Doig AT: Baritosis: A benign pneumoconiosis. *Thorax* 1976;31:30–39.

Pendergrass EP, Greening RR: Baritosis. Report of a case. *Arch Ind Hyg Occup Med* 1953;7:44–48.

5 • Beryllium

Industrial Uses

The element beryllium is extracted from beryl ore ($3BeO \cdot Al_2O_3 \cdot 6SiO_2$), which is mined in Brazil, Germany, Russia, India, and in the United States in Utah, South Dakota, and in the past in the New England states. Beryllium is the fourth lightest element, with an atomic weight of 9.02, and has been known to chemists since Vauquelin recognized it as a distinct element early in the 19th century. Great interest in beryllium has developed since the early 1930s when metallurgists promoted for industrial use the marvelous properties of alloys of beryllium in combination with copper, aluminum, nickel, magnesium, silver, and iron. Beryllium alloys are light and remarkably resistant to stress and strain. A wide, recent use for beryllium was as a phosphor in the manufacture of fluorescent lamps and neon signs, a practice discontinued in 1949. Beryllium was, and is, used in atomic energy development and nuclear reactor research since, when bombarded with alpha particles, beryllium releases neutrons. In addition, beryllium and its compounds are used in making radio and electronic tubes, electric heating elements, and x-ray tube windows. Because of its heat resistance, beryllium oxide is used as a refractory in work requiring high temperatures. Beryllium compounds in small amounts have been used in making Welsbach lamp mantles for years, and they have also been used in preparing ceramics and crystals for radio use.

Since the preparation of the second edition of this book in 1949, a number of different uses for beryllium and its compounds have been introduced. As a result, the amount of industrial beryllium in the United States increased from roughly 500 tons in 1950 to 8500 tons in 1969, although worldwide usage fell to 2200 metric tons in 1977–78. Beryllium in various forms is used by the military and for space exploration in the struc-ture of vehicles, guidance systems, radar devices, nose cones, jet plane brakes, and in missiles. In 1972 there were 8000 workplaces in the United States using beryllium (Hasan and Kazemi, 1973), and it has been estimated that 30,000 persons have a potential occupational exposure to dusts or fumes of beryllium in this country (NIOSH, 1972).

Industrial Illness

European physicians incriminated beryllium compounds as the cause of pulmonary disability of occupational origin since the early 1930s. Weber and Engelhardt (1933) in Germany de-scribed cases of bronchitis and bronchiolitis in workers extracting beryllium from ore. In 1936, Gelman and his colleagues in Moscow presented a description of "Occupational Poisoning by Oxy-fluoride of Beryllium" that consisted of an irritant action on the skin, mucous membranes, and con-junctivae, rarely serious in character, that was followed in some patients by a pulmonary disorder consisting of cough and moist râles, and an x-ray picture resembling miliary tuberculosis. Subsequently, according to Gelman, broncho-alveolitis appeared. Berkovitz and Izrael (1940) described in detail the x-ray observations and physical findings in 46 patients with what they called fluorine beryllium intoxication. Meyer (1942) presented a series of cases he had observed in Germany of a unique pulmonary disease suf-fered by men engaged in beryllium extraction and exposed to silicates, hydroxide, sulfate, and chloride of beryllium. Fifty percent of the workers suffered dyspnea on exertion, irritating cough, and chest pain. A few of the workers died after a prodromal period of mild dyspnea and cough lasting two weeks, with x-ray and physical find-ings indicating severe pulmonary disease. Most of the workers gradually recovered, but a year after the acute illness, hard work produced symptoms of respiratory insufficiency that suggested chronic disease. Wurm and Rüger (1942) described the pathologic lesion in fatal cases as a large-celled carnifying alveolitis. When the lesion became extensive in a given case, Wurm called it chronic large-celled pneumonia. These European reports were summarized in a monograph by Tepper et al. in 1961.

The first report of disease in the beryllium industry in the United States came from the Cleveland Clinic in 1943 when Van Ordstrand et al. presented the case reports of three workers exposed in the manufacture of beryllium oxide from beryl ore. They had a chemical pneumonia with progressive dyspnea and dry cough, followed by x-ray changes that were bilateral and diffuse. Recovery occurred after an average illness of three months' duration. Shilen et al. (1944) concluded that fluorine compounds were responsible for the disability reported from the beryllium industry in Pennsylvania. This conclusion, which stated flatly that beryllium itself was nontoxic, proved to be a serious deterrent to understanding the risks of beryllium exposures.

Kress and Crispell (1944) published reports of four beryllium-exposed workers who suffered from a chemical pneumonitis caused by exposure to beryllium-containing fluorescent powder. Two complained of increasing dyspnea and cough followed after three to four weeks by the development of a chest x-ray picture described as a fine diffuse pulmonary fibrosis. The other two had similar x-ray findings.

In 1945, Van Ordstrand et al. published an extensive account of the acute illness seen in the beryllium industry. Here, the disability was encountered in the course of the processing of beryl ore for the production of beryllium oxide. As in the European reports, high operating temperatures and acid compounds of beryllium such as the sulfate, fluoride, and oxyfluoride were considered of etiologic importance. Thirty-eight cases with five deaths were reported. Symptoms included cough, dyspnea, substernal pain, anorexia, increasing fatigue, and weight loss. Three weeks after an insidious onset a characteristic diffuse bilateral haziness appeared in the chest radiographs. Elevation of body temperature appeared only terminally in the few fatal cases. If the patients were kept in bed, recovery took place in one to four months. Return of the worker to the same beryllium exposure produced a second

bout of chemical pneumonitis. The necropsy findings were described as bilateral acute organizing atypical bronchopneumonia. It is certain that a number of cases of acute and subacute beryllium pneumonitis were not identified because of the similarity of the clinical picture to that of viral pneumonia.

Van Ordstrand also described 42 cases of dermatitis and conjunctivitis encountered in the same industry, while 90 patients were depicted as having chemical nasopharyngitis and, or separately, chemical tracheobronchitis. These findings were very much like those of Shilen of Pennsylvania from very similar beryllium operations. Since the number of irritating materials to which these workers could have been exposed is large, it seems not unlikely that there may have been more than one etiologic agent in these reported cases of "beryllium poisoning." Nevertheless, the cases of chemical pneumonitis reported by Van Ordstrand are so very like those described in the 1943 Cleveland Clinic report, the Pennsylvania report of Kress and Crispell (1944), and the European reports that one is forced to accept a common etiologic background involving beryllium in some form.

Hardy and Tabershaw (1946) described the case records of 17 workers in the Massachusetts fluorescent lamp manufacturing industry who suffered from what they termed "delayed chemical pneumonitis." The material involved was a mixture of zinc and manganese beryllium silicates. The clinical picture was characterized by delayed onset in half of the workers six months to three years after they had left the common environment, plus severe dyspnea, great weight loss, and a poor prognosis. These 17 patients shared a unique x-ray picture that involved both lungs and was characterized early by a fine granularity and later by a snowstorm appearance with hilar node enlargement in many cases and varying amounts of emphysema. Total serum proteins were elevated with relative increase in the globulin fraction. Clubbed fingers and marked cyanosis were seen in one third of the patients. Those patients who lived for more than two years with the disease developed right heart enlargement. Skin lesions (nontraumatic) in three cases were biopsied and were thought to be sarcoid or chronic inflammation. One liver biopsy done in the absence of abnormal liver function tests, according to Mallory, showed tubercle-like collections of histiocytes between strands of normal hepatic cells. All studies for tubercle bacilli were negative. These findings helped to group the cases of delayed chemical pneumonitis together and to separate them from Boeck's sarcoid and miliary tuberculosis. At the time of that report, six of the 17 workers had died and eleven remained disabled with no case of recovery. The pathologic picture in the lungs was described as a granulomatous process replacing normal tissue. Lesions of a similar nature were found in liver, spleen, and hilar nodes.

Jackson (1950) described the illness of workers exposed in the casting shop of a metallurgy plant using alloys of copper that contained beryllium in amounts averaging under 4%. Seven men suffering for periods of from one to three years with dyspnea, cough, and some weight loss were noted to have extensive diffuse haziness on chest x-ray. Five of these men came to autopsy and a pulmonary granulomatous lesion identical with that seen in the Massachusetts cases of delayed chemical pneumonitis was found. That this casting shop first used copper beryllium alloys in 1931 and the first death occurred in 1938 further emphasized the delay in onset of the disease. Machle et al. (1948) reported that workers engaged in the manufacture of fluorescent powders, after one or more episodes of illness clinically similar to acute chemical pneumonitis, developed chronic pulmonary disability with an x-ray picture similar to that seen in the Massachusetts fluorescent lamp workers. Aub and Grier (1949) cared for research workers who were exposed to beryllium oxides and who developed dyspnea, weight loss, and x-ray changes, which cleared when the men ceased all activity. This is the picture of acute and subacute chemical pneumonitis. It is important to remember that this group was exposed to beryllium metal and beryllium oxide rather than silicates and acid compounds, as was the case in earlier reports of illness in the beryllium industry.

Since 1950 the findings of the many reports of the 1940s of illness in the beryllium industry have been confirmed. On the basis of data in the U.S. Beryllium Case Registry begun in 1962, it is known that in the absence of engineering controls, beryllium metal and all of its compounds have caused disease.

Reports of beryllium poisoning correlated with workroom air levels are of importance. A few examples help to illustrate the problem of low beryllium alloy exposures. Chamberlin et al. (1957) studied an operation involving a copper alloy containing 1% beryllium from which the final castings were machined. Drossing and casting gave levels of 3.55 to 21.20 mg/m³ and dry surface grinding produced 87 to 194 μg/m³; the two men on this job developed chronic beryllium disease. Sneddon (1958) reported two cases of chronic poisoning after exposure to 2% beryllium alloy dust.

Gelman's report (1936) of Russian experience with occupational beryllium poisoning gave air levels of 0.05 to 0.72 mg Be/m³. Eisenbud et al. (1948) measured beryllium in air in an extraction plant immediately after an accidental overexposure that led to acute beryllium poisoning. He concluded that an intake of 45 μg of beryllium inhaled in 20 minutes or less can cause acute disease. Griggs (1973) reported finding potentially harmful amounts of beryllium in the fumes from mantle-type camp lanterns. Also, the fact, for example, that clips of many modern pens contain small amounts of beryllium illustrates the need to take a careful work history in considering beryllium poisoning as the diagnosis in a case of sarcoid-like illness.

Not only the fact of beryllium use but the character of the operation needs attention in making a correct diagnosis. Heating, surface grinding, machining, or any work that can produce fumes or finely divided dust must be judged a hazardous job unless enclosure or proper ventilation is used. In foundries, machine shops, and research laboratories where beryllium or its compounds are worked only intermittently, a significant risk may arise because of careless housekeeping allowing beryllium to accumulate in workroom air. There is ignorance of the possible danger in many instances, and there is downgrading of the risk by those fearing litigation or union demands for extra hazard pay for work with beryllium. Present evidence makes it certain that beryllium can be used safely when conventional industrial hygiene controls are in place (Tepper et al., 1961). However, if large quantities of beryllium were to be released in rocket firing, it would be necessary to consider the hazards to the potentially exposed population.

Claims have been made on the basis of experiments with small animals that oxides of beryllium formed at high temperatures are not toxic. There have been no worker groups exposed solely to high fired oxides where this observation could be tested. Furthermore, because beryllium is excreted slowly and has proved to be carcinogenic in animals, risk of exposure to any beryllium compound must be controlled (Gardner and Heslington, 1946; Stokinger, 1966). Wagner et al. (1969) reported malignancies in animals after exposure to certain beryllium ores. There may be small amounts of beryllium compounds known to be toxic occurring with beryl to account for this observation, since workers handling naturally occurring beryl ores have not been ill. Men working with such ores are few and may have been exposed to other minerals and to uncertain silica levels.

Terminology

An array of terms describing the occupational disease associated with harmful beryllium exposure is to be found in the medical literature (Hardy, 1962). The preferred names are *beryllium poisoning, beryllium intoxication,* or *beryllium disease,* to be supplemented, as appropriate, with the adjectives *acute, subacute,* or *chronic,* or with terms such as *pneumonitis* or *hepatitis,* as examples, to indicate the affected organ. The term *berylliosis* was coined by Fabroni in 1935 (Tepper et al., 1961) and has been widely used. This term has unfortunately been defined as a pneumoconiosis. Because harmful beryllium exposures cause systemic damage that may involve a number of organs rather than localized pulmonary effects exclusively, the term beryllium disease is more accurate. Berylliosis has frequently been misspelled as berylosis or beryllosis, terms that suggest a pneumoconiosis due to the inhalation of beryl ore particulates. Such a disease is not known to exist. Earlier designations are of historical interest but have no use today. "Salem sarcoid" and "miliary sarcoid" implied that chronic beryllium disease was sarcoidosis. The term "delayed chemical pneumonitis" neglected the systemic nature of the disease that was demonstrated later, as did Gardner's (1946) term "generalized pulmonary granulomatosis" and the official Saranac Symposium (1947) term "pulmonary granulomatosis of beryllium workers." Granulomatosis is, in addition, a pathologic designation and does not indicate other aspects of the disease that have proved to be of functional importance.

Clinical Syndromes of Beryllium Disease

The physician may be helped by a summarizing discussion of present knowledge of the clinical patterns associated with harmful beryllium exposures. A few European reports dating from 1933–1942 and the United States literature since 1943 support the fact that, depending on duration and level of exposure, the metal and all industrially encountered beryllium compounds except the naturally occurring ore, beryl, cause illness.

Acute beryllium poisoning Acute beryllium poisoning may be defined arbitrarily to include those beryllium-induced disease patterns of less than one year's duration and to exclude those syndromes lasting more than one year. In most series of cases the acute forms of beryllium disease – if not fatal – are of several months' duration, while the chronic disease, with no known exception, has to date never resolved. The diagnosis of acute beryllium poisoning rests on the character of the patient's work history. There are no unique signs and symptoms in cases of beryllium dermatitis, conjunctivitis, bronchitis, or pneumonitis, with the possible exception of the weight loss described by Van Ordstrand et al. (1945). Abnormal chest x-ray findings vary with the severity of the clinical picture. Roentgenologic changes mimic viral pneumonia and, in fatal cases, pulmonary edema of any cause. There are reports that beryllium is present in urine during and after exposure, but the level is poorly correlated with active disease. If beryllium exposure is suspected and is difficult to document in a sick person with clinical evidence that is consistent with acute poisoning, finding beryllium in the urine can establish the diagnosis. Serious drawbacks, however, result from the fact that beryllium is excreted slowly, the assay is technically difficult, and only a few research laboratories are prepared to carry out such a test (Tepper et al., 1961).

In the middle 1940s an important series of mild but definite beryllium pneumonitides was studied and later reported by Aub and Grier (1949). Dyspnea, hacking cough, some weight loss, and mild chest x-ray changes very much like those of viral pneumonia comprised the clinical picture. After exposure to beryllium stopped, an interval of three to 12 months passed before all evidence of the disease disappeared. Of great importance is the fact that 10 of the 27 workers diagnosed as suffering from subacute beryllium poisoning subsequently, after varying periods of time, developed chronic disease without further exposure to beryllium. Experience with cases of acute beryllium poisoning and in taking histories of patients with chronic disease from beryllium exposure make plain the fact that progression from acute to chronic disease, with and without known further beryllium exposure, is a far more frequent occurrence than is generally recognized. The very slow excretion of beryllium from the body may help to explain this clinical experience. Careful treatment of mild manifestations of beryllium toxicity and exclusion from further beryllium exposure, however minor, may control this problem.

X-ray changes in acute and subacute beryllium poisoning may vary from hardly recognizable densities in several, but rarely all, lung fields to bilateral apex-to-base changes. The few postmortem studies of patients dying from acute beryllium disease reported from Cleveland (Hazard, 1959) demonstrated that the acute pulmonary lesion is a chemical pneumonitis or bronchoalveolitis characterized by nonspecific intra-alveolar edema and inflammatory infiltrates throughout the lung parenchyma. Although the lesions described by Hazard were nongranulomatous in character, HLH has held the view that acute, subacute, and chronic beryllium disease are varying clinical responses to beryllium. This concept is contrary to the notion that acute and chronic beryllium poisoning are different diseases caused by specific identifiable beryllium compounds. This point is stressed because of the hazard to the patient of further beryllium exposure after acute or subacute poisoning.

Chronic beryllium disease The clinical character of the chronic illness differs from that of the acute in that the former is 1) frequently separated by a period of years from the time of the etiologic beryllium exposure, 2) prolonged in duration with no evidence of lasting cure, 3) commonly progressive in severity, especially if untreated, in spite of cessation of exposure, and 4) a disease that may affect organs other than the lung and may involve several biochemical systems. The lung is usually the organ attacked first with varying clinical, x-ray, and pathologic patterns, but it is rarely, if ever, the only organ or system affected by harmful beryllium exposure. Hilar, scalene, and abdominal lymph nodes, lung, pleura, spleen, liver, myocardium, muscle, skin, salivary glands, kidney, and bone have, to differing extents, been found to contain significant amounts of beryllium and evidence of associated pathologic change. In addition, calculi of lung, salivary glands (both rare), and kidney (up to 30% in one series), and changes in serum proteins and uric acid metabolism support the concept of beryllium poisoning as a body-wide, not a local lung, disease. A few postmortem studies of human cases with chronic disease have shown that beryllium in significant quantities may be found in the liver and be barely detectable in the lung or vice versa. This observation suggests that beryllium is translocated among various organs and is slowly excreted in accordance with biological patterns that are not now fully understood.

As might be expected with chronic lung disease, pulmonary hypertension with cor pulmonale, ultimate right heart failure, and pulmonary insufficiency are sequelae of progressive beryllium intoxication. There have been deaths from overwhelming cachexia, renal failure, and cardiac standstill associated with myocarditis. Registry experience indicates that chronic beryllium disease carries a poor prognosis. Mortality rates have been 26% in 1969 and 30% in 1972. In patients in whom abnormal lung function indices were established, there have been no complete recoveries although Sprince et al. (1978) reported improvement in gas exchange and radiographic findings of interstitial disease among a group of workers after engineering and ventilation controls reduced the peak air concentrations of beryllium. There are a few cases of chest x-ray changes being the sole evidence of toxic beryllium effect. Diagnosis was established by elimination of other causes for the radiographic changes and by knowledge of beryllium disease in fellow workers. In one well-studied case, the roentgenographic densities persisted for 20 years with no other sign or symptom of illness.

Of special interest and importance is the character of onset of chronic beryllium poisoning and its delay, which in many cases has led to mistaken diagnosis. Wood (1964) pointed out that half of the Massachusetts fluorescent lamp workers became ill with weight loss and dyspnea while at work. Some indication of the extent of delay in onset can be gleaned from Beryllium Case Registry data (Hardy et al., 1967):

Time after exposure	No. of cases
1 month	126
1 month to 1 year	27
1 to 5 years	89
5 to 10 years	56
10 years or more	12

In most cases, intercurrent illness, other toxic exposure, surgery, pregnancy, and a variety of other stresses, including military combat duty, appear to have acted as precipitating factors influencing the onset of symptoms. Clary and Stokinger (1973) studied adrenal imbalance in small animals as an explanation of these clinical findings of latency in chronic beryllium disease. Severe cases in man, thought to follow high-level beryllium exposure, present themselves with little or no delay in onset, with the patient suffering striking weight loss, dyspnea on effort, and chronic nonproductive cough so violent as to cause vomiting. In less severe cases, the patient usually complains only of shortness of breath on exertion. Very mild disease may be discovered on a chest x-ray done for other purposes. Unusual onsets of well-studied cases include joint pains suggestive of rheumatic fever, sarcoid-like skin lesions, and renal calculi. The most valuable diagnostic clue is the history of significant beryllium exposure. Reports of beryllium disease after exposure to broken fluorescent lamps have proven to be false, especially since beryllium has no longer been used in the phosphors since 1949. Help of a chemist, engineer, or industrial hygienist trained in the field may be required to assess the extent and importance of exposure in research laboratories or industrial operations using alloys containing small quantities of beryllium.

The clinical course of chronic beryllium poisoning is, in all but very mild cases, one of exacerbation and remission over a long period of time. Some cases, usually severe in character from the outset, suffer periods of fever and chills controlled by steroids but not by antibiotics, signs of a poor prognosis. Availability of steroids has improved the patient's chance of survival and such therapy may delay the development of right heart failure but does not cure the disease.

Chest x-ray studies show that chronic beryllium disease in most cases produces densities of different sizes in all lung fields and hilar adenopathy in about half of the cases. Unusual and important are three cases known to HLH that showed a large area of x-ray density in an upper lobe that was thought to be either a malignancy or a tuberculous infection. In one of these cases, densities appeared in all lung fields shortly after surgery. The single lesion contained beryllium and characteristic pathologic changes. The patient proved to have had moderately heavy beryllium exposure in 1944–46 and became ill after a pregnancy in 1952. In the other two cases, similar findings on biopsy demonstrated that chronic beryllium poisoning may present as a solitary lung lesion.

Pulmonary function studies originally showed that chronic beryllium disease causes a diffusion defect without changes in the other indices. As pa-

tients live longer with steroid therapy and milder disease, beryllium intoxication has been shown to affect all lung function values in spite of reasonable control with steroids of complaints and physical findings (Andrews et al., 1969). Laboratory results that have been shown to be abnormal at differing times in different cases are: increased total protein due to elevated globulin, increased serum uric acid (Kelley et al., 1969), abnormal liver function tests, and increased urinary calcium excretion. Elevated hematocrit and changes in the electrocardiogram and the vectorcardiogram have been seen in surprisingly few cases, even in those of progressive chronic beryllium disease in patients receiving steroid therapy.

Curtis (1959) developed a patch test for use in the diagnosis of beryllium disease that used solutions of soluble salts, with the results read after 48 hours. For a number of reasons this test is seldom used now, especially since beryllium proved to be a skin sensitizer in 50% of normal cases tested. A few carefully studied cases with negative patch tests were shown by beryllium assay and pathologic findings on biopsy to have the occupational disease. Waksman (1959) argued on theoretical grounds that such testing would exacerbate the disease if beryllium poisoning is a result of an abnormal host response.

Sterner and Eisenbud (1951) had suggested that certain manifestations of beryllium disease, such as granuloma formation and varying susceptibility to exposure, did not conform to the usual concept of acute or chronic chemical intoxication and might be better explained by hypersensitivity and a modified immunologic reaction. This concept was resisted because of evidence that beryllium poisoning was essentially a systemic disease that affected many tissues in the body. New interest in hypersensitivity as the explanation for some cases of beryllium poisoning has been stimulated by Deodhar et al. (1973) and Reeves (1976). It has again been proposed that the pathogenesis of pulmonary beryllium disease may depend upon certain immunologic reactions of the host (Reeves et al., 1971). Support for this concept has come from Resnick and Morgan (1971) who found marked hypergammaglobulinemia with significantly increased IgG levels in a group of symptomatic beryllium workers as well as in some with long exposure to the metal but with no clinical evidence of beryllium toxicity.

The pathologic changes of beryllium intoxication have been summarized by Tepper et al. (1961) and by Freiman and Hardy (1970). The acute disease presents changes similar to those of any acute chemical pneumonitis, while the chronic form is characterized by a noncaseating granulomatous lesion containing mononuclear cells and usually, but not always, giant cells. Asteroid bodies are often seen. Blood vessels are involved when pulmonary hypertension develops, and emphysema and pneumothorax are frequently present. A single case of maxillary salivary gland disease with stone formation is well documented but no cases of parotitis are known. In some cases it has been impossible to tell the difference between chronic beryllium disease and sarcoidosis.

A number of diseases may have to be considered in the differential diagnosis of chronic beryllium disease. Sarcoidosis and tuberculosis have been the chief problems. The latter is ruled out by appropriate study of sputum or gastric washings. In HLH's experience, skin testing with tuberculin, when used to the second strength, is positive in about the same percentage of persons as that found in the general population. Negative fungal tests may mean only that the residence and health of the victims of beryllium poisoning rule out these diseases. Chronic beryllium disease, in contrast to Boeck's sarcoid, has not to date attacked eye or tonsil. Skin lesions in the two diseases are identical in appearance, but beryllium is detectable in biopsies of the industrial disease in samples of 0.5 g or more. The Kveim test has been uniformly negative in beryllium case studies (Israel and Sones, 1959). In general, beryllium disease has proved to be a more serious problem than sarcoidosis for, although it is responsive to steroids, there have been no recoveries as is often true in Boeck's disease. The problems of differentiating between these two diseases were summarized by Sprince et al. in 1976.

A few cases of hemosiderosis secondary to heart disease were considered to be beryllium disease prior to biopsy because of the patients' work history. Experience suggests that an unknown number of cases of beryllium disease have been listed under the diagnoses of chronic nonspecific pulmonary disease (Hamman-Rich) or idiopathic pulmonary fibrosis. Without attention to work history, tissue assay, and search for other manifestations of toxic beryllium effect, this situation will continue to be true.

Carcinoma of the lung in beryllium workers, especially in heavy cigarette smokers, will be an etiologic problem because of beryllium-induced lung malignancy in rats. In addition, cohort studies by Mancuso (1970, 1980), Wagoner et al. (1980) and Beryllium Case Registry analyses by Infante et al. (1980) suggest that beryllium may be responsible for increased risk of lung cancer in exposed humans.

Treatment

The history of therapeutic trials has been described by Tepper et al. (1961). The chelating agents that are used for the treatment of heavy metal poisoning are useless in beryllium disease. Aurintricarboxylic acid (ATA) was tried, at the suggestion of White, Finkel, and Schubert (1951), as a laking agent to sequester the beryllium stored in the body. This compound proved to be ineffective in a few attempts to treat patients. In addition, pure ATA was nephrotoxic to laboratory animals.

Adrenocorticotropic hormone (ACTH) in 1949 and steroids subsequently have been useful in controlling disabling dyspnea and in delaying the onset of pulmonary insufficiency and right heart failure. Other manifestations of beryllium disease such as pleuritis, pneumothorax, weight loss, elevated serum protein and uric acid, and calculus formation also appear to be favorably influenced in most cases. An every-other-day single-dose regimen ranging from 20 to as high as 80 mg of prednisone for short periods, averaging from 20 to 40 mg over the years, has proved to be remarkably successful in clinical practice, with rare complications.

The use of sodium fluoride by mouth to control steroid-induced osteoporosis was tried in five patients (Tepper et al., 1961; Schepers, 1961; Stokinger, 1966; Nichols, Flanagan, and Hardy, unpublished data, 1971). By 1973 none of the five patients had suffered a bone fracture although osteoporosis was seen on x-ray (Stoeckle, personal communication to HLH, 1973). Only four recorded cases of steroid-induced bone fractures have been recorded, and these were associated with long periods in bed with daily cortisone doses at the level of 250 mg. Ferris (1962) showed that such doses favorably influence the diffusion defect of moderately severe beryllium disease after a two-week course. It has been felt that the risks are too great to continue such courses for longer periods. Appropriate diuretics have been used especially in menstruating women to prevent fluid retention. Care of right heart disease of any cause is difficult and has proved to be so in chronic beryllium disease. Very rarely, in long-standing cases, bronchodilators have been helpful. Inhalation of oxygen, once the only therapy, still has a place in the care of anoxia of beryllium disease. Because the disease process results in a shrunken lung bound down by thickened pleurae, cough is a problem that requires restriction of physical activity and has a risk of codeine addiction. Pneumothorax occurs in many cases, and as more patients live longer as a result of steroid therapy, emphysema is a serious complication.

Animal Studies

Experimental animal work that demonstrated a number of reproducible toxic beryllium effects similar to those seen in man has been summarized by Tepper et al. (1961) and by Groth (1980). Acute beryllium disease was studied experimentally by Scott (1950). Various investigators could, and others could not, produce in animals the recognizable forms of the chronic disease of humans. Gardner and Heslington's (1946) production of osteosarcoma in rabbits has been repeated by many. Vorwald (1953) produced lung neoplasia in rats and monkeys as a result of beryllium exposure. Pulmonary tumors have been reported to be caused by beryl ores containing 4% beryllium (Wagner et al., 1969), an effect not known in humans.

Aldridge et al. (1950) and Caccuri (1941) reported liver damage in animals. Inhaled 5µm Teflon particles coated with beryllium have been found to be highly toxic for rabbit alveolar macrophages (Camner et al., 1974). Of great interest is work done first by Grier et al. (1949), repeated and extended by DuBois et al. (1949), showing that beryllium replaces magnesium in certain enzyme systems and acts to inhibit alkaline phosphatase. Electron microscopic studies by Goldblatt et al. (1973) showed that beryllium may induce changes in fundamental structure of both the intact and regenerating liver. These studies followed those of Witschi and Marchand (1971) demonstrating that beryllium interferes with enzyme induction in rat liver. The findings of Aldridge et al. (1949) that intravenously injected soluble beryllium salt forms a stable complex with plasma proteins was thought by some to support the concept that beryllium disease was a systemic, not a local, lung ailment. Later work by Reeves and Vorwald (1961), however, indicated that the transport of soluble beryllium salts in the blood

principally involves the colloidal form of orthophosphate. All studies have shown that beryllium is so poorly absorbed through the gut that ingestion is not a hazard (Reeves, 1965; Stokinger, 1966).

Control

Since the early 1950s industrial hygiene controls of beryllium operations have been well understood, and where correctly applied no new cases have developed (Tepper et al., 1961; Stokinger, 1966). The threshold limit values (TLV) in use at the present time are 25 µg/m³ of beryllium for any exposure, however short; 2 µg/m³ for 40 hours a week and 0.01 µg/m³ averaged over a 30-day period for community air. NIOSH (1972) has recommended essentially the same values for occupational exposure. Attempts to set separate standards for quantity and duration of exposure for different compounds should be vigorously opposed on the basis of experience with beryllium disease in humans. The current use of animal data derived after exposure to beryllium oxides fired at various temperatures in order to form estimates of risk to the general population in connection with the use of beryllium in solid fuel for rocket firing is a dangerous practice.

In May, 1949 the three United States fluorescent lamp manufacturers agreed to stop using beryllium in phosphors. It is ironic that a harmless compound, calcium phosphate, was substituted. There is little knowledge of how long danger will exist from finely divided beryllium allowed to go up the stacks of beryllium-using plants. The discovery of 5 to 14 ppm beryllium in soil in the neighborhood of a beryllium-producing plant in contrast to 0.2 ppm in soil in a Boston suburb raises the possibility of an unknown risk of beryllium disease to persons living nearby. So-called "neighborhood" cases have occurred, but the routes of contamination have been other than by ambient air pollution (NIOSH, 1972). It has been established that lungs and hilar nodes of city dwellers and coal miners contain beryllium in detectable amounts. These findings are accounted for by the presence of beryllium compounds in certain fossil fuels.

There are several reasons why beryllium disease and its control are of importance to the physician. Because of delay in onset, cases of chronic beryllium disease from old exposures may continue to appear. Since it is likely that beryllium is also a

34

carcinogen, and because beryllium leaves the body slowly, cases of malignancy resulting from beryllium inhalation many years earlier may begin to appear in significant numbers. The U.S. Beryllium Case Registry listed 55 new cases of beryllium disease admitted between 1973 and 1977 (Sprince and Kazemi, 1980). At the end of 1977, there were 887 cases registered, 675 of which were chronic and 212 acute. Of the total, 46% were known to be dead and 40% were known to be alive. Of the 55 new cases added to the Registry between 1973 and 1977, 22 had exposures after 1950, three as late as 1970. These findings confirm the impression that new uses of beryllium are not always controlled. Ignorance and apathy on the part of those unaware of the epidemic of disease in the beryllium industry in the decade between 1940 and 1950 indicate that beryllium toxicity requires continuing attention (Hardy, 1965, 1980).

Thirty-five years of experience with occupational exposure to beryllium in industry has shown that medical control rests chiefly on regular monitoring of personnel by use of large-size chest radiographs. Small films are useless, as are lung function tests of ventilatory capacity only. Early changes of chronic beryllium disease are detected by indices of gas diffusion, and such changes may be present in overexposed beryllium workers who still have normal chest films. Tissue biopsies are best done by obtaining mediastinal nodes. Except for workers with established chronic lung disease, no pre-employment exclusion is required. After accidental exposure, removal from further beryllium exposure, frequent chest x-ray examinations, and daily weighings will help detect beryllium damage.

In summary, beryllium disease has been shown by the experience of chest and occupational physicians, by the 1977 data of the U.S. Beryllium Case Registry of 887 case reports (Sprince and Kazemi, 1980), by its frequent delay in onset, its mimicry of sarcoidosis, and by the difficulties of engineering control, to be a continuing occupational hazard and a problem in differential diagnosis.

References

Aldridge WN, Barnes JM, Denz FA: Biochemical changes in acute beryllium poisoning. *Br J Exp Pathol* 1950;31:473–484.

Andrews JL, Kazemi H, Hardy HL: Patterns of lung dysfunction in chronic beryllium disease. *Am Rev Respir Dis* 1969;100:791–800.

Aub JC, Grier RS: Acute pneumonitis in workers exposed to beryllium oxide and beryllium metal. *J Ind Hyg Toxicol* 1949;31:123–133.

Berkovitz M, Izrael B: Changes in the lungs caused by beryllium oxyfluoride intoxication (in Russian). *Klin Med (Mosk)* 1940;18:117–122.

Caccuri S: Sulle alterazioni del fegato e del rene nell'intossicazione da berillio. *Rass di Med Indust* 1941;11:307–314.

Camner P, Lundborg M, Hallström PA: Alveolar macrophages and 5 μm particles coated with different metals. *Arch Environ Health* 1974;29:211–213.

Chamberlin GW, Jennings WP, Lieben J: Chronic pulmonary disease associated with beryllium dust. *Penn Med J* 1957;60:497–503.

Clary JJ, Stokinger HE: The mechanism of delayed biologic response following beryllium exposure. *J Occup Med* 1973;15:255–259.

Curtis GH: The diagnosis of beryllium disease, with special reference to the patch test. *Arch Ind Health* 1959;19:150–153.

Deodhar SD, Barna B, Van Ordstrand HS: A study of the immunologic aspects of chronic berylliosis. *Chest* 1973;63:309–313.

DuBois KP, Cochran KW, Mazur M: Inhibition of phosphatases by beryllium and antagonism of the inhibition by manganese. *Science* 1949;110:420–422.

Eisenbud M, Berghout CF, Steadman LT: Environmental studies in plants and laboratories using beryllium; the acute disease. *J Ind Hyg Toxicol* 1948;30:281–285.

Ferris BC Jr: Chronic beryllium intoxication treated with corticosteroids and corticotropin. *Am Rev Respir Dis* 1962;85:583.

Freiman DG, Hardy HL: Beryllium disease: The relation of pulmonary pathology to clinical course and prognosis based on a study of 130 cases from the U.S. Beryllium Case Registry. *Human Pathol* 1970;1:25–44.

Gardner LU: Generalized pulmonary granulomatosis occurring among workers believed to be exposed to beryllium or its compounds. *Trans 11th Annual Mtg Ind Hyg Foundation,* 1946; 89–94.

Gardner LU, Heslington HF: Osteosarcoma from intravenous beryllium compounds in rabbits. *Fed Proc* 1946;5:221.

Gelman I: Oxyfluoride poisoning by vapors of beryllium oxyfluoride. *J Ind Hyg Toxicol* 1936;18:371–379.

Goldblatt PJ, Lieberman MW, Witschi H: Beryllium-induced ultrastructural changes in intact and regenerating liver. *Arch Environ Health* 1973;26:48–56.

Grier RS, Hood MB, Hoagland MB: Observations on the effects of beryllium on alkaline phosphatase. *J Biol Chem* 1949;180:289–298.

Griggs K: Toxic metal fumes from mantle-type camp lanterns. *Science* 1973;181:842–843.

Groth DH: Carcinogenicity of beryllium: Review of the literature. *Environ Res* 1980; 21:56–72.

Hardy HL: Reaction to toxic beryllium compounds: Terminology. *J Occup Med* 1962; 4:532–534.

Hardy HL: Beryllium poisoning—lessons in the control of man-made disease. *N Engl J Med* 1965; 273:1188–1199.

Hardy HL: Beryllium disease: A clinical perspective. *Environ Res* 1980;21:1–9.

Hardy HL, Rabe EW, Lorch S: United States Beryllium Case Registry (1952–1966): Review of its methods and utility. *J Occup Med* 1967;9:271–276.

Hardy HL, Tabershaw IR: Delayed chemical pneumonitis occurring in workers exposed to beryllium compounds. *J Ind Hyg Toxicol* 1946; 28:197–211.

Hasan FM, Kazemi H: Progress Report, U.S. Beryllium Case Registry, 1972. *Am Rev Respir Dis* 1973;108:1252–1253.

Hazard JB: Pathologic changes of beryllium disease; the acute disease. *Arch Ind Health* 1959;19:179–183.

Infante PF, Wagoner JK, Sprince NL: Mortality patterns from lung cancer and nonneoplastic respiratory disease among white males in the Beryllium Case Registry. *Environ Res* 1980;21: 35–43.

Israel HL, Sones M: The differentiation of sarcoidosis and beryllium disease. *Arch Ind Health* 1959;19:160–163.

Jackson AJ: Beryllium alloys, in Vorwald AJ (ed): *Pneumoconiosis: Beryllium, Bauxite Fumes, Compensation.* New York, Hoeber, 1950, pp 20–27.

Kelley WN, Goldfinger SE, Hardy HL: Hyperuricemia in chronic beryllium disease. *Ann Intern Med* 1969;70:977–983.

Kress JE, Crispell KR: Chemical pneumonitis in men working with fluorescent powders containing beryllium. *Guthrie Clin Bull* 1944;13:91–95.

Machle W, Beyer E, Gregorius F: Berylliosis; acute pneumonitis and pulmonary granulomatosis of beryllium workers. *Occup Med* 1948;5: 671–683.

Mancuso TF: Relation of duration of employment and prior respiratory illness to respiratory cancer among beryllium workers. *Environ Res* 1970;3:251–275.

Mancuso TF: Mortality study of beryllium industry workers' occupational lung cancer. *Environ Res* 1980;21:48–55.

Meyer HE: Über Berylliumer Krankungen der Lunge. *Beitr Klin Tuberk* 1942;98:388–395.

NIOSH: *Criteria for a Recommended Standard. . . . Occupational Exposure to Beryllium.* Washington, DC, National Institute for Occupational Safety and Health (NIOSH 72-10268), 1972.

Reeves AL: The absorption of beryllium from the gastrointestinal tract. *Arch Environ Health* 1965; 11:209–218.

Reeves AL: Berylliosis as an auto-immune disorder. *Ann Clin Lab Sci* 1976;6:256–262.

Reeves AL, Swanborg RH, Busby EK, et al: The role of immunologic reactions in pulmonary berylliosis. *Inhaled Particles III* 1971; pp 599–608.

Reeves AL, Vorwald AJ: The humoral transport of beryllium. *J Occup Med* 1961;3:567–574.

Resnick H, Morgan WKC: Immunoglobulin levels in berylliosis. *Inhaled Particles III* 1971; pp 589–598.

Sixth Saranac Symposium (1947), in Vorwald AJ (ed): *Pneumoconiosis: Beryllium, Bauxite Fumes, Compensation.* New York, Hoeber, 1950.

Schepers GWH: Neoplasia experimentally induced by beryllium compounds. *Prog Exper Tumor Res* 1961;2:203–244.

Scott JK: Pathology of acute beryllium poisoning, in Vorwald AJ (ed): *Pneumoconiosis: Beryllium, Bauxite Fumes, Compensation.* New York, Hoeber, 1950, pp 267–282.

Shilen J, Galloway AE, Mellor JF Jr: Beryllium oxide from beryl. Health hazards incident to extraction. *Ind Med* 1944;13:464–469.

Sneddon IB: Beryllium disease. *Postgrad Med J* 1958;34:262–267.

Sprince NL, Kazemi H, Hardy HL: Current (1975) problem of differentiating between beryllium disease and sarcoidosis. *Ann NY Acad Sci* 1976;278:654–662.

Sprince NL, Kanarek DJ, Weber AL, et al: Reversible respiratory disease in beryllium workers. *Am Rev Respir Dis* 1978;117:1011–1017.

Sprince NL, Kazemi H: U.S. Beryllium Case Registry through 1977. *Environ Res* 1980;21:44–47.

Sterner JH, Eisenbud M: Epidemiology of beryllium intoxication. *Arch Ind Hyg Occup Med* 1951;4:123–151.

Stokinger HE: *Beryllium, Its Industrial Hygiene Aspects.* New York, Academic, 1966.

Tepper LB, Hardy HL, Chamberlin RI: *Toxicity of Beryllium Compounds.* New York, Elsevier, 1961.

Van Ordstrand HS, Hughes R, Carmody MG: Chemical pneumonia in workers extracting beryllium oxide. *Cleve Clin Q* 1943;10:10–18.

Van Ordstrand HS, Hughes R, DeNardi JM, et al: Beryllium poisoning. *J Am Med Assoc* 1945;129:1084–1090.

Vorwald AJ: Adenocarcinoma in the lung of albino rats exposed to compounds of beryllium: Cancer of the lung; an evaluation of the problem. *Proc Sci Session, Am Cancer Soc Ann Mtg,* November 3–4, 1953.

Wagner WD, Groth DH, Holtz JL, et al: Comparative chronic inhalation toxicity of beryllium ores, bertrandite, and beryl, with production of pulmonary tumors by beryl. *Toxicol Appl Pharmacol* 1969;15:10–29.

Wagoner JK, Infante PF, Bayliss DL: Beryllium: An etiologic agent in the induction of lung cancer, nonneoplastic respiratory disease, and heart disease among industrially exposed workers. *Environ Res* 1980;21:15–34.

Waksman BH: The diagnosis of beryllium disease, with special reference to the patch test. *Arch Ind Health* 1959; 19:154–156.

Weber HH, Engelhardt WE: Anwendung bei der Untersuchungen von Stauben aus der Berylliumgewinnung. *Zentralbl Gewerbehyg* 1933;10:41–47.

White MR, Finkel AJ, Schubert J: Protection against experimental beryllium poisoning by aurin tricarboxylic acid. *J Pharmacol Exp Ther* 1951;102:88–93.

Witschi HP, Marchand P: Interference of beryllium with enzyme induction in rat liver. *Toxicol Appl Pharmacol* 1971;20:565–572.

Wood CH: *Observations on the Natural History of Beryllium Disease.* Massachusetts Institute of Technology Dissertation, Cambridge, MA, 1964.

Wurm H, Rüger H: Untersuchungen zur Frage der Berylliumstaubpneumonie. *Beitr Klin Tuberk* 1942;98:396–404.

6 • Boron

Boron is used chiefly in high-energy fuels and in nuclear reactors as a shielding material to absorb neutrons. In addition, boron is used for hardening of steel alloys, as an abrasive, for fireproofing, and in the textile and glass industry (Browning, 1969).

Worker illness has been associated with hydrides of boron, called boranes. Of the three boranes—diborane, decaborane, and pentaborane—the latter is the most hazardous and is the only compound of the three that is detectable by odor in concentrations that are not acutely toxic (Lowe and Freeman, 1957). Diborane (B_2H_6) is a colorless gas at ordinary temperatures and pressures, and is rapidly hydrolyzed by water to form boric acid and hydrogen along with release of heat. Toxic effects are largely the result of bronchopulmonary involvement with tightness of the chest, dyspnea, and nonproductive cough as the presenting symptoms (Rozendaal, 1951; Cordasco et al., 1962; Lowe and Freeman, 1957).

Pentaborane (B_5H_9) and decaborane ($B_{10}H_{14}$) exposures, in contrast, lead to fewer respiratory tract symptoms, but produce unusual neurological disturbances. Low-level exposures have been followed by drowsiness, nausea, headache, and vertigo. Severe pentaborane intoxication has been reported to lead to generalized muscle spasms, clonic movements of neck and limbs, diffuse fasciculations, opisthotonus, and catatonia. Decaborane exposures produce gross tremors of the extremities, bizarre positioning of hands and feet, and hypoglossal spasms (Cordasco et al., 1962). Abnormalities of hepatic and renal function tests have been reported (Rozendaal, 1951; Krackow, 1953; Lowe and Freeman, 1957).

Toxic effects of boron on the gonads of male experimental animals have been reported (Krasovskii et al., 1976; Lee et al., 1978) but no comparable effect on human spermatogenesis has been recorded from occupational exposure to boron or its compounds.

References

Browning E: *Toxicity of Industrial Metals,* ed 2. New York, Appleton-Century-Crofts, 1969, pp 90–97.

Cordasco EM, Cooper RW, Murphy, JV, et al: Pulmonary aspects of some toxic experimental space fuels. *Dis Chest* 1962;41:68–74.

Krackow EH: Toxicity and health hazards of boron hydrides. *Arch Ind Hyg Occup Med* 1953; 8:335–339.

Krasovskii GN, Varshavskaya SP, Borisov AI: Toxic and gonadotropic effects of cadmium and boron relative to standards for these substances in drinking water. *Environ Health Perspectives* 1976;13:69–75.

Lee IP, Sherins RJ, Dixon RL: Evidence for induction of germinal aplasia in male rats by environmental exposure to boron. *Toxicol Appl Pharmacol* 1978;45:577–590.

Lowe HJ, Freeman G: Boron hydride (borane) intoxication in man. *Arch Ind Health* 1957; 16:523–533.

Rozendaal HM: Clinical observations on the toxicology of boron hydrides. *Arch Ind Hyg Occup Med* 1951;4:257–260.

7 • Cadmium

Industrial Uses

Cadmium, which was for a long time a rare metal in industry, has become widely used in the manufacture of alloys and for electroplating. When imports are necessary, the United States obtains cadmium chiefly from Canada and Mexico. Cadmium is extracted from zinc sulfide ores in the course of smelting and is a constituent of the so-called "blue powder," a condensation product that has up to 4 or 5% of cadmium. Cadmium is also found in sludge after the electrolytic recovery of zinc. It is used in silver, copper, and other alloys, but about half the amount produced is used in the electroplating of metals since it resists corrosion better than nickel or steel. It is also used extensively as a stabilizer in plastics and in pigments (cadmium "lithopone" as well as the cadmium yellows). Minor uses include nickel–cadmium storage batteries, fungicides and insecticides, photography, television picture tubes, and as a neutron absorber in nuclear reactors (Browning, 1969; NIOSH, 1976). Other uses for cadmium are in bearing metals, in ceramics, in process engraving, in cadmium vapor lamps, and for rustproofing tools and other iron and steel articles previously coated with zinc. Although in France ferronickel storage batteries have an anode made of cadmium, there is little manufacture of cadmium storage batteries in the United States.

The presence of cadmium has to be considered, not only in the manufacture of paints, but in the spraying of pigments and in welding processes when the metal or the welding rod contains cadmium. Photoelectric cells, made by coating small steel plates with selenium, are sprayed with metallic cadmium. Cadmium may be sprayed onto graphite or may be used in rods as neutron absorbers in nuclear reactors. Stokinger (1981) reported the use of diethyl cadmium in the manufacture of tetraethyl lead as an additive to gasoline.

Prodan (1932) stated that the greatest industrial hazards involving cadmium were in the smelting of ores, the working up of residues, the handling of "blue powder," production of compounds, spraying of pigments, welding alloys, and melting the metal. Fairhall (1945) considered that industrial cadmium poisoning was not due for the most part to the electroplating process but rather it was the subsequent firing or welding of cadmium-plated material leading to the overheating and oxidation of cadmium metal that was an important source of occupational intoxication.

Recently, solders containing cadmium in varying amounts with copper, lead, tin, zinc, and silver, especially silver solders, have been a source of poisoning. Remelting of scrap and the use of a blowtorch in working cadmium-plated steel pipes are dangerous, often because of the presence of potentially toxic cadmium that is not suspected.

Industrial and experimental evidence has shown cadmium to be one of the most hazardous metals. It has a significant vapor pressure at its melting point (320.9°C), at which point an air concentration many times the safe limit can be produced. Freshly generated fumes of cadmium have been shown to be more acutely poisonous than "old" settled fumes that are inhaled as dust.

Metabolism

Cadmium and its compounds may be inhaled or ingested. Piscator and Pettersson (1977) have pointed out that in industry exposure is mainly via air, while for the general population exposure is through food. Smoking of tobacco may provide additional exposure in both groups. Inhaled cadmium may be absorbed to the extent of 10 to 50%, but some is undoubtedly swallowed after clearance from the lung by the ciliary ladder in the bronchi and trachea. About 5% of ingested cadmium is absorbed through the gut.

38

Absorbed cadmium is bound and transported by metallothionein, a low molecular weight compound that appears to be induced protein (Cousins, 1979). Cadmium is deposited in the liver from which it is slowly released and subsequently deposited in the kidney, which is the critical organ in long-term exposure. Renal tubular damage is estimated to occur when cadmium concentration reaches 200 μg/g wet weight in the cortex. Excretion of cadmium from the body is very slow, the biological half-time in humans being 10 to 40 years; calculations by Tsuchiya et al. (1976) put it at about 13 years. When cadmium exposure has been at low levels for a prolonged period, urine cadmium values reflect the body burden of cadmium. When, however, exposure is more intense, urine cadmium levels may be as high as 50 μg/g creatinine and will indicate recent exposure rather than body burden. Blood cadmium levels largely indicate the extent of recent exposure since they measure cadmium in transport rather than cadmium deposited in body tissues (Friberg et al., 1974).

Cadmium is thought to act biochemically by competing with and displacing other metals, especially zinc, and by reacting with −SH groups in enzymes (Vallee and Ulmer, 1972; Buell, 1975). Davis and Avram (1978) found that cadmium activated δ-aminolevulinic acid dehydratase (ALAD), which is very rich in sulfhydryl groups, at very low concentrations but inhibited blood ALAD at higher concentrations. They also found that this inhibition, unlike that readily caused by lead, is not reversed by the *in vitro* addition of zinc.

Worker Illness: Early Reports

Although cadmium poisoning was not generally recognized as an occupational disease until the 1940s, there are earlier reports of adverse effects. There is the old observation of Stockhusen in 1656 (*Public Health Rep,* 1942) describing gastrointestinal disturbances in foundry workers exposed to cadmium fumes. Sovet (1858) reported on three servants who inhaled cadmium carbonate dust from a silver polish, with subsequent severe abdominal cramps, vomiting, and diarrhea, characteristic symptoms of acute poisoning from the ingestion of cadmium. Tracinski (1888) described the industrial diseases of zinc smelters in Upper Silesia in whom upper respiratory tract irritation, as well as indigestion, vomiting, and

diarrhea occurred. The chief exposure, poorly controlled, was to 5% cadmium as a fume with some SO_2.

Stephens (1920) drew attention to cadmium poisoning in Welsh zinc smelters that was also characterized by gastrointestinal symptoms. He reported the recovery of cadmium but no lead from the liver of an aged smelter-worker whose necropsy showed marked evidence of chronic interstitial nephritis as well. A case reported by Schwartz (1930) was caused by inhaling the fumes of melting cadmium with subsequent chronic respiratory symptoms diagnosed as bronchitis with bouts of bronchopneumonia.

Acute cadmium poisoning Ross (1944) reported an accident in England that affected 23 workers at once. Since finely divided cadmium is inflammable and will produce cadmium oxide fumes when ignited, smoking is strictly forbidden in industries where such materials are handled in quantity. As a result of breaking this rule, cadmium dust was ignited by a lighted cigarette with resultant dangerous exposure of the workers to cadmium oxide. The victims complained of irritation of the eyes, headache, vertigo, dryness of the throat, cough, and chest constriction. After three hours, the exposed workers complained of nausea, epigastric pain, and dyspnea.

Severe acute cadmium poisoning, caused by the fumes produced by the use of a propane–oxygen blowtorch on cadmium-plated steel pipe, was reported by Spolyar et al. in 1944. After using the torch for four hours, five workmen became violently ill with nausea, sore throat, severe chest pains, cough, dyspnea, chills, and fever. One man died after a total exposure of eight hours. Chest radiographs of three of the survivors taken four weeks after exposure showed that they were free of residual chest pathology. Another fatal case of cadmium poisoning was investigated by the Massachusetts Division of Occupational Hygiene (Elkins, in a personal communication to HLH). The victim was a helper in a brass foundry who, with a fellow employee, melted cadmium to be poured into molds and small castings without protection or warning of the dangers involved. The metal became overheated and gave off dense fumes that filled the shop. Both employees and two onlookers began to cough, but the worker who died had stayed on to skim the metal after it was removed from the fire. In spite of coughing and bouts of vomiting that continued through the night after the exposure, the sick worker went back to his job the next day. He died six days after the incident from what the attending physician called "bronchial pneumonia."

More recently, Beton and his associates (1966) described the accidental poisoning of five workers by cadmium oxide fumes produced by dismantling a girder frame with an oxyacetylene torch. The men were not aware that the bolts were cadmium-plated. The initial symptoms were mild, consisting of throat irritation and an unpleasant taste in the mouth. After two hours symptoms developed that resembled acute upper respiratory infection: cough, throat discomfort, general malaise, shivering and sweating, with body pains and headache. While these manifestations are similar to metal fume fever from zinc, the latter usually subsides within 12 hours while cadmium fume disease progresses to a prolonged pulmonary phase with severe pulmonary edema lasting up to seven days, and bronchopneumonia. The fatal case in this group died on the fifth day and necropsy revealed alveolar metaplasia of the lung and bilateral cortical necrosis of the kidneys. Similar fatalities with death on the fifth day after oxyacetylene burning of silver solder were reported by Winston (1971) and by Lucas et al. (1980).

Subacute cadmium intoxication in jewelry workers was described by Baker et al. (1979) when a cadmium-containing brazing alloy ("silver solder") was used in the production of handmade silver jewelry. The prevalence of dyspnea, chest pain, dysuria, and dizziness was correlated with blood cadmium levels. Although symptoms subsided after the cadmium alloy was replaced, elevated cadmium levels in the urine persisted in four workers. No significant renal or pulmonary dysfunction was noted.

Chronic cadmium poisoning   Until relatively recently, it was not generally recognized that there was evidence for the existence of a clinical picture of chronic cadmium poisoning of occupational origin. However, the history of Stephen's (1920) aged smelter-worker, whose liver at necropsy contained 130.0 mg/kg, provided evidence that disability may arise from industrial exposures too slight to produce the violent symptoms of acute poisoning. In 1942, Nicaud et al. described a series of cases in workers exposed to unstated amounts of cadmium whose clinical complaints were felt to present a unique clinical syndrome due to chronic cadmium intoxication. After periods of exposure varying from eight to 16

years, these workers of both sexes developed pain in the lower back and legs. Without treatment and with continued exposure, the workers became unable to walk. X-rays of the scapula, femur, and ilium showed lines of pseudofracture known as Milkman's syndrome. The only other regular finding was an anemia of the iron-deficiency type. Treatment with Vitamin D, calcium, and parathyroid extract resulted in cure. A similar report was made by Barthelemy and Moline (1946), from France, where the anode of ferronickel batteries is made of cadmium. Workers in this industry, after exposure to operations involving cadmium for more than six years, presented a clinical picture resembling that described by Nicaud et al. Prior to the onset of signs and symptoms, the teeth of the workers exposed in this way to cadmium had a characteristic appearance that may serve as a warning that the workers are absorbing dangerous amounts of cadmium. The enamel of the teeth took on a yellow color that also discolored the tartar but not the gingiva. Princi (1947), in the United States, also reported cadmium in discolored teeth of workers exposed to cadmium in smelting after ten years.

Gervais and Delpech (1963) reported detailed clinical findings in eight cases of cadmium workers with evidence of abnormalities of the skeleton. Exposure to cadmium lasted from 12 to 30 years. Several cases suffered pathological fractures, and in all cases bone changes were visible in the radiographs. In the absence of any other etiology, the authors concluded that the cadmium had produced serious metabolic changes. These French reports are of great interest in light of cadmium-induced disease of bone in Japan, named "Itai-itai disease," that occurred in workers in rice fields near a mine producing zinc, lead, and cadmium (Kobayashi, 1971). This condition is characterized by hypercalciuria, resulting from inhibition of proximal tubular reabsorption, leading to osteomalacia and painful fractures. Similar cases have been reported in cadmium workers by Adams et al. (1969) and Kazantzis (1979).

Hardy and Skinner (1947), in the United States, reported worker illness that followed exposure to cadmium during the covering of large steel parts for protection against rust. Air studies for a six-year period showed exposure varying from 0.06 to 0.68 mg/m^3. The work period was lengthened during the war years. Urine values in the five cases varied from a trace of cadmium to 0.05 mg/L. The five men reported that they had sternal pain, throat irritation, and cough. Four had gastrointestinal complaints of varying severity, ranging from anorexia to nausea, vomiting, and epigastric pain that, in one worker, led to the diagnosis of peptic ulcer. Two of the men had hemoglobin values that were consistent with those found in iron deficiency.

Support for the concept of chronic cadmium poisoning in workers has derived from reports of illness among those exposed in storage battery and alloy manufacture in Sweden and England. Friberg described loss of weight, pulmonary disease, and the appearance of a low molecular weight protein in the urine as evidence of chronic disease. Friberg's first reports appeared in 1948 and 1950, and his observations have been amply confirmed, among others by Lane and Campbell (1954), Bonnell (1955), King (1955), Kazantzis (1956), Piscator (1966), Meerkin et al. (1976), and Lauwerys et al. (1979). Kidney stones and nephrocalcinosis are established complications of cadmium poisoning (Piscator and Pettersson, 1977).

Of unusual interest is the finding of Friberg of low molecular weight proteins in the urine of cadmium workers who are otherwise free of symptoms or detectable signs of illness. The molecular weights are from 20,000 to 30,000, lower than any known serum protein, and are now known to consist mainly of β_2-microglobulin, along with ribonuclease, muramidase, and immunoglobulin chains (Piscator and Pettersson, 1977). This cadmium proteinuria is not usually demonstrable by the methods routinely used to detect albuminuria. Electrophoresis of concentrated urine proteins, gel filtration, ion exchange chromatography, and immunological methods are used to detect and characterize these substances. Shiroishi et al. (1977) concluded from a cooperative Japanese-Swedish study that radioimmunoassay (RIA) of β_2-microglobulin is a sensitive indicator of cadmium-induced proteinuria. Tsuchiya (1976) reported that this proteinuria was reversible in some workers and that in some workers, while this proteinuria subsided after cessation of exposure, there was no decrease in cadmium urine levels. The presence of certain globulins in the serum proteins of workers with long-term cadmium exposure led to the suggestion that an abnormal antigen–antibody reaction had been provoked (Piscator, 1966; Vigliani et al., 1966). Buchet et al. (1980) put forward the hypothesis that the glomerular dysfunction might result from an autoimmune mechanism.

Piscator (1966) stated that the amount of cadmium in urine is a reflection of the extent of renal tubular damage. Excess excretion of amino acids is considered to be due to the same cause rather than a result of metabolic abnormalities. Clarkson and Kench (1956) had found aminoaciduria (threonine and serine) in workers exposed to cadmium oxide dust. Swedish workers similarly exposed were shown by Ahlmark et al. (1960) to have low insulin clearance values and an inability to concentrate urine. These abnormalities were shown to increase with length of time and level of cadmium exposure.

Several authors (Schroeder and Nason, 1969; Petering et al., 1973; Brancato et al., 1976) have studied hair for metal content hoping to discover useful correlations with exposure and body burdens. Variables such as age, sex, and handling of the sample have proved cadmium values in hair to be unreliable as a monitoring technique.

Chronic pulmonary insufficiency characterized by emphysema is a significant risk in continued uncontrolled cadmium exposure. There are a few reports of lung function abnormalities. Bonnell (1955) described a cadmium worker under his care who had evidence of severe airway obstruction. According to Buxton (1956), men suffering from the emphysema of chronic cadmium poisoning do not show the increase in total lung volume characteristic of the emphysema of chronic bronchitis. Several reports include anosmia, excess fatigue, and anemia as a result of cadmium exposure. An important feature of chronic cadmium poisoning, emphasized by Bonnell et al. (1959) is the delay in onset of clinical illness in some cases, an indication that cadmium disease progresses even though exposure has ceased. Lane and Campbell (1954) considered cadmium emphysema to be unique, with postmortem evidence of a narrow zone of normal lung under the pleura and no bullae at the periphery. Spencer (1962) did not agree but did note the absence of severe fibrosis in the presence of advanced emphysema. Hirst et al. (1973) assayed emphysematous lungs with age-matched controls, and found that only cadmium was elevated among the metals that were tested; they suggested that cigarettes were the source of cadmium in the lungs.

Decreased α_1-antitrypsin in plasma is thought to be an important factor in the pathogenesis of pulmonary emphysema. Chowdhury and Louria (1976) found that cadmium alone of several trace elements reduced the α_1-antitrypsin content of human plasma *in vitro* as well as its trypsin inhibitory capacity (TIC). However, Bernard et al. (1977) could not confirm these results at blood cadmium levels found in cadmium workers, nor was there a reduction of α_1-antitrypsin and TIC in the blood of workers exhibiting chronic cadmium intoxication. They attributed obstructive pulmonary disease in these workers to smoking rather than to occupational exposure to cadmium.

Kipling and Waterhouse (1967) raised the question as to whether lifelong exposures to cadmium might be associated with a significant increase in prostatic cancer. However, no prostate changes were seen after repeated subcutaneous injections of $CdSO_4$ or its long-term administration in drinking water in rats (Levy et al., 1973). Kjellström et al. (1979) found that there was a tendency for increased mortality from prostate, lung, and colon–rectum cancers in cadmium-nickel battery and cadmium-copper alloy workers, but these were not statistically significant. Lemen et al. (1976) studied 292 cadmium smelter workers with more than two years of exposure and found a significantly increased risk of prostatic cancer (4 observed vs. 0.88 expected) 20 years after the onset of cadmium exposure as well as a significant excess of respiratory tract and total malignancies. Kolonel (1976) found an association of exposure to cadmium and renal cancer with a strong suggestion of interaction between occupational exposure and smoking.

In summary, it is established that intense exposures to cadmium oxide can cause fatal pulmonary edema. Repeated exposures may damage the kidneys, and the respiratory and gastrointestinal tracts, including the liver (Kazantzis et al., 1963). Lauwerys et al. (1974) studied three groups of workers exposed to cadmium dust and found that kidney damage was more prevalent than pulmonary changes, and suggested that the lesion is glomerular at first and later becomes tubular. This mixed-type proteinuria has been confirmed in cadmium-treated rats by Bernard et al. (1978). These job-related illnesses become more important as cadmium pollution of the air as well as tobacco smoking in industrialized countries expose general populations to unknown quantities of this toxic material.

Animal Studies

The literature describing animal experimentation with cadmium has increased considerably in recent years. Various aspects of the problem of cadmium poisoning and its treatment were studied during the Second World War (Tobias et al.,

1946; Gilman et al., 1946). There has been a renewed interest in the biological behavior of cadmium since the studies of Friberg (1948). Many animal studies have been reported, and only a summary of some of them will be attempted here. Animal investigations have corroborated the gastrointestinal effects seen in man after the ingestion of cadmium. Prodan's studies (1932) showed that changes in the liver vary from generalized inflammation to pronounced fatty infiltration. Pathological changes were also seen in the kidneys, especially in the convoluted tubules, findings confirmed by Itokawa et al. (1974). Numerous studies have explored the role of metallothionein in the transport of cadmium (Kägi and Vallee, 1960; Foulkes, 1978, and Nordberg, 1978, among others). Shaikh and Hirayama (1979) reported that the appearance of metallothionein in plasma and urine of rats provided specific indices of cadmium exposure. Probst et al. (1977) suggested that a threshold dose of cadmium must be exceeded in order to induce concentrations of metallothionein adequate to ameliorate acute cadmium toxicity.

Cadmium storage in liver, kidneys, and bones is of interest since some of the gastrointestinal symptoms of subacute illness may be due to the toxic effect of cadmium on liver function. Prodan (1932) reported that the kidneys in his experimental animals retained much of the administered cadmium and excreted it very slowly. Johns et al. (1923) had also found that the kidney retains more cadmium than any other organ, while more recently Klaassen and Kotsonis (1977) have shown in rats, rabbits, and dogs that bile is the main route for cadmium elimination, a result that amplified earlier knowledge that the major path of cadmium excretion is fecal (Decker et al., 1957; Burch and Walsh, 1959; Caujolle et al., 1971; Ogawa et al., 1972). On the other hand, Cikrt and Tichý (1974) concluded from their studies on rats that more cadmium is excreted by the intestinal wall than in bile.

Acute injury to rat lungs by inhalation of cadmium chloride aerosols damages peribronchiolar alveoli by producing epithelial cell and interstitial edema and proliferation of cuboidal epithelium lining the alveoli. These changes parallel those of occupational cadmium fume toxicity in man where there is centrilobular emphysema around the respiratory bronchioles (Strauss et al., 1976).

The effect of cadmium on iron metabolism has been studied in feeding experiments in which cadmium chloride given to rats resulted in severe anemia (Wilson et al., 1941). According to Granick and Michaelis (1942), cadmium is capable of precipitating iron-containing protein, and it may be that, by so doing, it produces the low hemoglobin reported in animal and human experience. Experimental cadmium poisoning of rabbits produced slight but consistent lowering of serum calcium (Kennedy, 1966), a finding that is undoubtedly related to the clinical picture of renal stones, hypercalciuria, and osteomalacia seen in some cadmium workers. Changes typical of osteomalacia have also been produced in rats fed cadmium on a long-term basis (Takashima et al., 1980).

Ingestion of cadmium chloride by male rats resulted in emphysema and reduced pulmonary function although these effects were ameliorated or delayed if dietary zinc concentrations were high (Petering et al., 1979). These results are consistent with the known interaction between cadmium and zinc in metabolic systems. Among the interactions of dietary cadmium and zinc in rats is a more severe anemia when these elements are fed together than when administered individually (Thawley et al., 1977).

The dental effects reported by Barthelemy and Moline (1946) and Princi (1947) have no exact counterpart in animal studies. Several investigators have looked into the effect of cadmium on rat teeth because, in common with fluorine, it has the property of bleaching. Cadmium increases the susceptibility of rat teeth to dental caries rather than increasing resistance to decay as fluorine does (Ginn and Volker, 1944).

Lung changes and the unusual proteinuria of cadmium workers also occur in exposed rabbits (Friberg, 1952). Abnormal serum proteins have been found in cadmium-poisoned animals (Axelsson and Piscator, 1966). In rats, cadmium was found to be highest in the kidney cortex; it was also present in liver, pancreas, thyroid, and spleen (Buxton, 1956; Kazantzis, 1956). Rats given cadmium by injection were found to have a correlation between elevated plasma enzyme activities and ultrastructural liver changes (Faeder et al., 1977).

Cadmium in high doses has been shown to produce testicular atrophy in several mammalian species, including the rhesus monkey. However, immature rats are resistant to testicular injury by cadmium given at levels that produce damage in adult animals (Wong and Klaassen, 1980). Interstitial cell tumors of the testes of rodents have been reported by Gunn et al. (1963) and Roe et al.

(1964), but Gilliavod and Léonard (1975) found no genetic effects of cadmium on male mouse germ cells. Other experimental findings include damage to the placenta, teratogenic effects, and hemorrhage in sensory nerves (Roe et al., 1964; Holmberg and Ferm, 1969). The inhibitory effect of cadmium on neuromuscular transmission in the rat appears to be largely due to inhibition of the role of calcium at presynaptic nerve terminals (Forshaw, 1977). Flick et al. (1971) and Buell (1975) reviewed the effects of cadmium toxicity on a wide variety of biological systems.

Treatment

After the discovery of the favorable effect of British antilewisite (BAL) in arsenic and mercury poisoning, the Chemical Warfare Service made extensive studies of this material in the treatment of acute cadmium intoxication (Gilman et al., 1946). This report and that of Dalhamn and Friberg (1955) showed the cadmium-BAL complex to be nephrotoxic. Moeschlin (1965) suggested that BAL be used for acute pneumonia due to cadmium. Because of the fact that urine cadmium levels are poorly correlated with toxic effects of cadmium, and because of Friberg's (1956) report that intravenous ethylenediaminetetraacetic acid (EDTA) produced renal damage if used for a prolonged period in animals, EDTA was also not recommended for therapy of chronic cadmium poisoning. However, Friberg found no kidney damage after a single dose of EDTA that resulted in cadmium excretion of up to 500-fold. On balance, the use of BAL or EDTA is not to be recommended for cadmium intoxication on the basis of current knowledge.

Schroeder et al. (1968), studying increase in body cadmium as a cause of hypertension in rats, proposed the use of a zinc chelate as a means of removing cadmium from the body. This procedure has been successful in cadmium poisoning in animals and a zinc chelate has been proposed for human use. Moeschlin (1965) suggested that, in addition to removing the worker from further cadmium exposure, the use of intravenous calcium gluconate (20 ml of a 10 to 20% solution) and subcutaneous Vitamin D (600,000 U at weekly intervals for six doses) be tried. He advised such treatment at the earliest stage of chronic cadmium intoxication — for example, when the "yellow ring" is seen on the teeth.

As with all chemical pneumonias that are symptomatic and show chest x-ray changes, complete

44

bed rest combined with oxygen therapy and the use of steroids will reverse the abnormalities of cadmium pneumonitis if used promptly in adequate doses.

Control of Toxic Exposures

The standards for allowable concentrations of cadmium have changed over the years and these trends have been summarized in NIOSH (1976). The current safe limits in the United States are 0.2 mg/m³ for cadmium dust and 0.1 mg/m³ for cadmium fume, although NIOSH (1976) recommends a limit of 40 μg Cd/m³ for both, determined as a time-weighted average for a 10-hour workday, 40-hour workweek, with a ceiling concentration of 200 μg Cd/m³ for any 15-minute sampling period. Because of prolonged cadmium retention in the body, these levels may not protect workers from the harmful effects arising from long-term exposure. Tsuchiya (1976) found that when the cadmium concentration in the working environment was decreased to 20 μg/m³ the general health of the workers improved noticeably.

Urine cadmium levels reflect absorption but are not correlated with disease or intensity of exposure. Tsuchiya et al. (1976) found that among workers exposed to cadmium fumes, protein in the urine increased when urine cadmium exceeded 50 μg/L and blood cadmium exceeded 4 to 6 μg/100 ml. Lauwerys et al. (1979) proposed a tentative threshold of 10 μg/g urine creatinine for adult males occupationally exposed to cadmium, since kidney damage was seen in some workers who excreted more than 15 μg Cd/g creatinine.

Periodic examination of workers exposed to a cadmium risk provides the opportunity to record vague gastrointestinal complaints, anosmia, and chronic rhinitis as evidence of early cadmium poisoning. Regular inspection of the teeth, routine hemoglobin determinations, and urine analyses for cadmium-induced proteinuria may be valuable means for recognizing a toxic cadmium effect. Pulmonary function tests (FVC and FEV$_1$) and blood pressure measurements are also recommended on a periodic basis. Plant sanitation and personal hygiene practices should be encouraged. In particular, food and drink should not be brought into cadmium-contaminated areas, nor should smoking be allowed where cadmium is handled.

References

Adams RG, Harrison JF, Scott P: The development of cadmium-induced proteinuria, impaired renal function, and osteomalacia in alkaline battery workers. *Q J Med* 1969;38:425–443.

Ahlmark A, Axelsson B, Friberg L, et al: Further investigations into kidney function and proteinuria in chronic cadmium poisoning. *Proc 13th Intnatl Cong Occup Health (1960)*. New York, Book Craftsmen, 1961, pp 201–203.

Axelsson B, Piscator M: Serum proteins in cadmium poisoned rabbits, with special reference to hemolytic anemia. *Arch Environ Health* 1966;12: 374–381.

Baker EL Jr, Peterson WA, Holtz JL, et al: Subacute cadmium intoxication in jewelry workers: An evaluation of diagnostic procedures. *Arch Environ Health* 1979;34:173–177.

Barthelemy P, Moline R: Intoxication chronique par l'hydrate de cadmium, son signe precoce: La bague jaune dentaire. *Paris Med* 1946; 1:7–8.

Bernard A, Roels HA, Buchet JP, et al: α_1-antitrypsin level in workers exposed to cadmium, in Brown SS (ed): *Clinical Chemistry and Chemical Toxicology of Metals*. New York, Elsevier, 1977, pp 161–164.

Bernard A, Goret A, Roels H, et al: Experimental confirmation in rats of the mixed type proteinuria observed in workers exposed to cadmium. *Toxicology* 1978;10:369–375.

Beton DC, Andrews GS, Davies HG, et al: Acute cadmium fume poisoning. Five cases with one death from renal necrosis. *Br J Ind Med* 1966; 23:292–301.

Bonnell JA: Emphysema and proteinuria in men casting copper–cadmium alloys. *Br J Ind Med* 1955;12:181–195.

Bonnell JA, Kazantzis G, King E: A follow-up study of men exposed to cadmium oxide fume. *Br J Ind Med* 1959;16:135–147.

Brancato DJ, Picchioni AL, Chin L: Cadmium levels in hair and other tissues during continuous cadmium intake. *J Toxicol Environ Health* 1976; 2:351–359.

Browning E: *Toxicity of Industrial Metals,* ed 2. New York, Appleton-Century-Crofts, 1969, pp 98–108.

Buchet JP, Roels H, Bernard A Jr, et al: Assessment of renal function of workers exposed to inorganic lead, cadmium or mercury vapor. *J Occup Med* 1980;22:741–750.

Buell G: Some biochemical aspects of cadmium

toxicology. *J Occup Med* 1975;17:189–195.

Burch GE, Walsh JJ: The excretion and biological decay rates of Cd[115m] with a consideration of space, mass, and distribution in dogs. *J Lab Clin Invest* 1959;54:66–72.

Buxton RS: Respiratory function in men casting cadmium alloys: II. The estimation of the total lung volume, its subdivisions, and mixing coefficient. *Br J Ind Med* 1956;13:36–40.

Caujolle F, Oustrin J, Silve-Mamy G: Fixation et circulation énterohépatique du cadmium. *Eur J Toxicol* 1971;4:310–315.

Chowdhury P, Louria DB: Influence of cadmium and other trace metals on human α_1-antitrypsin: An in vitro study. *Science* 1976; 191:480–481.

Cikrt M, Tichý M: Excretion of cadmium through bile and intestinal wall in rats. *Br J Ind Med* 1974;31:134–139.

Clarkson TW, Kench JE: Urinary excretion of amino acids by men absorbing heavy metals. *Biochem J* 1956;62:361–372.

Cousins RJ: Metallothionein synthesis and degradation: Relationship to cadmium metabolism. *Environ Health Persp* 1979;28:131–136.

Dalhamn T, Friberg L: Dimercaprol (2,3-Dimercaptopropanol) in chronic cadmium poisoning. *Acta Pharmacol Toxicol* 1955;11:68–71.

Davis JR, Avram MJ: A comparison of the stimulatory effects of cadmium and zinc on normal and lead-inhibited human erythrocytic δ-aminolevulinic acid dehydratase activity *in vitro*. *Toxicol Appl Pharmacol* 1978;44:181–190.

Decker CF, Byerrum RJ, Hoppert CA: A study of the distribution and retention of cadmium-115 in the albino rat. *Arch Biochem Biophys* 1957; 66:140–145.

Faeder EJ, Chaney SQ, King LC, et al: Biochemical and ultrastructural changes in livers of cadmium-treated rats. *Toxicol Appl Pharmacol* 1977;39:473–487.

Fairhall LT: Inorganic industrial hazards. *Physiol Rev* 1945;25:182–202.

Flick DF, Kraybill HF, Dimitroff JM: Toxic effects of cadmium: A review. *Environ Res* 1971;4:71–85.

Forshaw PJ: The inhibitory effect of cadmium on neuromuscular transmission in the rat. *Eur J Pharmacol* 1977;42:371–377.

Foulkes EC: Renal tubular transport of cadmium-metallothionein. *Toxicol Appl Pharmacol* 1978;45:505–512.

Friberg L: Proteinuria and kidney injury among workmen exposed to cadmium and nickel dust: Preliminary report. *J Ind Hyg Toxicol* 1948;30:32–36.

Friberg L: Health hazards in the manufacture of alkaline accumulators with special reference to chronic cadmium poisoning. *Acta Med Scand* 1950;138(suppl 240).

Friberg L: Further investigations on chronic cadmium poisoning. A study of rabbits with radioactive cadmium. *Arch Ind Hyg Occup Med* 1952;5:30–36.

Friberg L: Edathamil calcium disodium in cadmium poisoning. *Arch Ind Health* 1956;13:18–23.

Friberg L, Piscator M, Nordberg GF, et al: *Cadmium in the Environment*, ed 2. Cleveland, CRC Press, 1974.

Gervais J, Delpech P: L'intoxication cadmique. *Arch Med Prof* 1963;24:803–816.

Gilliavod N, Léonard A: Mutagenicity tests with cadmium in the mouse. *Toxicology* 1975; 5:43–47.

Gilman A, Philips FS, Allen RP, et al: The treatment of acute cadmium intoxication in rabbits with 2,3-dimercaptopropanol (BAL) and other mercaptans. *J Pharmacol Exp Ther* 1946; 87(suppl 7):85–101.

Ginn JT, Volker JF: Effect of cadmium and fluorine on rat dentition. *Proc Soc Exp Biol Med* 1944;57:189–191.

Granick S, Michaelis L: Ferritin and apoferritin. *Science* 1942;95:439–440.

Gunn SA, Gould TC, Anderson WA: Cadmium induced interstitial cell tumors in rats and mice and their prevention by zinc. *J Nat Cancer Inst* 1963;31:745–759.

Hardy HL, Skinner JB: The possibility of chronic cadmium poisoning. *J Ind Hyg Toxicol* 1947;29:321–324.

Hirst RN Jr, Perry HM Jr, Cruz MG, et al: Elevated cadmium concentration in emphysematous lungs. *Am Rev Resp Dis* 1973;108:30–39.

Holmberg RE Jr, Ferm VH: Interrelationships of selenium, cadmium and arsenic in mammalian teratogenesis. *Arch Environ Health* 1969;18:873–877.

Itokawa Y, Abe T, Tabei R, et al: Renal and skeletal lesions in experimental cadmium poisoning. Histological and biochemical approaches. *Arch Environ Health* 1974;28:149–154.

Johns CO, Finks AJ, Alsberg CL: Chronic intoxication by small quantities of cadmium chloride in the rat. *J Pharmacol Exp Ther* 1923; 21:59–64.

Kägi JHR, Vallee BL: Metallothionein—a

cadmium- and zinc-containing protein from equine renal cortex. *J Biol Chem* 1960;235:3460-3465.

Kazantzis G: Respiratory function in men casting cadmium alloys: I. Assessment of ventilatory function. *Br J Ind Med* 1956;13:30-36.

Kazantzis G: Renal tubular dysfunction and abnormalities of calcium metabolism in cadmium workers. *Environ Health Persp* 1979;28:155-159.

Kazantzis G, Flynn FV, Spowage JS, et al: Renal tubular malfunction and pulmonary emphysema in cadmium pigment workers. *Q J Med* (New Series) 1963;32:165-192.

Kennedy A: Hypocalcemia in experimental cadmium poisoning. *Br J Ind Med* 1966;23:313-317.

King E: An environmental study of casting copper-cadmium alloys. *Br J Ind Med* 1955;12:198-205.

Kipling MD, Waterhouse JAH: Cadmium and prostatic carcinoma. *Lancet* 1967;1:730-731.

Kjellström T, Friberg L, Rahnster B: Mortality and cancer morbidity among cadmium-exposed workers. *Environ Health Persp* 1979;28:199-204.

Klaassen CD, Kotsonis FN: Biliary excretion of cadmium in the rat, rabbit, and dog. *Toxicol Appl Pharmacol* 1977;41:101-112.

Kobayashi J: Relation between the "Itai-Itai" disease and the pollution of river water by cadmium from a mine. *Proc 5th Intnatl Water Pollution Res Conf* 1971;I-25:1-7.

Kolonel LN: Association of cadmium with renal cancer. *Cancer* 1976;37:1782-1787.

Lane RE, Campbell HCB: Fatal emphysema in two men making a copper cadmium alloy. *Br J Ind Med* 1954;11:118-122.

Lauwerys RB, Buchet JP, Roels HA, et al: Epidemiological survey of workers exposed to cadmium. Effect on lung, kidney, and several biological indices. *Arch Environ Health* 1974;28:145-148.

Lauwerys RB, Roels HA, Buchet JP, et al: Investigations on the lung and kidney function in workers exposed to cadmium. *Environ Health Persp* 1979;28:137-145.

Lauwerys RB, Roels HA, Regniers M, et al: Significance of cadmium concentration in blood and in urine in workers exposed to cadmium. *Environ Res* 1979;20:375-391.

Lemen RA, Lee JS, Wagoner JK, et al: Cancer mortality among cadmium production workers. *Ann NY Acad Sci* 1976;271:273-279.

Levy LS, Roe FJC, Malcolm D, et al: Absence of prostatic cancer changes in rats exposed to cadmium. *Ann Occup Hyg* 1973;16:111-118.

Lucas PA, Jariwalla AG, Jones JH, et al: Fatal cadmium fume inhalation. *Lancet* 1980;2:205.

Meerkin M, Clarke R, Oliphant R: Chronic cadmium poisoning. *Med J Aust* 1976;1:23-24.

Moeschlin S: *Poisoning: Diagnosis and Treatment.* New York, Grune & Stratton, 1965.

Nicaud P, Lafitte A, Gros A: Les troubles de l'intoxication chronique par le cadmium. *Arch Mal Prof* 1942;4:192-202.

NIOSH: *Criteria for a Recommended Standard . . . . Occupational Exposure to Cadmium.* Washington, DC, National Institute for Occupational Safety and Health (NIOSH 76-192), 1976.

Nordberg M: Studies on metallothionein and cadmium. *Environ Res* 1978;15:381-404.

Ogawa E, Suzuki S, Tsuzuki H: Radiopharmacological studies on the cadmium poisoning. *Jpn J Pharmacol* 1972;22:275-281.

Petering HG, Chowdhury H, Stemmer KL: Some effects of the oral ingestion of cadmium on zinc, copper, and iron metabolism. *Environ Health Persp* 1979;28:97-106.

Petering HG, Yeager DW, Witherup SO: Trace metal content of hair: II. Cadmium and lead of human hair in relation to age and sex. *Arch Environ Health* 1973;27:327-333.

Piscator M: Proteinuria in chronic cadmium poisoning: III. Electrophoretic and immunoelectrophoretic studies on urinary proteins from cadmium workers. *Arch Environ Health* 1966;12:335-344.

Piscator M: Proteinuria in chronic cadmium poisoning: IV. Gel filtration and ion exchange chromatography of urinary proteins from cadmium workers. *Arch Environ Health* 1966;12:345-359.

Piscator M, Petterson B: Chronic cadmium poisoning—diagnosis and prevention, in Brown SS (ed): *Clinical Chemistry and Chemical Toxicology of Metals.* New York, Elsevier, 1977, pp 143-155.

Princi F: A study of industrial exposures to cadmium. *J Ind Hyg Toxicol* 1947;29:315-320.

Probst GS, Bousquet WF, Miya TS: Correlation of hepatic metallothionein concentrations with acute cadmium toxicity in the mouse. *Toxicol Appl Pharmacol* 1977;39:61-69.

Prodan L: Cadmium poisoning: I. The history of cadmium poisoning and uses of cadmium. *J Ind Hyg* 1932;14:132-155.

Prodan L: Cadmium poisoning: II. Experimental cadmium poisoning. *J Ind Hyg* 1932;14:174-196.

Roe FJC, Dukes CE, Cameron KM, et al: Cadmium neoplasia: Testicular atrophy and Leydig cell hyperplasia and neoplasia in rats and mice following the subcutaneous injection of cadmium salts. *Br J Cancer* 1964;18:674–681.

Ross P: Cadmium poisoning. *Br Med J* 1944; 1:252–253.

Schroeder HA, Nason AP, Mitchener M: Action of a chelate of zinc on trace metals in hypertensive rats. *Am J Physiol* 1968;214:796–800.

Schroeder HA, Nason AP: Trace metals in human hair. *J Invest Dermatol* 1969;53:71–78.

Schwartz L: Kleine Mittheilungen: Gewerbliche Cadmium Vergiftung. *Zeit Gewerbehyg* 1930;36:190.

Shaikh ZA, Hirayama K: Metallothionein in the extracellular fluids as an index of cadmium activity. *Environ Health Persp* 1979;28:267–271.

Shiroishi K, Kjellström T, Kubota K, et al: Urine analysis for detection of cadmium-induced renal changes, with special reference to β_2-microglobulin. *Environ Res* 1977;13:407–424.

Sovet: Empoisonnement par une poudre à écurer l'argenterie. *Presse Med Belge* 1858;10:69–70.

Spencer H: *Pathology of the Lung.* New York, Macmillan, 1962.

Spolyar LW, Keppler JF, Porter HG: Cadmium poisoning in industry: Report of five cases, including one death. *J Ind Hyg Toxicol* 1944; 26:232–240.

Stephens GA: Cadmium poisoning. *J Ind Hyg* 1920;2:129–132.

Stockhusen, cited by *Public Health Rep* 1942; 57:601–612.

Stokinger HE: The metals, in Clayton GD, Clayton FE (eds): *Patty's Industrial Hygiene and Toxicology,* ed 3. New York, John Wiley, 1981, vol. 2A, pp 1563–1583.

Strauss RH, Palmer KC, Hayes JA: Acute lung injury induced by cadmium aerosol: I. Evolution of alveolar cell damage. *Am J Pathol* 1976;84:561–578.

Takashima M, Moriwaka S, Itokawa Y: Osteomalacic change induced by long-term administration of cadmium to rats. *Toxicol Appl Pharmacol* 1980;54:223–228.

Thawley DG, Willoughby RA, McSherry BJ, et al: Toxic interactions among Pb, Zn, and Cd with varying levels of dietary Ca and vitamin D: Hematological system. *Environ Res* 1977;14:463–475.

Tobias JM: The pathology and therapy with 2,3-dimercaptopropanol (BAL) of experimental cadmium poisoning. *J Pharmacol Exp Ther* 1946; 87(suppl 7):102–118.

Tracinski: Die oberschlesische Zinkindustrie. *Vrtljrschr öffentl Gesundspflg* 1888;20:59. (Also in *Ann d'Hyg* 1888;19:399–412.)

Tsuchiya K: Proteinuria of cadmium workers. *J Occup Med* 1976;18:463–466.

Tsuchiya K, Seki Y, Sugita M: Biological criteria for exposures to lead and cadmium. *Keio Med J* 1976;25:91–100.

Tsuchiya K, Sugita Y, Seki M: Mathematical derivation of the biological half-time of cadmium in human organs based on the accumulation of the metal in the organs. *Keio Med J* 1976;25:73–82.

Vallee BL, Ulmer DD: Biochemical effects of mercury, cadmium, and lead. *Ann Rev Biochem* 1972;41:91–128.

Vigliani EC: The biopathology of cadmium. *Am Ind Hyg Assoc J* 1969;30:329–340.

Wilson RH, DeEds F, Cox AJ Jr: Effects of continued cadmium feeding. *J Pharmacol Exp Ther* 1941;71:222–235.

Winston RM: Cadmium fume poisoning. *Br Med J* 1971;1:401.

Wong KL, Klaassen CD: Age difference in the susceptibility to cadmium-induced testicular damage in rats. *Toxicol Appl Pharmacol* 1980; 55:456–466.

8 • *Chromium*

Uses

Metallic chromium is relatively inert but its surface is oxidized in damp air and it burns readily in the finely powdered state. Its bivalent salts (e.g., chromous oxide, CrO) are unstable. The trivalent compounds that are important in industry are chromic oxide (Cr_2O_3) and chromic sulfate ($Cr_2(SO_4)_3$). The most important industrial compounds are the hexavalent (e.g., chromic acid, CrO_3, the chromates, $CrO_4{}^{2-}$, and the dichromates, $Cr_2O_7{}^{2-}$, and these are also the most toxic (Browning, 1969; Tandon et al., 1978).

Metallic chromium is alloyed with iron, nickel, molybdenum, and manganese to produce a series of stainless steels that are resistant to corrosion and inert to nitric acid. Chromic acid and the dichromates are familiar occupational hazards because of their wide use in industry. The acid is used in chrome plating of a great variety of objects, such as household appliances and automobile trim, where brightness, beauty, and resistance to wear and rust are advantageous. Chromium plated directly on aluminum is used in the chemical, food, aviation, and electronic industries. The dichromates (potassium, sodium, and ammonium) are used as mordants in dyeing and in the quick tanning of leather, the method used almost exclusively in the United States. The cement industry uses chromium compounds, magnesium foundries use chromic acid solution to give weather resistance, and the forestry industry impregnates some timbers with chromium salts. Chromates are also employed in making coal-tar dyes, in photography and in photoengraving, and chromic acid is used in lithography.

A source of chromic acid poisoning arises from exposure to the mist formed in anodizing, an operation whereby a corrosion-resistant coating is formed on aluminum and its alloys. The anodizing solution contains up to 10% chromic acid.

The protection of workers against the fine sprays of chromic acid has engaged the best efforts of ventilation engineers. One wishes that lead, mercury, manganese, and silica had such irritating effects as has the far less harmful chromic acid.

Toxic Effects

Chromic acid and the chromates are oxidizing agents and are irritating to exposed tissues. Consequently, the harmful effects of chromium are largely confined to dermatitis, ulceration of the skin and nasal mucosa, and effects on the lungs, principally cancer.

Chromium is a common cause of contact dermatitis, both as a result of irritation and, more frequently, from sensitization. Occupations known to have a risk of chromium dermatitis are cement workers, chromium platers, dyers, and persons working in printing, photography, and with antirust agents and with wood impregnated with chromium (Burrows, 1978). A great variety of additional occupations have been incriminated in chromium dermatitis and have been listed by Burrows and by NIOSH (1976). Chromium dermatitis is typically eczematous and previous contact with chromium can be verified by the proper history of exposure and by patch tests.

For many years it was thought that cutaneous allergy is common with hexavalent chromium compounds and extremely rare with trivalent chromium exposure. There is no question that hexavalent compounds will cause dermatitis but the experience with tannery operations is instructive since it is the trivalent compound that tans the hide. Patch testing with the trivalent compounds, chromic acid and chromic chloride, proves that chrome dermatitis in tanneries is the result of exposure to these compounds. Burrows (1978) pointed out that while it is commonly difficult to sensitize with trivalent chromium, immunological

48

methods of detection of such sensitization, apart from patch testing and macrophage migration, indicate that Cr^{3+} is the valence form involved. It would appear that hexavalent chromium, which does not complex readily with organic compounds, does readily penetrate the epidermis to the dermis. Trivalent chromium, on the other hand, does not penetrate the epidermis readily, perhaps because it does form complexes with protein, possibly after it is formed by reduction from the hexavalent form (Polak et al., 1973).

The lesions caused by chromic acid have had an amount of attention paid to them that is out of proportion to their real importance, for in spite of their conspicuous character, they are not painful and do little, if any, permanent damage. But, as in phosphorus poisoning, the lesions develop in places where they are easily seen, so that from early days they have attracted the attention of physicians. In 1827 Cumming of Glasgow wrote about "chrome holes," the name workmen still use for indolent ulcers that developed chiefly on the hands and arms of men working with dichromates. These skin lesions caused by the caustic nature of the acid and the dichromate heal with difficulty but with little pain and do not spread. The term "holes" was given to the ulcers because they are penetrating. Yet, while such lesions may penetrate, suppuration rarely occurs even though there is every opportunity for infection. The commonest sites are around fingernails, surfaces of exposed finger joints, or the eyelids, sometimes the forearms, rarely the toes. Newhouse (1963) reported dermatitis due to chromate-containing paint among workers in automobile production.

The lesions of the nasal mucosa are the ones that give the most trouble and usually are the basis for compensation claims made by chrome workers. The chromate dust or the chromic acid spray that is inhaled causes irritation of the nasal mucosa, with inflammation, purulent discharge, formation of crusts, and some difficulty in breathing. Painless and chronic ulcers may form and are confined to the cartilaginous portion of the septum, never causing periostitis or deformity. This process ends in perforation of the septum that is often detected only by physical examination, but in some cases it causes real discomfort and makes mouth breathing necessary. Crusts form continually in many cases, and in others breathing through the nose makes an audible whistling sound because of the septal perforation, both of which are troublesome complications.

The report of Bloomfield and Blum (1928) on six chromium plating plants reflects earlier United States experience with this industrial hazard. The exposure in these plants ranged from 0.1 to 5.6 mg/m³ chromic acid. Among the persons examined, 16% had perforation of the nasal septum, 21% ulcerated septum, 89% inflamed nasal mucosa, and 58% a history of frequent nosebleed. Of 14 workers directly engaged in plating work, 43% had from one to five chrome holes. This study showed that, wherever the concentration consistently exceeds 0.1 mg/m³, nasal involvement may be expected. More recently, Edmundson (1951) found that 69.5% of 285 workers in a United States chromate manufacturing plant had chrome ulcers or scars and 61.4% had perforations of the nasal septum. Royle (1975) reported that the risk of skin and nasal ulceration increases progressively with the length of chromic acid exposure.

Dichromates, used in the chemical industry at temperatures of 80° to 100°C, are readily absorbed through skin burned by the chemical and can lead, as in two documented cases, to renal shutdown and death. Fatal nephritis has occurred in a man due to use of chromium (VI) oxide to cauterize a wound (Major, 1922). Renal damage by chromium has been confirmed in animal and *in vitro* studies (Berndt, 1976).

Since chromates and chromic acid are irritating to skin and to mucous membranes of the upper respiratory tract, it is likely that these chemicals can act alone or with infection and cigarette smoking to cause bronchial disease. Mancuso (1951) did describe a higher rate of bronchitis among chromate workers. Both length and level of exposure are critical factors and, because United States workers in general change jobs more often than do Europeans, it is difficult in this country to pinpoint bronchitis as a result of chromate exposure.

Mancuso and Hueper (1951) also described acute chromium pneumonia and Sluis-Cremer and DuToit (1968) wrote of chronic chromate lung. Royle (1975) found a higher incidence of respiratory symptoms (e.g., productive cough, asthma) in chromium platers than in a control group, but apparently both dust and chromic acid were involved. Earlier, Reggiani et al. (1973) reported that 60% of a group of 101 workers exposed to chromic acid inhalation had subjective symptoms of chronic bronchitis, although spirometry was not sufficiently sensitive to detect these changes. Metal-fume fever in 70 ferrochrome workers was attributed by Stoke (1977) to inhalation of freshly prepared chromium oxide. Chronic exposure to mixed metal dusts that include chromium may occur in many occupations such as metal dressers in steel works (Jones and Warner, 1972) and automobile repairmen (Clausen and Rastogi, 1977), sometimes with resultant pneumoconioses. Bovet et al. (1977) reported a correlation between lowered spirometry values and increased urine chromium in 44 workers in 17 electroplating plants, and they suggested that these persons were at increased risk in developing chronic obstructive respiratory disease.

Systemic effects of chromium are not often encountered, but Pascale et al. (1952) reported a case of acute hepatitis with jaundice as a result of chromium exposure in a chrome-plating plant.

Carcinogenic Action of Chromates

For many years there was a general conviction among industrial toxicologists that chromates had no carcinogenic action. Legge (1934) in England stated that chrome ulcers do not undergo malignant change, and American experience seemed to support this view. However, in the 1930s reports of respiratory cancers affecting workers in the chromate-producing and chrome pigment industries began to be published in the German literature.

Machle and Gregorius (1948) published the results of the first United States study of the incidence of lung cancer in workers exposed to dusts in the course of producing chromates, dichromates, and chromic acid. This study was made of the five companies in the country that were extracting chromates from ore in seven plants employing 1445 men. In this population there were 193 deaths of which 21.8% were from respiratory cancer while only 1.4% of 733 deaths in a control group died with this disease. The incidence of nasal irritation and perforation did not run parallel with lung cancer. In two plants belonging to the same company there was a marked difference in the occurrence of lung cancer, although the plant populations were demographically similar and had comparable lengths of exposure. The first plant, with a 17% death rate from lung cancer, handled sodium chromate and dichromate; the second, where there were no deaths from this cause, handled only sodium dichromate, chromic acid, and basic chromic sulfate, a trivalent compound. These findings suggested that the monochromates might be the compounds responsible for the lung cancer.

The British chromate industry, studied by Bidstrup (1951) showed no increase in lung malignancy. But when Bidstrup and Case (1956) restudied the same industry five years later, they found a significant risk of lung cancer. There has been considerable discussion in the literature as to the variations in industrial operations in England, Germany, and the United States that would account for the differing cancer experience (Mancuso, 1951; Gafafer, 1953; Goldblatt and Goldblatt, 1956). Respiratory tract cancers have now also been reported among workers in chromate-producing or processing plants in a wide range of industrial countries that include Italy, Japan, Norway, Czechoslovakia, and the Soviet Union (Sunderman, 1976). A decade earlier, Hueper (1966) had collected 187 respiratory tract cancers worldwide among chromate workers, of which 180 were lung cancers, mainly anaplastic and squamous-cell carcinomas.

The monochromates have been suggested as the active carcinogen. However, it appears that chromium and all its compounds, as well as chrome ore dust, should be regarded as potential carcinogens. HLH knows of a small group of workers exposed to chrome dust in which half of the workers suffered neoplasia of the respiratory tract. Unfortunately, precise data are not available because of litigation. The malignant lung lesion in chromate workers is no different in location or cell character from other respiratory tract cancers.

Hueper and Payne (1962) concluded from their studies with animals that both trivalent and hexavalent chromium possess carcinogenic properties. Local sarcomas have been produced in rodents by injections of chromium powder and hexavalent chromium compounds. Calcium chromate, in particular, has been shown to be the most potent respiratory carcinogen in rats (Hueper and Payne, 1959; Roe and Carter, 1969; Laskin et al., 1970). While the mechanism of chromium carcinogenesis has not been elucidated, Schoental (1975) has made the interesting suggestion that epoxyaldehydes, specifically glycidal (a known carcinogen for rats and mice), are derived from tissue lipids when cells are damaged by hexavalent chromium.

Treatment and Control

Beyond removal from exposure to chromium there is no specific therapy. Chromium compounds spilled on the skin should be flushed off with copious amounts of water and the same advice applies to the eyes (NIOSH, 1976). British antilewisite (BAL) and calcium sodium ethylene-diaminetetraacetic acid (CaNa₂ EDTA) have no effect. Penicillamine is unlikely to be of benefit if CaNa₂ EDTA is not. For treatment of skin ulcers several specific forms of therapy have been suggested. Johnstone and Miller (1960) recommended mild ointments or wet dressings incorporating citric or tartaric acid. Moeschlin (1965) suggested using wet dressings of 5 to 10% sodium citrate to remove necrotic tissue. Maloof, in a personal communication to HLH (1971), uses a 10% Ca EDTA ointment, which makes it easy to remove the scab formed by the action of chromates on the skin.

The prevention of injury from chromic acid and the chromates depends upon prevention of skin contact and the escape of dust into the air. It may be necessary to provide rubber gloves, boots, and an apron for a person working around chromic acid tanks. But these do not provide complete protection since the solution may drip onto upraised arms and run down inside the gloves. Solutions may also run down inside the boots if they are loose at the top. The rubber apron should cover the back as well as the front for splashing of the back may occur. A bland ointment lightly smeared over the exposed skin may act as protection. White petrolatum applied to the nasal septum has proved to be useful. Nasal passages should be inspected regularly and careful attention should be given to trivial injuries of the skin since they may lead to serious chrome ulcers.

The permissible exposure limits recommended by NIOSH (1976) vary with the form of chromium. Exposure limits for carcinogenic chromium (VI) compounds are 0.001 mg/m³. For noncarcinogenic chromium (VI) NIOSH recommends reduction of the permissible exposure limit to 0.025 mg Cr/m³ averaged over a work shift of up to 10 hours a day, 40 hours per week, with a 15-minute ceiling level of 0.05 mg Cr/m³. The chromium (VI) compounds currently believed to be noncarcinogenic are the monochromates, the dichromates of hydrogen, lithium, sodium, potassium, rubidium, cesium, and ammonium, and chromic acid anhydride.

For chromic acid (defined as chromium trioxide and its aqueous solutions), NIOSH (1973) recommended an occupational exposure limited to 0.05 mg as chromium oxide per m³ determined as a TWA for an 8-hour workday, 40-hour week, or a ceiling value of 0.1 mg/m³ in a 15-minute sample.

References

Berndt WO: Renal chromium accumulation and its relationship to chromium-induced nephrotoxicity. *J Toxicol Environ Health* 1976;1:449–459.

Bidstrup PL: Carcinoma of the lung in chromate workers. *Br J Ind Med* 1951;8:302–305.

Bidstrup PL, Case RAM: Carcinoma of the lung in workmen in the bichromates-producing industry in Great Britain. *Br J Ind Med* 1956;13:260–264.

Bloomfield JJ, Blum W: Health hazards in chromium plating. *Public Health Rep* 1928;43:2330–2347.

Bovet P, Lob M, Grandjean M: Spirometric alterations in the chromium electroplating industry. *Int Arch Occup Environ Health* 1977;40:25–32.

Browning E: *Toxicity of Industrial Metals,* ed 2. New York, Appleton-Century-Crofts, 1969, pp 119–131.

Burrows D: Chromium and the skin. *Br J Dermatol* 1978;99:587–595.

Clausen J, Rastogi SC: Heavy metal pollution among auto workers: II. Cadmium, chromium, copper, manganese, and nickel. *Br J Ind Med* 1977;34:216–220.

Edmundson WF: Chrome ulcers of the skin and nasal septum and their relation to patch testing. *J Invest Dermatol* 1951;17:17–19.

Gafafer WM: Health of workers in the chromate industry. *Public Health Serv Publ* No. 192, 1953.

Goldblatt MW, Goldblatt J: Industrial carcinogenesis and toxicology: Part 1. Occupational carcinogenesis, in Merewether ERA (ed): *Industrial Medicine and Hygiene.* London, Butterworth, 1956, vol 3, pp 188–196.

Hueper WC: *Occupational and Environmental Cancers of the Respiratory System.* New York, Springer, 1966, pp 57–85.

Hueper WC, Payne WW: Experimental cancers in rats produced by chromium compounds and their significance to industry and public health. *Am Ind Hyg Assoc J* 1959;20:274–280.

Hueper WC, Payne WW: Experimental studies in metal carcinogenesis—chromium, nickel, iron, arsenic. *Arch Environ Health* 1962;5:51–68.

Johnstone RT, Miller SE: *Occupational Diseases and Industrial Medicine.* Philadelphia, Saunders, 1960.

Jones JG, Warner CG: Chronic exposure to iron oxide, chromium oxide, and nickel oxide

52

fumes of metal dressers in a steelworks. *Br J Ind Med* 1972;29:169–177.

Legge TM: *Industrial Maladies*. London, Oxford, 1934.

Laskin S, Kuschner M, Drew RT: Studies in pulmonary carcinogenesis, Hanna MG Jr, Nettesheim P, Gilbert JR (eds): in *Inhalation Carcinogenesis*. Washington, DC, U.S. Atomic Energy Commission, 1970, pp 321–351.

Machle W, Gregorius F: Cancer of the respiratory system in the United States chromate-producing industry. *Public Health Rep* 1948;63:1114–1127.

Major RH: Studies on a case of chromic acid nephritis. *Johns Hopkins Hosp Bull* 1922;33:56–61.

Mancuso TF: Occupational cancer and other health hazards in a chromate plant: A medical appraisal: II. Clinical and toxicologic aspects. *Ind Med Surg* 1951;20:393–407.

Mancuso TF, Hueper WC: Occupational cancer and other health hazards in a chromate plant: A medical appraisal: I. Lung cancers in chromate workers. *Ind Med Surg* 1951;20:358–363.

Moeschlin S: *Poisoning: Diagnosis and Treatment*. New York, Grune & Stratton, 1965.

Newhouse ML: A cause of chromate dermatitis among assemblers in an automobile factory. *Br J Ind Med* 1963;20:199–203.

NIOSH: *Criteria for a Recommended Standard . . . .Occupational Exposure to Chromic Acid*. Washington, DC, National Institute for Occupational Safety and Health, (NIOSH 73-11021) 1973.

NIOSH: *Criteria for a Recommended Standard . . . . Occupational Exposure to Chromium (VI)*. Washington, DC, National Institute for Occupational Safety and Health, (NIOSH 96-129) 1976.

Pascale LR, Walderstein SS, Engloring G, et al: Chromium intoxication with special reference to hepatic injury. *J Am Med Assoc* 1952;149:1385–1389.

Polak L, Turk JL, Frey JR: Studies on contact hypersensitivity to chromium compounds. *Prog Allergy* 1973;17:145–226.

Reggiani A, Lotti M, DeRosa E, et al: Respiratory functional changes in subjects exposed to chromium: I. Spirographic changes. *Lavoro Umano* 1973;25:23–27.

Roe FJC, Carter RL: Chromium carcinogenesis: Calcium chromate as a potent carcinogen for the subcutaneous tissues of the rat. *Br J Cancer* 1969;23:172–176.

Royle H: Toxicity of chromic acid in the chromium plating industry (2). *Environ Res* 1975;10:141–163.

Schoental R: Chromium carcinogenesis, formation of epoxyaldehydes and tanning. *Br J Cancer* 1975;32:403–404.

Sluis-Cremer GK, DuToit RSJ: Pneumoconiosis in chromite miners in South Africa. *Br J Ind Med* 1968;25:63–67.

Stoke J: Metal fume fever in ferro-chrome workers. *Central African J Med* 1977;23:25–28.

Sunderman FW Jr: A review of the carcinogenicities of nickel, chromium and arsenic compounds in man and animals. *Prevent Med* 1976;5:279–294.

Tandon SK, Saxena DK, Gaur JS, et al: Comparative toxicity of trivalent and hexavalent chromium. Alterations in blood and liver. *Environ Res* 1978;15:90–99.

9 • Cobalt

Uses

Cobalt is extracted from copper-cobalt ores found in Zaire, Canada, and the United States. It is used in alloys to produce high-speed steel and to give permanent magnets greater lifting power. It is also used as a pigment in glass, china, and paint, and as a catalyst in the oil and chemical industries. Its principal use, however, is in the manufacture of hard metal, which is a man-made product consisting of metal carbide powders (usually tungsten) cemented by cobalt binder. Hard metal has unusual properties of heat resistance, wear resistance, and its hardness approaches that of diamond. It becomes harder when the temperature increases so that hard-metal tipped machine tools remain sharp up to 1700°C (Browning, 1969; Payne, 1976, 1977).

Industrial Exposure

Workers in hard metal are exposed to a number of carbides including titanium, tantalum, and vanadium. Cobalt is used in all of the processes, the quantity usually varying from 5 to 12% (Fairhall et al., 1949), but it may be as high as 25% (Payne, 1977). A pulmonary disease associated with this work is referred to as "hard-metal disease." The jobs in the manufacture of hard metal associated with illness are milling, mixing, and pressing the fine powder. The report of Miller et al. (1953) is important, for although the affected men were grinders in tungsten tool manufacture and may have been exposed to other dusts, cobalt is incriminated as the likely cause of the disease.

Reports of symptoms and signs of respiratory disease among hard-metal workers appeared first in 1947 and to date descriptions of such industrial illness have come from Sweden, Germany, Great Britain, the United States, and other industrial countries (Bech, 1974). Because of exposures to dust other than hard-metal dust, several authors were uncertain of the precise etiology (Ahlmark et al., 1960; Bech et al., 1962), although Payne (1977) states that it is now generally accepted that the cobalt content is the responsible factor in the development of the disease.

There appear to be two clinical patterns, both with chest x-ray abnormalities and complaints of cough, dyspnea, and expectoration. The acute form appears to be a hypersensitivity reaction with wheezing and nonproductive cough, with complete relief of symptoms on removal from exposure. The chronic form is frequently delayed in onset, is progressive, and leads to chronic pulmonary insufficiency, cor pulmonale, and eventually, death. Descriptions of chest x-ray changes vary from increase of linear markings with small nodular densities to conglomerate opacities, or notable evidence of shrinking of the lungs and emphysema. Bech et al. (1962), reporting relatively mild cases, found, on lung function study, significant diffusion defects. A few postmortem studies describe varying degrees of interstitial pulmonary fibrosis and, in severe cases, marked emphysema. Electron microscopy of fibrotic lungs demonstrates crystals associated with these areas of interstitial cellular reaction and while analyses by x-ray diffraction confirms the presence of tungsten and titanium, there is no trace of cobalt. This surprising finding was attributed by Payne (1977) to the high degree of solubility of cobalt in protein-containing fluids such as plasma and lung surfactant, so that the other components of hard metal remain in the lung while cobalt is not present in the alveolar macrophages. Case reports of severe hard-metal pneumoconiosis continue to appear (Coates and Watson, 1971; Bech, 1974; Siegesmund et al., 1974; Bartl and Lichtenstein, 1976; Forrest et al., 1978).

54

Cobalt has been incriminated in "beer-drinker's cardiomyopathy" reported from Omaha (McDermott, 1966), Quebec City (Morin and Daniel, 1967), and Brussels (Kesteloot et al., 1968) as a result of cobalt chloride having been used as an additive to stabilize beer foam that was otherwise impaired by traces of detergents on incompletely rinsed beer glasses. The cardiomyopathy in beer drinkers and in experimental animals consisted of noninflammatory thickening and vacuolar degeneration of myocardial fibers, and interstitial edema. Pericardial effusion also occurred and distinguished this form from other types of alcohol cardiomyopathy. Cardiac muscle pathology from industrial exposure to cobalt is not common, but a fatal case in a metal worker was reported by Barborik and Dusek (1972).

Cobalt dermatitis has been reported frequently in association with chromium exposure. Frequently, this skin problem has been the result of cross-reactions as a result of haptene similarities between chromium, cobalt, and nickel (Cohen, 1976). Although cobalt oxides in cement, for example, are not water soluble, Co may form complexes with amino acids, especially in eczematous skin, and this phenomenon may thus explain cobalt sensitization in persons with cement eczema due to chromium sensitivity (Fregert and Gruvberger, 1978). Contact urticaria from cobalt chloride is well-known, but usually occurs after its use as an indicator of sweat production (Smith et al., 1975). Lymphocyte transformation tests are significantly higher in patients with cobalt-induced contact dermatitis and positive cobalt patch tests than in controls (Veien and Svejgaard, 1978).

Hazard Control

The TLV for pure cobalt is 0.1 mg/m³ of air while the maximum allowable concentration is 0.5 mg/m³ in the U.S.S.R. Ventilation measures for control of cobalt exposures during tungsten carbide grinding are discussed by Lichtenstein et al. (1975). Workers found to be hypersensitive to cobalt by demonstration of contact dermatitis or asthmatic symptoms should be removed from actual or potential exposure to cobalt.

References

Ahlmark A, Bruce T, Nyström A: *Silicosis and Other Pneumoconioses in Sweden.* Stockholm, Svenska Bokförlaget, 1960.

Barborik M, Dusek J: Cardiomyopathy accompanying industrial cobalt exposure. *Br Heart J* 1972;34:113–116.

Bartl F, Lichtenstein ME: Tungsten carbide pulmonary fibrosis — A case report. *Am Ind Hyg Assoc J* 1976;37:668–670.

Bech AO, Kipling MD, Heather JC: Hard metal disease. *Br J Ind Med* 1962;15:239–252.

Bech AO: Hard metal disease and tool room grinding. *J Soc Occup Med* 1974;24:11–16.

Browning E: *Toxicity of Industrial Metals,* ed 2. New York, Appleton-Century-Crofts, 1969, pp 132–142.

Coates EO Jr, Watson JHL: Diffuse interstitial lung disease in tungsten carbide workers. *Ann Intern Med* 1971;75:709–716.

Cohen HA: The role of carrier in sensitivity to chromium and cobalt. *Arch Dermatol* 1976;112:37–39.

Fairhall, LT, Keenan RG, Brinton HP: Cobalt and the dust environment of the cemented tungsten carbide industry. *US Pub Health Serv Rep* 1949;64:485.

Forrest ME, Skerker LB, Nemiroff MJ: Hard metal pneumoconiosis: Another cause of diffuse interstitial fibrosis. *Radiology* 1978;128:609–612.

Fregert S, Gruvberger B: Solubility of cobalt in cement. *Contact Dermatitis* 1978;4:14–18.

Kesteloot H, Roelandt J, Willems J, et al: An enquiry into the role of cobalt in the heart disease of chronic beer drinkers. *Circulation* 1968;37:854–864.

Lichtenstein ME, Bartl F, Pierce RT: Control of cobalt exposures during wet process tungsten carbide grinding. *Am Ind Hyg Assoc J* 1975;36:879–885.

McDermott PH, Delanoy RL, Egon JD, et al: Myocardosis and cardiac failure in men. *J Am Med Assoc* 1966;198:253–256.

Miller CW, Davis MW, Goldman A, et al: Pneumoconiosis in the tungsten-carbide tool industry. *Arch Ind Hyg Occup Med* 1953;8:453–465.

Morin Y, Daniel P: Quebec beer-drinkers' cardiomyopathy: Etiological considerations. *Can Med Assoc J* 1967;97:926–928.

Payne LR: Hard metal. *J Soc Occup Med* 1976;26:141–142.

Payne LR: The hazards of cobalt. *J Soc Occup Med* 1977;27:20–25.

Siegesmund KA, Funahashi A, Pintar M: Identification of metals in lung from a patient with interstitial pneumonia. *Arch Environ Health* 1974;28:345–349.

Smith JD, Odom RB, Maibach HI: Chronic urticaria from cobalt chloride. *Arch Dermatol* 1975; 111:1610–1611.

Veien NK, Svejgaard E: Lymphocyte transformation in patients with cobalt dermatitis. *Br J Dermatol* 1978;99:191–196.

10 • *Copper*

Copper occurs widely in nature, both in free form as native copper and in a variety of ores. Extraction from ores involves crushing, roasting, and smelting to produce "matte," a mixture in varying proportions of copper and iron sulfides that is further refined to remove sulfur and iron. Copper is used in an extensive range of alloys to which it imparts hardness, principally brass (with zinc) and bronze (with tin), as well as special mixtures with other metals such as nickel, beryllium, and cobalt. Copper is used in wires, pipes, roof sheeting, and vessels, and copper salts are used as insecticides, algicides, and parasiticides.

Copper is an essential element and because of its distribution in nature, it is normally found in all diets. The daily United States dietary intake of copper ranges from 2 to 5 mg, almost all of which is excreted in the feces. Minute amounts of cupric ion are absorbed and stored mainly in liver, blood, and brain. Copper balance is maintained by an efficient homeostatic mechanism that involves the intestine as a barrier and organ of excretion and the liver for storage (Schroeder, 1966).

Copper is a component of a number of cuproenzymes that catalyze important biochemical and physiological reactions that include iron absorption and heme biosynthesis. Copper deficiency consequently leads to anemia, neutropenia, and eventually to bone lesions resembling scurvy and to pathological fractures without hemorrhage (Prasad, 1978).

Copper poisoning, on the other hand, leads to a variety of toxic effects that include metallic taste, ptyalism, nausea, vomiting, epigastric burning, diarrhea, hemolysis, hepatic necrosis, gastrointestinal bleeding, oligiura, azotemia, hemoglobinuria, hematuria, hypotension, tachycardia, convulsions, coma, and death (Prasad, 1978).

Mallory (1925) published a famous paper on chronic copper poisoning as the cause of hemochromatosis. He held that the disease is much more common than supposed, the source of copper being, in most cases, alcoholic drinks contaminated with copper from stills. Interest in the question of chronic copper poisoning in industry was aroused by Mallory's publication, and the British Factory Inspection Service made a search for cases of cirrhosis among copper workers, but found evidence of such disease in only one case.

Schroeder (1966) and Browning (1969) reviewed reports of the controversial question as to whether there is evidence to support the diagnosis of chronic industrial copper poisoning. The green coloration of skin, hair, and teeth after intense exposure of long duration was first thought to be evidence of a toxic effect. However, the coloring came to be regarded as harmless, except for painful gums that occur in severe cases.

The effect of the fumes of copper oxide is described in the section on metal fume fever. Since the vaporization point of copper is high — about 2350°C — it is very rare that fumes of this sort are encountered in industry.

Workmen often speak of copper poisoning as they do of brass poisoning when they mean infected cuts resulting from the handling of sharp-edged copper plates or fragments. It is improbable that copper has any chemical action in such cases, the metal acting as a foreign body only. There are a few reports of copper neuritis and sympathetic nervous symptoms including one case of Raynaud's disease developing after fragments of copper became imbedded in a worker's hand. Such reports are hard to assess.

The green carbonate of copper is irritating to the skin and to the eyes. A troublesome skin eruption accompanied by much swelling and itching among workmen is due to finely divided "cement copper" obtained from the precipitation of the metal from solution by metallic iron. The effect on the nasal passages and throat is irritating and the worker notices a sweetish taste in his mouth with excess salivation. The presence of 0.1% of arsenic in the dust may influence this picture.

However, the 1967 report of Saury et al. (1967) makes clear the fact that high-level industrial copper exposure can cause disabling illness. After six years of recovering copper waste from a furnace at 1000°C, a worker suffered diarrhea and vomiting. This man and seven others on the same job excreted excessive amounts of copper (66 to 104 μg/L). The patient's symptoms reversed after a week of no copper exposure. Gleason (1968) reported general malaise and "head stuffiness" in workers polishing copper plates. When local exhaust ventilation reduced the copper dust concentrations of 0.75 to 1.20 mg/m³ down to 0.008 mg/m³, the complaints disappeared.

Pimentel and Menezes (1977) have described "vineyard sprayer's lung" in rural workers in Portugal who applied sprays of Bordeaux mixture (a mixture of aqueous $CuSo_4$ and CaOH that involves precipitates of CuOH and several basic sulfates of copper). There were interstitial pulmonary lesions consisting of copper-containing histiocytic granulomas and nodular fibrohyaline scars that either regressed, remained stationary, or progressed to diffuse pulmonary fibrosis, suppuration, and lung cancer. Copper-containing lesions were also found in the nasal mucosa, liver, kidney, spleen, and lymph nodes. Copper-related liver lesions included sarcoid-like granulomata, fibrosis, cirrhosis, and angiosarcoma, along with idiopathic portal hypertension.

Hypersensitivity skin reactions to copper in a welder have been described by Förström et al. (1977), and by Dhir et al. (1977) in furniture polishers who used commercial spirit colored blue with $CuSO_4$.

There are reports of ulcerated lesions of the nose as a result of inhaling copper dust. Fine fragments of copper penetrating the eye during certain industrial operations can give rise to severe ocular damage. The deposit of copper in the vitreous body, retina, and cornea is known as chalcosis (Moeschlin, 1965). Wilson's disease, a hereditary copper storage illness, has not been described as a result of chronic industrial exposure to copper.

Study of the literature describing the symptoms occasionally observed in copper and brass workers does not allow one to conclude that copper intoxication is a widespread occupational disease. Such symptoms may be due to poor working conditions, the presence of arsenic and lead as impurities, or some other reason. However, the published reports suggest the possibility that copper may act with other exogenous agents or subclinical metabolic disorders to produce, in some workers, an industrially acquired atypical Wilson's disease or, as Mallory postulated and Pimentel proposes, chronic liver disease. Further carefully controlled studies of copper workers are required. Reviews on the health hazards from copper exposure are provided by Browning (1969) and Cohen (1974).

The United States' so-called threshold limit values for copper exposure for a 40-hour workweek are 0.1 mg/m³ for fumes and 1.0 mg/m³ for the dusts and mists of copper.

References

Browning E: *Toxicity of Industrial Metals,* ed 2. New York, Appleton-Century-Crofts, 1969, pp 145–152.

Cohen SR: A review of the health hazards from copper exposure. *J Occup Med* 1974;16:621–624.

Dhir GG, Rao DS, Mehrotra MP: Contact dermatitis caused by copper sulfate used as coloring material in commercial alcohol. *Ann Allergy* 1977;39:204.

Förström L, Kiistala R, Tarvainen K: Hypersensitivity to copper verified by test with 0.1% $CuSO_4$. *Contact Dermatitis* 1977;3:280–281.

Gleason RP: Exposure to copper dust. *Am Ind Hyg Assoc J* 1968;29:461–462.

Mallory FB: The relation of chronic poisoning with copper to hemachromatosis. *Am J Pathol* 1925;1:117–133.

Moeschlin S: *Poisoning: Diagnosis and Treatment.* New York, Grune & Stratton, 1965.

Pimentel JC, Menezes AP: Liver disease in vineyard sprayers. *Gastroenterol* 1977;72:275–283.

Prasad AS: *Trace Elements and Iron in Human Metabolism.* New York, Plenum, 1978.

Saury A, Girard R, Rouzioux JM: Intoxication professionelle par le cuivre. *Arch Mal Prof* 1967; 28:696–698, abstracted in *Abs Hyg* 1968;43:748.

Schroeder HA, Nason AP, Tipton IH, et al: Essential trace metals in man: Copper. *J Chron Dis* 1966;19:1007–1034.

11 • *Germanium*

While this element and its industrially used compounds have not caused recognizable occupational illness (Browning, 1969), mention of germanium is included because of its value in the electronics industry. Germanium diodes were developed for rectification of microwaves for use in radar. Later, the invention of germanium transistors had a marked influence on many electronic applications such as portable radios, hearing aids, and television sets. Certain electroplating operations involve exposure to germanium dioxide, and some alloys are made with germanium combined with aluminum or tin. Germanium lenses and filters are used in optical instruments that operate in the infrared region of the spectrum.

The hydride of germanium is known to be a hemolytic poison. Hueper (1947) discussed the relative toxicity of metal hydrides and concluded that the germanium hydride (monogermane, GeH_4) is the least toxic, arsenic hydride (arsine, AsH_3) and antimony hydride (stibine, SbH_3) more toxic, and tin hydride (SnH_4) the most toxic. Germanium tetrachloride and tetrafluoride are considered mucous membrane irritants (Harrold et al., 1944).

Some attempts have been made to use germanium as an anticoagulant for human disease, but desired pharmacological and toxic effects are too close together. Germanium tried as a drug for various anemias proved useless (Rosenfeld and Wallace, 1953). The literature on animal studies of germanium toxicity does not present a clear picture of pathologic effect (Schroeder and Balassa, 1967; Hueper, 1947; Dudley, 1953). The best studied compound, germanium dioxide, is rapidly excreted and in moderately large doses produces no damage in inhalation experiments (Rosenfeld and Wallace, 1953). Germanium trioxide administered intravenously to pregnant hamsters did not produce malformations in the fetuses, although earlier investigators had reported that dimethyl germanium oxide was teratogenic in chick embryos (Ferm and Carpenter, 1970).

References

Browning E: *Toxicity of Industrial Metals,* ed 2. New York, Appleton-Century-Crofts, 1969, pp 158–163.

Dudley HC: Pharmacological studies of radiogermanium (Ge[71]). *Arch Ind Hyg Occup Med* 1953;8:528–530.

Ferm VH, Carpenter SJ: Teratogenic and embryopathic effects of indium, gallium, and germanium. *Toxicol Appl Pharmacol* 1970;16:166–170.

Harrold GC, Meek SF, McCord CP: The physiological properties of germanium. *Ind Med* 1944;13:236–238.

Hueper WC: Germanium. *Occup Med* 1947;4:208–227.

Rosenfeld G, Wallace ED: Studies of acute and chronic toxicity of germanium. *Arch Ind Hyg Occup Med* 1953;8:466–479.

Schroeder HA, Balassa JJ: Abnormal trace metals in man: Germanium. *J Chron Dis* 1967;20:211–224.

12 • *Indium*

Industrial use of the rare metal indium has increased remarkably since the 1930s, with consequent lowering of its once fabulous cost of $87 per gram. It is used in industry in dental alloys, both in gold and in mercury amalgams; in bearings to improve strength, hardness, and corrosion resistance; in low-melting fusible alloys that are used to seal metals to glass and ceramics; in electronics in semiconductors and solar cells; in nuclear reactor control rods; and in lubrication of moving machine parts. Its use in tarnish protection of silverplate has declined (Smith et al., 1978). Several thousand tons of indium are available each year as a by-product in the zinc and coal industries. Extraction of indium carries the risk of exposure to lead and tin.

Although McCord et al. (1942) speculated that indium plating may be harmful because of the presence of cyanide, there are no reports of indium-related human illness in industry. In part, this absence is because occupational exposures to indium alone have not been studied, probably because mineral acid aerosols and/or compounds of lead, arsenic, mercury, cadmium, zinc, and other metals are present during smelting operations in amounts greater than indium (Smith et al., 1978). Patch testing of workers has shown no irritant properties nor evidence of sensitization.

A number of toxicity studies in animals have been done that have shown indium to be essentially nontoxic to animals when given by mouth; when given by injection, it caused damage chiefly to liver and kidneys (Stokinger, 1963; Browning, 1969; Smith et al., 1978). Large doses (> 1 mg In/kg) of indium nitrate given to pregnant hamsters intravenously are embryocidal, while lower doses are teratogenic (Ferm and Carpenter, 1970). Indium chloride given intraperitoneally to rats led to rapid and pronounced changes in hepatic heme metabolism, mainly by depression of crucial rate-limiting enzymes (Woods et al.,

1979). Because indium compounds are used as diagnostic radiopharmaceuticals, Castronovo and Wagner (1973) studied the toxic effects of ionic indium chloride and hydrated indium oxide on mice and found that the latter was 40 times more toxic than $InCl_3$ and primarily affected the reticuloendothelial system, while the ionic form caused acute kidney tubule necrosis.

References

Browning E: *Toxicity of Industrial Metals,* ed 2. New York, Appleton-Century-Crofts, 1969, pp 164–168.

Castronovo FP, Wagner HN: Comparative toxicity and pharmacodynamics of ionic indium chloride and hydrated indium oxide. *J Nucl Med* 1973;14:677–682.

Ferm VH, Carpenter SJ: Teratogenic and embryopathic effects of indium, gallium, and germanium. *Toxicol Appl Pharmacol* 1970;16:166–170.

McCord CP, Meek SF, Harrold GC, et al: The physiological properties of indium and its compounds. *J Ind Hyg Toxicol* 1942;24:243–254.

Smith IC, Carson BL, Hoffmeister F: *Trace Metals in the Environment–Indium,* vol 5. Ann Arbor, MI, Ann Arbor Science Publishers, Inc, 1978.

Stokinger HE: The metals (excluding lead), in Patty FA (ed): *Industrial Hygiene and Toxicology,* ed 2. New York, John Wiley, 1963, vol 2.

Woods JS, Carver GT, Fowler BA: Altered regulation of hepatic heme metabolism by indium chloride. *Toxicol Appl Pharmacol* 1979;49:455–461.

13 • *Iron*

Uses

Iron is the fourth most abundant element in the earth's crust (5%) and is mainly extracted from hematite (Fe_2O_3) and limonite ($Fe_2O_3 \cdot 3H_2O$) although other ores such as magnetite (Fe_3O_4), siderite ($FeCO_3$), and taconite (an iron silicate) also serve as sources. Iron is used mainly for structural materials, principally in steel, an iron-carbon alloy. Iron is also used in magnets, dyes, pigments, abrasives, and polishing compounds (rouge).

Results of Exposure

Occupational siderosis is caused by exposure to iron oxide, such as in paint pigments and jeweler's rouge. Other causes of siderosis include the manufacture of iron oxide, iron shot, sieving and bagging of powder from emery rock, and grinding with an emery wheel. Chest x-ray changes of this benign pneumoconiosis are easily confused with those of silicosis, hemosiderosis, and a number of diseases that produce bilateral densities. Workers using electric arc or oxyacetylene equipment in welding, cutting, grinding, or polishing are at risk, especially when working in closed spaces such as boilers, tanks, and below decks of ships. The high temperatures of welding operations produce a fume of iron oxide that is readily inhaled in the absence of respiratory protection. Because of the heat and the physical effort required, it is often impossible for a worker to wear a useful mask except for very short periods.

Guidotti et al. (1978) distinguish between *arc welders' siderosis* from inhalation of iron oxide particles alone and *arc welders' pneumoconiosis* from inhalation of mixed dusts generated by welding that include silica, flux, and traces of other metals. The former is a pure siderosis while the latter is primarily a sidero-silicosis with a fibrotic component (see entry on Silica). Indeed, iron oxides may inhibit or delay silicotic fibrosis from the inhalation of quartz (Reichel et al., 1977). If exposure ceases, the dramatic chest x-ray changes of pure siderosis disappear (Sander, 1944; Morgan and Kerr, 1963). The few autopsy reports confirm the fact that the nodules of siderosis are collections of iron particles with no fibrosis.

Well-studied series of workers with siderosis show no increase in morbidity or mortality from respiratory disease (Stanescu et al., 1967; Kleinfeld at el., 1969). Albu and Popescu (1973) found no impairment in pulmonary blood flow in 12 iron oxide pigment workers with radiographic nodular opacities who were studied with macro-aggregated albumin-^{131}I lung scans. Morgan (1978) reported a case of pneumoconiosis in a worker who was exposed for nine years to very dusty atmospheres in a mill that pulverized magnetite that had a negligible silica content. The primary complaints were of cough and sputum. Although the chest film showed multiple rounded opacities throughout both lung fields, pulmonary function tests were normal.

The amount of welding fume contaminants (mainly iron oxide) has been determined *in vivo* in arc welders by magnetic measurements by Kalliomäki et al. (1978), who followed a suggestion of Cohen (1973). Mössbauer spectroscopy promises to provide a useful tool in distinguishing between different iron compounds in dried lung samples. This technique can differentiate endogenous blood and storage iron from exogenously acquired inhaled hematite (Guest, 1976, 1978).

Considerable iron oxide dust may be caught in the respiratory tract defenses and expectorated in sputum, a process well-known to exposed workers because of the rust color of the phlegm. The remaining iron oxide accumulates in lymphoid tissue along the bronchi, especially at the bifurcation. If a worker exposed to iron oxide is short of breath or has abnormal lung function indices, it is important to discover whether or not he has inhaled a fibrogenic dust such as silica in addition to the iron (Charr, 1956; Graham-Jones and Warner, 1972). HLH cared for a patient who developed disabling respiratory disease as a result of sandblasting rust from locomotive engines. At autopsy the presence of both severe silicosis and siderosis was confirmed. Meyer et al. (1967) point out that silica in coated electrodes and metals in materials being welded may produce pathological changes that overshadow the benign changes of siderosis.

The study of Faulds and Stewart (1956) revealed a significant increase in lung cancer among hematite ore miners in England. In contrast to other occupational lung tumors, these arose not in the larger bronchi but in scar tissue of siderosilicosis. Boyd et al. (1970) raised the possibility that the radioactive gas, radon, was responsible for these malignant changes since it is held, with its radioactive daughters, to be the etiologic carcinogen for lung tumors among other metal miners in Canada and the Colorado Plateau. On the other hand, Axelson and Sjöberg (1979), after a study of workers in a plant producing H_2SO_4 from pyrite (FeS_2), found no association between elevated exposures to iron oxides, mainly hematite, and the development of cancer.

References

Albu A, Popescu HI: Lung scanning in occupational siderosis. *Am Rev Resp Dis* 1973;107:291–294.

Axelson O, Sjöberg A: Cancer incidence and exposure to iron oxide dust. *J Occup Med* 1979; 21:419–422.

Boyd JT, Doll R, Faulds JS, et al: Cancer of the lung in iron ore (haematite) miners. *Br J Ind Med* 1970;27:97–105.

Charr R: Pulmonary changes in welders: A report of three cases. *Ann Intern Med* 1956;44: 806–812.

Cohen D: Ferromagnetic contamination in the lungs and other organs of the human body. *Science* 1973;180:745–748.

Faulds JS, Stewart MJ: Carcinoma of the lung in haematite miners. *J Pathol Bact* 1956;72:353–366.

Graham-Jones J, Warner CG: Chronic exposure to iron oxide, chromium oxide, and nickel oxide fumes of metal dressers in a steelworks. *Br J Ind Med* 1972;29:169–177.

Guest L: Investigation into the endogenous iron content of human lungs by Mössbauer spectroscopy. *Ann Occup Hyg* 1976;19:49–62.

Guest L: The endogenous iron content, by Mössbauer spectroscopy, of human lungs: II. Lungs from various occupational groups. *Ann Occup Hyg* 1978;21:151–157.

Guidotti TL, Abraham JL, DeNee PB, et al: Arc welders' pneumoconiosis: Application of advanced scanning electron microscopy. *Arch Environ Health* 1978;33:117–124.

Kalliomäki PL, Alanko K, Korhonen O, et al: Amount and distribution of welding fume lung contaminants among arc welders. *Scand J Work Environ Health* 1978;4:122–130.

Kleinfeld M, Messite J, Kooyman O, et al: Welders' siderosis: A clinical, roentgenographic and physiological study. *Arch Environ Health* 1969;19:70–73.

Meyer EC, Kratzinger SF, Miller WH: Pulmonary fibrosis in an arc welder. *Arch Environ Health* 1967;15:462–469.

Morgan WKC: Magnetite pneumoconiosis. *J Occup Med* 1978;20:762–763.

Morgan WKC, Kerr HD: Pathologic and physiologic studies of welders' siderosis. *Ann Intern Med* 1963;58:293–304.

Reichel G, Bauer H-D, Bruckmann E: The action of quartz in the presence of iron hydroxides in the human lung. *Inhaled Particles IV, Part I:* 1977;403–411.

Sander OA: Further observations on lung changes in electric arc welders. *J Ind Hyg Toxicol* 1944;26:79–85.

Stanescu DC, Pilat L, Gavrilescu N, et al: Aspects of pulmonary mechanics in arc welders' siderosis. *Br J Ind Med* 1967;24:143–147.

14 • *Lead*

Despite the antiquity of knowledge about lead poisoning, interest in problems of lead toxicity continues to be great. In recent years there has been a special concern about lead in air, water, and soil from leaded gasoline as well as from uncontrolled industrial sources. Awareness that paint and putty in old and in some new homes, contaminated street dirt, and playground soil are responsible for childhood lead poisoning that could be prevented has justifiably produced angry reactions (Hardy et al., 1971; Lin-Fu, 1972). Furthermore, occupational lead intoxication continues to be a problem in the United States and elsewhere. This chapter, while concerned chiefly with industrial disease, will also deal to some extent with current knowledge of the lead hazard in the general environment. Alice Hamilton's published work from 1910 to 1949, which was based on a wealth of experience with cases of lead poisoning as well as familiarity with clinical and experimental work throughout the world, provides a background and understanding of present problems. Subsequently, McCord (1953–1954) published an interesting and detailed account of lead poisoning in the early days of the United States.

History

Lead came into use very early in the history of civilization, and its poisonous effects were soon discovered. Greek, Roman, and Arabian physicians knew that lead would cause colic if swallowed. Dioscorides, in the first century of the present era, accurately described not only lead colic but also paralysis that developed after the swallowing of lead; he also knew that breathing lead fumes would cause the same disorder. Dioscorides wrote of the mechanical devices used in his day by workmen to protect themselves from lead fumes. His "molybdania" is supposed to have been litharge (lead monoxide). Pliny used the term "minium" in its present meaning of red lead oxide, and white lead (the basic carbonate) was known to the famous Arabian alchemist, Geber.

It was the widespread use of lead for cooking vessels and other household articles that caused the most notorious outbreaks of lead poisoning. In France, moreover, it was the custom to promote acid fermentation in wine by adding lead to it. Since Poitou was the region where this custom prevailed, the name "colic of Poitou" was given to lead colic. Stockhausen in 1656 published a treatise declaring that Poitou colic was caused by lead, and he accurately described clinical plumbism. The principal source of this condition in early days in England was lead-contaminated cider, and in Spain there was much poisoning from the use of lead to line cooking vessels. The outstanding work on the subject was written by Tanquerel des Planches, the "Columbus of lead poisoning," in the mid-19th century. His clinical observations on 1217 cases of plumbism were accurate and not much of importance has been added to them. He also noted what has escaped many industrial physicians since his day: that severe poisoning could always be traced to lead vapors or emanations. Only relatively mild and slow poisoning followed exposure to solid lead or lead paint. He also confirmed Bright's observation that there is a cause and effect relationship between chronic plumbism and renal disease, a subject still under discussion.

The potters' trade was for centuries a notorious source of lead poisoning. In Britain, France, Germany, and Hungary, the early literature paints shocking pictures of palsy in potters, of insanity, blindness, cachexia, and sterility. In several European countries pottery work was a home industry; whole villages were given over to it in Russia as late as 1924. Even in the large and well-managed potteries of England and Germany the rate of lead poisoning was high. The lead palsy described in H. G. Wells' *"New Machiavelli"* led to English housewives demanding "fritted ware." The government prescribed such strict regulations for users of soluble glaze as to force pottery manufacturers to go over to fritted glaze. In fritted glaze, lead is added before fusing and, when fused, forms poorly soluble silicate and borosilicate. Fritted glaze was slow in reaching American potteries, and the rate of plumbism in the first two decades of this century was alarmingly high. At the present time, however, tableware and toiletware are covered with fritted lead glaze, and, when lead is used in color spraying, proper precautions can be taken to carry off the spray. Despite this knowledge, various glazes again contain enough harmful amounts of lead in the finished products to cause illness (Klein et al., 1970; Browder, 1972).

Toxicity of Lead Compounds Used in Industry

In industry, the toxicity of a given lead compound depends on 1) its solubility in body fluids, and 2) the size of the particles, for the finer they are, the more quickly they are absorbed. Lead acetate, for instance, which when swallowed is very toxic, may not be an industrial hazard because it is not dusty. On the other hand, freshly sublimed lead suboxide is hazardous because of its physical character as a fume.

Lead is a heavy metal (specific gravity, 11.34; atomic weight, 207.21) that has a bluish color that tarnishes to a dull gray. It is amphoteric, forming lead salts of acids and metal salts of plumbic acid. In addition to alloys, the important industrial uses of lead are as inorganic compounds and tetraethyl lead. The lead compounds of importance in industry are the black, amorphous suboxide (Pb_2O); the red and yellow monoxides (PbO); the higher oxides (bronze PbO_2, orange-yellow Pb_2O_3, red Pb_3O_4); the basic carbonate ($2PbCO_3 \cdot Pb(OH)_2$), known as white lead or Old Dutch process; orange mineral, derived by roasting white lead; and the carbonate ($PbCO_3$), the black sulfide (PbS, galena), the white sulfates ($PbSO_4$, $PbSO_4 \cdot PbO$), the red and yellow chromates, the disilicates, and borosilicate. These compounds differ decidedly in their solubility and toxicity (Fairhall and Sayers, 1940). It is far less necessary, for example, to guard against dust in

the lead mines of Missouri where the ore is lead sulfide, which is very slightly soluble in human gastric juice and is poorly absorbed when inhaled (Carlson and Woelfel, 1913), than in the mines of Utah that contain the more soluble carbonate and sulfate. Pottery glaze gave rise to much plumbism as long as raw white lead, the soluble basic carbonate, was used; but when the white lead was changed by fritting (i.e., fusing and granulating) to the insoluble disilicate, the danger disappeared. The basic carbonate, the monoxide, and the basic sulfate are more toxic than metallic lead or other less soluble compounds. Lead arsenate is very toxic, in part due to the arsenic radical. The insoluble lead chromate used in paint was found by Harrold and his co-workers (1944) to be of low toxicity to man, principally because of poor absorption. Lead azide ($Pb(N_3)_2$), an explosive, can cause an acute toxic effect due to the azide radical rather than to the lead. Lead acetate, nitrate, and chloride are highly soluble but fortunately they do not form dusts readily, nor are they industrially important. Several compounds that are of industrial importance are worth discussing in some detail.

Lead oxide Metallic lead produced from ore is used in a wide variety of industries where it is cast or molded into shape or used as a solder. The danger comes from the suboxide, a fine grayish powder that makes a coating on solid lead and forms dross on the surface of molten lead. This is the form of lead found in the dust of casting rooms, printing plants, wherever solid lead is handled, and in the fumes from molten lead. It is important to remember that the danger of contaminating the air from lead depends not only on the temperature at which lead vaporizes, but at much lower points, for whenever molten lead is agitated, such as in skimming off dross, dropping in pigs of lead, ladling or pouring, the delicate coating of gray suboxide is detached and floats up with the waves of heat. This oxide, a fine powder, is easily soluble in weak acids. Exposure to lead suboxide occurs in zinc smelting when the ore contains lead. It also occurs in typefounding (unless it is completely mechanized), in founding brass, railway bronze, and bearing metal when a high proportion of lead is present in the alloy. There is risk in making molded lead goods and finishing them.

In those printing establishments where lead is still used there should be no risk at all of plumbism if precautions against fumes and dust are taken. Of commonly used lead alloys, type metal contains tin, antimony, and 60 to 90% lead, while bearing bronzes contain antimony, tin and 15 to 25% lead. Where large quantities of molten lead and scrap are handled, the hazard can be reduced to a minimum by controlling the pot temperatures, and on the whole, the printers' trade carries with it less danger of plumbism than do any of the other lead-using trades. On the other hand, photoengraving is one branch of the printing industry in which there is not only a long list of possibly dangerous chemicals, but such continual changes in methods that it is difficult to know to which of these chemicals an individual photoengraver has been exposed. The list includes mineral and organic acids, alkalis, ammonium, chromium, and bromine compounds, aniline, benzene, naphtha, chlorinated compounds, cyanides, sulfides, formaldehyde, nitric acid, and nitric oxides. Hayhurst (1915) stated many years ago that photoengravers are probably exposed to a greater number of poisonous substances than any other industrial group (Queries and Minor Notes, *J Am Med Assoc* 1946;132:753).

The lack of evident danger in the use of metallic lead seems to induce neglect of ordinary precautions. As a result, in many plants where soldering or remelting used metal or casting is carried on, there may be more lead poisoning than in a very well managed white lead plant. A greater danger from lead suboxide exists in the smelting and refining of lead because fumes from the furnaces carry both the suboxide and the sulfate of lead. Severe poisoning can result from exposure to lead furnaces if the fumes are allowed to escape and from the dust from drossing. Next to the smelting industry in point of danger from suboxide fumes and dust is lead burning. Using a heat source applied to a lead surface and brushing the fine oxide coating from the tempered part after it has cooled are operations that give rise to hazardous lead exposures. Two occupations in shipbuilding that carry a decided hazard from lead suboxide are welding and cutting metal sheets that contain lead or are covered with red lead paint. The latter source of often acute and severe plumbism came into prominence in the early 1920s when, in accordance with the international naval disarmament agreement of 1921, warships were scrapped on a large scale. During the Second World War similar reports came from shipyards and from such work as the destruction of the New York City elevated railways.

It is common practice in the United States for skilled structural steel workers to be hired for work in different locations that present varying risks of lead exposure. These men repair bridges often covered with many layers of lead-containing paint as protection against wear and weather and they weld new steel so painted in new construction. HLH studied such workers and found evidence of excess body lead apparently acquired from a series of jobs with few intervals free of exposure.

A modern hazard arises from the use of very large spray guns to apply leaded paint to new structures. Inhalation of the finely divided lead droplets may cause poisoning. Due to the physical effort required and the tent-like booths used to confine such spray, a worker finds it impossible to wear a protective respirator. While such exposures are intermittent, they are usually high and occur in combination with prior exposures. Also, because of the risks of falling, workmen discard protective face masks. Such men endure poor living conditions, often are heavy drinkers of alcohol, and their lead absorption or poisoning is rarely recognized.

The use of lead solder is another familiar source of lead poisoning. This solder contains tin and 50 to 80% lead, and when melted at high temperatures creates hazardous amounts of fumes of lead suboxide. Brass founding may be attended with the production of lead fumes because an appreciable quantity of lead may be added to the alloy and it is then volatilized at the temperature at which pouring is done. A brass founder who complains of "chronic" brass poisoning may be found to be suffering from chronic plumbism. Few of the studies of relative toxicities include metallic lead dust, and it may be that the plumbism that occurs in such trades as printing and plumbing is caused by lead suboxide. These occupations seem to carry with them a lead hazard that is not found in smelting, refining, oxide roasting, lead burning, and the like, where the amount of suboxide produced is far greater.

Oxides, such as litharge, red lead, and orange mineral, are used extensively in industry. They are not as soluble as the basic carbonate (white lead), but operations involving their use are often dusty and hard to control. They are produced by the oxidation of lead in furnaces, and the roasting, grinding, and packing of oxides are notoriously dangerous occupations. Litharge (PbO) is used in rubber manufacture and in making glazes for pottery and tiles, in storage batteries, leaded glass, and varnish. Red lead (Pb_3O_4) is used in making some glazes and enamels, in making cast iron and sheet iron, and in paint. Most of these uses involve occupations attended with a high rate of plumbism. Storage battery manufacture and reclamation head the list of dangerous lead trades in some countries and, although there are no reliable statistics, they are among the most prolific sources of industrial plumbism in the United States. The red lead used in battery manufacture is often scattered widely on benches and floors where the dried plates are handled. Elkins (1959) considered storage battery manufacture in Massachusetts as a moderate risk among industrial causes of lead poisoning contrasted with high risks in such operations as spraying red or molten lead, and sanding or scraping lead paint.

Next to these industries as a source of lead poisoning comes enameling. Sanitary ware, such as bathtubs and sinks, which are made of cast iron, are first heated to red heat in a furnace and then scattered over with powdered enamel that melts and flows to form a smooth surface. This work is very dusty, and when there is lead in the enamel the rate of poisoning is likely to be high. Of late, enameled sanitary ware has given place to clay ware with a leadless coating. Some, if not all, pottery glaze is usually lead-free, but that used for tiles and for terra cotta may contain litharge or red lead (Browder, 1972). Lead glass is made with litharge, but the hazard is in the mixing room. Litharge was formerly used in compounding rubber, and some of the severest cases of lead poisoning reported in the literature occurred in compounders and mixers of rubber when lead was the accelerator. Red lead and orange mineral are not so often constituents of paints as was formerly the case, but red lead is still used on ships, especially battleships, on structural-iron bridges, and on railway cars, since it has the property of expanding and contracting with the underlying metal as the temperature changes. Lead oxide is also used in the so-called doctor treatment for "sour" petroleum crudes to remove sulfur and sulfur compounds, especially mercaptans.

Basic carbonate The basic carbonate $(2PbCO_3 \cdot Pb(OH)_2)$, white lead, is the most notorious source of industrial plumbism, although not now the most prolific one. It is an old pigment and is still made in part by the Old Dutch process, which was used for many centuries. This method consists of burying metallic lead strips in spent tan bark with acetic acid and waiting several months for the slow change, "cor-rosion," to take place, first to lead acetate and then to the basic carbonate under the action of the acetic acid and the carbon dioxide and heat produced by the fermentation of the tan bark. A quicker process, the Carter, has been increasingly popular and depends on the exposure of finely divided lead to acetic acid and CO_2 in rotating wooden barrels. White lead is readily soluble in human gastric juice, to the extent of over 60% (Carlson and Woelfel, 1913). It is responsible for the plumbism of painters, of most pottery workers, and of lithotransfermakers; it is also responsible, in part, for the poisoning of plumbers who used white lead for joint-wiping. Dust is the great danger in dry sandpapering of painted surfaces, handling of dry glazed ware, and in scattering finely ground lead colors onto lithotransfer paper. Some of the large American white lead works are now models of industrial sanitation, with the work almost wholly mechanized. But the introduction of machinery, enclosed and ventilated by suction, has not completely controlled the hazardous exposures involved in the making of lithotransfer paper.

Basic sulfate The basic sulfate, $PbSO_4 \cdot PbO$, known as sublimed blue or sublimed white lead, was actively promoted some 30 years age as a non-poisonous substitute for Old Dutch white lead, but the claims were soon disproved. Sublimed blue lead has a fairly wide use as a pigment (the "blue" is really a steel-gray), and the white is sometimes used as a rubber accelerator. Risk during manufacture arises as a result of fumes when the lead is heated to high temperatures in an oxidizing atmosphere.

Chromates The chromate, $PbCrO_4$, a yellow pigment, is used in paints along with the green chromate, which is made by mixing the yellow with Prussian blue. Both give little trouble since they are insoluble.

Lead sulfate The risk of lead poisoning in the mining of lead ores depends on the character of the ore. Old, deep mines, such as those in southwestern Missouri, yield only galena, which contains lead sulfide, a poorly soluble compound. Lead poisoning is rare among miners of galena. The mines of the western states are nearer the surface and contain oxidized ores, sulfates and carbonates, and hence the work exposures are far more hazardous. Lead mining is one of the chief sources of industrial plumbism in Utah. Dreessen et al. (1942) found that among nonferrous miners lead poisoning was second only to silicosis as an occupational disease.

Fate of Lead in the Body

Absorption In the mid-1920s, Aub et al. (1925) established the basic facts regarding the absorption of lead: ingested lead is usually only 5 to 10% absorbed, and the balance is excreted in the feces, in contrast to inhaled lead, 35 to 50% of which enters the blood. There may, however, be large biological variations from person to person in the gastrointestinal absorption of lead (Blake, 1976). Excess of phosphate ions in the gut keeps the lead insoluble. Some of the absorbed lead is taken up by the liver and is re-excreted into the intestinal tract in the bile. In childhood poisoning, ingestion has been considered to be the main route of lead absorption, although evidence has accumulated that inhalation of lead in urban air is also of importance (Hardy et al., 1971). Substantiation of these ideas come from the work of Kehoe et al. (1933b) who fed an adult healthy male volunteer lead for 39 months and found that practically all of the ingested lead was recovered from the feces. Ingestion of lead occurs in industry when workers handle their food, cigarettes, or chewing tobacco with lead-smeared fingers. This route is a relatively unimportant cause of lead poisoning and the clinical syndrome that results is neither so severe nor so rapid as when lead enters the body through the respiratory tract. It is, however, important enough to make provision of proper washing facilities essential in all of the lead industries.

Absorption from the respiratory tract in contrast is very rapid. The absorption begins in the upper respiratory tract as shown by Blumgart (1923) who produced experimental poisoning by tying off the esophagus, and spraying dust of basic lead carbonate into the nose. Lead was later recovered from various organs. Aub and his co-workers (1925) further showed that injection of lead into the trachea causes rapid intoxication. Currently, it is thought that 35 to 50% of the lead that reaches the lower respiratory tract is absorbed into the blood stream. The greater rapidity of absorption from the respiratory tract is due to prompt phagocytosis; also, by this route, lead enters directly into the general circulation instead of passing through the liver as it does in gastrointestinal absorption. The fact that lead

poisoning is brought about far more rapidly and intensely by inhalation of lead-laden air than by ingestion is of the greatest practical importance. There can be no intelligent control of the lead hazard in industry unless it is based on the principle of keeping the air clean from lead-containing dusts and fumes.

Skin absorption, except in the case of tetraethyl lead, is of very slight importance (Laug and Kunze, 1948). It is possible that lead pigments incorporated in oil may enter through the skin, but the danger is ordinarily negligible. An unusual case of lead poisoning by way of skin absorption was found in an actress to be due to theatrical grease paint that contained 40% lead oxide (Bartleman and Dukes, 1936). Stippled red blood cells, anemia, and excess lead in the urine supported the diagnosis. Various other aspects of lead and skin have been reviewed by Allen et al. (1975).

Transportation and distribution After lead is absorbed into the body, more than 90% is carried in the blood in nondiffusible form bound to dibasic phosphate and glycerophosphate in the erythrocyte membranes (Aub et al., 1925; Clarkson and Kench, 1958). The remainder is bound to microligands in the plasma and does cross cell membranes (Castellino and Aloj, 1969). If large quantities of lead enter the body over a short period of time, the lead is promptly distributed generally throughout the body and causes symptoms of acute poisoning. In this case the amount of lead stored in the skeleton is less; but, when absorption is slow, by far the greater portion is distributed to the skeleton. After lead enters the bloodstream it comes in contact with all of the body tissues and can produce local damage if it is present in sufficient quantity. Liver, spleen, lungs, and kidneys may retain lead in amounts that depend on the rate and intensity of exposure. During the period of early high exposure the excretion rate is highest; subsequently, considerable amounts continue to appear in feces and urine even after cessation of exposure. Redistribution results in the shift of most of the remaining lead to the skeleton, with small amounts retained in the liver and spleen.

Aub et al. (1932) showed, and all studies since have confirmed the fact, that lead is deposited in the same manner as is calcium, as the very poorly soluble phosphate, at first chiefly in the bone trabeculae, with a gradual redistribution to the cortex. Aub and his colleagues (1924, 1938) emphasized the mobilization of inorganic lead salts into and out of trabeculae relatively easily under certain conditions. Once it is deposited in the cortex, the lead is less easily mobilized. The deposition and elimination of calcium and lead are influenced chiefly by high or low intake of calcium and by changes in the acid-base equilibrium in the blood. Both acidity and alkalinity of sufficient degree have been shown experimentally to be capable of dissolving the relatively insoluble tribasic phosphate of lead, the form in which lead is deposited in bone (Cantarow and Trumper, 1944).

Although it is still a matter of controversy, clinical experience supports the claim that infection or alcoholism may precipitate episodes of acute lead poisoning in workers chronically exposed to lead in industry. HLH, studying storage battery workers, found, as older texts describe, that on Mondays symptoms of acute lead colic appear apparently after excessive eating or alcohol intake. So striking is that phenomenon that, if one is alert to this experience with lead workers, it is possible to identify such cases in hospital emergency rooms where patients are awaiting surgery for acute appendicitis or are scheduled for x-ray studies with a diagnosis of renal colic or gallstones. Shufflebotham (1915) found that British army recruits from the lead-using potteries suffered attacks of typical colic as a result of an exhausting military drill. Aub demonstrated that such clinical events are best explained by acidosis, accompanied by a negative calcium balance, although Kehoe (1963) did not agree on the basis of his experimental studies. However, the variables of clinical events cannot be reproduced experimentally, and it is clear from experience that intercurrent stress can produce damage because stored lead returns to the circulation in toxic form.

Lead in blood and excreta The apparent value of finding lead in feces and urine was lessened when control groups of non-lead workers were also found to be excreting lead (Webster, 1941). The precise level of lead in blood, urine, and feces that may be considered to be "safe" has received a great deal of attention in the past 30 years and is still under discussion (Chamberlain and Massey, 1972; Vitale et al., 1975, and subsequent Letters to the Editor; Posner, 1977). Benson et al. (1976) found that blood levels of lead (Pb-B) in lead workers began to increase within one week after starting employment. However, the studies by

King et al. (1979) failed to establish a close correlation between blood lead levels and dust exposure over a wide range of particle sizes. In general, blood lead levels are a poor index of stored lead, and because the blood is cleared promptly of circulating lead, a single value is rarely of help in diagnosis. Goldwater and Hoover (1967) and Schroeder and Tipton (1968) reported "normal" blood lead to be from zero to 50 μg/100 ml. Kehoe (1963) insisted that no intoxication occurs until the level reaches 0.08 mg/100 g of blood.

In practice it is not possible to make a diagnosis of lead poisoning on a blood lead determination alone. Lead assay is a difficult laboratory exercise. Lead is so ubiquitous that contamination is a problem, and unless lead determinations are done by well-trained individuals using frequent blanks and spiked samples as correctives, serious errors can occur. In addition, the method of assay is critical. Since over 90% of the lead in circulating blood is fixed to red blood cell surfaces, it is critical that the determination of lead be done on whole blood, although Cavalleri et al. (1978) found that plasma lead, which is the biologically active pool, is a constant percentage of whole blood lead. The dithizone method of analysis is generally considered best if the lead contamination of the sample can be controlled (Elkins, 1959; Kehoe, 1963; Morgan and Burch, 1972; NIOSH, 1978). A recently recognized problem in assessing levels of lead in blood is the increase in lead in air, soil, and water that add to the body burden as a result of the ever increasing industrial waste and smoking habits (Patterson, 1965; McLaughlin and Stopps, 1973).

Lead ingested in small quantities is excreted almost quantitatively by the gastrointestinal tract in the feces. According to Kehoe et al. (1933a), average fecal lead above 1.1 mg per day is indicative of harmful levels of absorption. A small amount in the feces of a person exposed occupationally can be accounted for by atmospheric lead dust that has been inhaled and/or swallowed. Fecal assays are not used as a means of medical control in industrial lead exposure because of problems of collection and chemical procedures.

The amount of lead in the urine may be a useful index of the amount to which a worker has been exposed since it reflects the air-lead level in the environment (Elkins, 1959). If lead exposure ceases, elimination of lead continues steadily with wide fluctuations in the daily urine values. Kehoe (1963) reported a level of 0.02 to 0.08 mg/L in the urine of healthy individuals in the United States with no occupational exposure to lead. The exact value that reflects a harmful lead burden or recent exposure varies in clinical practice. Some organizations, such as the Massachusetts Division of Occupational Hygiene, have used 0.20 mg/L of lead in urine as the level beyond which a hazardous exposure exists. Levels as high as 0.30 to 0.50 mg/L of lead, however, have been recorded in the urine of individuals having no symptoms. The level of lead in the urine, which is dependent on the state of kidney function, is only one piece of evidence, although an important one, in making a diagnosis of lead poisoning. Routine assay of urine for lead is widely and successfully used for medical control in industries where engineering techniques and job rotation or vacations can be used to offset chronic as well as acute intoxication. Only in the case of tetraethyl lead poisoning does lead become fixed in the body, chiefly in the central nervous system.

Toxic Effects of Lead

Lead produces a damaging effect on the tissues and organs with which it comes in contact and yet there are no characteristic specific lesions that are universally accepted. This situation may be because methods of examination lack sophistication or because of the nonspecificity of the body's response to injury. There is a literature on the biological effects of lead that is too vast to condense for this text, which is intended to serve as a clinical manual. Because of the great experience of Alice Hamilton, some of her early reports, often missing in other reviews, are included as helpful background.

Gastrointestinal tract The most common syndrome of plumbism in adults is gastrointestinal. After a prodromal stage that varies in duration and that consists of increasing anorexia, vague dyspepsia, and constipation, there is an attack of colic. This colic is severe and paroxysmal, and is accompanied by a rigid retracted abdomen that is sometimes tender on pressure, but more often the pain is relieved by the pressure. There is rarely any temperature elevation and leukocytosis is usually lacking. Occasionally, however, the white cell count is over 20,000, and a relative lymphocytosis, which is usual, is a decided aid in diagnosis. The skin is usually pale, the blood pressure may be increased, and the pulse rate may

be slow. All of these, including the colic and constipation, are results of the underlying pathological condition: the spasmodic contraction of smooth muscle of the intestine caused by the direct action of lead (Aub, 1931). The pain is due to reflex contraction as in intestinal obstruction. The German reports cited by Hamilton (1934), in contrast, hold that vagal irritation is the basis of lead colic. They explain not only the spasmodic pain but also the formation of peptic ulcer, which has been known to be strikingly prevalent among sufferers from plumbism, by this action of the vagus nerve. Lead thus acts like pilocarpine, which causes vagal irritation that results in spastic ischemia of the intestinal tract. In addition to the risk of peptic ulcer, other observers have described chronic gastritis as a common complication of long-standing excess exposure to lead. Improved control of lead exposures may explain the fact that gastritis and peptic ulcer are not notable clinical problems in cases of plumbism in the United States.

Kidney When it comes to the effect of lead poisoning on the human kidney, there is a wide difference of opinion. It was the belief of earlier pathologists, who had extensive clinical experience and far more pathologic material to deal with than is possible for anyone at the present time, that the contracted kidney of Bright is the typical kidney of chronic plumbism (Oliver, 1891; Osler, 1911). Most authorities, especially in the United States, refuse to accept a direct connection between chronic glomerulonephritis and plumbism, but in the older industrial countries such a connection is regarded as long proven. Vigdortschik (1935) found kidney damage three times more often in lead workers than in a control group. The changes that were reported were those of the later stages of glomerulonephritis developing slowly over 20 to 30 years. Perhaps the most striking evidence of chronic nephritis following long after an acute attack of plumbism is to be found in the reports from Queensland, Australia. Gibson (1908), in his studies of optic neuritis among children, traced this toxic effect to white lead paint on the verandas where the children played, paint that cracks and powders under the very hot sun. Some years later it was found that deaths from chronic interstitial nephritis in people between 10 and 40 years of age of both sexes were strikingly more frequent in Queensland hospitals than in those of other states (Nye, 1929). Finding excess amounts of lead in bone many years after cessation of exposure established the etiology (Henderson and Inglis, 1957). The clinical picture resembled the Fanconi syndrome caused by acute renal damage incurred years earlier. Emmerson (1968) reported that these Queensland cases of childhood plumbism have developed renal gout with serious disability. Tepper (1963) tried without success to similar cases among American adults known to have had acute childhood lead poisoning.

Lead-containing solder in copper tubing of stills used in the preparation of "moonshine" liquors in certain southern U.S. states has been found to be the cause of prolonged lead poisoning giving rise to progressive renal disease, moderate hypertension, and "saturnine" gout (Morgan et al., 1966). These authors have stressed the potentiating effects of alcohol and pre-existing hypertension on the development of lead nephropathy (Morgan and Hartley, 1976), a view also proposed by Campbell et al. (1979).

Lane (1949) presented an explanation of the difference between British and American experience in the lead trades, especially with respect to kidney damage. He referred to earlier studies by Legge and Goadby (1912) showing that during a two-year period, among British workers with many years of exposure, the death rate from Bright's disease among male lead workers was 160 compared with 35 for all males. In the United States, great labor turnover made the number of cases of prolonged exposure far smaller than in Britain. Lane also reported that nine lead workers, who had been exposed to 0.5 mg/m³ of lead for many years, all died from hypertension and renal failure between the ages of 42 and 52 years. In these chronic cases, the glomeruli were affected with hyaline sclerosis of the arterioles. In contrast, rapidly progressive cases of lead poisoning showed changes similar to those seen in malignant hypertension with arteriolar necrosis. Cooper and Gaffey (1975) studied the mortality of 1032 men employed in lead production facilities or battery manufacture, and they found an excess of deaths from hypertensive disease and from "unspecified nephritis or renal sclerosis," but these involved only 3% of the death certificates. Recent findings by Wedeen et al. (1979) of tubular and glomerular immunoglobulin deposition, along with reduced glomerular filtration rates, in lead workers led them to suggest that an autoimmune mechanism may contribute to the pathogenesis of the interstitial nephritis of occupational lead poisoning.

It seems likely that workers exposed acutely or at high levels for long periods will suffer renal changes frequently not recognized. Use of a provocative dose of a chelating agent or of a bone biopsy for lead assay should be considered as diagnostic procedures when the occupational history suggests a past intense or chronic high exposure to lead (Westerman et al., 1965). HLH studied a small group of lead workers aged 65 to 70 years who had impaired kidney function. In several cases, after a single intravenous dose of calcium sodium ethylenediaminetetraacetic acid (CaNa₂ EDTA), the amount of lead excreted increased to 0.75 to 1.0 mg/L in contrast with the 0.35 to 0.45 mg/L excreted by nonexposed city dwellers after a similar dose of the chelating agent (Hardy et al., 1954). In individual cases the concept of lead acting alone or with other causes of renal damage is important in clinical management. Because intravenous chelation therapy offers a chance to remove lead from the body safely, the prognosis may be favorably influenced.

In clinical practice, during an acute attack of lead poisoning an increase of blood pigments may be found in the urine due to the rapid destruction of red blood cells. Transient albuminuria, aminoaciduria, and glycosuria have been reported as toxic effects of lead. In long-standing chronic plumbism, the fixed specific gravity of the urine may signify the establishment of irreversible renal damage. On the other hand, moderate exposure to lead evidenced by blood levels less than 62 μg/100 ml does not alter renal function (Buchet et al., 1980). These investigators suggest that renal dysfunction in more highly exposed workers might result from cadmium contamiraation rather than lead.

In summary, evidence at hand supports the view that kidney damage can be caused by lead and, when it occurs, is related to the extent of exposure. With modern industrial control of harmful operations, chronic renal damage should rarely be seen in lead workers, and only after long-standing excess exposure.

Heme synthesis Of the many deleterious biochemical effects of lead, its action on the enzymes of heme biosynthesis are most important. These changes, summarized by Moore et al. (1980), include an increase in δ-aminolevulinic acid (ALA) synthase and in heme oxygenase along with an inhibition of ALA dehydratase. The net effect of these changes is excessive production and excretion of ALA. Other changes induced by lead are a decrease in coproporphyrinogen III oxidase, evidenced by increased urinary excretion of coproporphyrin, and an inhibition of ferrochelatase that may contribute to the anemia of lead poisoning and to the rise in protoporphyrin synthesis.

Much attention has been devoted to ALA levels in blood and urine in lead poisoning, both of which are related to each other and are substantially elevated (Meredith et al., 1978). It turns out that at higher blood levels of ALA a greater proportion is excreted in the urine so that there is a plateau of ALA concentration in blood when the blood lead level exceeds 3 μmol/L (60 μg/100 ml). At this level there is an increase in ALA excretion in urine attributable to reduced renal tubular reabsorption (Druyan et al., 1965).

Protoporphyrin accumulates in the erythrocytes as a result of inhibition by lead of ferrochelatase in the bone marrow. So-called "free erythrocyte protoporphyrins" (FEP) exist as zinc protoporphyrin IX (ZPP), which is readily assayed in dilute whole blood (Lamola and Yamane, 1974; Joselow and Flores, 1977; Blumberg et al., 1977; Hernberg, 1980; among others).

The anemia of lead poisoning is the combined result of depression of heme biosynthesis, altered globin synthesis, and red cell hemolysis due to increased fragility (Moore et al., 1980). Dose-dependent inhibition of globin synthesis occurs independently of disturbances in heme synthesis and takes place at levels of blood lead below the accepted safe upper limits of 70 to 80 μg/100 ml (Ali and Quinlan, 1977). Elevated concentrations of lead in bone marrow compared to circulating blood as a result of uptake by bone may thus adversely affect erythropoiesis (Albahary, 1972; Landaw et al., 1973), along with inhibition of utilization of iron as a result of lead-induced reduction of ferrochelatase.

Liver The liver unquestionably plays an important role in the temporary storage and elimination of lead, but the direct effect of lead on liver is not clearly understood. Some pathologists hold that injury to the liver is the same as that found generally in plumbism: namely, vascular spasm leading to arteriosclerotic changes. Lewin (1928) reported two patients and Oliver (1891) a single case with fatal yellow atrophy of the liver associated with severe plumbism. Lewin considered the direct action of lead on the liver to be supported by the fact that there is no parallel between the degree of anemia and the extent of liver disturbance. Koelsch (1927) reported finding an enlarged

tender liver in cases of clinically acute plumbism. These and other early reports were summarized in Hamilton and Hardy (1949). Many writers have emphasized the difficulty in determining how much liver cirrhosis is to be attributed to alcoholism and how much to lead because of the custom of many laborers doing heavy work drinking large amounts of alcohol daily.

Icterus may occur as a result of red blood cell destruction after intense lead exposure. HLH has seen three cases of jaundice in workers with chronic lead poisoning associated with heavy exposure over a short period of time. One worker, who had been using a fast rotary sander on lead-soldered auto body parts, was at first diagnosed as having viral hepatitis. A second, after sanding painted surfaces, had such an abrupt drop in red blood cell count that he rapidly developed a deep jaundice, which led to an initial diagnosis of hemolytic anemia. The third, a storage battery worker, presented with slight icterus and was thought to have alcoholic cirrhosis of the liver. Hemolysis correlated with intense lead exposure led to the correct diagnosis. In current clinical experience, liver disease due to lead toxicity is not ordinarily recognized. However, Butt et al. (1960) showed that excess lead accumulates in the liver in cases of iron storage disease. It is reasonable to conclude that lead can have a damaging effect on hepatic cells under certain circumstances.

Vascular lesions Not only glomerulonephritis but general arteriosclerosis with high blood pressure was attributed by earlier authorities to the action of lead in persons exposed for a long period. This view remains a disputed point. There are several studies of groups of lead workers performed to determine the part played by lead in the causation of hypertension and arteriosclerosis. Among 381 lead workers, Mayers (1927) found 98 with hypertension, 32 of whom showed other evidence of arteriosclerosis. However, when she compared these with a control group of workmen in similar occupations, but free from lead, she found a similar rate. Belknap (1936) also could find no difference in the blood pressures of otherwise comparable lead and nonlead exposed groups, but the period of lead exposure for most of these persons was short. Lane (1949) found no evidence of hypertension in 56 storage battery workers, even in those working as long as 20 years under modern conditions. However, he reversed this opinion in 1964 when he found a significant increase in cerebrovascular disease among lead workers as a result of arteriosclerosis. In a study from Russia, Vigdortschik (1935) examined 2769 hospital records, 1437 of which were of workers exposed to lead. He found 15.7% with hypertension, chronic nephritis, and cerebral hemorrhage, compared to 7.4% among the controls. These lead workers may have been exposed for many years to excessive amounts of lead, for industrial hygiene was slow in developing in Russia.

Statistics published by the sickness insurance bureaus of European countries from 1910 to 1930 show a high rate of cerebrovascular accidents in certain groups of lead workers. In the United States a similar risk existed among printers in the early decades of the 20th century before the lead hazard was properly understood and controlled. The English have had no hesitation in accepting chronic plumbism as the cause of death in aged lead workers, especially the potters of Staffordshire, men and women who began their working life under very bad factory conditions. Such workers suffered typical plumbism in early life, and then were apparently free from it, but years later succumbed to what the English accept as a typical manifestation of chronic plumbism — namely, chronic nephritis with or without generalized arteriosclerosis. Support for the fact that excess lead is required to cause such disease is found in a 20-year study by Cramér and Dahlberg (1966) of a storage battery plant with ideal engineering controls where no hypertension was found among the workers. Voors et al. (1973) found that lead levels in the aorta in 79 noncancer cases was positively correlated with the degree of arteriosclerosis. They suggested that in the presence of vascular wall disease lead behaves as a chemical congener of calcium and is deposited in the wall of the aorta.

Joint involvement   That variety of plumbism in which the most conspicuous symptom is pain in the joints or muscles, or both, usually known as lead arthralgia, is either much rarer than other forms or is much more infrequently recognized. Tanquerel des Planches (1839) listed 755 out of his 1217 patients with lead poisoning as suffering from joint pain; of these, 525 also had colic. Among more recent observers who have seen large numbers of cases of plumbism, Linenthal (1924) and others laid stress on the frequency of pains simulating rheumatism or lumbago. In Mayers' study of 381 lead workers (1927), arthralgia or myalgia was present in 42, with laboratory evidence of plumbism in all but four. Arthralgia and myalgia are found in chronic lead poisoning rather than in the acute form, and the pain may be very severe and accompanied by muscular cramps.

Lead gout was first described in England by Garrod (1854). Many reports of gout associated with lead gave rise to the term "saturnine" gout (Cantarow and Trumper, 1944). This term is again in use in the United States as a result of excessive lead absorption from drinking moonshine whiskey (Ball and Sorensen, 1969). British authorities (Oliver, 1891; Prendergast, 1910) reported no gout even in heavily exposed women workers with a high incidence of plumbism, while more recently Talbott (1957) concluded from the low incidence of gout among exposed workers that there is no causal relationship. Emmerson's report, in 1968, of gout with bone destruction and deformity in patients who suffered Queensland lead poisoning in childhood demonstrates that lead damage to the kidney can lead to gout. Campbell et al. (1978) suggested that symptomless hyperuricemia in subclinical lead poisoning may result in gout.

Palsy   Although generalized paralysis is seen only in rare cases, there are five varieties of local paralysis that may be caused by lead. These include 1) the antebrachial type, involving the extensors of the wrists and fingers, but not the supinator or flexors; 2) the brachial or Duchenne-Erb type, which involves the deltoid, biceps, brachialis, and supinator; 3) the Aran-Duchenne type, involving the small muscles of the hand; 4) the peroneal type, involving the extensors of the toes and foot, the peroneal muscles, and sometimes the tibialis anterior; 5) the laryngeal type, which is very rare, described only some five or six times.

Lead-induced pathologic change is an atrophic degenerative neuritis, with subsequent fibrosis. It must be distinguished from paralysis resulting from lesions of the spinal cord, although degeneration of the anterior horn cells with typical Wallerian changes in the nerves supplying the paralyzed muscle was described by many of the earlier pathologists. Injured Schwann cells are primarily involved in the lead neuropathy of rats (Dyck et al., 1977) and studies of endoneurial edema by Myers et al. (1980) suggested that extravasated lead in the interstitial fluid injures the Schwann cells sufficiently to result in demyelination. That the lesion in the nerve is periaxial, and not in the axis cylinder, explains why lead palsy is reversible. Atrophy of the affected muscles is a consequence of sustained or repeated exposure.

The localization of lead palsy was long a puzzle to students, for the groups of muscles affected are not supplied by the same nerve, nor are all the muscles that a single nerve supplies affected. Thus, in the commonest form of occupational lead palsy, the so-called wristdrop, the muscles that are affected are supplied by the radial nerve, but so is the supinator, a muscle that escapes involvement. It is evident that use of muscles is the determining factor, a theory first proposed by Edinger in 1908. It explains why painters and printers suffer from wristdrop, children and laborers from ankledrop, and smelters and kilnmen from the scapulohumeral type. In the occupations where the usual type of lead palsy is found, the flexors are bulkier and stronger than the extensors and are aided by gravity. Reznikoff and Aub (1927) were inclined to find the cause of lead palsy in the metabolism of muscles. Contractility is lost, and recovery from fatigue is impaired, only if both lead and fatigue are present, the latter apparently increasing the toxic action of the metal. Exposure to lead results in reduction of motor nerve conduction velocity that is demonstrable even in the absence of clinical evidence of nerve damage (Araki and Honma, 1976; Buchtal and Behse, 1979; Ashby, 1980); Silbergeld et al. (1974) have presented experimental evidence from their studies of rat phrenic nerves that lead interferes with either the release of acetylcholine at the neuromuscular junction or with its subsequent resynthesis.

Lead palsy develops slowly. It is rarely a feature of plumbism that follows a short severe exposure. In the neuritis and paralysis of alcohol or arsenic there is usually a much greater prominence of sensory symptoms than in lead palsy. Lead-induced palsy tends to improve; there is even complete recovery unless lead exposure is too long continued. The earliest sign of wristdrop is the dropping of the middle fingers when the hands are stretched out with the fingers extended and separated. At this stage, freedom from lead exposure for a month or six weeks will probably be enough to clear up the weakness. If actual wristdrop develops, it may last six months; if it has lasted two years, it may never be cured. HLH has seen two cases of lead palsy treated successfully with chelating agents even after recurrence on return to lead exposure.

Lead encephalopathy Tanquerel des Planches (1850) gave the name "encephalopathia saturnina" to the cerebral form of plumbism, at once the most dramatic and the rarest variety in adults of this many-sided disease. He described a number of syndromes that included coma, delirium, and convulsions with partial preservation of consciousness. Westphal in 1888 added to Tanquerel's description the clinical pictures of progressive general paralysis, bulbar paralysis, disseminated sclerosis, laryngeal paralysis, and choreic movements. This rare and dramatic form of lead intoxication has almost completely disappeared. Strict control and disappearance of some industries with excess lead hazard explains the fact that occupational lead encephalopathy is rare at the present time. An acute attack of encephalopathy is usually preceded by other symptoms of lead poisoning, by headache and disturbed sleep, increasing irritability, attacks of excitement or (in women) hysteria, and sometimes disorders of vision. These symptoms increase and finally explode in a sudden attack of unconsciousness, with convulsions, or of delirium. Recovery from such an attack is slow, and it may be months before the victim recovers, if indeed he ever returns to normal health, for he may be left with permanent mental deterioration, with blindness, partial or total, or with motor paralysis.

Less typical are saturnine pseudoparalysis, indistinguishable clinically from progressive paralysis of the insane (Oliver, 1914), with or without a tendency to epileptiform or maniacal attacks, or a lasting epilepsy after a typical attack of encephalopathy. The slowly progressing form of encephalopathy involves mental deterioration that resembles general paralysis with arteriosclerosis, and usually follows a more prolonged but less severe exposure to lead.

The most prominent changes in the brain are cerebral edema, increase in cerebrospinal fluid pressure, proliferation and swelling of endothelial cells, dilatation of arterioles and capillaries, proliferation of glial cells, focal necrosis, and neurone degeneration (Goyer and Rhyne, 1973). Lead may also induce focal anatomic lesions in the cranial nerves, especially the optic. In slowly developing cases the changes are typical of what used to be called dementia paralytica — namely, atrophy of the cortex, chronic inflammation of the meninges with adhesions, and external and internal hydrocephalus. Early in the 20th century, reports of lead meningitis associated with acute lead poisoning appeared in France (Mosny and Malloizel, 1907; Loeper and Pinard, 1911). Their work was confirmed in this country by Aub et al. (1925) and Weller (1925). Gradually the idea has prevailed that the pathologic condition in lead encephalopathy is essentially a meningoencephalopathy or a lead meningitis. Furthermore, Pentschew (1965) has suggested that the astrocytic and microglial proliferations may be primary toxic reactions rather than results of neuronal degeneration.

Lumbar puncture in patients with acute lead poisoning having severe headache and exaggeration of tendon reflexes will show a clear sterile cerebrospinal fluid under increased pressure, with a cell count, usually lymphocytes, of about 300/mm³. Lead is found in the spinal fluid of most patients with lead poisoning. HLH cared for a lead worker with headache as the only clinical complaint. Elevated levels of lead were present in urine and spinal fluid, and there were definite abnormalities in the electroencephalogram. Even without the discovery of lead in the cerebrospinal fluid, it is easy to differentiate lead meningitis from the bacterial disease, but it is more difficult to separate the former from luetic meningoencephalopathy.

Electroencephalographic changes are usual in childhood lead poisoning and it is likely that EEG abnormalities would be found in adult lead poisoning if this test were regularly performed. In 1972, Whitfield et al. reported lead encephalopathy in 54 adults, 23 of their own cases, of which only four were workers. The source of the lead was solder and old automobile radiators. Confusion, seizures, coma, and death were reported. All responded favorably to treatment with CaNa₂ EDTA if treated promptly. Powers et al. (1977) reported a case of "moonshine" alcoholism in which the focal edema of lead encephalopathy led to an incorrect clinical diagnosis of cerebral glioma. Focal cortical necroses and widespread cerebral edema were found by Hopkins and Dayan (1974) in baboons intoxicated by intratracheal injections of lead carbonate.

Impaired psychological performances, especially those dependent on visual intelligence and visual motor functions, were found in workers with low exposure to lead (Haenninen et al., 1978). Similar findings were reported by Grandjean et al. (1978) who noted decreased performance in tests of long-term memory, verbal and visual–spatial abstraction, and psychomotor speed in a group of 42 lead workers. These decrements were correlated with blood lead and zinc protoporphyrin levels so that these analyses can be used as good predictors of the neurotoxic effects of lead.

Lesions involving the nuclei of cranial nerves have been reported to be caused by lead (Westphal, 1888; von Monakow, 1880; Remak, 1899). These have included involvement of the optic, auditory, olfactory, and glossopharyngeal nerves. Toxic effects of lead on the nuclei of the third, fourth, and sixth nerves, the fifth and seventh, and the vagus and hypoglossal have also been recorded. Lead blindness, which has as its basis an optic neuritis followed by atrophy, has rarely been described in the United States (Pedley, 1930), but many cases have been reported from Britain and Australia. Prendergast (1910) found that no less than 7.7% of the women potters who had lead poisoning became totally blind, while 10.2% had some loss of vision and 14% had a slighter loss. Among the men the percentages were lower. Gibson (1908) saw 54 cases of lead amblyopia in Australia in 15 years. HLH has seen two cases of amblyopia in adult lead workers, but because these men were also heavy cigarette smokers and there were no precise measurements of the lead exposure, the toxic influence of the lead was uncertain. Baghdassarian (1968) reported a case of bilateral optic neuropathy in a painter in Baltimore. Vision returned to normal as blood lead levels declined to normal as a result of penicillamine therapy. Sonkin (1963) described stippling of the retina as an early sign of lead intoxication but this observation has not been confirmed.

Chromosome changes   Whether the chromosome changes sometimes seen in lymphocytes of persons occupationally exposed to lead are of significance has not yet been established. Deknudt et al. (1973, 1977) and Forni et al. (1976), among others, have reported chromosome aberrations in lead workers, but such changes were not seen by O'Riordan and Evans (1974) or Schmid et al. (1972). The explanation may lie in variations in technique or, as Deknudt et al. (1977) suggest, in concomitant subclinical disturbances in calcium metabolism. Since cytogenetic changes have now been reported in women occupationally exposed to lead (Forni et al., 1980), these findings may be significant in supporting the warnings raised by

Bridbord (1978) concerning the possible effects of occupational lead exposure on fetuses.

Diagnosis of Lead Poisoning

The literature on the diagnosis of lead poisoning is voluminous and reflects the importance of the subject. Of greatest value is the patient's occupational history — whether the patient has been exposed to lead, and the intensity, duration, and character of that exposure. In addition, whether the exposure was recent or some years ago, and whether the lead compound was readily or poorly soluble will influence the clinical picture of the toxic effect. A brief, intense exposure will produce a clinical appearance quite different from that following prolonged exposure to low levels. Currently, it is the latter that chiefly concerns the physician and often presents him with puzzling problems. One after another, diagnostic signs and laboratory tests that have been hailed as unfailing have proved to be far from reliable because they are also found in workers not exposed to lead. Indeed, instead of growing simpler, the problem of diagnosis seems to become more difficult the more it is studied. A slow, banal clinical syndrome presenting gastrointestinal disturbances but no typical colic, perhaps with pain in joints and muscles, perhaps with tremors, rarely with palsy, often with headache and disturbed sleep, is what one looks for in persons working with metallic lead and bearing metals, in workers with molten lead with good engineering controls, in painters doing exterior work or interior work with sandpaper, in plumbers and makers of plumbing goods. On the other hand, persons exposed to fairly large quantities of soluble lead will probably suffer from colic, while arthritic and central nervous system lesions will be in the background, unless the dose is excessive, in which case symptoms of encephalopathy may be expected. Such hazards exist in lead smelting, lead burning, production of white lead and oxides, pasting and finishing storage battery plates, making lithotransfer paper, sanding lead-painted surfaces, chipping off lead paint, or burning through lead-painted steel with acetylene torches.

After the facts of lead exposure, its character and duration, are established, the next step is the medical examination plus assay of blood and urine. Here the divergence of opinion begins to appear, for there is little agreement as to the relative importance of certain signs and certain groupings of symptoms.

Lead line   If a lead line is present, it is a great help in establishing lead exposure. But its presence does not mean that lead is being absorbed at that time. Mayers (1927) found a typical lead line in only 31 of 381 lead workers examined, but in 10 of them there was no evidence of active lead absorption, as shown by blood and urine levels, so that the line reflected lead deposited at some earlier time. The line is a bluish-black stippling that appears along the margin of the gums, usually most clearly evident along the lower incisors but in some cases on the lining of the cheeks. It cannot be rubbed off since it lies within the tissues. It is composed of irregular amorphous granules deposited in the walls of blood vessels and in connective tissue, especially in the dermal papillae that reach upward to the base of the epithelium. These granules consist of black lead sulfide produced by contact of the absorbed lead with the hydrogen sulfide produced by the decay of proteinaceous material between the teeth. Aub et al. (1924, 1938) observed that rabbits fed lead while on a vegetable diet never develop a lead line, while cats eating meat invariably show it. The lead line was given great prominence in the earlier literature. However, modern dental hygiene has reduced oral decay processes that are basic to the formation of the black sulfide of lead, while dentures preclude finding a lead line. HLH has continued to use the lead line, if present, as a diagnostic clue. It is best demonstrated by using the sharp edge of an applicator or broken tongue blade to scrape a sample of the alveolar tissue around incisors. This tissue, unstained on a glass slide, will show a black bead of lead sulfide under the low power of a light microscope. It must be remembered, however, that any heavy metal will combine with sulfur to form a black sulfide and thus confuse the diagnosis.

Weakness in the hands   Great stress has been put on the diagnostic importance of weakened extensors of the wrist and fingers of the hand most used in work. Some observers believe that even a slight difference in strength between the two hands is the best early diagnostic sign of plumbism. The usual objection to this test is that a person can easily simulate weakness if he wishes to claim compensation or disguise it if he is afraid of losing his job. The same may be said of muscular tremors of the fingers and lips. However, a carefully executed test should reveal the slight extensor weakness of the middle and ring fingers when the hand is held out in pronation.

Lewy and Weiss (1928) advocated the use of "chronaxie" to demonstrate the "larval" (i.e., the subclinical) stage of lead intoxication. Chronaxie is the minimal length of time that a galvanic current of standard strength takes to induce muscular contraction. Increased chronaxie signifies a reaction slower than normal and a fall in muscle excitability, and is the danger signal. HLH has found that patients with documented occupational lead poisoning do have muscle weakness demonstrable by electromyography but not discovered on physical examination. Seppäläinen and Hernberg (1972) have confirmed these observations, and a neuropathy may precede all other signs of lead poisoning. Feldman and his colleagues (1977) have suggested that measurements of motor nerve conduction velocity would be useful in the diagnosis of subliminal or otherwise unrecognized toxic effects of lead.

Red blood cell abnormalities The appearance of basophilic granules in the red blood cells was described as an infallible diagnostic sign of lead poisoning at the turn of the century. This sign, objective, impossible to simulate, easy to demonstrate, was for years greatly depended upon by industrial physicians. Even workmen talked about "stippled cells." But before long doubt began to be cast on the specific character of this change in the red cells, for it was found in other diseases — for example, malaria, severe secondary anemias, malignant disease. There are also other forms of chronic intoxication, such as from benzene, carbon monoxide, and aniline, in which stippling of the red cells may appear during the stage of marrow stimulation. But in these cases stippling is accompanied by a low red cell count and a reduction of hemoglobin. It is the distinctive feature of plumbism that the number of stippled cells is vastly out of proportion to the degree of anemia.

There has been a long controversy over the number of stippled erythrocytes that can be regarded as significant. For many years the standard was at least 100 stippled cells per million, preferably 300, but these figures were soon considered too low. Badham and Taylor (1925) used 500 per million as the lowest figure but Sanders (1943) held that any number under 5000 per million was dubious because he found stippled cells in the blood smears of over 30% of 2231 individuals not in lead work. Qualitatively, therefore, stippled cells are not significant; quantitatively, roughly 5000 per million or more may be taken to show lead absorption; over 9000, lead in-toxication. European observers with wide experience reported that stippled cells are absent in mild chronic cases, and they concluded that varying results published in the literature must be attributed in part to variations in the methods used for demonstrating stippled cells. Lehmann (1933) simplified the procedure by assuming that there will be about 200 red cells in each microscopic field so that a blood smear is diagnostic of lead poisoning if there is one stippled cell in every field or several in each third field. Repeated observations of lead workers along with appropriate controls make stippling counts combined with hemoglobin determinations a reasonably precise, though time consuming, method of medical control. Because increase of reticulocytes coincides with the appearance of stippled cells in peripheral blood, McCord et al. (1935) urged counting these immature cells. He developed a technique that caused clumping of cell reticulum that he called "basophilic aggregations," and this he considered both an earlier and more dependable sign than stippled cell counts.

Destruction of red blood cells of varying degree depends on the character of the lead exposure. In chronic lead poisoning the blood picture is that of mild secondary anemia. Too little attention has been paid to the value of repeated hematocrit determinations correlated with data on the amount of lead to which a worker has been exposed. A downward trend of hematocrit readings provides a warning of harmful lead exposure that usually antedates symptomatic illness. An example is found in Belknap's study in 1958 in which he reported hemoglobin values of 9.8 to 13.7 g in workers who were not ill and excreting 0.12 to 0.39 mg/L of lead in urine. HLH's experience with storage battery workers has been similar.

The evidence of erythrocyte regeneration reflected in stippling and reticulocyte counts is often out of proportion to the anemia. The destruction of red blood cells, however, may be marked, with profound anemia. HLH has seen, as have others, cases of severe anemia with counts of less than 3 million and occasionally, because of the speed of the red cell destruction, clinical jaundice that led to errors in diagnosis. Marrow examination in cases of subacute and chronic plumbism reveals that the anemia of plumbism has definite characteristics that include erythroblast hyperplasia and presence of granuloblasts, accelerated in subacute poisoning, delayed in chronic. Stippling may be present in the marrow smear and absent in the peripheral blood, especially after brief, high level exposure.

It is known that lead interference with red blood cell permeability causes potassium loss. Aub et al. (1925) demonstrated that lead acting on the surface of the red cells causes physical changes resulting in their destruction and removal by the reticuloendothelial system. Genetic defects of red blood cells, such as the sickle cell trait, increases the danger of exposure to lead.

In modern experience there are no reports of consistent changes in the white blood cells. In individual cases abnormalities have been found to be related to other causes such as bacterial infection. Early reports (Legge and Goadby, 1912), now thought to be erroneous, described both relative lymphocytosis and monocytosis as diagnostic features in lead poisoning. A more recent report has made several new points on the damage to hematopoiesis by lead (Albahary, 1972). The mitochondria and ribosomes of the erythroblasts are damaged so that abnormal heme synthesis results. This effect along with the toxic action of lead on liver and kidney causes secondary porphyria, poor utilization of iron, and a globinopathy similar to that of thalassemia minor.

Porphyrinuria in lead poisoning There are many references in the literature to porphyrinuria as reflecting lead absorption or intoxication. The irregularity with which it appears and the fact that intoxication due to arsenious acid, cresol, benzene, and barbiturates also produces porphyrinuria has discouraged its general use as a diagnostic aid in lead poisoning. Kark and Meiklejohn (1942) suggested that the anemia of plumbism is not hemolytic in nature but due to a disturbance in hemoglobin formation. They postulated that lead takes the place of iron in heme synthesis and made the interesting speculation that this disturbance in porphyrin metabolism may explain symptoms of lead poisoning such as colic, encephalopathies, and palsies. Dagg et al. (1965) maintained that the changes in porphyrin metabolism produced by lead may be comparable to the clinical picture of acute idiopathic porphyrinuria. Considerable work has supported the idea that lead causes a defect in hemoglobin synthesis that leads to excretion of excess porphyrins. Reliable methods of assay for the amount of coproporphyrin III excreted in urine are available and have proven to be a useful survey test as shown by Maloof (1950) and Pinto et al. (1952). Excretion of increasing amounts of porphyrin may be an early warning of potentially harmful lead exposure. Boyett and

Butterworth (1962) described a significant effect of lead that produces a defect in the synthesis of porphyrobilinogen from δ-aminolevulinic acid (ALA) so that an increase in the excretion of the latter results. A great deal of work has been done on this aspect of lead metabolism, especially in the study of childhood lead poisoning. Hernberg et al. (1970) described an inverse correlation between levels of lead in the blood and red cell δ-aminolevulinic acid dehydratase (ALAD) activity. However, both ALAD levels and porphyrin excretion values can be influenced by other metabolic disturbances and cannot serve as unique evidence of lead toxicity in an individual patient. They can be sensitive indicators if occupational levels of lead exposure are known. The large literature on this subject has recently been reviewed by Hernberg (1980).

Lead in hair Assay of the amount of lead in hair by atomic absorption spectrophotometry (Kopito et al., 1969) has been proposed as an index of the threat of lead poisoning. Boylen's studies of college students' hair with the dithizone method led him to conclude that, since hair close to the scalp contains 3.3 to 12.5 ppm, a significant value would be in excess of 20 ppm (Hardy et al., 1971). Hair more than 5 cm from its root in the scalp contains 7.5 to 36 ppm and a significant value would be in excess of 50 ppm. Since the lead concentration of hair increases with distance from the roots, Renshaw et al. (1972) have suggested that lead enters the hair by surface deposition from the environment. However, Clarke and Wilson (1974) found that when hair samples are adequately washed with ethylenediaminetetraacetic acid to remove surface contamination, absorption of surface lead into the hair shaft was not observed. Moreover, Schroeder and Nason (1969) pointed out that hair is a poor organ of excretion and is not a reliable index of tissue lead. Nevertheless, a study of large groups has shown that the amount of lead in or on hair is significantly higher in city dwellers or in those living near a lead smelter than it is in those living in rural areas, a finding that reflects the amount of lead in the air from which the hair adsorbs lead (Hammer et al., 1971).

Lead absorption and lead intoxication In understanding occupational lead poisoning, it is important to distinguish lead absorption from lead intoxication. To prove the presence of lead in the body is not to prove that it has produced actual injury. The presence of lead in urine and blood in excess of normal demonstrates lead absorption, not intoxication. Lead in the feces does not prove even that, for the lead may have passed through the intestinal tract without being absorbed at all. The proof of lead absorption is a matter of great importance for the industrial physician since it constitutes grounds for keeping the worker under special observation, if not for transferring him, at least for a time, to other work while control of lead levels in workroom air is established.

A single intense exposure may be followed by the picture of chronic lead intoxication within weeks or months if sufficient lead is retained. Depending upon freedom from further lead exposure and on therapy, an episode of acute poisoning may subside completely. To prove that lead intoxication has actually occurred may be easy or it may be very difficult. Typical lead colic and typical lead palsy are easy to recognize, but in the absence of these well-known symptoms it may be hard to establish the diagnosis. In well-managed industrial plants lead workers are given medical examinations on a regular, periodic schedule. Careful questioning elicits such complaints as loss of appetite, disturbed sleep, constipation, and malaise. The added risk to the lead worker who lives in industrial cities results from heavy motor traffic and lead in urban air, as do self-imposed habits of smoking and drinking wine and beer (Hardy, 1966). Studies of postmortem tissues by Schroeder and Tipton (1968), Horiuchi (1965), Henderson (1954), and Ingalls et al. (1961) support the view that city dwellers and those with a history of acute lead poisoning in childhood carry a burden of lead greater than the excretory system has been able to handle. Such studies make it clear that blood and urine do not reflect accurately the quantity of potentially harmful lead in the tissues.

Since the middle 1950s it has been possible to assess the difference between lead absorption and intoxication by using a single dose of a chelating agent such as CaNa₂ EDTA to provoke excretion (Hardy et al., 1954; Teisinger, 1971). There are data to show that, without work exposure, healthy adults living in industrial cities excrete about 0.5 mg Pb/L of urine after such a challenge. City dwellers, heavy smokers, and wine and beer drinkers may excrete somewhat more but experience shows that lead workers, even after long periods since exposure, excrete about 1 mg/L to as high as 30 or even 40 mg/L after a single dose of 1.5 to 5 mg of CaNa₂ EDTA, the adult dose

range. These high levels of excretion may be recovered with this drug challenge even though pretreatment levels are as low as 0.03 mg Pb/L and blood levels 0.05 mg%. Ohlsson (1962) maintained that oral N-acetyl-D-penicillamine will also chelate stored lead. The amounts of lead excreted with this provocative maneuver with EDTA make it possible to detect exposed workers and make an accurate diagnosis of mild illness attributable to the toxic effects of lead.

It is generally conceded that in the absence of a typical acute attack the diagnosis of plumbism must be made on the basis of a composite picture, the elements of which will vary in individual cases. One or more objective signs should be present: lead line, tremors of fingers and tongue, demonstrable extensor muscle weakness, blood cell stippling and reticulocytosis, excess lead in blood and/or urine, porphyrinuria, elevated δ-aminolevulinic acid (ALA) in the urine, along with depression of ALA dehydratase and elevation of zinc protoporphyrin in the blood. Together with such signs must go clinical symptoms that involve the gastrointestinal tract (anorexia, abdominal pain, constipation), less often the nervous system (insomnia, headache), and least often symptoms simulating arthritis or myositis. Mayers (1927) and Belknap (1936), both of whom have had wide practical experience, warned against relying too much on laboratory tests. Although such tests accurately performed provide values that are helpful in assessing lead exposures, no single one is decisive and both the occupational history and the clinical picture must be considered. Studies using more sophisticated biochemical techniques support this conclusion (Cramér and Selander, 1965; Ellis, 1966; de Bruin, 1971). Consideration of nonindustrial lead exposure, adequate medical study to rule out or include diseases of other causes, and establishing the character and duration of lead exposure are required to make a correct diagnosis.

Treatment

Until the 1950s, the only treatment for occupational lead poisoning was freedom from exposure to lead. Although this is still the ideal treatment, often it is not possible for economic reasons or in small plants where no other worker is at hand to take the sick worker's place.

Based on Aub's finding that lead follows calcium into bone, a high intake of milk used to be prescribed for the treatment of acute plumbism. A cathartic was given to hasten the excretion of any lead in the gut. There is still wide use of milk in lead-using industries to prevent poisoning, but students of the subject do not agree that one or two quarts of milk a day has a place in the medical control or treatment of toxic lead effect. An important argument against the value or use of milk is the fact that calcium drives absorbed lead into the skeleton. Excretion is thus delayed and the total body burden of lead may be increased. Furthermore, the belief that milk intake prevents poisoning may postpone engineering control of lead in workroom air.

Aub's theory that acidosis causes mobilization of stored lead led to attempts to hasten excretion by this method. The danger of a sudden increase in circulating lead in toxic form was soon discovered and emphasized in the writings of Aub, Kehoe, and Belknap, and such therapy is no longer used. Others with considerable experience believe that intravenous calcium acts to force free lead out of the circulation into bone and thus relieve the symptoms of acute colic. Johnstone (1941) first pointed out that intravenous calcium brings prompt relief from the pain of lead colic by action on the smooth muscle of the intestine, not as a result of forcing lead into bone. So dramatic is the effect of calcium that there is no need to use morphine or atropine.

During the early 1950s, following a suggestion by Kety and Letonoff (1943), Hardy et al. (1951) attempted to use citrates and citric acid to increase lead excretion safely by the formation of a harmless complex. Such therapy increased both urine and fecal lead levels but not enough lead was excreted at doses of citric acid that the patient would tolerate to make this treatment worthwhile. In 1954 the powerful chelating agent calcium ethylenediaminetetraacetic acid (Ca EDTA) was introduced. In laboratory animals, children, and industrial workers poisoned with lead, this agent proved to be of therapeutic benefit (Hardy et al., 1954; Rieders, Dunnington, and Brieger, 1955). This drug increases lead excretion dramatically, returns porphyrin excretion and hemoglobin levels to normal in a matter of days, and relieves the clinical signs and symptoms of lead toxicity. Maximum excretion is obtained by a course of four to seven consecutive days of intravenous administration of Ca EDTA followed by a rest of at least two days. The number of such courses that may be required is judged by the relief of symptoms, the reversal of wristdrop, and the normal

laboratory indices. Critical factors in treatment plans are duration of past exposure to harmful amounts of lead and whether or not a patient must return to poorly controlled lead operations. If the chelating agent is given on more than 10 consecutive days without interruption, excretion of lead returns to pretreatment levels. This phenomenon apparently reflects the complex equilibria that exist among soft tissue and skeletal lead deposits and the transport system in the body.

The literature on dosage and modes of treatment with Ca EDTA contains a variety of suggestions. The drug is best given by vein in 500 ml of normal saline as slowly as can be tolerated. As little as 1.5 g for a 70 kg adult up to 4 g in one day is the recommended dose. A flurry of papers, especially one by Dudley et al. (1955), and reports from Europe collected by Moeschlin (1965) warned of renal toxicity and interference with blood coagulation caused by EDTA. Some of these reports were of cases of malignant disease with high blood calcium levels in which very large doses, up to 100 g of the drug per day, were used for clinically desperate problems. Moeschlin (1965) reported that as little as 6 g caused renal toxicity in cases of lead poisoning, and Foreman et al. (1956) reported transient albuminuria at a similar dose level. HLH believes that it is reasonable to state from experience and the literature that there is no demonstrable danger to adults not suffering from renal disease or hypercalcemia from daily doses of 1.5 to 4 g of $CaNa_2$ EDTA given intravenously in series of four to seven days with two intervening days in which the drug is withheld. Studies to date do not show that other essential metals are chelated by this treatment in amounts sufficient to cause undesirable side effects.

The use of oral preparations of Ca EDTA is to be condemned because of evidence that the ability to chelate is lost after it is absorbed through the intestinal wall. In addition, the oral drug has been used by some as a cheap substitute for engineering control of industrial lead exposures. Intramuscular preparations have been used successfully but are not acceptable because the injections are painful.

N-acetyl-D-penicillamine will also bind lead, but not to the extent that Ca EDTA does, although both fecal and urine lead levels are increased by its use (Hardy et al., 1971). This drug, which can be given by mouth, has come into use especially in childhood poisoning once the episode of acute poisoning is controlled (Chisholm, 1968).

However, an unwanted effect of this chelating agent is to bind iron, and when it is used over a period of time it should be supplemented with an iron preparation such as ferrous gluconate.

The use of British antilewisite (BAL) is contra-indicated in adult lead poisoning on the basis of present knowledge. Although it increases lead excretion, some authors suggest that it increases lead toxicity. Chisholm (1968) found that the use of BAL along with Ca EDTA improves the prognosis in severe cases of acute lead poisoning in children.

Moeschlin (1965) reported that European physicians with wide experience with lead poisoning recommend the use of intramuscular B_{12} in cases with elevated porphyrin excretion. Others suggest giving folic acid and yeast, the cystine thought to act as a detoxifying agent. In cases of lead palsy, daily intramuscular injections of vitamin B_1 (40 mg) are prescribed in addition to conventional physiotherapy and specific therapy with Ca EDTA. Treatment of lead encephalopathy is directed toward the reduction of intracranial pressure. There is a favorable report by Mehbod (1967) on the value of peritoneal dialysis plus Ca EDTA for lead-induced central nervous system involvement.

Worth mentioning, because it is often forgotten, is the need to use purgatives to enhance the excretion of lead from the intestinal tract. In childhood poisoning this is a critical part of the therapy prior to the use of specific chelating agents to avoid a sudden increase in the level of circulating toxic lead.

Control

The first attempt to provide a standard for the control of air contamination by lead was made by Legge and Goadby in 1912. These authors held that if workers breathe no more than 2 mg of lead during their 8-hour work day there will rarely be any cases of colic and there will be no palsy or encephalopathy. The levels of lead in air that are currently considered safe are based on a great deal of experience accumulated over many years. The present United States permissible exposure limits for a 40-hour workweek are as follows: lead and inorganic lead compounds, 0.05 mg/m³; lead arsenate, 0.15 mg/m³; tetraethyl lead, 0.075 mg/m³ and tetramethyl lead, 0.07 mg/m³ (NIOSH/OSHA, 1978).

Organolead Compounds

Tetraethyl lead (TEL) and, to a lesser extent, tetramethyl lead (TML), are added to gasoline in order to eliminate the "knock" or detonation in the internal combustion engine. One part of TEL is added to 1300 parts of gasoline together with some organic halogen compound, usually ethylene dibromide, which is introduced in order to assist in the removal of lead from the engine after combustion. Combustion in the engine changes TEL to a solid compound, the exact composition of which depends on the halogen carrier used. The solid compounds collect in the engine and are also discharged with the exhaust gases. About 95% of the deposit in the engine head, pipe, crankcase, and drip pan consists of lead, 55% of which is in the form of chloride or bromide, both of which are highly soluble compounds. The particle sizes of these compounds makes it possible for them to be inhaled and retained.

TEL and TML are lipid soluble and are absorbed through the skin and in vapor form are readily taken up by the lungs. In blood they are transported to a much larger extent by the lipid fraction in the blood than is the case with inorganic lead (Beattie et al., 1972). Conversion to the tri-alkyl form and to inorganic lead occurs in the liver, and Cremer (1959) suggested that the tri-alkyl form is the toxic agent. Since TEL is converted more rapidly than is TML, the former is considered to be more toxic (Davis et al., 1963). Organolead compounds also cross the blood-brain barrier readily, and become concentrated in the central nervous system and in other lipid-rich tissues, such as bone marrow (Waldron, 1978). Their metabolites are water soluble and are excreted by the kidney. Although TEL and TML decrease erythrocyte ALA-dehydrase activity, they do not appreciably affect heme synthesis (Millar et al., 1972).

Worker illness The persons exposed to the effects of organolead compounds are those who produce them and those who blend them with gasoline. Tetraethyl lead is probably the only compound that can cause acute plumbism when absorbed through the skin. Far more serious is the risk from inhalation of organolead vapors. In 1923–24 a number of cases of severe poisoning from TEL occurred in men engaged in producing or blending this compound; there were at least 100 cases with 11 deaths. Eldridge (1924) published histories of some of the severest cases, and Kehoe

80

et al. (1925, 1936) added records of milder forms of intoxication. The victims were not only workmen engaged in blending and quite ignorant of any danger but also experimental chemists who handled the liquid recklessly, for there was general ignorance of its extreme toxicity and of the ease with which it enters the body. According to Machle (1935), slight and brief exposure may cause insomnia, anorexia, and fall in blood pressure. Such symptoms increased with longer and more severe exposures. The earliest symptom, and one of the most troublesome, is insomnia with restless and excited dreams. Vomiting, especially in the morning, may be brought on by the odor of TEL. Loss of strength as a result of loss of sleep and appetite is a common complaint. Machle described tremors, coarse and well defined, with exaggerated reflexes and sudden violent twitchings, which were sometimes continual and made worse by efforts to control them.

In contrast with inorganic lead poisoning, there are no complaints of severe gastrointestinal cramps or constipation. The lead line is not an early sign nor is stippling usually found. According to Hamilton (1925), the observers who saw the first cases of severe and fatal poisoning noted that symptoms were those of profound cerebral involvement and finally maniacal attacks like those of delirium tremens. Death came apparently from exhaustion. At necropsy, the microscopic features were congestion of the visceral and cerebral vessels with thrombi. A volatile lead compound was found by assay of the brains of those men who died within the first 24 hours after admission. Excess lead in nonvolatile form was also found. But volatile lead disappeared from brain, viscera, and the blood within a few hours. Contrary to the usual findings in death from lead poisoning, the amount of lead in the brain and liver exceeded that in the bones. That all organs contained significant levels of lead pointed to a very recent intake. The danger to men producing and blending TEL was thus demonstrated with devastating clearness (Kehoe et al., 1934, 1936).

A secondary danger exists in connection with the use of leaded gasoline, namely from the carbonized products found in the engine (Waniek, 1941) that may give rise to the more common forms of plumbism and thereby mask the cerebral symptoms from TEL. A serious hazard arises when workmen clean sludge from storage tanks or railway tank cars that have held TEL (Bruusgaard, 1946; Beattie et al., 1972). Chronic poisoning due to TEL does not occur and a subacute

form is considered to be a prodromal stage of the acute (Taeger, 1944).

Case reports of intoxication from TEL and TML have continued to appear sporadically. Gething (1975) described an industrial accident in which a young adult worker was exposed to a high level of TML but no symptoms or signs of lead poisoning appeared although the blood levels of lead were elevated for six months. HLH has seen two cases of serious renal disease associated with the practice of stealing leaded gasoline from parked cars by siphoning by mouth. Gasoline sniffing has given rise to serious lead encephalopathy in children and adults (Law and Nelson, 1968; Boeckx et al., 1977). On the other hand, Robinson (1974) concluded from a 20-year mortality study of TEL workers that in his experience such workers did not have a shortened life-span as a result of their work.

During the 1920s there was a question of the danger to garage employees, especially repair men, and to the general public from the soluble lead compounds that collect in the engine and are discharged with the exhaust gases. The Surgeon-General of the United States Public Health Service convened a conference in 1925 to determine what steps were needed for the protection of workers and the public. Evidence of toxic lead effect was reported from the industries producing TEL and absorption of lead was noted in certain garage workers, but not in chauffeurs and nonexposed garage workers. In view of these findings an expert committee reported that no menace to the public had been revealed. The producers and blenders of TEL agreed to sell only blended gasoline to retail dealers and to label supply pipes in filling stations with warning signs stating that the gasoline contains lead, must not be used for cleansing, and is dangerous if spilled on the skin. During the subsequent years, illnesses thought to be due to lead were investigated by Leake (1926) and by Kehoe, but in no instance was a diagnosis of plumbism supported except in the producing industries.

It is over a half century since the 1925 inquiry into the hazard due to leaded fuel. In the past ten years there has been a new wave of concern that lead in air, water, and soil is an ever-increasing threat to humans, especially children, animals, and vegetation. A higher percentage of TEL was added to gasoline after a report to the government, named the "Tri-Urban Survey" (U.S. Public Health Service, 1965) that concluded that lead in gasoline presents no risk to the public. At the same time, industrial uses of lead increased with little attention paid to lead in air from junk-yards, salvage operations, and the many lead-producing and lead-using operations. Stimulus for new investigations was provided by Patterson (1965) whose studies showed that industrial use of lead and leaded fuel added to the biosphere 250 times the amount of lead found naturally. Urban risk from lead exposure has meant that those who work in lead-using industries and who live in or near cities are, as a result, a population at double risk from lead toxicity. This added hazard may now decline with the gradual discontinuation of leaded gasoline and the promulgation of more stringent air quality standards.

Congenital Lead Poisoning

In the 19th and early 20th centuries it was a matter of common knowledge among women who worked in lead industries, such as pottery and white-lead production, that lead has an abortifa-cient action. The usually accepted theories as to the mode of action were that lead kills the fetus either by its effect on the maternal germ cell or directly through the maternal blood. Bell (1924) concluded from his studies on the action of lead on malignant cells that lead first injures the chorionic epithelium and thus indirectly injures the fetus and leads to its expulsion. When many women were employed in English potteries and white-lead works and when the exposure to lead was excessive, Reid, according to Oliver (1911), was able to collect data on the effect of plumbism on childbearing. A woman in lead work, as com-pared to one not employed in this work, was more likely to be sterile, and if she became pregnant, to miscarry. If a pregnancy went to term, it was more likely to end in stillbirth; and if a child was born living, death was more likely to come in the first year of life.

In the United States, where the danger of lead poisoning in childbearing women was thought to be unimportant, the possible effect of plumbism in the father became of greater interest. As long ago as 1860 Constantin Paul published figures that indicated a profound effect of paternal plum-bism on sterility and on the viability of the off-spring. Torelli (1930) reported that in the printing trade in Milan, where the abortion rate in general was 4 to 4.5%, among the wives of printers the rate was 14% and among women printers 24%. The average death rate in 1930 in all Italy for the

first year of life was 150 per 1000 births but for this group it was 320 per 1000. Earlier, Rennert (1881) found an impressive prevalence of convul-sions and a peculiar form of macrocephaly among the children of a German village where pottery glazing was at that time a home industry. He stated that the fetus is apparently more susceptible to lead than is the mother, being affected by quantities too small to injure her.

Chyzer (1908) published a description of the pottery villages of Hungary, where conditions were much the same as those found by Rennert, and where the same peculiar form of macro-cephaly prevailed among the children. His find-ings were confirmed by Oliver who made a special journey to Hungary to study this form of con-genital plumbism. The opportunities for actual lead poisoning were present in those cottages where lead glaze was in constant use, and indeed Rennert found some children with typical plum-bism, with palsy of the peroneal muscles and the toes. Koinuma (1926) compared the marital life records of workmen exposed to lead in storage battery plants in Japan with the histories of those working in nonlead occupations. Sterile marriages constituted 24.7% for the lead group and only 14.8% for the nonlead group. The percentage of pregnancies ending prematurely or in stillbirth was 8.2 for the lead group and 0.2 for the control population. Lancranjan et al. (1975) found decreased reproductive ability and increased fre-quency of spermatozoal abnormalities in 150 men occupationally exposed to lead in Rumania. Since 17-ketosteroid excretion was not impaired, these authors concluded that lead acts directly on the gonads.

From these data it is reasonable to conclude that lead is a poison to the germ cells, male as well as female. Lead poisoning in the mother means in-jury not only to the germ cell but also to the fetus during intrauterine life by the lead circulating in the mother's blood. Gilfillan (1965) presented an interesting hypothesis that the fall of Rome was caused by sterility due to leaded wine. While the reports of "hereditary" lead poisoning by Oliver (1914) are hard to judge and depend upon uncon-trolled lead exposures, they deserve attention. Can lead at low levels, such as protracted ex-posure to city air, cause fetal damage? Boylen found lead in bone, kidney, liver, and lung of five stillborn infants delivered in Massachusetts in 1971 (Hardy et al., 1971). Investigators in many countries are actively pursuing this question because of the increase of lead in air due to leaded gasoline and the continuing rise of industrial use of lead. The increasing use of unleaded gasoline to control the emission of lead in automobile exhausts may alleviate this problem.

The U.S. National Academy of Sciences published a summary study entitled *Lead, Airborne Lead in Perspective* in 1972 that covered most of the data concerning recent lead contamination in this country. Various aspects of lead poisoning have recently been summarized in a collection of papers published under the editorship of Singhal and Thomas (1980).

References

Albahary C: Lead and hemopoiesis. The mechanism and consequences of the erythropathy of occupational lead poisoning. *Am J Med* 1972;52:367-378.

Ali MAM, Quinlan A: Effect of lead on globin synthesis *in vitro*. *Am J Clin Pathol* 1977;67:77-79.

Allen BR, Moore MR, Hunter JAA: Lead and the skin. *Br J Dermatol* 1975;92:715-717.

Araki S, Honma T: Relationships between lead absorption and peripheral nerve conduction velocities in lead workers. *Scand J Work Environ Health* 1976;4:225-231.

Ashby JAS: A neurological and biochemical study of early lead poisoning. *Br J Ind Med* 1980;37:133-140.

Aub JC: Lead poisoning in the individual, in *Oxford Medicine*. New York, Oxford Univ Press, 1931, vol 4, chap XVIII-B.

Aub JC, Evans, RD, Gallagher DM, et al: Effects of treatment on radium and calcium metabolism in the human body. *Ann Intern Med* 1938;11:1443-1463.

Aub JC, Fairhall LT, Minot AS, et al: Lead poisoning. *Medicine* 1925;4:1-250.

Aub JC, Minot AS, Fairhall LT, et al: Recent investigations of absorption and excretion of lead in the organism. *J Am Med Assoc* 1924;83:588-591.

Aub JC, Robb GP, Rossmeisl E: The significance of bone trabeculae in the treatment of lead poisoning. *Am J Pub Health* 1932;22:825-830.

Badham C, Taylor HB: Lead poisoning: Standards of diagnosis, in *Studies in Industrial Hygiene, No. 7*. New South Wales, Sydney, Report of the Director General of Public Health, 1925.

Baghdassarian SA: Optic neuropathy due to lead poisoning. *Arch Ophthalmol* 1968;80:721-723.

Ball GV, Sorensen LB: Pathogenesis of hyperuricemia in saturnine gout. *N Engl J Med* 1969;280:1199-1202.

Bartleman EL, Dukes C: Chronic lead poisoning due to theatrical grease paint. *Br J Med* 1936;1:528-530.

Beattie AD, Moore MR, Goldberg A: Tetraethyl lead poisoning. *Lancet* 1972;2:12-15.

Belknap EL: Clinical studies on lead absorption in the human: Blood pressure observations. *J Ind Hyg Toxicol* 1936;18:380-390.

Belknap EL: Clinical control of health in the storage battery industry. *Proc Lead Hygiene Conference*. Chicago, Lead Industries Assoc, 1958.

Bell WB: Influence of lead on normal and abnormal cell growth and on certain organs. *Lancet* 1924;1:267-276.

Benson GI, George WHS, Litchfield MH, et al: Biochemical changes during the initial stages of industrial lead exposure. *Br J Ind Med* 1976;33:29-35.

Blake KCH: Absorption of [203]Pb from gastrointestinal tract of man. *Environ Res* 1976;11:1-4.

Blumberg WE, Eisinger J, Lamola AA, et al: Zinc protoporphyrin level in blood determined by a portable hematofluorometer: A screening device for lead poisoning. *J Lab Clin Med* 1977;89:712-723.

Blumgart HL: Lead studies: VI. Absorption of lead by the upper respiratory passages. *J Ind Hyg* 1923;5:153-158.

Boeckx RL, Postl B, Coodin FJ: Gasoline sniffing and tetraethyl lead poisoning in children. *Pediatrics* 1977;60:140-145.

Boyett JD, Butterworth CD Jr: Lead poisoning and hemoglobin synthesis. Report of a study of fifteen patients with chronic lead intoxication. *Am J Med* 1962;32:884-890.

Bridbord K: Occupational lead exposure and women. *Prevent Med* 1978;7:311-321.

Browder A: Lead poisoning from glazes. *Ann Intern Med* 1972;76:665.

Bruusgaard A: Three cases of intoxication with cleavage products of tetraethyl lead. *Nordisk Med* 1946;32:2644-2648, abstracted in *J Ind Hyg Toxicol* 1947;29:97.

Buchet JP, Roels H, Bernard A, et al: Assessment of renal function of workers exposed to inorganic lead, cadmium, or mercury vapor. *J Occup Med* 1980;22:741–750.

Buchtal F, Behse F: Electrophysiology and nerve biopsy in men exposed to lead. *Br J Ind Med* 1979;36:135–147.

Butt EM, Nusbaum RE, Gilmour TC, et al: Trace metal patterns in disease states: Hemachromatosis, Bantu siderosis and iron storage in Laennec's cirrhosis and alcoholism, in Seven MJ, Johnson LA (eds): *Metal-Binding in Medicine.* Philadelphia, J.B. Lippincott, 1960.

Campbell BC, Beattie AD, Elliott HL, et al: Occupational lead exposure and renin release. *Arch Environ Health* 1979;34:439–443.

Campbell BC, Moore MR, Goldberg A: Subclinical lead exposure: A possible cause of gout. *Br Med J* 1978;2:1403.

Cantarow A, Trumper M: *Lead Poisoning.* Baltimore, Williams & Wilkins, 1944.

Carlson AJ, Woelfel A: The solubility of lead salts in human gastric juice, and its bearing on the hygiene of the lead industries. *J Am Med Assoc* 1913;61:181–184.

Castellino N, Aloj S: Intracellular distribution of lead in the liver and kidney of the rat. *Br J Ind Med* 1969;26:139–143.

Cavalleri A, Minoia C, Pozzoli L, et al: Determination of plasma lead levels in normal subjects and in lead-exposed workers. *Br J Ind Med* 1978; 35:21–26.

Chamberlain MJ, Massey PMO: Mild lead poisoning with an excessively high blood lead. *Br J Ind Med* 1972;29:458–461.

Chisholm JJ Jr: The use of chelating agents in the treatment of acute and chronic lead intoxication in childhood. *J Pediatr* 1968;73:1–38.

Chyzer A: Les intoxications par le plomb se présentant dans le céramique en Hongrie. *Chir Presse* (Budapest) 1908;44:906–909.

Clarke AN, Wilson DJ: Preparation of hair for lead analysis. *Arch Environ Health* 1974;28:292–296.

Clarkson TW, Kench JE: Uptake of lead by human erythrocytes *in vitro. Biochem J* 1958; 69:432–439.

Cooper WC, Gaffey WR: Mortality of lead workers. *J Occup Med* 1975;17:100–107.

Cramér K, Dahlberg L: Incidence of hypertension among lead workers. A follow-up study based on regular control over 20 years. *Br J Ind Med* 1966;23:101–104.

Cramér K, Selander S: Studies in lead poisoning: Comparison between different laboratory tests. *Br J Ind Med* 1965;22:311–314.

Cremer JE: Biochemical studies on the toxicity of tetraethyl and other organo-lead compounds. *Br J Ind Med* 1959;16:191–199.

Dagg JH, Goldberg A, Lochhead A, et al: The relationship of lead poisoning to acute intermittent porphyria. *Q J Med* 1965;34:163–175.

Davis RK, Horton AW, Larson EE, et al: Inhalation of tetramethyl lead and tetraethyl lead. *Arch Environ Health* 1963;6:473–479.

Deknudt Gh, Léonard A, Ivanov B: Chromosome aberrations observed in male workers occupationally exposed to lead. *Environ Physiol Biochem* 1973;3:132–138.

Deknudt Gh, Manuel Y, Gerber GB: Chromosome aberrations in workers professionally exposed to lead. *J Toxicol Environ Health* 1977;3: 885–891.

de Bruin A: Certain biological effects of lead upon the animal organism. *Arch Environ Health* 1971;23:249–264.

Dreessen WC, Page RT, Hough JW, et al: Health and working environment of non-ferrous metal mine workers. *Publ Health Bull No. 277,* U.S. Public Health Service, 1942.

Druyan R, Haeger-Aronsen B, von Studnitz W, et al: Renal mechanism for excretion of porphyrin precursors in patients with acute intermittent porphyria and chronic lead poisoning. *Blood* 1965; 26:181–189.

Dudley HR, Ritchie AC, Schilling A, et al: Pathologic changes associated with the use of sodium ethylene diamine tetraacetate in the treatment of hypercalcemia: Report of two cases with autopsy findings. *N Engl J Med* 1955;252:331–337.

Dyck PJ, O'Brien PC, Ohnishi A: Lead neuropathy: 2. Random distribution of segmental demyelination among "old internodes" of myelinated fibers. *J Neuropathol Exp Neurol* 1977;36:570–575.

Edinger L: *Der Anteil der Funktion an der Entstehung von Nervenkrankheiten.* Wiesbaden, Bergman, 1908.

Eldridge WA: A study of the toxicity of lead tetraethyl. Rep. E.A.M.R.D. 29, Chemical Warfare Service, October 5, 1924.

Elkins HB: *The Chemistry of Industrial Toxicology,* 2nd ed, New York, John Wiley, 1959.

Ellis RW: Urinary screening tests to detect excessive lead absorption. *Br J Ind Med* 1966;23: 263–275.

Emmerson BT: The clinical differentiation of lead gout from primary gout. *Arthritis Rheum* 1968;11:623–634.

84

Fairhall LT, Sayers RR: The relative toxicity of lead and some of its compounds. *Public Health Bull No. 253,* U.S. Public Health Service, 1940.

Feldman RG, Hayes MK, Younes R, et al: Lead neuropathy in adults and children. *Arch Neurol* 1977;34:481–488.

Foreman H, Finnegan C, Lushbaugh CC: Nephrotoxic hazard from uncontrolled edathamil calcium-disodium therapy. *J Am Med Assoc* 1956;160:1042–1046.

Forni A, Cambiaghi G, Secchi GC: Initial occupational exposure to lead. Chromosome and biochemical findings. *Arch Environ Health* 1976; 31:73–78.

Forni A, Sciamé A, Bertazzi PA, et al: Chromosome and biochemical studies in women occupationally exposed to lead. *Arch Environ Health* 1980;35:139–145.

Garrod AB: *On Gout and Rheumatism: Their Differential Diagnosis, and the Nature of the So-called Rheumatic Gout.* London, Adlard, 1854.

Gething J: Tetramethyl lead absorption: A report of human exposure to a high level of tetramethyl lead. *Br J Ind Med* 1975;32:329–333.

Gibson JL: Plumbic ocular neuritis in Queensland children. *Br Med J* 1908;2:1488–1490.

Gilfillan SC: Lead poisoning and the fall of Rome. *J Occup Med* 1965;7:53–60.

Goldwater LJ, Hoover AW: An international study of "normal" levels of lead in blood and urine. *Arch Environ Health* 1967;15:60–63.

Goyer RA, Rhyne BC: Pathological effects of lead. *Intern Rev Exp Pathol* 1973;12:1–77.

Grandjean P, Arnvig E, Beckmann J: Psychological dysfunctions in lead-exposed workers. Relation to biological parameters of exposure. *Scand J Work Environ Health* 1978;4:295–303.

Haenninen H, Hernberg S, Mantere P, et al: Psychological performance of subjects with low exposure to lead. *J Occup Med* 1978;20:683–689.

Hamilton A: *Industrial Poisons in the United States.* New York, MacMillan, 1925.

Hamilton A: *Industrial Toxicology.* New York, Harper, 1934.

Hamilton A, Hardy HL: *Industrial Toxicology,* ed 2. New York, Hoeber, 1949; ed 3, Acton, MA, Publishing Sciences Group, 1974.

Hammer DI, Finklea JF, Hendricks RH, et al: Hair trace metal levels and environmental exposure. *Am J Epidemiol* 1971;93:84–92.

Hardy HL: What is the status of knowledge of the toxic effect of lead on identifiable groups in the population? *Clin Pharmacol Therap* 1966;7: 713–722.

Hardy HL, Bishop RC, Maloof CC: Treatment of lead poisoning with sodium citrate. Report of four cases. *Arch Ind Hyg Occup Med* 1951;3: 267–278.

Hardy HL, Chamberlin RI, Maloof CC, et al: Lead as an environmental poison. *Clin Pharmacol Therap* 1971;12:982–1002.

Hardy HL, Elkins HB, Ruotolo PW, et al: Use of monocalcium disodium ethylene diamine tetra-acetate in lead poisoning. *J Am Med Assoc* 1954; 154:1171–1175.

Harrold GC, Meek SF, Collins GR, et al: Toxicity of lead chromate. *J Ind Hyg Toxicol* 1944; 26:47–54.

Hayhurst ER: *A Survey of Industrial Health-Hazards and Occupational Diseases in Ohio.* Columbus, Ohio, Heer, 1915.

Henderson DA: A follow-up of cases of plumbism in children. *Australasian Ann Med* 1954;3: 219–224.

Henderson DA, Inglis JA: The lead content of bone in chronic Bright's disease. *Australasian Ann Med* 1957;6:145–154.

Hernberg S: Biochemical and clinical effects and responses as indicated by blood concentration, in Singhal RL, Thomas JA (eds): *Lead Toxicity.* Baltimore, Urban & Schwarzenberg, 1980, pp 367–399.

Hernberg S, Nikkanen J, Mellin G, et al: δ-aminolevulinic acid dehydrase as a measure of lead exposure. *Arch Environ Health* 1970;21: 140–145.

Hopkins AP, Dayan AD: The pathology of experimental lead encephalopathy in the baboon (*Papio anubis*). *Br J Ind Med* 1974;31: 128–133.

Horiuchi K: Sixteen years' experiences in the research on industrial lead poisoning. *Osaka City Med J* 1965;2:225–256.

Ingalls TH, Tiboni EA, Werrin M: Lead poisoning in Philadelphia, 1955–1960. *Arch Environ Health* 1961;3:575–579.

Johnstone RT: *Occupational Diseases, Diagnosis, Medico-Legal Aspects and Treatment.* Philadelphia, WB Saunders, 1941.

Joselow MM, Flores J: Application of the zinc protoporphyrin (ZP) test as a monitor of occupational exposure to lead. *Am Ind Hyg Assoc J* 1977;38:63–66.

Kark R, Meiklejohn AP: The significance of porphyrinuria in lead poisoning. *J Clin Invest* 1942;21:91–99.

Kehoe RA: Tetra-ethyl lead poisoning. Clinical analysis of a series of nonfatal cases. *J Am Med Assoc* 1925;85:108–110.

Kehoe RA: Industrial lead poisoning, in Irish DD, Fassett DW (eds): *Patty: Industrial Hygiene and Toxicology,* rev ed 2. New York, Interscience, 1963, pp 941–985.

Kehoe RA, Thamman F, Cholak J: On normal absorption and excretion of lead: Lead absorption and lead excretion in modern American life. *J Ind Hyg* 1933a;15:273–288.

Kehoe RA, Thamman F, Cholak J: Lead absorption and excretion in relation to the diagnosis of lead poisoning. *J Ind Hyg* 1933b;15:320–340.

Kehoe RA, Thamman F, Cholak J: An appraisal of the lead hazards associated with the distribution and use of gasoline containing tetraethyl lead. *J Ind Hyg* 1934;16:100–128.

Kehoe RA, Thamman F, Cholak J: An appraisal of the lead hazards associated with the distribution and use of gasoline containing tetraethyl lead: Occupational lead exposure of filling station attendants and garage mechanics. *J Ind Hyg Toxicol* 1936;18:42–68.

Kety SS, Letonoff MS: Treatment of lead poisoning by sodium citrate. *Am J Med Sci* 1943;205:406–414.

King E, Conchie A, Hiett D, et al: Industrial lead absorption. *Ann Occup Hyg* 1979;22:213.

Klein M, Namer R, Harpur E, et al: Earthenware containers as a source of fatal lead poisoning. *N Engl J Med* 1970;283:669–672.

Koelsch F: Beiträge zur Arbeitsmedizin; die Bleischaden der Leber und der Nieren und ihre arbeits- und versicherungs medizinische Bedeutung. *Jahresb f ärtzl Fortbild* 1927;18:35–42.

Koinuma S: Impotence of workmen. (Foreign letter). *J Am Med Assoc* 1926;86:1924.

Kopito L, Briley AM, Shwachman H: Chronic plumbism in children. Diagnosis by hair analysis. *J Am Med Assoc* 1969;209:243–248.

Lamóla AA, Yamane T: Zinc protoporphyrin in the erythrocytes of patients with lead intoxication and iron deficiency anemia. *Science* 1974;186:936–938.

Lancranjan I, Popescu HI, Găvănescu O, et al: Reproductive ability of workmen occupationally exposed to lead. *Arch Environ Health* 1975;30:396–401.

Landaw SA, Schooley JC, Arroyo FL: Decreased erythropoietin (ESF) synthesis and impaired erythropoiesis in acutely lead-poisoned rats. *Clin Res* 1973;21:559.

Lane R: The care of the lead worker. *Br J Ind Med* 1949;6:125–143.

Lane R: Health control in inorganic lead industries. A follow-up of exposed workers. *Arch Environ Health* 1964;8:243–250.

Laug EP, Kunze FM: The penetration of lead through the skin. *J Ind Hyg Toxicol* 1948;30:256–259.

Law WR, Nelson ER: Gasoline-sniffing by an adult. Report of a case with the unusual complication of lead encephalopathy. *J Am Med Assoc* 1968;204:1002–1004.

Leake JP: Text of full report of investigation of health hazards from tetraethyl lead. *Public Health Serv,* 1926.

Legge TM, Goadby KW: *Lead Poisoning and Lead Absorption.* New York, Longman, 1912.

Lehmann H: Über den Wert der basophilgranulierten Erythrozyten für Frühdiagnose der gewerblichen Bleivergiftung. *Arch f Hyg* 1933;111:49–56.

Lewy FH, Weiss S: Ergebnisse eine neuen exakten Methode zum Nachweis der Bleischädigung (Chronaxie). *Med Klin* 1928;14:1505–1506, abstracted in *J Ind Hyg* 1929;11:181.

Lewin C: Bleivergiftung, Ikterus und Leberschädigung. *Deutsche med Wchnschr* 1928;54:1450–1453.

Linenthal H: Early diagnosis of lead poisoning, in Kober GM, Hayhurst ER (eds): *Industrial Health.* Philadelphia, Blakiston, 1924.

Lin-Fu JS: Undue absorption of lead among children—A new look at an old problem. *N Engl J Med* 1972;286:702–710.

Loeper M, Pinard M: Méningite saturnine aiguë précoce (forma méningitique complète). *Bull et mém Soc med d hôp de Paris* 1911;31:226–239.

Machle W: Tetraethyl lead intoxication and poisoning by related compounds of lead. *J Am Med Assoc* 1935;105:578–585.

Maloof CC: Role of porphyrins in occupational diseases: I. Significance of coproporphyrinuria in lead workers. *Arch Ind Hyg Occup Med* 1950;1:296–307.

Mayers MR: A study of the lead line, arteriosclerosis and hypertension in 381 lead workers. *J Ind Hyg* 1927;9:239–250.

McCord CP: Lead and lead poisoning in early America. *Ind Med Surg* 1953;22:393–399, 534–539, 573–577; 1954;23:27–31, 75–80, 120–125, 169–172.

McCord CP, Holden FR, Johnston J: The basophilic aggregation test for lead poisoning and lead absorption: Ten years after its first use. *Ind Med* 1935;4:180–185.

McLaughlin M, Stopps GJ: Smoking and lead. *Arch Environ Health* 1973;26:131–136.

Mehbod H: Treatment of lead intoxication. Combined use of peritoneal dialysis and edetate calcium disodium. *J Am Med Assoc* 1967;201:972–974.

Meredith PA, Moore MR, Campbell GG, et al: Delta-aminolevulinic acid metabolism in normal and lead exposed humans. *Toxicology* 1978;9:1–9.

Millar JA, Thompson GG, Goldberg A, et al: δ-aminolevulinic acid dehydrase activity in the blood of men working with lead alkyls. *Br J Ind Med* 1972;29:317–320.

Moeschlin S: *Poisoning: Diagnosis and Treatment.* New York, Grune & Stratton, 1965.

Moore MR, Meredith PA, Goldberg A: Lead and heme synthesis, in Singhal RL, Thomas JA (eds): *Lead Toxicity.* Baltimore, Urban & Schwarzenberg, 1980, pp 79–117.

Morgan JM, Burch HB: Comparative tests for diagnosis of lead poisoning. *Arch Intern Med* 1972;130:335–340.

Morgan JM, Hartley MW, Miller RE: Nephropathy in chronic lead poisoning. *Arch Intern Med* 1966;118:17–29.

Morgan JM, Hartley MW: Etiologic factors in lead nephropathy. *South Med J* 1976;69:1445–1449.

Mosny E, Malloizel L: La meningite saturnine. *Rev de Med* 1907;27:505, 659.

Myers RR, Powell HC, Shapiro HM, et al: Changes in endoneurial fluid pressure, permeability, and peripheral nerve structure in experimental lead neuropathy. *Ann Neurol* 1980;8:392–401.

NIOSH: *Criteria for a Recommended Standard . . . .Occupational Exposure to Inorganic Lead* (Revised Criteria, 1978). Washington, DC, National Institute for Occupational Safety and Health, NIOSH 78-158, 1978.

NIOSH/OSHA: *Pocket Guide to Chemical Hazards.* Washington, DC, National Institute for Occupational Safety and Health (NIOSH 78-210), 1978.

Nye LJJ: An investigation of the extraordinary incidence of chronic nephritis in young people in Queensland. *Med J Austral* 1929;2:145–159.

Ohlsson WT: Penicillamine as lead-chelating substance in man. *Br Med J* 1962;1:1454–1456.

Oliver T: *Lead Poisoning in its Acute and Chronic Forms.* Edinburgh, Pentland, 1891.

Oliver T: A lecture on lead poisoning and the race. *Br Med J* 1911;1:1096–1098.

Oliver T: Lead poisoning from industrial and medical points of view. *Clin J* 1914;43:417–424.

O'Riordan ML, Evans HJ: Absence of significant chromosome damage in males occupationally exposed to lead. *Nature* 1974;247:50–53.

Osler W: *Principles and Practice of Medicine.* New York, Appleton-Century-Crofts, 1911.

Patterson CC: Contaminated and natural lead environments of man. *Arch Environ Health* 1965;11:344–360.

Paul C: Étude sur l'intoxication lente par les préparations de plomb et son influence sur le produit de la conception. *Arch gén de Med* 1860;15:513.

Pedley FG: The effects of lead on the vision: A case of subhyoid hemorrhage. *J Ind Hyg* 1930;12:359–363.

Pentschew A: Morphology and morphogenesis of lead encephalopathy. *Acta Neuropathol* 1965;5:133–160.

Pinto SS, Einert C, Roberts WJ, et al: Coproporphyrinuria. Study of its usefulness in evaluating lead exposure. *Arch Ind Hyg Occup Med* 1952;6:496–507.

Posner HS: Indices of potential lead hazard. *Environ Health Persp* 1977;19:261–284.

Powers JM, Rawe SE, Earlywine GR: Lead encephalopathy simulating a cerebral neoplasm in an adult. Case report. *J Neurosurg* 1977;46:816–819.

Prendergast WD: The classification of the symptoms of lead poisoning. *Br Med J* 1910;1:1164–1166.

Remak R: Neuritis and polyneuritis. *Nothnagel's Spez. Therapie* 1899;11(Pt 3):279.

Rennert O: Über eine hereditäre Folge der chronischen Bleivergiftung. *Arch f Gynäk* 1881;18:109–131.

Renshaw GD, Pounds CA, Pearson EF: Variations in lead concentration along single hairs as measured by non-flame atomic absorption spectrophotometry. *Nature* 1972;238:162–163.

Reznikoff P, Aub JC: Lead studies: XIV. Experimental studies of lead palsy. *Arch Neurol Psychiatr* 1927;17:444–465.

Rieders F, Dunnington WG, Breiger H: The efficacy of edathamil calcium disodium in the treatment of occupational lead poisoning. *Ind Med Surg* 1955;24:195–202.

Robinson TR: Twenty-year mortality of tetraethyl lead workers. *J Occup Med* 1974;16:601–605.

Sanders LW: Measurement of industrial lead exposure by determination of stippling of the erythrocytes. *J Ind Hyg Toxicol* 1943;25:38–46.

Schmid E, Bauchinger M, Pietruck S, et al: Die cytogenetische Wirkung von Blei in menschlichen peripheren Lymphocyten *in vitro* und *in vivo*. *Mutat Res* 1972;16:401–406.

Schroeder HA, Nason AP: Trace metals in human hair. *J Invest Dermatol* 1969;53:71–78.

Schroeder HA, Tipton IH: The human body burden of lead. *Arch Environ Health* 1968;17:965–978.

Seppäläinen AM, Hernberg S: Sensitive technique for detecting subclinical lead neuropathy. *Br J Ind Med* 1972;29:443–449.

Shufflebotham F: The effects of military training on lead workers. *Br Med J* 1915;1:672.

Silbergeld EK, Fales JT, Goldberg AM: Evidence for a junctional effect of lead on neuromuscular function. *Nature* 1974;247:49–50.

Singhal RL, Thomas JA (eds): *Lead Toxicity*. Baltimore, Urban & Schwarzenberg, 1980.

Sonkin N: Stippling of the retina. A new physical sign in the early diagnosis of lead poisoning. *N Engl J Med* 1963;269:779–780.

Taeger H: Subakute Bleitetra-äthylvergiftungen durch Bleibenzin. *Deutsch med Wchnschr* 1944;70:186–188, abstracted in *J Ind Hyg Toxicol* 1945;27:114.

Talbott JH: *Gout*. New York, Grune & Stratton, 1957.

Tanquerel des Planches L: *Traité des Maladies du Plomb ou Saturnisme,* Paris, 1839, translated by Dana SL: *Lead Diseases, a Treatise from the French of L. Tanquerel des Planches,* 1850.

Teisinger J: Biochemical responses to provocative chelation by edetate disodium calcium. *Arch Environ Health* 1971;23:280–283.

Tepper LB: Renal function subsequent to childhood plumbism. *Arch Environ Health* 1963;7:76–85.

Torelli G: L'influenza dell'avvelenamento cronico da piombo (saturnismo sulla discendenza). *Med Lavoro* 1930;21:110–121.

U.S. Public Health Service: Survey of lead in the atmosphere of three urban communities. Publ 999-AP-12, Washington, DC, 1965.

Vigdortschik NA: Lead intoxication in the etiology of hypertonia. *J Ind Hyg Toxicol* 1935;17:1–6.

Vitale LF, Joselow MM, Wedeen RP, et al: Blood lead—An inadequate measure of occupational exposure. *J Occup Med* 1975;17:155–162.

von Monakow C: Zur pathologischen Anatomie der Bleilähmung und der saturninen Encephalopathie. *Arch f Psychiatr* 1880;10:495–526.

Voors AW, Shuman MS, Woodward GP, et al: Arterial lead levels and cardiac death: A hypothesis. *Environ Health Persp* 1973;4:97.

Waldron HA: Health care of people at work. Workers exposed to lead: 2. Organic lead. *J Soc Occup Med* 1978;28:109–110.

Waniek H: Zur Frage der Bleigefährdung durch die Bleimischung von Bleitetraäthyl zu Kraftsstoffen als Antiklopfmittel. *Arch f Gewerbepathol u Gewerbehyg* 1941;11:165–169, abstracted in *J Ind Hyg Toxicol* 1943;25:62.

Webster SH: The lead and arsenic content of urines from 46 persons with no known exposure to lead or arsenic. *Publ Health Rep* 1941;56:1953–1961.

Wedeen RP, Mallik DK, Batuman V: Detection and treatment of occupational lead nephropathy. *Arch Intern Med* 1979;139:53–57.

Weller CV: Some clinical aspects of lead meningo-encephalopathy. *Ann Clin Med* 1925;3:604–613.

Westerman MP, Pfitzer E, Ellis LD, et al: Concentrations of lead in bone in plumbism. *N Engl J Med* 1965;273:1246–1250.

Westphal A: Über Encephalopathia saturnina. *Arch f Psychiatr* 1888;19:620–666.

Whitefield CL, Ch'ien LT, Whitehead JD: Lead encephalopathy in adults. *Am J Med* 1972;52:289–298.

15 • Lithium

Lithium and its salts are used in industry as constituents in alloys, as coolants in nuclear reactors, and as additives in alkaline storage batteries. Lithium stearate is an important thickener in lubricating greases, especially those used in the automobile industry. Lithium salts used in the therapy of mental illness and in place of sodium are known to physicians because of their toxic effects. Such effects are not experienced in industry, perhaps because lithium and its salts are not used in large amounts nor are they ingested or inhaled. Lithium hydride, on the other hand, is corrosive and would be a respiratory hazard if inhaled (Spiegl et al., 1956).

Reference

Spiegl CJ, Scott JK, Steinhardt H, et al: Acute inhalation toxicity of lithium hydride. *Arch Ind Health* 1956;14:468–470.

16 • *Manganese*

Uses

Manganese is in demand for the production of alloys, especially manganese steel, and the making of dry batteries. In the latter, the negative pole consists of a zinc container into which is placed a mixture of coke, sal ammoniac, and manganese dioxide, the latter intended to prolong the life of the battery. The positive pole is a carbon electrode placed in the center of the receptacle. Such batteries are widely used for flashlights and radios. Manganese is also used in making chlorine gas and potassium permanganate, in the manufacture of paints, varnish, enamel, and linoleum, in marbling soap, in coloring glass and ceramics, and in making matches and fireworks (Browning, 1969).

Industrial Hazards

Manganese poisoning was described first in five workers in a pyrolusite mill in 1837 by Couper. It was rediscovered in 1901 by von Jaksch and by Emden who separately reported cases of central nervous system disease that resembled multiple sclerosis (National Academy of Sciences, 1973). Friedel in 1903 described a case and rightly attributed it to manganese dust (Hamilton and Hardy, 1949, p. 166). The first American report of manganese poisoning was made by Casamajor (1913) who reported nine cases, all in men working in the same mill. The cases reported by Edsall et al. (1919) brought the number in America up to 39. Since the 1930s, reports of manganese poisoning have come from all over the world and have been summarized in the National Academy of Sciences monograph (1973).

The most hazardous manganese exposures occur in mining and in smelting of ores. Braunite (a mixture of Mn_2O_3 and $MnSiO_3$) is reported to be more harmful than pyrolusite (MnO_2) (Rodier, 1955). Harmful levels may exist in plants manufacturing alloys of manganese and steel. Less dangerous industrial uses of manganese occur in dry battery manufacture, electric arc welding (where the rods contain manganese), as well as to some extent in the production of paints, varnishes, enamels, linoleum, fireworks, ceramic glazes, and fertilizers.

Potential occupational hazards also exist in the manufacture of manganese tricarbonyl compounds that are used as additives to fuel oil for inhibiting smoke formation and to gasoline as supplementary antiknock compounds. Inhalation hazard is low because of the slight volatility of these substances but there is some danger from skin contact (Hinderer, 1979).

Harmful Effects

The whole subject of the toxic action of manganese, the mode of entry, the clinical history, and the diagnosis and prevention of manganese poisoning has been dealt with at length by Edsall et al. (1919), Fairhall and Neal (1943), Cotzias (1958), and the National Academy of Sciences monograph (1973). Recent reports of this clinical problem include those of Peñalver (1957), Schuler et al. (1957), Suzuki et al. (1960), Stokinger (1963), Whitlock et al. (1966), Tanaka and Lieben (1969), Rosenstock et al. (1971), Smyth et al. (1973), Cook et al. (1974), Hine and Pasi (1975), and Šarić et al. (1977).

The industrial cause of manganism is considered to be the inhalation of dust of manganese ore, or the dioxide, or the fumes from the fusing of manganese in steel manufacture. The following symptoms of manganese poisoning are listed in the approximate order of appearance after a history of exposure to manganese dust for at least three months: 1) apathy, anorexia, and somnolence, sometimes preceded by a transitory phase of psychomotor excitement ("manganese madness"); 2) stolid, masklike face; 3) low, monotonous voice with economical speech; 4) muscular twitching, varying from a fine tremor of the hands to gross rhythmical movements of the arms, legs, trunk, and head; 5) stiffness of the leg muscles and cramps in the calves that usually come on at night and are worse after a day of exertion; 6) retropulsion and propulsion in walking, with a peculiar slapping gait as the patient keeps as broad a base as possible, endeavoring involuntarily to avoid propulsion; 7) uncontrollable laughter, less frequently crying. Additional manifestations of manganism include speech difficulties, impaired ability to arise and to maintain postural stability, diminished libido, dysdiadochokinesia and difficulty with fine movements (such as writing), memory loss, dysphagia, and urinary bladder disturbances. Some neurological signs stabilize, and speech difficulties and tremor may subside after exposure ceases but gait disturbances persist.

In addition to the signs and symptoms of central nervous system involvement, several authors report hematological changes of uncertain importance such as anemia, leukopenia, neutropenia, and monocytosis. Browning (1969, p. 221) summarized these reports and concluded that there are no blood count changes diagnostic of manganese intoxication. According to Horiuchi et al. (1970), the interpretation of elevated levels of manganese in body fluids is difficult and Browning states that there is poor correlation between urinary manganese levels and the severity of the acute disease. Smyth et al. (1973) found that urine manganese concentrations were about three times higher in dust-exposed workers in a ferromanganese processing facility than in an unexposed group. Since manganese can be found in the hair, the study of hair levels associated with manganese in the air may prove to be a useful method of control (Rodier, 1955; Balani et al., 1967; Rosenstock et al., 1971), provided that surface contamination is removed.

It is significant that, unlike lead, manganese produces no life shortening, but seriously poisoned workers are lifelong cripples. According to Cotzias (1962), manganese toxicity is due to an active depot in the lungs that releases manganese to the extracellular fluid. Homeostatic mechanisms keep tissue concentrations under control, but the constant perfusion of the brain with manganese leads to the appearance of extrapyramidal disease, which may be reversed if the lung depot is exhausted or if there is chemical sequestration of circulating manganese. The neurological lesions in manganism are found mainly within the striatum and pallidum, and these pathological changes distinguish this disorder from parkinsonism where the damage is classically in the substantia nigra (Barbeau et al., 1976).

Two other clinical syndromes can be caused by excessive industrial manganese exposure. Metal fume fever can follow inhalation of finely divided manganese. Manganese pneumonitis has been reported among workers handling manganese ores (Rodier, 1955), and in workers exposed to manganese dioxide in dry battery manufacture and those in the chemical industry making potassium permanganate (Davies, 1946). Pneumonitis has also been reported in basic slag workers who process, bag, and load Thomas slag or Thomas meal that contains 6 to 8% manganese (National Academy of Sciences, 1973). Davies concluded from clinical and experimental animal studies that manganese dust injures the respiratory epithelium. Bergström (1977) stated from animal studies that a temporary inflammatory reaction occurs in the respiratory tract after exposure to MnO_2 and that this is accompanied by a depression of the phagocytic capacity of alveolar macrophages. None of the reported cases of manganese pneumonitis has also had central nervous system involvement.

Treatment and Control

Because manganese poisoning is a crippling disease, sometimes with a delay in onset after exposure has ceased, treatment with chelating agents was for some time the therapy of choice when the diagnosis was suspected. British antilewisite (BAL) is reported as being useless. Peñalver (1957) reported success with calcium ethylenediaminetetraacetic acid (EDTA) in at least one case. In animal studies, diethylenetriaminepentaacetic acid (DTPA) was found to be more effective than EDTA. In the experience of Smyth et al. (1973), EDTA in doses of 2 g daily by vein mobilized large amounts of manganese, and they concluded that the enhanced urinary excretion after EDTA reflected prior accumulation of stored manganese, but they do not urge its use as therapy. Obviously, early freedom from exposure is the method of choice for prevention.

Absence of benefit from chelation therapy in chronic manganese poisoning affecting the nervous system suggested that the treatment used for parkinsonism be tried. Cotzias and his colleagues (Mena et al., 1970; Cotzias et al., 1971) have changed the previously hopeless prognosis of chronic manganese poisoning, since treatment with slowly increasing oral doses of L-dopa usually results in prompt improvement without the side effects of hypotension and of choreoathetoid movements so troublesome in the therapy of patients with Parkinson's disease. Rosenstock et al. (1971) found that many neurological abnormalities were improved by this therapy although the marked dystonia in their patient was unaffected.

Reports of the air concentrations of manganese resulting in poisoning have been recorded as 100 to 900 mg/m³ (Rodier, 1955), 40 to 174 mg/m³ (Flinn et al., 1941), 10 mg/m³ (Davies, 1946), and 7 to 63 mg/m³ (Kesic and Häusler, 1954). There are reports summarized by Stokinger (1963) that cases have occurred at manganese levels averaging as low as 3 to 9 mg/m³. These values suggest that the present United States safe level of 5 mg/m³ for continued exposure may be too high. By contrast, the maximum allowable concentration (MAC) in Yugoslavia, for example, is 2 mg/m³ (Šarić et al., 1977).

Since neither blood nor urinary manganese levels are correlated with the presence or severity of disease, physical examinations of potentially exposed workers are required at regular intervals to detect any slight and incipient neurological abnormalities.

References

Balani SG, Umarji GM, Bellare RA, et al: Chronic manganese poisoning. *J Postgrad Med* 1967;13:116–122.

Barbeau A, Inoué N, Cloutier T: Role of manganese in dystonia. *Adv Neurol* 1976;14:339–351.

Bergström R: Acute pulmonary toxicity of manganese dioxide. *Scand J Work Environ Health* 1977;3(suppl 1):1–41.

Browning E: *Toxicity of Industrial Metals,* ed 2. New York, Appleton-Century-Crofts, 1969, pp 213–225.

Casamajor L: An unusual form of mineral poisoning affecting the nervous system: manganese? *J Am Med Assoc* 1913;60:646–649.

Cook DG, Fahn S, Brait FA: Chronic manganese intoxication. *Arch Neurol* 1974;30:59–64.

Cotzias GC: Manganese in health and disease. *Physiol Rev* 1958;38:503–532.

Cotzias GC: Manganese, in Comar CL, Bronner F (eds): *Mineral Metabolism, An Advanced Treatise.* New York, Academic Press, 1962.

Cotzias GC, Papavasiliou PS, Ginos J, et al: Metabolic modification of Parkinson's disease and of chronic manganese poisoning. *Ann Rev Med* 1971;22:305–326.

Davies TAL: Manganese pneumonitis. *Br J Ind Med* 1946;3:111–135.

Edsall DL, Wilbur FP, Drinker CK: The occurrence, course and prevention of chronic manganese poisoning. *J Ind Hyg* 1919;1:183–193.

Fairhall LT, Neal PH: Industrial manganese poisoning. *National Institute of Health Bulletin No. 182,* Washington, DC, 1943.

Flinn RH, Neal PA, Fulton WB: Industrial manganese poisoning. *J Ind Hyg Toxicol* 1941;23:374–387.

Hamilton A, Hardy HL: *Industrial Toxicology,* ed 2. New York, Paul B. Hoeber, 1949, pp 166–171.

Hinderer RK: Toxicity studies of methylcyclopentadienyl manganese tricarbonyl. *Am Ind Hyg Assoc J* 1979;40:164–167.

Hine CH, Pasi A: Manganese intoxication. *West J Med* 1975;123:101–107.

Horiuchi K, Horiguchi S, Shinagawa K, et al: On the significance of manganese contents in the whole blood and urine of manganese handlers. *Osaka City Med J* 1970;16:29–37.

Kesic B, Häusler DN: Hematological investigation after manganese exposure. *Arch Ind Hyg Occup Med* 1954;10:336–341.

Mena I, Court J, Fuenzalida S, et al: Modification of chronic manganese poisoning: Treatment with L-dopa or 5-OH tryptophane. *N Engl J Med* 1970;282:5–10.

National Academy of Sciences: *Manganese.* Washington, DC, 1973.

Peñalver R: Diagnosis and treatment of manganese intoxication. Report of a case. *Arch Ind Health* 1957;16:64–66.

Rodier J: Manganese poisoning in Moroccan mines. *Br J Ind Med* 1955;12:21–35.

Rosenstock HA, Simons DG, Meyer JS: Chronic manganism. *J Am Med Assoc* 1971;217:1354–1358.

Šarić M, Markićević A, Hrustić O: Occupational exposure to manganese. *Br J Ind Med* 1977;34:114–118.

Schuler P, Oyanguren H, Maturana V, et al:

Manganese poisoning: Environmental and medical study at a Chilean mine. *Ind Med Surg* 1957; 26:167–173.

Smyth LT, Ruhf RC, Whitman NE, et al: Clinical manganism and exposure to manganese in the production and processing of ferromanganese alloy. *J Occup Med* 1973;15:101–109.

Stokinger HE: The metals (excluding lead), in Patty FA (ed): *Industrial Hygiene and Toxicology,* ed 2. New York, John Wiley, 1963.

Suzuki Y, Nishiyama K, Doi M, et al: Studies on chronic manganese poisoning. *Tokushima J Exp Med* 1960;7:124–132.

Tanaka S, Lieben J: Manganese poisoning and exposure in Pennsylvania. *Arch Environ Health* 1969;19:674–684.

Whitlock CM Jr, Amuso SJ, Bittenbender JB: Chronic neurological disease in two manganese steel workers. *Am Ind Hyg Assoc J* 1966;27:454–459.

17 • *Mercury*

Sources of Occupational Poisoning

Mining Mercury is one of the oldest industrial poisons. It was known to the Romans who included mercurialism among the diseases of slaves, for only slave labor was used in the great Spanish mines of Almaden. So terrible was the poisoning in those mines that Justinian wrote that a sentence to work there was almost equal to a death sentence, and Plutarch blamed a mine owner because he employed slaves who were not criminals. After slavery was abolished, the mines were worked by convicts, and when free labor was introduced it was found necessary to limit the hours of work because there was so much incapacitating illness among the men.

Other countries have added to our knowledge of severe disease among mercury miners. The Austrian mines at Idria, a mining town north of Trieste (given to Italy after the First World War and to Yugoslavia after the Second), have been worked for more than four centuries. The first description that we have of the symptoms of chronic mercurialism was written during the first half of the 16th century by Andrea Mattioli of Siena, who had observed it among the miners at Idria. Some 200 years later, in 1761, Giovanni Scopoli wrote a remarkably clear description of mercurial tremors in Idria miners. There are no longer any severe cases of mercurialism among miners or furnace men and few cases that are even moderately severe, but there are many that are mild. A system of alternation of work has been in force in Idria since 1897 and the men work a six-hour day. The institution of this short working day in April, 1665 in what was then the province of Friuli, is said to be the first legislative measure of industrial hygiene known to history.

The Italian mines of Monte Amiata were evidently worked with highly primitive methods, for the description of mercurialism as it was found in the early years of this century includes forms as severe and dramatic as any to be found in the literature. The United States has held third place in world production of quicksilver, by far the greatest part of the metal coming from California (the area named New Idria), with Texas following with a much lower output. Most of these mines yield cinnabar (sulfide) ore only, but in some there is also metallic mercury — "the silver runs free," as the miners say. Mexico, several South American countries, Yugoslavia, and the Philippines all produce mercury at the present time.

The hatter's trade Second to the mining of mercury as a classic source of mercurialism has been the hatter's trade, the treatment of fur to make felt hats. This is an old industry whose age is not known. There is a legend that St. Clement the Roman, the patron saint of hatters, when on a pilgrimage to Jerusalem, lined his sandals with camel's hair to ease his feet; the combined action of heat, pressure, and sweat produced a sheet of felt. Similar primitive methods were used, even in recent times, in the Orient. Fine, soft hairs were cut by hand, blown onto a cone-shaped form, and pressed with a hot, wet cloth. These processes — cutting, blowing, coning, and shrinking (sizing) with hot water — are still in use but have been largely mechanized in industrial countries.

At some time before 1685 mercury nitrate entered the hatter's trade in France and its use was kept a valuable trade secret by the hatter's guild. The French still call the liquid "le secret" and the process "secretage." The use of mercury nitrate makes felting much easier, for it softens the stiff hairs, and makes them limp, twisted, and rougher. The English word for this process is "carrotting" and the nitrate solution is called "carrot" because it turns white fur a reddish-brown color. The French had a monopoly of felt-hat manufacture until the Revocation of the Edict of Nantes

(1685) drove the Huguenot hatters, who took their secret with them, over to England. The use of mercury carrot persisted to the 20th century in all industrial countries, but in Russia, after the Revolution of 1917, the use of mercury was abandoned and a nonmercurial method, devised in France, was gradually substituted. Felt production had been a home industry in Russia and whole families suffered from the effects of exposure to mercury (Hamilton, 1922a,b). The hatter's trade, which was notoriously unhealthful in every country, as the terms "hatter's shakes" and "mad as a hatter" show, had an especially bad reputation in France and Belgium. The French paid little attention to the sanitation of their plants, but set about to develop a method of felting without the use of mercury, an endeavor that resulted in a number of usable, nontoxic mixtures to replace the carrot. But to introduce a new carrotting fluid meant a change in many processes that had become standardized through the years, and even the French kept to the old ways.

The first mention of the manufacture of felt hats in the United States was in 1662, when the Virginia Assembly offered a reward of 10 pounds of tobacco for every good felt hat produced from the fur of native animals. The earliest American study of mercurial poisoning in the making of hats was made by Freeman in 1860 who reported that during the winter of 1858–59 and the following spring there prevailed among the hatters of New Jersey a disease showing all the characteristics of mercury poisoning: swelling and ulceration of the gums, loosening of the teeth, fetid breath, abnormal flow of saliva, and a shaking palsy of the limbs. Dennis, a public health physician working in New Jersey, published a paper on the health of hatters in 1878. This report is admirably complete and deserves far more attention than it has ever received. Conditions in the industry at that time seem to have been very bad. In some instances "all hands in the shop within a few days were rendered unfit for work or had their health impaired." Harris (1915) found 47 incontestable and 51 probable cases of mercurialism among 347 hatters and hat furriers. Wright (1922) examined 108 hatters and found that 53 showed at least two of the three classic symptoms: erethism, tremor, gingivitis.

Studies made by the U.S. Public Health Service (Neal et al., 1937, 1941) reported 59 of 534 hatters suffering from chronic mercury poisoning. Those afflicted had worked in air containing from 0.21 to 0.50 mg Hg/m³ of air. The outstanding clinical findings in these reports included irritability, timidity, apprehension, restlessness, vasomotor disorders (shown by readiness to blush, sweating, and dermographia), increased reflexes, gingivitis, and slight abnormalities in speech. Psychic disturbances were detected more often than they were reported by the men, a phenomenon that is typical of this form of intoxication. Instead of dwelling on or exaggerating his trouble, the victim of mercurialism seemed eager to hide it. Increase in systolic blood pressure, albuminuria, and hematuria were also noted.

These reports had very important consequences, for in 1941 the Connecticut Commissioner of Health convened a conference on mercury poisoning in the hatter's trade. Participants included the Surgeon General and representatives of the hatting industry. It was decided to forbid the use of mercury carrot in the preparation of hatter's fur or the use of such carrotted fur in the making of felt hats. Several states at first did not prohibit the use of mercury in felt hat manufacture but did develop successful medical and engineering controls. Today, there are a relatively small number of cases of occupational mercurialism. HLH saw one case of classic chronic mercury poisoning in Boston in 1947 and one while visiting Italy in 1963, both hatters. Baldi et al. (1953) reported more than 300 cases of mercurialism among felt hat workers during the period from 1942 through 1952 in Italy. Even at the present time mercury may still be used in fur processing and hat manufacture in some parts of the world.

Other Uses Associated with Illness

Second in toxic importance to mercury nitrate is the fulminate of mercury ($Hg(CNO)_2$) used in detonator manufacture. Knowledge of its harmful effects became known in England and the United States during World War I. The clinical descriptions included dermatitis, eczematous ulceration of the face, neck, arms, hands, and genitals, and, in some cases, conjunctivitis, rhinitis, and laryngitis. Painful, so-called "powder holes" were the result of necrotic lesions when the fulminate became lodged in a crack of skin. Mercurial stomatitis from fulminate powder appears to be rare. Jordi (1947) reported on fulminate poisoning in a Swiss factory where ventilation was poor because of war-time blackout. Nervous system symptoms and nephrosis predominated, but salivation and hyperhidrosis also occurred.

Another formerly important use for mercury has gradually been abandoned: mercury pumps to exhaust the air in incandescent lamp bulbs to produce the necessary vacuum. These pumps often broke, so that mercury was scattered about. The foreign literature on industrial mercurialism had a great deal about this problem and the risk to workers in the lamp industry, but in this country such pumps were rarely used.

Cinnabar, the ore containing mercury sulfide, is insoluble in body fluids and there is no trouble mining it, but miners often pass back and forth between mining and metallurgy, for the condensing plants are situated close to the mines. The metallurgy of cinnabar reduction is simple for it decomposes at a low heat, 338° to 420°C, into metallic mercury and SO_2, and the former is usually collected in condensers made of tile or wood. Quicksilver penetrates such substances and works its way through the lining of the furnace, iron pipes, fire bricks, terra cotta, and, by impregnation, the sides of a wooden condenser. Mercury has been recovered from the ground 30 feet (over nine meters) under an old furnace. Severe cases of mercurialism were common some 30 years ago, but mechanization and fume control have made great strides in recent years (West and Lim, 1968). Mercury amalgam is still used for extracting gold and silver from the richer ores.

A great deal of metallic mercury is used in the manufacture of thermometers and barometers. This procedure is potentially hazardous because mercury volatilizes at room temperature. Because of the nonspecificity of the symptoms of subacute mercury poisoning, there are few reports of illness that is bound to occur in small plants with poor housekeeping. HLH knows of one such shop where the control was so good that in ten years transient albuminuria in a few workers was the only evidence of possible toxic mercury effect. On the other hand, Vermeiden et al. (1980) reported a case of vesicular exanthem resembling erythema multiforme in a man who had spent a week cleaning up broken thermometers. Joselow and Goldwater (1967) reported a weak correlation between proteinuria and urinary mercury level in healthy workers exposed to mercury. This finding suggests that low-level mercury exposure may produce unrecognized renal damage.

Solder for dry batteries contains mercury, and the making and use of this solder is productive of a form of mercurialism that is likely to be unusually acute, for the heat used in melting and soldering volatilizes the mercury quickly. Another unusually dangerous job is that of repairing, with an acetylene torch, high-frequency induction furnaces or mercury boilers. Although death from industrial mercurialism is very rare now, a case was reported in which the source was vapor escaping from a high-frequency induction furnace with a mercury seal (Jordan and Barrows, 1924). A similar danger is found in what is known as the "constant potential" department of electric works, when alternating current is changed to direct current by passage through a large flask of mercury. HLH found transient hematuria in four of six men so exposed while repairing an electron accelerator for which mercury was used as a heat-transfer liquid. There is also the risk of overexposure to mercury in the modern method of chlorine manufacture (Smith et al., 1970). El-Sadik and El-Dakhakhny (1970) reported that signs of mercurialism appeared in workers in a sodium hydroxide manufacturing plant who were intermittently exposed to mercury in the electric cells. Calomel (HgCl) is said to cause typical mercury poisoning when it is inhaled in small amounts as a dust by workers handling tracer ammunition.

The occurrence of chronic mercurialism among dentists as a result of continual handling of amalgam may occur and go unrecognized. Gronka et al. (1970) studied 59 dental offices in which 98 persons working in these places showed elevated levels of urine mercury up to 0.33 mg/L. Exposures arose from the preparation of amalgams, the use of excess mercury and spillage. Joselow et al. (1968a) reported that 14% of the dentists and dental assistants that they studied were exposed to potentially harmful levels of mercury vapor. A serious occupational epidemic of mercury poisoning affected 22 of 36 workers exposed in handling a mercury-copper amalgam. A three-year follow-up showed improvement in both mildly and severely affected workers (Benning, 1958). This report illustrates both the consistent hazard of mercury and the fact that toxicity will reverse when exposure ceases.

Smith (1978), in discussing his cases of mercury poisoning in three dentists, pointed out that of the approximately 110,000 dentists in the United States about 70% work with amalgam almost daily, and these each use from 1 to 5 kg of mercury annually. Battistone et al. (1976) concluded from their studies of 1555 dentists evaluated at an annual session of the American Dental Association in 1972 that American dentists as a group practice good mercury hygiene. Those general practitioners with higher blood mercury values tended to show dental practice characteristics, such as mixing their own amalgam and expressing the mercury from the amalgam, that were conducive to producing the higher values (hr > 10 ng/ml blood) that were found. Rothwell et al. (1977) reported that mercury vapor hazards result from the use of hot air sterilizers in dental practice because amalgam-contaminated instruments are subjected to twice the temperatures reached in boiling water sterilizers.

Laboratories using mercury are notorious for their carelessness in handling this potentially dangerous metal. After 20 years' experience with this potential risk at a hospital and a large academic community with many research laboratories, HLH found it striking that few instances of mercury poisoning were discovered. Goldwater et al. (1956) reported the case of a student exposed to mercury vapors who suffered from salivation, colicky pains, irritability, and loss of memory but who had no neurological changes. The air mercury level averaged 0.5 mg/m³ and the urine levels 0.45 mg Hg/L. HLH studied a professor who augmented his income by cleaning mercury and who, as a consequence, suffered true chronic poisoning with nervous system effects. Three men engaged in a similar task for a shorter time in a government laboratory suffered excessive salivation, bleeding gums, hematuria, and albuminuria. Removal from mercury exposure led to complete recovery. Intermittent exposure and rapid excretion probably explain those cases where urine mercury levels indicate unsafe exposures but no clinical manifestations appear. Danziger and Possick (1973) studied 75 workers exposed to mercury vapors in the manufacture of scientific glassware, particularly in the calibration of vessel volumes. Despite the poor workroom hygiene, only one of the employees exhibited signs of mercury poisoning. Stewart et al. (1977) found increased urine mercury levels and proteinuria among the staff of a pathology laboratory until routine control measures reduced the exposures to within acceptable limits.

Vigliani (1946) described an unusual case of acute mercury poisoning that followed the introduction of metallic mercury under the skin with a fragment of broken capillary tube. A radiograph showed that droplets of mercury were scattered through the finger. An intense tremor developed, but this subsided when the inflamed area was incised and the mercury removed. There have been several cases in recent years of mercury introduced accidentally into the lungs or blood-stream during medical procedures. Buxton et al. (1965) reviewed the subject and reported nine cases occurring during blood sampling, a finding suggesting that mercury embolism occurs more often than is realized. Popper (1966) reported the death of a student nurse following empyema secondary to chronic lung damage due to mercury in her left lower lobe. Six years prior to her death she had broken a clinical thermometer and wounded her hand.

Organic compounds of mercury have been used extensively since 1914 as fungicides, most often as the dimethyl compound. Hunter and his colleagues (1940) described four severe cases of mercurialism that originated in a factory producing fungicides. The symptoms were not those of poisoning by inorganic mercury, for the central nervous system alone was affected. There were tremor, ataxia, dysarthria, and gross constriction of visual fields, but no changes in memory or intelligence. Serious mercury intoxication has occurred in Japan among fish-eating people as a result of contamination of fish, largely in Minamata Bay, by industrial discharges of methyl mercury. Poisoning by methyl and ethyl mercury that were used as fungicides has also occurred when treated seed grain was used instead as food. Such cases have occurred in Iraq, Iran, Pakistan, Ghana, and Guatemala, and total about 8000 (Clarkson, 1977). Dales (1972) discussed in detail the neurotoxicity of alkyl mercury compounds. As a result, records of industrial intoxication of workers handling organic mercury compounds in drug and pesticide manufacture, seed treating, and farming have become of real interest. Bidstrup (1964) collected case data of 45 workers suffering from varying degrees of mercury poisoning associated with exposure to a number of different organic compounds. These reports, which came from a number of countries, all confirm Hunter's observation that organic mercurials in toxic doses produce central nervous symptoms only.

Uses of mercury requiring small numbers of workers are mentioned because it is known that careless handling has caused poisoning (see Browning, 1969, for additional details). Manufacture of tungsten and molybdenum wires and rods for electrical contacts, filaments, and radio tube heaters requires the use of metallic mercury and heat (Lewis, 1945). Mercuric oxide is used for making dry batteries for use in hearing aids, small flashlights, and a variety of electronic products. A report by Williams et al. (1947) of experience with this industrial use claimed that mercuric oxide is far less hazardous than mercury vapor and that air levels up to 0.42 mg/m³ were not associated with illness except for "a few acute accidents." Without more information mercuric oxide must be considered hazardous.

Mercury can enter the body by way of the skin as well as the lungs. Mercury inunctions for medicinal purposes were used for many years because mercury penetrates intact skin. It is, however, the vapor that causes the most trouble in industry and that must be guarded against, especially if heat is used. This hazard is well illustrated by the report of Tennant et al. (1961) of five cases of acute pneumonitis, with one death, in workers exposed to high concentrations of mercury vapor as a result of the rupture of a boiler used for generating electricity. Symptoms began four hours after the accident. Necropsy of the fatal case showed interstitial pneumonitis without damage to liver or kidneys. Similar cases of acute mercury pneumonitis were reported by Seaton and Bishop (1978) after an industrial accident during the repair of a condenser in a power station.

Both the chemical and drug industries make mercury-containing compounds. Contraceptives, bacteriostatic agents, diuretics, and antiseptics make use of both inorganic and organic mercury salts. It is not surprising, then, that there are records of mercury illness among workers in drug manufacture. Cotter (1947) mentioned a variety of abnormal laboratory findings in asymptomatic workers exposed to organic mercurials in the drug industry. This report is hard to assess without further details of the industrial exposure.

Mercury is widely used in photoengraving and the paint industry uses mercury as an antifouling ingredient. A curious outbreak of transient neurological symptoms in a factory population was found by Miller et al. (1967) to be associated with mercury-containing paint, freshly applied to a heating system that was turned on before the paint was thoroughly dry. An unusual episode of mercury poisoning was reported by Agate and Buckell (1949) among British police who used gray powder (mercury with chalk) for fingerprint detection. Seven of 32 men developed classic chronic poisoning affecting the central nervous system. Elkins' (1959) experience is that in fluorescent lamp assembly there may be considerable absorption of mercury, but he reports no cases of poisoning. The history of occupational mercury poisoning has been recounted by Bidstrup (1964) and Goldwater (1972).

Metabolism

Mercury freezes at −39°C and vaporizes even at the temperature at which water turns to ice. Vapor pressure increases rapidly with increase in temperature so that at 24°C (75.2°F) the mercury concentration in the air can reach 18.3 mg Hg/m³.

Occupational exposure is usually to inorganic mercury by the inhalation of elemental mercury vapor or to aerosols of mercuric salts that are readily reducible. Elemental mercury can also enter the body by percutaneous absorption, although the rate of penetration is slow. Exposure may also occur to organic mercury compounds, typically the monoalkyl compounds (methyl and ethyl mercury), the salts of phenyl mercury, and methoxyethyl mercury (Report of an International Committee, 1969). In the body, metallic mercury is rapidly oxidized to divalent ionic mercury while methyl mercury undergoes biotransformation to Hg^{++} slowly, less than 1% per day (Clarkson, 1977). Other organic mercury compounds, such as phenyl mercury and mercurial diuretics, are rapidly converted to inorganic mercury in the body.

Clarkson also pointed out that the toxic effects of inhaled mercury vapor are probably attributable to the divalent mercury ion formed by oxidation, since the unchanged atomic form would not be expected to react with proteins and other cell constituents. It is of interest that the retention of inhaled mercury vapor is less in persons who previously consumed moderate amounts of alcohol (Nielsen-Kudsk, 1965).

Depending on the compound, mercury can be locally irritating or corrosive, and damaging to skin and mucous membranes. Mercury toxicity depends on a single basic mechanism: the mercuric ion acts to precipitate protein and to inhibit enzymes containing sulfhydryl groups. This inhibition of sulfhydryl enzymes is reversible after removal of the heavy metal, and this reversibility is the basis for the success of British antilewisite (BAL) in treating mercury poisoning.

Mercury vapor is absorbed readily and almost completely across the alveolar membranes of the lung and is cleared from the blood with a half-time of two to three days. Once mercury enters the circulation it is rapidly taken up, although the form of the mercuric ion circulated and deposited is not known. Mercury in tissue is found in varying quantities with the largest amount in the kidneys and decreasing amounts in liver, spleen, intestinal wall, heart, skeletal muscle, and lung.

Excretion starts immediately through kidney and colon and whole-body clearance has a half-time of 60 days (Hursh et al. 1976). Clearance from the kidneys in two cases of accidental inhalation of radioactive mercuric oxide aerosol ranged from half-times of 37 to 60 days (Newton and Fry, 1978). Clarkson (1968), in a helpful review, pointed out that there is a large area of ignorance of the precise biochemical mechanism of the action of mercury.

Workers exposed occupationally to mercury vapor as a group show a correlation between urine mercury levels and time-weighted averages of air concentration (Smith et al., 1970; Lindstedt et al., 1979). Blood mercury levels are indicative of recent exposure only in view of the rapid clearance of mercury from blood. Although oxidation is rapid, dissolved metallic mercury may persist in the bloodstream long enough to cross blood-brain and placental barriers. Once metallic mercury enters brain or fetal tissues, it is oxidized to the ionic form (Clarkson, 1977).

Mercury Poisoning in Industry

Industrial mercurialism is characterized by three features: inflammation of the mouth, muscle tremors, and psychic irritability — sometimes all three together, sometimes only two or even one. The picture of mercury poisoning found in toxicology textbooks is not what is usually seen in industrial poisoning. The severe gastrointestinal symptoms caused by the ingestion of mercury bichloride with nausea, vomiting, pain, purging, and bloody stools, and the severe involvement of the kidneys with scanty urine loaded with albumin and casts, form a picture almost never seen in industry. Lesions of the skin, which the textbooks give as a fairly common symptom, are also rare in industrial poisoning.

Older authorities such as Lehmann, Teleky, and Koelsch distinguished between the typically slow chronic form of industrial mercurialism and a subacute form that develops comparatively rapidly as a result of exposure to relatively large doses. For the latter, Kussmaul's classic description in 1861 still remains the most vivid and detailed picture in the literature. His observations were made among the Nuremberg-Furth mirror makers in the days when the method of backing mirrors involved the application of silver-mercury amalgam and driving off the mercury with heat. Similar methods were used for gold and silver plating. Now, of course, electroplating is used so

that cases of such severity are rare and are usually accidental.

Inflammation of the mouth   The changes in the mouth, consisting of inflammation of the gums (which become soft and spongy), loosening of the teeth, swelling of the salivary glands, and excessive flow of saliva are so well known as to give a name to the disease. Workers speak of "salivation" when they mean mercury poisoning, and the term has nothing to do with excess saliva, for it may be applied to a case where there have been no mouth symptoms at all. A man who has had an attack of "hatter's shakes" may tell you that he has been "salivated" even though his mouth and throat have been uncomfortably dry. The mouth is more likely to be affected in cases that develop fairly quickly from exposure to vapors of heated mercury. But hatters and hatters' furriers, metallurgists, and laboratory workers contract the slower form of poisoning, with little or no salivation, although some gingivitis with pyorrhea is common. A blue-gray line of mercury sulfide is sometimes visible along the gum margins. Stomatitis may be so severe as to interfere with speaking or chewing, but ptyalism is not a marked feature of chronic mercury poisoning.

Muscular tremors   The tremor of mercurialism is known as "hatters' shakes" because the hatters' trade was once the most notorious source of chronic mercurialism. It usually comes on slowly and first affects the muscles of the eyelids, tongue, and fingers. It is a typical intention tremor, increasing with the effort to control it and to make unusual motions, and dying down when the victim goes back to his accustomed work, or when he no longer feels himself under observation. The tremor is cerebellar in character, an uncontrollable ataxic motion, and with it go scanning speech and a handwriting like that in paralysis agitans. However, the tremor of mercurialism is not as regular as that of paralysis agitans, and it affects the whole hand, while in the latter each separate finger has its own tremor. Mercurial tremor is always lessened by repose and solitude, and disappears in sleep, even in severe cases. As it grows worse it spreads to the arms and legs, and jerky movements are added so that walking is difficult. The trembling causes changes in handwriting, and so characteristic is the jerky scrawl that periodic recording of writing is used to detect early evidence of chronic mercury poisoning. Men can keep on with the automatic motions involved in the making of felt hats even after they have reached the point of being unable to button their clothes, lace their boots, walk to their work-benches, or carry a cup of coffee to their mouths.

Usually, removal from exposure to mercury vapor results in recovery, although AH saw a case of apparently irreversible tremor in an old Danbury hatter who had been away from work for ten years. There are also a few reports from France of tremors persisting more than 30 years. Obviously, the duration and intensity of mercury exposure are critical factors in the persistence of tremors after exposure ceases. While mercury is steadily excreted from the body, distribution and storage in tissues other than the central nervous system influence the clinical picture. Chang (1977) pointed out, in his review of the neurotoxic effects of mercury, that vacuolar degeneration of neurons is a lesion mainly associated with inorganic mercury poisoning. Mercury penetrates the cytoplasm of neurons to produce degradation of cellular organelles but apparently does not enter the nucleus.

Psychic irritability   Mercurial tremor is closely associated with the psychic irritability that has been called *erethism,* from the Greek word for irritation, since it was first used by Pearson in London early in the 19th century (Buckell et al., 1946). There is an apprehensive timidity and shrinking from observation, a sense of discouragement, a loss of self-confidence, a fear of ridicule or criticism and of losing one's job, and loss of joy in life. Loss of memory is the commonest complaint, often associated with torpor from which, if the patient is roused, he shows great irritability. The affected workers have no tendency to exaggerate their symptoms; on the contrary, they are timid and diffident.

Erethism of mercurialism was very familiar among the miners and metallurgists in California, and the men recognized it in themselves as well as in others. They described an increasing shyness, anxiety, embarrassment at being noticed, loss of self-confidence, or irritability that was very marked if the victim was spoken to suddenly or asked to do something unusual. Some men were obliged to give up work because they could no longer take orders without losing their tempers, or, if they were foremen, they had no patience with the men they supervised. Sometimes, insomnia was the chief complaint, or bad dreams, or depression. Other men became drowsy and fell asleep as soon as they sat down.

Other Toxic Effects of Mercury

Skin lesions due to mercury are more commonly associated with organic (especially mercury fulminate) than with inorganic mercury exposures. Manifestations include erythema, intense itching, edema, papules, pustules, and, when mercury penetrates a skin abrasion, deep ulcers. Vermeiden's case of a vesicular eruption from inhalation of metallic mercury vapor has already been referred to. Kennedy et al. (1977) found electron-dense aggregates of mercury in dermal macrophages in a man whose facial pigmentation resulted from industrial inorganic mercury exposure.

Variations in the response of skin to mercury, both in industry and from the medicinal use of mercury compounds, is strong evidence of the sensitizing ability of mercury. Dental students have been found to have significant increases in the incidence of mercury sensitivity as they progressed through school, presumably from exposure to mercury in the preparation of silver amalgam (White and Brandt, 1976). HLH saw a chemistry student who developed such a severe reaction to metallic mercury that she was forced to abandon laboratory work. The same was true of a technician whose reaction was so violent that his skin was an exquisite monitor of mercury vapor, discovering its presence when those in charge of the laboratory considered it to be free of the element.

Severe mercury poisoning is reported to cause disabling constriction of the peripheral visual fields (Hunter et al., 1940). Atkinson's (1943) finding of a "brownish-coloured lustreless" reflex from the anterior capsule of the lens that was thought to be due to mercury was confirmed by Lockett and Nazroo (1952). These observers found that length of exposure was correlated with this mercurialentis. Most important, however, they found that the mercury-related phenomenon and the fine lens opacities seen in the same workers had no effect on vision.

Kantarjian (1961) reported six cases of farmers using material containing organic mercury compounds who developed a syndrome like progressive amyotrophic lateral sclerosis similar to the tragic disease associated with the ingestion of mercury-contaminated food. Friberg et al. (1953) believed that two workers, exposed to organic mercurials at levels considered safe but who developed nephrosis and recovered when exposure ceased, were suffering unusual sensitivity to mercury.

100

Diagnosis of Mercury Poisoning

The diagnosis of industrial mercury poisoning is not easy. Well-documented, high-level exposures associated with salivation, stomatitis, tremors, and psychic irritability have been rare in the mercury-using industry in recent years. Nonspecificity of spongy gums, transient proteinuria, and vague neurasthenic complaints make a diagnosis of toxic mercury effect difficult. There must be knowledge of the kind and amount of mercury absorbed by inhalation or through the skin and the amount excreted in the urine in order to make a presumptive diagnosis of mercury poisoning. A dose of N-acetyl-D-penicillamine to provoke an increase in mercury excretion is a useful diagnostic tool. Atkinson's (1943) brownish reflex from the anterior capsule of the lens may also be helpful, although it may be absent in some workers exposed to mercury (Lovejoy et al., 1973). Hair content of mercury has been studied by a number of laboratories and a variety of methods (Nord et al., 1973; Hefferren, 1976), but this analysis has offered no help in the diagnosis of occupational mercury intoxication.

Apparently, the kidney can eliminate mercury at low levels for a long period without damage, and urinary changes may be absent in cases of undoubted chronic mercurialism. Urinary abnormalities due to mercury are not specific although albuminuria was found in a fairly large proportion of hatters with chronic poisoning. Both polyuria and oliguria have been described in hatters, and proteinuria and hematuria have been recorded in cases of industrial mercury exposures of relatively high level and short duration.

Control

There are published reports of the quantities of mercury associated with worker illness. Göthlin (1909) examined himself and his fellow laboratory workers and decided that the danger line for causing chronic poisoning began at a daily absorption of 0.4 mg per day. Up to that point, excretion by the kidneys kept pace with absorption. Such a daily dose would take many years to bring about mercurialism. The amount of mercury in the air that is capable of causing severe, even fatal, poisoning was found by Jordan and Barrows (1924) to be 0.7 mg/m³ of air if breathed steadily in a 40-hour workweek. They recorded seven cases of poisoning with one death. Hill (1943)

estimated, on the basis of two deaths, that the fatal level is 1.04 mg/m³ breathed over a period of three months. Shepherd et al. (1941) examined 38 laboratory workers who were exposed to mercury vapors. They concluded that there was no medical evidence of mercurialism for those workers who were exposed to concentrations ranging from less than 0.4 to 0.7 mg Hg/m³ of air. Only with exposures to more than 1.0 mg Hg/m³ were cases of mercurialism found.

The question of how much mercury produces damage was further clarified by studies made in the two allied trades, fur-cutting and felt-hat manufacture (Neal et al., 1937, 1941). As noted above, they found 59 cases of mercurialism among 534 hatters who had worked in atmospheres containing from 0.2 to 0.5 mg Hg/m³ of air. They concluded that 0.1 mg Hg/m³ probably represents the upper limit of safety. In 1969 an International Committee decided that accumulated knowledge required that the safe level be lowered to 0.05 mg/m³, except for alkyl compounds for which the safe level was set at 0.01 mg/m³ because of their greater hazard. NIOSH (1973) has agreed with the International Committee and has recommended that workers not be exposed to concentrations of inorganic mercury greater than 0.05 mg Hg/m³ determined as a time-weighted average (TWA) exposure for an 8-hour workday. Nevertheless, the current OSHA ceiling limit for quicksilver is 0.1 mg Hg/m³ of air. In this connection, Bell et al. (1973) found, in their study of workers in a mercury-cell facility, that there was a close correspondence between the mercury contained in a 16-hour composite urine sample and measured TWA air exposures.

Prevention of toxic mercury damage in industry depends upon proper engineering control with enclosure or ventilation as necessary to keep the amount inhaled or absorbed below the level of 0.05 mg/m³ of air and below 0.2 mg Hg/L of urine for steady exposure. Goldwater and his colleagues, beginning in 1962, published a series of studies on the mercury contained in the biological fluids of workers (Goldwater et al., 1962; Jacobs et al., 1963; Ladd et al., 1963). They concluded that blood and urine excretion levels are poorly correlated with clinical evidence of intoxication, although Joselow et al. (1968b) reported that the mercury content of saliva is correlated with blood mercury levels. Lovejoy et al. (1973) published interesting data showing that mercury leaves the body first and significantly by sweating. They suggest that the old saying of mercury miners, "sweating them out," was the method of choice in healthy workers before chelating agents were used.

Wada and associates (1969) found a significant correlation in 47 healthy workers between urine mercury and decrease in activity of δ-amino-levulinic acid dehydratase (ALAD) and cholinesterase. This correlation was especially true in cases of long-term mercury exposure in the presence of renal disease. However, since exposures to vapor and dust differ and since mercury may be absorbed through unbroken skin and the biological indices are not unique for mercury, there is no thoroughly dependable mercury excretion level that may serve as a precise measure of mercury body burden. Because of physiological variations, unusual sensitivity, or disease processes in individual cases, signs of poisoning may appear at urine levels higher or lower than those published as indices of safety.

On the basis of knowledge of industrial mercury poisoning, it is common sense not to expose to mercury those workers who have nervous system disease, impaired renal function, or a history of unusual sensitivity to drugs or chemicals. Routine and repeated urinalyses, renal function tests, and a record of periodic handwriting samples provide helpful warnings in jobs where air concentrations of mercury are difficult to control. Such steps should be supplemented by examination of the skin and mouth and interviews with workers and foremen to detect signs of mercury effect on the nervous system.

Urinalyses for mercury levels should be done on a regular schedule by an experienced laboratory. The several methods available have not produced consistently accurate and reproducible results. As much as 100% loss of volatile mercury from urine has been reported. Dinman (1958) studied published reports of poisoning at low levels of mercury and concluded that in these cases the measurements of air and urine mercury were in error. Many reports fail to take account of skin and gastrointestinal tract as portals of entry and excretion of organic mercury compounds. Without industrial exposure, as much as 100 μg of mercury may be excreted in the urine in 24 hours. Dental amalgam may also give surprisingly high temporary urine mercury levels. Depending on the dose and duration of exposure, organic mercurials (diuretics or industrial) may cause continuing excretion of mercury for long periods after exposure.

It is important to remember that mercury-soiled clothing or floor covering may be the cause of poisoning, for the continual vaporization of the metal will lead to inhalation of small quantities even when the person is not at work, or the conditions may be ideal for skin absorption. Some years ago several miners' wives became poisoned as a result of washing their husbands' work clothes that contained metallic mercury. The children of Idria miners were said to acquire mercurialism if they slept in the same bed with their fathers. Indication of the importance of skin absorption was shown by Buckell et al. (1946), who found that 72 mercury workers making thermometers were excreting up to 10 times as much mercury as they could possibly absorb from the atmosphere. Washings from the hands indicated that absorption from the skin was the explanation. Because mercury penetrates many materials, including rubber, adequate protective gloves must be provided.

Mercury miners have definite ideas as to the proper way to prevent poisoning. They believe that the practice, prevalent among the Spanish miners, of rolling their own cigarettes is dangerous because it requires only a little over 300°C to reduce cinnabar and produce mercury vapors, and they believe that this occurs when cinnabar dust is mixed with the tobacco or is smeared on the cigarette paper, and the cigarette is then lighted and smoked. This danger is even greater when the worker is handling pure quicksilver. Old hands always advise a new man to give up smoking and begin chewing tobacco instead, believing, as most workers in dusts and vapors do, that constant spitting gets rid of much of the inhaled poison. They also believe, with good reason, that if a man takes a shower bath and puts on fresh clothing, not his work clothes, at the end of his shift, he can protect himself against an attack.

Treatment of Mercury Poisoning

The treatment of industrial mercury poisoning has been dramatically changed with the introduction of such agents as British antilewisite (BAL; 2,3-dimercaptopropanol) and a chelating compound, N-acetyl-D-penicillamine. Treatment with BAL should be reserved for acute poisoning, while penicillamine is useful for chronic intoxication, although Gledhill and Hopkins (1972) disagreed on the basis of their experience. The currently suggested treatment schedule for BAL is 5 mg/kg injected intramuscularly initially, followed by 2.5 mg/kg one or two times daily for 10 days (*AMA Drug Evaluations,* 1980). Variations in both the patient's clinical status and the estimate of total amount of mercury absorbed will dictate changes in this regimen. The D isomer of penicillamine is available in 125 and 250 mg capsules and is given orally. It is given in four doses per day up to a total of 1 to 4 g daily, depending on the age and size of the patient, as well as on the clinical picture and knowledge of the duration and intensity of mercury exposure (Hirschman et al., 1963). Calcium ethylenediaminetetraacetic acid (EDTA) is contraindicated according to experimental studies of Glömme and Gustavson (1959). Penicillamine chelates iron and copper as well as mercury so that long-term oral therapy may require, according to Moeschlin (1965), the addition of potassium sulfide (49 mg with meals) to reduce copper absorption, as well as an iron preparation. He also suggested the addition of a stabilized hydrogen sulfide preparation after a course of BAL as well as injection of 20 ml of a 10% solution of calcium gluconate during the clinically acute period of heavy metal poisoning. Large infusions of isotonic sodium chloride are suggested to produce diuresis and thus protect the kidney from high concentrations of mercury. Such vigorous therapy is reserved for very acute poisoning or if BAL or N-acetyl-D-penicillamine are not immediately available. Treatment of suicidal, homicidal, or accidental intake of large amounts of mercury require early heroic measures by gastric lavage with milk.

When the diagnosis of mercury poisoning is uncertain because of inadequate history or relatively low urine mercury, the use of a one-day course of oral penicillamine has been found to be useful by HLH as a diagnostic device. Tandon and Magos (1980) have found that 2,3-dimercaptosuccinic acid (DMSA) is the most successful of the thiol-complexing agents in the treatment of chronic mercury poisoning in rats. Contrary to the experience of Sanchez-Sicilia et al. (1963), hemodialysis has been successful in removing relatively large amounts of mercury in cases of renal shutdown due to mercury.

References

Agate JN, Buckell M: Mercury poisoning from fingerprint photography: Occupational hazard of policemen. *Lancet* 1949;2:451–454.

AMA Drug Evaluations. Chicago, American Medical Association, 1980.

Atkinson WS: A colored reflex from the anterior capsule of the lens which occurs in mercurialism. *Am J Ophthalmol* 1943;26:685–688.

Baldi G, Vigliani EC, Zurlo N: Il mercurialismo cronico nei cappellifici. *Med lavoro* 1953;44:161–198, abstracted in *Arch Ind Hyg Occup Med* 1953;8:847.

Battistone GC, Hefferren JJ, Miller RA, et al: Mercury: Its relation to the dentist's health and dental practice characteristics. *J Am Dent Assoc* 1976;92:1182–1188.

Bell ZG Jr, Lovejoy HB, Vizena TR: Mercury exposure evaluations and their correlation with urine mercury excretions: 3. Time-weighted average (TWA) mercury exposures and urine mercury levels. *J Occup Med* 1973;15:501–508.

Benning D: Outbreak of mercury poisoning in Ohio. *Ind Med Surg* 1958;27:354–363.

Bidstrup PL: *Toxicity of Mercury and its Compounds.* New York, Elsevier, 1964.

Browning E: *Toxicity of Industrial Metals,* ed 2. New York, Appleton-Century-Crofts, 1969, pp 226–242.

Buckell M, Hunter D, Milton R, et al: Chronic mercury poisoning. *Br J Ind Med* 1946;3:55–63.

Buxton JT Jr, Hewitt JC, Gadsden RH, et al: Metallic mercury embolism: Report of cases. *J Am Med Assoc* 1965;193:573–575.

Chang LW: Neurotoxic effects of mercury—A review. *Environ Res* 1977;14:329–373.

Clarkson TW: Biochemical aspects of mercury poisoning. *J Occup Med* 1968;10:351–355.

Clarkson TW: Mercury poisoning, in Brown SS (ed): *Clinical Chemistry and Chemical Toxicology of Metals.* New York, Elsevier, 1977, pp 189–200.

Cotter LH: Hazard of phenylmercuric salts. *Occup Med* 1947;4:305–309.

Dales LG: The neurotoxicity of alkyl mercury compounds. *Am J Med* 1972;53:219–232.

Danziger SJ, Possick PA: Metallic mercury exposure in scientific glassware manufacturing plants. *J Occup Med* 1973;15:15–20.

Dennis L: Hatting as affecting the health of operatives. *Rep Board Health New Jersey* 1878; iii:67–85.

Dinman DB, Evans EE, Linch AL: Organic mercury: Environmental exposure, excretion, and prevention of intoxication in its manufacture. *Arch Ind Health* 1958;18:248–260.

Elkins HB: *The Chemistry of Industrial Toxicology,* ed 2. New York, John Wiley, 1959.

El-Sadik YM, El-Dakhakhny AA: Effects of exposure of workers to mercury at a sodium hydroxide producing plant. *Am Ind Hyg Assoc J* 1970;31:705–710.

Freeman JA: Mercurial disease among hatters. *Trans Med Soc New Jersey* 1860; pp 61–64.

Friberg L, Hammarström S, Nyström A: Kidney injury after chronic exposure to inorganic mercury. *Arch Ind Hyg Occup Med* 1953;8:149–153.

Gledhill RF, Hopkins AP: Chronic inorganic mercury poisoning treated with N-acetyl-D-penicillamine. *Br J Ind Med* 1972;29:225–228.

Glömme J, Gustavson KH: Treatment of experimental acute mercury poisoning by chelating agents BAL and EDTA. *Acta Med Scand* 1959; 164:175–182.

Goldwater LJ: *Mercury, A History of Quicksilver*. Baltimore, York, 1972.

Goldwater LJ, Jacobs MR, Ladd AC: Absorption and excretion of mercury in man: I. Relationship of mercury in blood and urine. *Arch Environ Health* 1962;5:537–541.

Goldwater LJ, Kleinfeld M, Berger AR: Mercury exposure in a university laboratory. *Arch Ind Health* 1956;13:245–249.

Göthlin GF: Kvicksilfverhaltig luft och fall af kronisk kvicksilfverförgiftning vid en medicinsk läroanstalt. *Hyg Tijdskr* 1909;138–181, abstracted in *Hyg Rundschau* 1911;21:390.

Gronka PA, Bobkoskie RL, Tomchick GJ, et al: Mercury vapor exposures in dental offices. *J Am Dent Assoc* 1970;81:923–925.

Hamilton A: Industrial hygiene of fur cutting and felt hat manufacture. *J Ind Hyg* 1922a;4: 137–153.

Hamilton A: Industrial diseases of fur cutters and hatters. *J Ind Hyg* 1922b;4:219–234.

Harris LI: A clinical and sanitary study of the fur and hatters' fur trade. Monograph series No. 12, Dept of Health, City of New York, 1915.

Hefferren JJ: Usefulness of chemical analysis of head hair for exposure to mercury. *J Am Dent Assoc* 1976;92:1213–1216.

Hill WH: A report on two deaths from exposure to the fumes of diethyl mercury. *Can J Publ Health* 1943;34:158–160.

Hirschman SZ, Feingold M, Boylen G: Mercury in house paint as a cause of acrodynia. Effect of therapy with N-acetyl-D,L-penicillamine. *N Engl J Med* 1963;269:889–893.

Hunter D, Bomford RR, Russell DS: Poisoning by methyl mercury compounds. *Q J Med* 1940; 9:193–213.

Hursh JB, Clarkson TW, Cherian MG, et al: Clearance of mercury (Hg-197, Hg-203) vapor inhaled by human subjects. *Arch Environ Health* 1976;31:302–309.

International Committee: Report of an International Committee. *Arch Environ Health* 1969;19: 891–905.

Jacobs MR, Ladd AC, Goldwater LJ: Absorption and excretion of mercury in man: III. Blood mercury in relation to duration of exposure. *Arch Environ Health* 1963;6:634–637.

Jordan L, Barrows WP: Mercury poisoning from electric furnaces. *Ind Eng Chem* 1924;16: 898–901.

Jordi A: Quecksilbervergiftungen bei Munitionsarbeitern. *Schweiz Med Wchnschr* 1947;77: 621–623, abstracted in *J Ind Hyg Toxicol* 1948; 30:77.

Joselow MM, Goldwater LJ: Absorption and excretion of mercury in man: XII. Relationship between urinary mercury and proteinuria. *Arch Environ Health* 1967;15:155–159.

Joselow MM, Goldwater LJ, Alvarez A, et al: Absorption and excretion of mercury in man: XV. Occupational exposure among dentists. *Arch Environ Health* 1968a;17:39–43.

Joselow MM, Ruiz R, Goldwater LJ: Absorption and excretion of mercury in man: XIV. Salivary excretion of mercury and its relationship to blood and urine mercury. *Arch Environ Health* 1968b;17:35–38.

Kantarjian AD: A syndrome clinically resembling amyotrophic lateral sclerosis following chronic mercurialism. *Neurology* 1961;11:639–644.

Kennedy C, Molland EA, Henderson WJ, et al: Mercury pigmentation from industrial exposure: An ultrastructural and analytic electron microscopic study. *Br J Dermatol* 1977;96:367–374.

Kussmaul A: *Untersuchungen über dem constitutionellen Mercurialismus*. Würzburg, 1861.

Ladd AC, Goldwater LJ, Jacobs MR: Absorption and excretion of mercury in man: II. Urinary mercury in relation to duration of exposure. *Arch Environ Health* 1963;6:480–483.

Lewis L: Mercury poisoning in tungsten-molybdenum rod and wire manufacturing industry. *J Am Med Assoc* 1945;129:123–129.

Lindstedt G, Gottberg I, Holmgren B, et al: Individual mercury exposure of chloralkali workers and its relation to blood and urine mercury levels. *Scand J Work Environ Health* 1979;5:59–69.

Lockett S, Nazroo IA: Eye changes following exposure to metallic mercury. *Lancet* 1952;1: 528–530.

Lovejoy HB, Bell ZG Jr, Vizena TR: Mercury

exposure evaluations and their correlation with urinary mercury excretions: Part 4. Elimination of mercury by sweating. *J Occup Med* 1973;15: 590–591.

Miller G, Chamberlin R, McCormack WM: An outbreak of neuromyasthenia in a Kentucky factory: The possible role of a brief exposure to organic mercury. *Am J Epidemiol* 1967;86:756–764.

Moeschlin S: *Poisoning: Diagnosis and Treatment*. New York, Grune and Stratton, 1965.

Neal PA, Jones RR, Bloomfield JJ, et al: A study of hatters' mercurialism in the hatters' fur cutting industry. *Public Health Bull* No. 234, Washington, DC, 1937.

Neal PA, Flinn RH, Edwards TI, et al: Mercurialism and its control in the felt hat industry. *Public Health Bull* No. 263, Washington, DC, 1941.

Newton D, Fry FA: The retention and distribution of radioactive mercuric oxide following accidental inhalation. *Ann Occup Hyg* 1978;21:21–32.

Nielsen-Kudsk F: The influence of ethyl alcohol on the absorption of mercury vapour from the lungs in man. *Acta Pharmacol* 1965;23:263–274.

NIOSH: *Criteria for a Recommended Standard . . . .Occupational Exposure to Inorganic Mercury*. Washington, DC, National Institute for Occupational Safety and Health (NIOSH 73-11024), 1973.

Nord PJ, Kadaba MP, Sorenson JRJ: Mercury in human hair. *Arch Environ Health* 1973;27:40–44.

Popper L: Tod nach Thermometerverletzung. *Wien Med Wchnschr* 1966;116:779–780, abstracted in *Can Med Assoc J* 1967;96:Adv 8, Jan 14.

Rothwell PS, Frame JW, Shimmin CV: Mercury vapour hazards from hot air sterilisers in dental practice. *Br Dent J* 1977;142:359–365.

Sanchez-Sicilia L, Seto S, Nakamoto S, et al: Acute mercurial intoxication treated by hemodialysis. *Ann Intern Med* 1963;59:692–706.

Seaton A, Bishop CM: Acute mercury pneumonitis. *Br J Ind Med* 1978;35:258–261.

Shepherd M, Schuhmann S, Flinn RH, et al: Hazard of mercury vapor in scientific laboratories. *J Res Natl Bur Stand* 1941;26:357–375.

Smith DL: Mental effects of mercury poisoning. *South Med J* 1978;71:904–905.

Smith RG, Vorwald AJ, Patil LS, et al: Effects of exposure to mercury in the manufacture of chlorine. *Am Ind Hyg Assoc J* 1970;31:687–700.

Stewart WK, Guirgis HA, Sanderson J, et al: Urinary mercury excretion and proteinuria in pathology laboratory staff. *Br J Ind Med* 1977; 34:26–31.

Tandon SK, Magos L: Effect of kidney damage on the mobilisation of mercury by thiolcomplexing agents. *Br J Ind Med* 1980;37:128–132.

Tennant R, Johnston HJ, Wells JB: Acute bilateral pneumonitis associated with the inhalation of mercury vapor: Report of five cases. *Conn Med* 1961;25:106–109.

Vermeiden I, Oranje AP, Vuzevski VD, et al: Mercury exanthem as occupational dermatitis. *Contact Derm* 1980;6:88–90.

Vigliani EC: Infortunio da penetrazione di mercurio metallico nel sottocutaneo e sue conseguenze. *Med lavoro* 1946;37:7–13 abstracted in *J Ind Hyg Toxicol* 1948;30:11.

Wada O, Toyokawa K, Suzuki T, et al: Response to a low concentration of mercury vapor: Relation to human porphyrin metabolism. *Arch Environ Health* 1969;19:485–488.

West I, Lim J: Mercury poisoning among workers in California's mercury mills. *J Occup Med* 1968;10:697–701.

White RR, Brandt RL: Development of mercury hypersensitivity among dental students. *J Am Dent Assoc* 1976;92:1204–1207.

Williams CR, Eisenbud M, Pihl SE: Mercury exposure in dry battery manufacture. *J Ind Hyg Toxicol* 1947;29:378–381.

Wright W: A clinical study of fur cutters and felt hatters. *J Ind Hyg* 1922;4:296–304.

18 • *Molybdenum*

Uses and Industrial Hazards

The principal use of molybdenum is in alloying ferrous and nonferrous metals. Molybdenum steel is very resistant to chemicals and has great hardness. Because of these properties, there are many military uses in armor plate and rifle linings and in peace-time industry in high pressure boiler plates. Additional uses of molybdenum are in the manufacture of glass, ceramics, and pigments and as lubricants and catalysts. Molybdenum wire is used by the radio and electrical industry. Because molybdenum is essential for the fixation of nitrogen in soil by bacteria, fertilizers contain this element (Browning, 1969). Two mammalian enzymes, both dehydrogenases, are dependent upon molybdenum as a co-factor: xanthine and aldehyde oxidases (Schroeder et al., 1970).

There have been no reports of ill effects in workers exposed to molybdenum dust in the crushing and milling of ore. This situation is also true in the case of workers exposed to the fumes of molybdenum oxide in rolling red-hot billets of molybdenum steel. However, exposure of workers to molybdenum dust in a molybdenite roasting plant was recently found to be accompanied by substantial elevations of serum ceruloplasmin and smaller increases in serum uric acid levels. The estimated daily intake of Mo inhaled as dust particles averaged 10.2 mg, and both plasma and urine molybdenum levels were significantly increased in these workers. Joint pains, backaches, headaches, and nonspecific hair and skin changes were the most frequent medical complaints, but no long-term adverse health effects have yet been demonstrated, perhaps because of the high turnover rate in employment at the plant (Walravens et al., 1979).

Animal Studies

Because of the importance of molybdenum in animal nutrition, there is a vast literature on the harmful effects in animals of both deprivation of molybdenum, an essential trace element, and excessive doses (Fairhall et al., 1945; Underwood, 1977; Schroeder et al., 1970; Pitt, 1976). Cattle, feeding in pastures where there is an excess of molybdenum in the soil, contract a disease known as "teart" characterized by anemia and diarrhea. Inhalation studies have shown the trioxide to be very irritating to guinea pigs.

Control

Recommended permissible exposure limits have been set, largely on the basis of experience with animals, at 5 mg/m³ and 15 mg/m³, respectively, for soluble and insoluble molybdenum compounds (NIOSH, 1978). Walravens et al. (1979) question whether the former value is safe, since their studies demonstrated systemic absorption of molybdenum from inhaled dusts.

References

Browning E: *Toxicity of Industrial Metals,* ed 2. New York, Appleton-Century-Crofts, 1969, pp 243–248.

Fairhall LT, Dunn RC, Sharpless NE, et al: The toxicity of molybdenum. *Public Health Service Bull* No. 293, 1945.

NIOSH/OSHA: *Pocket Guide to Chemical Hazards.* Washington, DC, National Institute for Occupational Safety and Health (NIOSH 78-210), 1978.

Pitt MA: Molybdenum toxicity: Interactions

106

between copper, molybdenum and sulphate. *Agents and Actions* 1976;6:758–769.

Schroeder HA, Balassa JJ, Tipton IH: Essential trace elements in man: Molybdenum. *J Chron Dis* 1970;23:481–499.

Underwood EJ: *Trace Elements in Human and Animal Nutrition,* ed 4. New York, Academic Press, 1977, pp 109–131.

Walravens PA, Moure-Erasco R, Solomons CC, et al: Biochemical abnormalities in workers exposed to molybdenum dust. *Arch Environ Health* 1979;34:302–308.

19 • Nickel

Occurrence and Uses

The name nickel originated in the Harz mountains among copper miners who, finding their ores contaminated, ascribed the mischief to Old Nick. The evil contaminant proved to be arsenic compounded with an element that later received the name nickel (Hunter, 1978, p. 445).

Canada supplies about 45% of all nickel; smaller amounts (16% to 18%) come from USSR and New Caledonia, while Cuba, Australia, and Indonesia contribute about 5% each to world production (National Academy of Sciences, 1975). The Mond process was developed in Wales for the industrial production of pure nickel and involves the exposure of nickel oxide to carbon monoxide to make nickel carbonyl, $Ni(CO)_4$, a gaseous compound that can be condensed by cold into a clear liquid volatilizing at room temperature. When heated to 180°C, it decomposes to deposit metallic nickel with release of carbon monoxide. As a gas, nickel carbonyl has a peculiar sooty odor at low concentrations.

Although it was once thought that of nickel exposures only the carbonyl was hazardous, Doll et al. (1977) state that epidemiologic evidence also incriminates nickel dust exposures in the preliminary refining processes such as calcining of impure nickel sulfide to nickel copper oxide. Apart from the several refining processes, summarized by Morgan (1979), potential exposure is widespread, since there are at least 3000 known nickel alloys. Monel metal, a widely used material, is an alloy containing 67% nickel and 27% copper.

Uses of nickel leading to industrial exposures include the following (Browning, 1969; National Academy of Sciences, 1975):

1. Pure nickel: plating anodes, radio and electronic parts
2. Nickel-cadmium: storage batteries
3. Nickel-iron: heavy machinery, automotive parts, electrical equipment parts, permanent magnets
4. Nickel-copper (Monel): food processing and chemical equipment, condenser plates, coins
5. Nickel-aluminum: auto and aircraft parts
6. Nickel-chromium: gas turbine and jet engine parts
7. Nickel-copper-zinc: jewelry, plumbing fixtures
8. Nickel-chromium-iron: stainless steel cooking utensils
9. Nickel salts: electroplating baths (accounts for 16% of U.S. nickel consumption) and catalysts in hydrogenation of fats and oils

Reports of Worker Illness

The occupational hazards from nickel can be grouped into those leading to dermatitis, those from acute exposure to nickel carbonyl, and the problems of lung and sinus cancer from inhalation of nickel dusts and compounds.

Nickel dermatitis due to wearing nickel-plated metal objects such as wristwatches, jewelry, and spectacle frames is well known to dermatologists. The offending nickel compound is produced by interaction with sweat and the diagnosis can be established by patch testing, or more recently by leukocyte migration inhibition assay (Jordan and Dvorak, 1976). The dermatitis is usually completely cured by removing contact with nickel-containing objects. Nickel and its compounds are not absorbed through unbroken skin, and epidermal binding of nickel has been demonstrated and attributed to carboxyl groups (Samitz and Katz, 1976).

So-called nickel eczema, or "nickel itch," is fairly common in nickel-plating plants. The eruption typically begins with itching, burning, and erythema of the worker's hands and arms, and, if he is not removed from exposure to nickel, will spread to his neck and legs or to the whole body. If a man has been once affected, he is practically sure to have another attack, which comes on more promptly than the first, with lesions that heal slowly. Cases in which the eruption extends over a considerable portion of the body can be extremely serious and may require hospital care. Even careful industrial control may not make it possible for a sensitized worker to continue work with nickel. Nickel dermatitis from occupational exposure appears to be declining in the major industries (Marcussen, 1960) but it remains a problem in electroplating shops and in minor occupations, probably from contact with costume jewelry and other common nickel-containing items. McConnell et al. (1973) described asthma as a manifestation of nickel sensitivity. In view of the widespread industrial use of nickel, such asthma must be rare or unrecognized.

The most important hazard in the nickel-using industry arises as a result of inhalation exposure to nickel carbonyl even in very low concentrations. Two phases of acute poisoning are described. Headache, dizziness, nausea, and vomiting appear first, usually immediately after exposure. After an interval of time, depending on the exposure dose and the physical activity of the worker, severe pulmonary symptoms develop with chest pain and tightness, dyspnea, and dry cough, and cyanosis and extreme weakness occur. Leukocytosis and fever may also be present. In heavily exposed unrecognized cases death may follow in four to 10 days, and may be preceded by mental confusion, delirium, and convulsions (Mastromatteo, 1967; National Academy of Sciences, 1975). Patients who recover from acute nickel carbonyl poisoning usually have a prolonged convalescence because of persistent pulmonary insufficiency. The chief pathologic findings in fatal cases are diffuse interstitial pneumonitis and cerebral hemorrhage or edema (Sunderman, 1977).

While chronic disease has not been reported, repeated attacks of acute chemical pneumonitis, however mild, must be considered responsible, alone or with factors such as cigarette smoking, for chronic disabling lung disease. The question of chronic damage to the central nervous system among nickel carbonyl workers has not been examined.

Malignancies of lung and nasal cavities among workers exposed in the Mond process to arsenic and nickel have been established as a significant risk (Doll, 1958; Morgan, 1958; Williams, 1958). Sunderman (1977) has collected from the world literature 447 cases of lung cancer and 143 cases of cancer of the nose and paranasal cavities among nickel workers, but many of these were also exposed to arsenic, chromium, and cobalt. Inhaled particles of metallic nickel dust, nickel oxide, and nickel subsulfide have been implicated as carcinogenic along with nickel carbonyl vapor (National Academy of Sciences, 1975; Sunderman, 1976) although one recent long-term study of workers exposed to metallic nickel dust showed no evidence of increased mortality from respiratory cancer (Godbold and Tompkins, 1979). There may be an important interaction between nickel and asbestos in the development of occupational cancers and Kreyberg (1978) continues to stress the importance of tobacco smoking in the etiology of lung cancer in nickel refinery workers.

Comprehensive summaries of the literature on nickel toxicity to humans and animals can be found in the National Academy of Sciences monograph (1975) and the NIOSH documents on inorganic nickel (1977) and nickel carbonyl (1977).

Toxicity to Animals

There are many studies of animal reactions to nickel and its compounds, in part because of their therapeutic use in the past and more recently in attempts to understand their biochemical and toxicologic behavior, including carcinogenesis. Hueper (1952) and Sunderman et al. (1959) produced malignant lesions experimentally with nickel compounds. Gilman (1962) showed that the subsulfide (Ni_2S_3), a major constituent of refinery flue dust, induces a higher incidence of tumors than does the oxide when injected into rats. Nickel subsulfide carcinogenicity in these rodents is inhibited by manganese (Sunderman et al., 1974). The metabolism and toxicology of nickel in experimental animals have been summarized by Sunderman (1977), and the large literature on experimental nickel carcinogenesis was reviewed by Sunderman (1976).

Therapy and Control

Acute lung reaction due to nickel carbonyl is treated as are all forms of chemical pneumonitis by complete rest and oxygen. Vuopala et al. (1970) have stressed the value of preventive antibiotics and steroids. Calcium sodium ethylenediaminetetraacetic acid ($CaNa_2$ EDTA) has proved to be useless. British antilewisite (BAL, dimercaprol) is of some value in promoting urinary excretion of nickel (Sunderman and Kincaid, 1954).

Sunderman and Sunderman (1958) reported the value of sodium diethyldithiocarbamate (dithiocarb), a drug that can be used orally, in cases of overexposure to nickel carbonyl. By 1971, 50 workers with acute nickel carbonyl poisoning had been successfully treated with this compound and all were able to return to work within three weeks (Sunderman, 1971). The dosage is regulated initially by the urinary nickel concentration. Since dithiocarb is an intermediary metabolite of disulfiram (Antabuse), patients receiving the former should abstain from alcoholic beverages during and for one week after therapy. Sedatives such as paraldehyde and chloral hydrate, tranquilizers, and other psychopharmacologic drugs should also be avoided. Oral disulfiram has been used successfully to treat dermatitis in nickel-hypersensitive patients (Kaaber et al., 1979), presumably by the chelating action of dithiocarb.

Since nickel carbonyl is excreted primarily in the urine (Tedeschi and Sunderman, 1957), the measurement of nickel in urine specimens of exposed workmen is important both for monitoring exposure and for guiding therapy. The normal concentration of nickel in urine does not exceed 6 µg/dl (Sunderman, 1970). Human exposure to nickel carbonyl is considered to be mild if the nickel concentration in the initial 8-hour specimen is less than 10 µg/dl, moderately severe if it is between 10–50 µg/dl, and severe if it is above the latter range (Sunderman and Sunderman, 1958). Toia et al. (1979) found close positive correlations between air nickel concentrations in an electroplating shop and urine and plasma nickel levels of the exposed workers. Plasma nickel values have been used to monitor exposure of nickel refinery workers in Norway (Høgetveit et al., 1978).

The toxic potential of industrial nickel exposure makes its control mandatory. The current (1980) U.S. standard for occupational exposure to nickel metal and soluble nickel salts measured as nickel is an 8-hour TWA concentration limit of 1 mg/m^3, although NIOSH (1977) has proposed a limit of 0.015 mg/m^3 for a 10-hour TWA. For nickel carbonyl the permissible exposure limit is 0.001 ppm (0.007 mg/m^3). Engineering controls and protective clothing are obviously needed to insure safe working conditions.

References

Browning E: Toxicity of Industrial Metals, ed 2. New York, Appleton-Century-Crofts, 1969, pp 249–260.

Doll R: Cancer of the lung and nose in nickel workers. Br J Ind Med 1958;15:217–223.

Doll R, Mathews JD, Morgan LG: Cancers of the lung and nasal sinuses in nickel workers: A reassessment of the period of risk. Br J Ind Med 1977;34:102–105.

Gilman JPW: Metal carcinogenesis: II. A study on the carcinogenic activity of cobalt, copper, iron and nickel compounds. Cancer Res 1962; 22:158–162.

Godbold JH Jr, Tompkins EA: A long-term mortality study of workers occupationally exposed to metallic nickel at the Oak Ridge Gaseous Diffusion Plant. J Occup Med 1979;21:799–805.

Hueper WC: Experimental studies in metal carcinogenesis. Nickel cancer in rats. Texas Rep Biol Med 1952;10:167–186.

Hunter D: Diseases of Occupations, ed 6. London, Hodder and Stoughton, 1978, p 445.

Høgetveit AC, Barton RT, Kostøl CO: Plasma nickel as a primary index of exposure in nickel refining. Ann Occup Hyg 1978;21:113–120.

Jordan WP Jr, Dvorak J: Leukocyte migration inhibition assay (LIF) in nickel contact dermatitis. Arch Dermatol 1976;112:1741–1744.

Kaaber K, Menne T, Tjell JC, et al: Antabuse treatment of nickel dermatitis. Chelation—A new principle in the treatment of nickel dermatitis. Contact Derm 1979;5:221–228.

Kreyberg L: Lung cancer in workers in a nickel refinery. Br J Ind Med 1978;35:109–116.

Marcussen PV: Ecological considerations on nickel dermatitis. Br J Ind Med 1960;17:65–68.

Mastromatteo E: Nickel: A review of its occupational health aspects. J Occup Med 1967; 9:127–136.

McConnell LH, Fink JN, Schlueter DP, et al:

Asthma caused by nickel sensitivity. *Ann Intern Med* 1973;78:888–890.

Morgan JG: Some observations on the incidence of respiratory cancer in nickel workers. *Br J Ind Med* 1958;15:224–234.

Morgan LG: Manufacturing processes. Refining of nickel. *J Soc Occup Med* 1979;29:33–35.

National Academy of Sciences: *Nickel*. Washington, DC, 1975.

NIOSH: *Criteria for a Recommended Standard . . . .Occupational Exposure to Inorganic Nickel*. Washington, DC, National Institute of Occupational Safety and Health (NIOSH 77-164), 1977.

NIOSH: *Special Occupational Hazard Review and Control Recommendations for Nickel Carbonyl*. Washington, DC, National Institute for Occupational Safety and Health (NIOSH 77-184), 1977.

Samitz MH, Katz SA: Nickel-epidermal interactions: Diffusion and binding. *Environ Res* 1976;11:34–39.

Sunderman FW: Nickel poisoning, in Sunderman FW, Sunderman FW Jr (eds): *Laboratory Diagnosis of Diseases Caused by Toxic Agents*. St Louis, Warren H. Green, 1970, pp 387–396.

Sunderman FW: The treatment of acute nickel carbonyl poisoning with sodium diethyldithiocarbamate. *Ann Clin Res* 1971;3:182–185.

Sunderman FW, Donnelly AJ, West B, et al: Nickel poisoning: IX. Carcinogenesis in rats exposed to nickel carbonyl. *Arch Ind Health* 1959;20:36–41.

Sunderman FW, Kincaid JF: Nickel poisoning: II. Studies on patients suffering from acute exposure to vapors of nickel carbonyl. *J Am Med Assoc* 1954;155:889–894.

Sunderman FW, Sunderman FW Jr: Nickel poisoning: VIII. Dithiocarb: A new therapeutic agent for persons exposed to nickel carbonyl. *Am J Med Sci* 1958;236:26–31.

Sunderman FW Jr: A review of the carcinogenicities of nickel chromium and arsenic compounds in man and animals. *Prev Med* 1976;5:279–294.

Sunderman FW Jr: A review of the metabolism and toxicology of nickel. *Ann Clin Lab Sci* 1977; 7:377–398.

Sunderman FR Jr, Lau TJ, Cralley LJ: Inhibitory effect of manganese upon muscle tumorigenesis by nickel subsulfide. *Cancer Res* 1974;34:92–95.

Tedeschi RE, Sunderman FW: Nickel poisoning: V. The metabolism of nickel under normal conditions and after exposure to nickel carbonyl. *Arch Ind Health* 1957;16:486–488.

Toia S, Kilpiö J, Virtamo M: Urinary and plasma concentrations of nickel as indicators of exposure to nickel in an electroplating shop. *J Occup Med* 1979;21:184–188.

Vuopala U, Huhti E, Takkunen J, et al: Nickel carbonyl poisoning. Report of 25 cases. *Ann Clin Res* 1970;2:214–222.

Williams WJ: The pathology of the lungs in five nickel workers. *Br J Ind Med* 1958;15:235–242.

20 • *Niobium and Tantalum*

These two materials are described in one section because they occur together in nature, are chemically similar, and are difficult to separate. Both niobium (formerly columbium) and tantalum are used in alloys with a variety of metals that includes aluminum, tungsten, titanium, and certain steels. The great strength at high temperatures of niobium and its alloys has led to their use in recent years in jet engines, nuclear reactors, and guided missiles. In addition, tantalum is used in rectifiers and capacitors, radio tubes, in the rayon and chemical industries, and as a catalyst in the manufacture of rubber (Browning, 1969). Many surgical implants and prosthetic devices are made of tantalum.

There are very few industrial hazards to workers that are associated with these two metals (Schroeder and Balassa, 1965). In the milling and extraction of the ore there may be exposure to such toxic materials as manganese and hydrofluoric acid. Stokinger (1981) abstracted a report from the Russian medical literature that described early chest x-ray changes in 22 welders and chemical workers handling niobium and tantalum. There is also one report of skin lesions in the tantalum industry of which the exact cause and character are uncertain (Wampler, 1943). An incident in which two workmen inhaled radioactive tantalum oxide was described by Sill and his colleagues (1969). Approximately 93% of the inhaled tantalum was eliminated in seven days, entirely in the feces. The remainder was lost by radioactive decay with a 115-day half-life. In another incident involving accidental inhalation of activated tantalum oxide by three nuclear reactor workers, whole body retention at seven days was only 1%, but further clearance had a biological half-time of 1400 days, a result that suggests that there may be a prolonged retention in the alveoli of a small fraction of the inhaled tantalum powder (Newton, 1977).

The few cases of respiratory tract lesions in animals reported by Schepers (1955) to be due to tantalum are hard to assess because massive doses were given by the intratracheal route. Indeed, administration of tantalum powder by inhalation was proposed by Nadel et al. (1968) for bronchography. Subsequent studies have shown this procedure to be without adverse effect on pulmonary function (Smith et al., 1979) or on the histological appearance of airway mucosa (Gamsu and Nadel, 1972). In contact with tissue, metallic tantalum is inert, as shown by animal experiment and human experience (Dales and Kyle, 1958). Cochran et al. (1950) reported extensive animal studies of the toxicity of niobium and tantalum.

References

Browning E: *Toxicity of Industrial Metals,* ed 2. New York, Appleton-Century-Crofts, 1969, pp 143–144, 307–309.

Cochran KW, Doull J, Mazur M, et al: Acute toxicity of zirconium, columbium, lanthanum, cesium, tantalum, and yttrium. *Arch Ind Hyg Occup Med* 1950;1:637–650.

Dales HC, Kyle J: Late results of using tantalum gauze in the repair of large hernias. *Surgery* 1958;43:294–297.

Gamsu G, Nadel JA: New technique for the roentgenographic study of airways and lungs using powdered tantalum. *Cancer* 1972;30:1353–1357.

Nadel JA, Wolfe WG, Graf PD: Powdered tantalum as a medium for bronchography in canine and human lungs. *Invest Radiol* 1968; 3:229–238.

Newton D: Clearance of radioactive tantalum from the human lung after accidental inhalation. *Am J Roentgenol* 1977;129:327–328.

Schepers GWH: The biological action of tan-

112

talum oxide. Studies on experimental pulmonary histopathology. *Arch Ind Health* 1955;12: 121–123.

Schroeder HA, Balassa JJ: Abnormal trace elements in man: Niobium. *J Chron Dis* 1965;18: 229–241.

Sill CW, Voelz GL, Olson DG, et al: Two studies of acute internal exposure to man involving cerium and tantalum radioisotopes. *Health Physics* 1969;16:325–332.

Smith P, Stitik F, Smith F, et al: Tantalum inhalation and airway responses. *Thorax* 1979;34: 486–492.

Stokinger HE: The Metals, in Clayton GD, Clayton FE (eds): *Patty's Industrial Hygiene and Toxicology,* rev ed 3. New York, John Wiley, 1981, vol IIA.

Wampler FJ (ed): *Principles and Practice of Industrial Medicine.* Baltimore, Williams and Wilkins, 1943.

21 • *Osmium*

Osmium is a hard white metal that is found in nature in association with iridium and is a by-product of platinum extraction. The solid metal is inert but its surface forms a blue oxide that is further oxidized when heated to form osmic tetroxide (OsO_4), also known as osmic acid. When spongy osmium, which is harmless, is exposed to air it also becomes slowly converted to osmic tetroxide. This irritating and toxic compound is encountered in the refining of osmiridium, the naturally occurring form of osmium.

The industrial uses of metallic osmium are as an exceptionally hard alloy that is used to tip fountain pens, as a catalyst for hydrogenation and in preparing synthetic ammonia, and in laboratory preparation of specimens for histologic study and for electron microscopy (Browning, 1969). Osmic acid turns black in contact with oils and fats. This effect was once utilized in taking fingerprints, but it is rarely used now because it can cause dermatitis. As is true of many metals, metallic osmium was tried as a drug for such varied diseases as lues, peripheral neuritis, and epithelioma with little success but with no toxic effects. Osmium salts, when ingested, react with the lipids of the mucosal wall and are not absorbed (Luckey and Venugopal, 1977). The only known harmful compound of osmium is the highly volatile tetroxide, osmic acid. Hunter (1978, p. 458) stated that tetroxide has an irritating odor very like bromine or chlorine with an effect alluded to by workmen as "the kick of a mule."

Browning (1969, p. 264) reviewed reports of toxic effects of osmic tetroxide starting in the mid-19th century, including postmortem findings from a fatal case of accidental inhalation of OsO_4 in 1874. The latter included bronchitis, suppurative bronchopneumonia, and fatty degeneration of the renal tubules. Eye symptoms and asthmatic breathing persisting for 12 to 24 hours after brief exposure by laboratory workers was noted by Fairhall (1945). Brunot (1933) described one group of workers who complained of lacrimation, of painful irritation of the eyes, and of seeing large halos around lights. Such eye symptoms disappeared in 24 hours but recurred within two hours on re-exposure. One worker, who had been working with osmiridium for three years, complained of chronic productive cough. Brunot personally found that inhalation of osmium tetroxide had a marked and immediate effect on the mucous membranes of nose, throat, and bronchi with a sense of constriction of the chest and inability to breathe. The irritation of the nose and throat persisted at least 12 hours after exposure ceased. While repeated exposures of small amounts of osmic acid inhaled over long periods are said to cause headache, insomnia, persistent irritation of pharynx and larynx, as well as gastrointestinal complaints, there are no reports of irreversible damage.

Because of the irritating effect that occurs immediately, exposed workers move away quickly from high concentrations of osmic acid. The air in the environment of seven workers was studied by McLaughlin et al. (1946) and concentrations of up to 640 $\mu g/m^3$ were recorded. When the osmium tetroxide vapors were removed from the workroom by proper exhaust ventilation, all symptoms disappeared.

The present safe working level for osmium tetroxide is 0.002 mg/m^3 for a 40-hour workweek.

References

Browning E: *Toxicity of Industrial Metals,* ed 2. New York, Appleton-Century-Crofts, 1969, pp 261–266.

Brunot FR: The toxicity of osmium tetroxide (osmic acid). *J Ind Hyg* 1933;15:136–143.

114

Fairhall LT: Inorganic industrial hazards. *Physiol Rev* 1945;25:182–202.

Hunter D: *Diseases of Occupations,* ed 6. London, Hodder & Stoughton, 1978.

Luckey TD, Venugopal B: *Metal Toxicity in Mammals: I. Physiologic and Chemical Basis for Metal Toxicity.* New York, Plenum, 1977.

McLaughlin AIG, Milton R, Perry KMA: Toxic manifestations of osmium tetroxide. *Br J Ind Med* 1946;3:183–186.

22 • Palladium

Palladium is a white metal that is the lightest in the platinum group. It is used in telephone parts, in dental alloys, as a chemical catalyst especially in automotive exhaust converters, in metal plating, and as an alloy with ruthenium in jewelry. Hunter et al. (1945) noted its presence in platinum refineries and remarked on its nontoxic effects on the workers. Meek et al. (1943) performed various studies with human and animal subjects and reported that only on intravenous injection does palladium chloride produce toxic effects. Later studies with rats showed that soluble platinum salts given orally at high levels were more toxic than those of palladium (Holbrook et al., 1975).

For reasons that are not clear, palladium in colloidal form was given orally for tuberculosis and gout without success. A similar preparation of $Pd(OH)_2$ was given by subcutaneous injection in 1913 for the control of obesity, in daily doses of 5 to 7 mg. This therapy, while resulting in dramatic weight loss, was used only briefly because of fever, local necrosis, and a hemolytic effect (Browning, 1969, p. 269).

Although exposure to platinum is known to result in respiratory and cutaneous hypersensitivities, there have been no reports of ill effects in workers exposed to palladium and its compounds.

References

Browning E: *Toxicity of Industrial Metals,* ed 2. New York, Appleton-Century-Crofts, 1969, pp 267–269.

Holbrook DJ Jr, Washington ME, Leake HB, et al: Studies on the evaluation of the toxicity of various salts of lead, manganese, platinum, and palladium. *Environ Health Perspect* 1975;10: 95–101.

Hunter D, Milton R, Perry KMA: Asthma caused by the complex salts of platinum. *Br J Ind Med* 1945;2:92–98.

Meek FF, Harrold CC, McCord CP: The physiological properties of palladium and its compounds. *Ind Med Surg* 1943;12:447–448.

23 • *Phosphorus*

Toxic effects of phosphorus and its inorganic compounds are limited to elemental phosphorus and phosphine, PH_3. The effects of tri-orthocresyl phosphate and organophosphorus insecticides are discussed elsewhere in this volume. Few workers are exposed to harmful inorganic phosphorus compounds in modern industry, although phosphoric acid and phosphates are used extensively. The history of phosphorus toxicity, however, illustrates the problems of diagnosis of previously unrecognized occupational disease and its control.

History

Phosphorus is one of the older industrial poisons and one of the most famous. Harmful effects were first reported in the manufacture of "congreve matches," which were made with white phosphorus, and were popularly known as "lucifer matches" after an earlier device that was made with potassium chlorate and contained no phosphorus. The first cases of so-called phossy jaw were described from Vienna and Boston in the mid-19th century. Because the disease is very slow in developing and since phosphorus only affects a minority of those exposed, a period of 15 years elapsed before a cause and effect relationship was recognized.

Industrial phosphorus poisoning is known as "phossy jaw" because of the swollen jaw that is so conspicuous a symptom in most cases. It is the most distressing of the occupational diseases, not because it is necessarily serious, for only a small proportion of the victims die, nor because its onset is violent and dramatic; on the contrary, it is slow and insidious, usually beginning with toothache. But, it is extremely painful and suppuration is accompanied by a foul, fetid discharge from the infection in the jaw that makes the victim unen-durable to others. It is a chronic disease and often results in distressing disfigurement. Probably the conspicuous disfigurement accounted for the wide publicity given to phosphorus poisoning in Europe that led to abolition of its industrial use.

The occurrence of phossy jaw in the United States was reported in 1902 by the Federal Bureau of Labor in the course of a survey of women and children in the match-making industry. Andrews (1910) made a national survey of this industry and secured the histories of 100 cases of phosphorus poisoning. Forty cases were found in a plant with careful engineering control, which was not sufficient at that time to prevent this disease. Although the nontoxic allotrope, red phosphorus, was discovered in 1845 by Schrötter in Austria and a safety match using this form of phosphorus was devised by Lundström in Sweden in 1855, strike matches continued to be made with white phosphorus for another half-century (Hunter, 1978). The discovery in 1898 by Sévène and Cahen in France of the nonpoisonous substitute, phosphorus sesquisulfide (P_4S_3) made it possible for the French government to give up the use of white phosphorus, and other European governments followed, joining in an agreement, the "Berne Convention" (1906), pledging themselves neither to manufacture nor to import white phosphorus matches. In the United States the Esch law made their manufacture as costly as that of sesquisulfide matches, and put an end to the use of white phosphorus in the match industry.

Worker Illness in the Twentieth Century

Between 1923 and 1926 a number of serious cases of phosphorus poisoning occurred among workers in the small United States fireworks industry after relatively short periods of exposure. The manufacturers of such fireworks were induced by the Secretary of Labor to agree to cease the manufacture. Heimann (1946) described jaw bone necrosis in men producing phosphorus and converting the dangerous white, occasionally referred to as yellow, compound to the harmless red allotrope. Preparation of phosphate fertilizer carries the risk of exposure to the harmful white phosphorus. Cases of phosphorus poisoning have been reported from other industries (Rubitsky and Myerson, 1949), chiefly in the production of phosphorus, in the chemical industry, in the manufacture of phosphor bronze, in making rat poison, and in making lights for miners' lamps.

In cases of chronic exposure, yellow phosphorus acts on the periosteum and the subperiosteal bone. Layers of very compact tissue form on the bone and there is an enormous thickening of the periosteum. This process, however, does not go on to necrosis unless an injury to the soft parts permits the entrance of bacteria. Thorpe, quoted by Hamilton (1934, p. 91), was able to show that phosphorus fumes, when dissolved in the saliva, exert a solvent action on human teeth and penetrate to the periosteum; more often, the tooth is extracted and the extraction cavity constitutes the portal of entry. In rare cases, similar changes occur in the periosteum of other bones, making them brittle and liable to fracture when subjected to slight violence. Sometimes the change in the periosteum persists a long time and necrosis develops years later. The dramatic bone destruction of workers with uncontrolled chronic inhalation exposure to yellow phosphorus should no longer be seen in industry.

If yellow phosphorus is ingested in amounts as small as a few milligrams, acute hepatic damage may occur with renal pathologic changes, hepatic encephalopathy, or death due to acute yellow atrophy of the liver. Much information on this toxic action of absorbed yellow phosphorus has come from the tragic suicidal deaths in Latin America following ingestion of local fireworks, so-called totes (Marin et al., 1971). Ingestion of rodenticides containing yellow phosphorus has resulted in accidental poisoning in children in recent years (Simon and Pickering, 1976). These cases have been characterized by smoking stools.

Severe burns follow skin contact with yellow phosphorus. Some compounds of phosphorus are said to be potent irritants, not only of skin but also of eyes, nose, throat, and respiratory tract (Gafafer, 1964, p. 203; Moeschlin, 1965, p. 181). Matches are now made with amorphous red phosphorus and the "strike anywhere" match is made with the sesquisulfide of phosphorus. Neither of these has the harmful properties of white phosphorus. However, Nicolas et al. (1930) reported rapidly developing erythema with formation of vesicles or pustules accompanied by pain and pruritis as a result of handling phosphorus sesquisulfide. Greasy skins were said to be most susceptible. A similar reaction was produced in volunteers by the use of the paste and also the powder.

There are reports that a number of other phosphorus compounds act as irritants to the respiratory tract. Inhalation of red phosphorus dust may cause acute chemical pneumonia. Phosphorus trichloride, PCl_3, used as a chlorinating agent, acts like chlorine gas. Other phosphorus compounds such as the oxychloride, $POCl_3$, and pentachloride, PCl_5, may behave in a similar fashion. At lower levels the direct irritant effect of these chemicals on repeated exposure can cause asthma-like symptoms with subsequent chronic chemical bronchitis.

Phosphine

A rare source of phosphorus poisoning is the accidental formation of a gas, phosphoretted hydrogen, phosphine, PH_3, in the production of acetylene gas from calcium carbide for use in autogenous welding. The spontaneously combustible character of phosphine liberated by the action of water on calcium phosphide is made use of in buoys and torpedos. Another source of poisoning from phosphoretted hydrogen is from the escape of phosphine from ferrosilicon, probably by the wetting of calcium phosphide, in the same way that the formation and escape of arsine occurs from arsenide. Either or both of these gases may be formed, but in the larger number of instances the latter has caused poisoning.

Phosphine is also produced in the preparation of flare mines using calcium phosphide, in the quenching of metal alloys with water, and in the accidental wetting of zinc phosphide rodenticides and of aluminum phosphide grain fumigants (Hunter, 1978). Phosphine poisoning produces abdominal pain, nausea and vomiting, severe diarrhea and, when overwhelming, gait disturbances, convulsions, coma, and rapid death from pulmonary edema. Completely pure phosphine is odorless, even up to 200 ppm (Fluck, 1976) and the lower odor thresholds, variously given at 0.02 to 3 ppm, that are characterized by a garlic-like smell, are attributed to higher phosphines and to

118

organic phosphine derivatives such as alkyl phosphines. The hemolytic action of arsine does not occur with phosphine exposure.

Control and Treatment

The present suggested safe level of white phosphorus for healthy workers is 0.1 mg/m³. The level of 0.4 mg/m³ (0.3 ppm) ppm of phosphine gas recognizes its potential danger (NIOSH, 1978). Because phosphorus ignites and burns on exposure to air, it must be handled under water to protect the worker. The exposure limits for phosphoric acid (H_3PO_4), phosphorus pentachloride (PCl_5), and phosphorus pentasulfide (P_2S_5 or P_4S_{10}) are each 1 mg/m³; for phosphorus trichloride it is 3 mg/m³ (0.5 ppm).

Careful and repeated medical examinations are required for all phosphorus exposed workers. Weight loss, jaundice, unexplained gastrointestinal symptoms, and albuminuria require study of liver and kidney function. Scrupulous care of the teeth and gums to prevent phosphorus effect on bone is required.

Phosphorus burns of the skin have been treated by washing the skin with a 2% to 5% solution of copper sulfate on the theory that metallic copper will coat the phosphorus and prevent further absorption and local corrosive action. Potassium permanganate and sodium bicarbonate in solution applied locally are reported as successful in therapy of skin reactions to phosphorus sesquisulfide. Treatment of phosphorus damage to bone, liver, and kidney is nonspecific. Heroic treatment of acute hepatic necrosis by cross-circulation has been proposed (Burnell et al., 1976) on the basis of experimental yellow phosphorus poisoning of dogs.

References

Andrews JB: Phosphorus poisoning. *U.S. Bureau of Labor Statistics Bull* No. 86, 1910.

Burnell JM, Dennis MB Jr, Clayson KJ, et al: Evaluation in dogs of cross-circulation in the treatment of acute hepatic necrosis induced by yellow phosphorus. *Gastroenterology* 1976;71: 827–831.

Fluck E: The odor threshold of phosphine. *J Air Pollut Cont Assoc* 1976;26:795.

Gafafer WM (ed): *Occupational Diseases: A Guide to Their Recognition*. U.S. Public Health Service Publ. No. 1097, 1964.

Hamilton A: *Industrial Toxicology*, New York, Harper, 1934, p 91.

Heimann H: Chronic phosphorus poisoning. *J Ind Hyg Toxicol* 1946;28:142–150.

Hunter D: *The Diseases of Occupations*, ed 6. London, Hodder and Stoughton, 1978.

Marin GA, Montoya CA, Sierra JL, et al: Evaluation of corticosteroid and exchange-transfusion treatment of acute yellow-phosphorus intoxication. *N Engl J Med* 1971;284:125–128.

Moeschlin S: *Poisoning: Diagnosis and Treatment*. New York, Grune and Stratton, 1965.

Nicolas J, Gate J, Rousset J: Phosphorus dermatitis. Abstracted in *Arch Dermatol Syph* 1930; 21:306.

NIOSH: *NIOSH/OSHA Pocket Guide to Chemical Hazards*. Washington, DC, National Institute for Occupational Safety and Health (NIOSH 78-210), 1978.

Rubitsky HJ, Myerson RM: Acute phosphorus poisoning. *Arch Intern Med* 1949;83:164–178.

Simon FA, Pickering LK: Acute yellow phosphorus poisoning. "Smoking stool syndrome." *J Am Med Assoc* 1976;235:1343–1344.

24 • *Platinum*

Platinum and its alloys are used in the jewelry, chemical, and electrical industries, in the manufacture of fiberglass, and in dentistry (Browning, 1969). Complex platinum salts are encountered in refining platinum, in photography, in manufacture of x-ray fluorescent screens, in electroplating, as catalysts in many chemical reactions, and recently in therapy of solid tumors.

Reports of Occupational Disease

Karasek and Karasek (1911) studied workers in 40 photographic studios in Chicago and described a specific clinical picture of rhinorrhea, sneezing, dyspnea, cyanosis, and skin irritation. Hunter et al. (1945) studied platinum refineries and reported no ill effects from exposure to platinum as the metal. When complex platinum salts were handled in dry operations, 57% of the workers exposed to such salts of platinum as a dust, or, in the wet handling, as a fine spray, experienced symptoms, the severity of which paralleled the degree and length of exposure. The syndrome reported by Hunter was very like that reported by Karasek and Karasek. This respiratory syndrome is now known as *platinum asthma*. About one hour after the men left the factory, all symptoms disappeared, but in an occasional case the worker was awakened by a bout of early morning coughing. Thirteen of the 91 men had skin lesions; in the majority of instances these were of the scaly erythematous type, in a few, urticarial. Laboratory studies on this group of asthma cases revealed nothing startling except for mild eosinophilia in 26%. Chest x-rays showed 11 workers (12%) to have emphysema. Skin tests were not helpful in evaluating unusual host repsonse.

Roberts (1951) described the harmful effects of exposure to complex platinum salts in workers in a platinum refinery and laboratory. He named such effects platinosis, reporting that 60% of the workers had skin and/or respiratory symptoms and the other 40% had inflammatory changes of conjunctivae and mucous membranes of nose and throat. Roberts considered that the platinum salt was acting as an allergen, although all workers were affected and relative lymphocytosis was found rather than eosinophilia. Reports of skin testing results in cases thought to be due to platinum exposure are conflicting. While Roberts said that scratch tests reactions to sodium chloroplatinate at high dilution ($1:10^{-3}$ to $1:10^{-8}$) correlated well with severe symptomatic platinosis, he also reported positive reactions in unexposed applicants at the level of $1:10^{-2}$. Hunter et al. (1945) had found such testing unreliable.

In contrast to the opinion of Hunter et al. (1945), Roberts held that chronic exposure to platinum salts may give rise to pulmonary fibrosis. He described increased bronchovascular markings seen on chest x-ray in 16 of 21 cases of platinosis and one case of definite pulmonary fibrosis. Reports from other countries (France, Switzerland, Spain, South Africa) reviewed by Browning (1969) and Hunter (1978) and listed by Parrot et al. (1969) confirm the occurrence of platinum dermatitis or asthma in a number of workers including solderers, electroplaters, and jewelers.

Freedman and Krupey (1968) pointed out that the syndrome of acute rhinitis, conjunctivitis, and bronchial asthma in platinum refinery workers is commonly caused by potassium tetrachloroplatinate (K_2PtCl_4) and potassium hexachloroplatinate (K_2PtCl_6), while ammonium chloroplatinate ((NH_4)$_2$ $PtCl_6$) and sodium chloroplatinate (Na_2PtCl_6) have also been incriminated. These low molecular weight substances are capable of inducing and evoking immediate type reagenic hypersensitivity although other transitional group VIII elements (ruthenium, rubidium, palladium) do not appear to have this allergenic property. Cleare et al. (1976) stated that the responses of platinum workers known to be sensitive to hexachloroplatinate salts demonstrate that the allergenicity is confined to those charged complexes that contain reactive halogen ligands, principally chloride. Passive transfer tests and a radioallergo-sorbent test (RAST) have shown the pressure of specific IgE antibodies to platinum salts in the sera of sensitized platinum workers (Pepys et al., 1979; Cromwell et al., 1979).

Hunter (1978) stated that it is advisable to wash the platinum salts away from the nose with water. Prompt withdrawal from exposure is the best treatment of platinum asthma. In severe attacks, recognized drug therapy used in asthma of any cause is required. Exhaust ventilation can completely prevent the occurrence of this asthmatic syndrome in the industrial handling of complex salts of platinum. Roberts, who had great experience with platinum exposures, believed that individuals with fine-textured skin, and light or red hair should not work with platinum salts, while Hunter (1978) maintained that persons who have acquired sensitivity will be unable to continue further exposure to the hazard of inhaling complex salts of platinum.

The permissible occupational exposure level for soluble salts of platinum is 0.002 mg/m³ (NIOSH, 1978).

References

Browning E: *Toxicity of Industrial Metals,* New York, Appleton-Century-Crofts, 1969, pp 270–275.

Cleare MJ, Hughes EG, Jacoby B, et al: Immediate (type I) allergic responses to platinum compounds. *Clin Allergy* 1976;6:183–195.

Cromwell O, Pepys J, Parish WE, et al: Specific IgE antibodies to platinum salts in sensitized workers. *Clin Allergy* 1979;9:109–117.

Freedman SO, Krupey J: Respiratory allergy caused by platinum salts. *J Allergy* 1968;42:233–237.

Hunter D, Milton R, Perry KMA: Asthma caused by the complex salts of platinum. *Br J Ind Med* 1945;2:92–98.

Hunter D: *The Diseases of Occupations,* ed 6. London, Hodder and Stoughton, 1978, pp 460–463.

Karasek, SR, Karasek M: The use of platinum paper. *Rep Illinois State Commission Occup Dis,* 1911, p 97.

NIOSH: *NIOSH/OSHA Pocket Guide to Chemical Hazards.* Washington, DC, National Institute for Occupational Safety and Health, (NIOSH 78-210), 1978.

Parrot JL, Hébert R, Saindelle A, et al: Platinum and platinosis. Allergy and histamine release due to some platinum salts. *Arch Environ Health* 1969;19:685–691.

Pepys J, Parish WE, Cromwell O, et al: Passive transfer in man and the monkey of Type I allergy due to heat labile and heat stable antibody to complex salts of platinum. *Clin Allergy* 1979;9:99–108.

Roberts AE: Platinosis. *Arch Ind Hyg Occup Med* 1951;4:549–559.

25 • *Rare Earths (Lanthanons)*

The term "rare earths" refers to a group of 14 elements from atomic numbers 58 through 71, to which element 57, lanthanum, is added; yttrium, element 39, is sometimes also included. Although they are not rare, these metallic elements are properly designated rare earth metals and their oxides, rare earths. They are found in nature in a number of common minerals, including monazite, but some are produced in radioactive form during nuclear fission of uranium, thorium, and plutonium. The rare earths, their symbols, and their atomic numbers, consist of

Yttrium, Y, 39	Gadolinium, Gd, 64
Lanthanum, La, 57	Terbium, Tb, 65
Cerium, Ce, 58	Dysprosium, Dy, 66
Praseodymium, Pr, 59	Holmium, Ho, 67
Neodymium, Nd, 60	Erbium, Er, 68
Promethium, Pm, 61	Thulium, Tm, 69
Samarium, Sm, 62	Ytterbium, Yb, 70
Europium, Eu, 63	Lutetium, Lu, 71.

Industrial Uses

The metals are readily oxidized and because of this avidity for oxygen, mixtures of these elements are used as "getters" in metallurgical operations. Many of them, especially cerium, produce an intense white light when heated and are used in cored arcs in motion picture work. Since cerium is very pyrophoric when it is slightly oxidized or when alloyed with iron, it is used in the manufacture of lighter flints. When alloyed with aluminum and magnesium, it has applications in pyrotechnics and tracer bullets. Cerium is also used as an opacifier and polisher in the glass industry while praseodymium and neodymium are used for coloring glass and ceramic glazes. Didymium, a mixture of Pr and Nd, is used in glassblowers' goggles because it absorbs the intense yellow line of flamed sodium. Lanthanon imparts a high refractive index to glass and is used in the manufacture of expensive lenses.

Some of the rare earths, particularly Sm, Eu, and Gd, absorb neutrons, and because of this property are used in control rods in nuclear reactors. Thulium[170] emits an 84 keV x-ray that is useful in portable units for medical and other radiography.

Toxic Effects

The rare earths are known to have anticoagulant and hepatotoxic properties. The light lanthanides are more effective in this regard than are the medium or heavy lanthanides. Nevertheless, the rare earths are relatively nontoxic when compared with other metals (Luckey and Venugopal, 1977, p. 174). Medical use for therapy of thrombotic disease and other conditions has been abandoned because of side effects that include headache, hematuria, hemoglobinuria, and chills and fever.

Animal studies have shown that intraperitoneal injections of cerium, lanthanum, neodymium, and praseodymium chlorides and citrate complexes produce local inflammatory changes followed by dyspnea, pulmonary edema, liver edema and portal congestion, pleural effusion, and pulmonary hyperemia. The local inflammation leads to peritonitis with serous or hemorrhagic ascites (Graca et al., 1957). Rare earth oxides introduced into the lungs of guinea pigs produce a fatal, delayed chemical hyperemia. Survivors developed isolated granulomata after a year, but no chronic cellular reaction or fibrosis developed in relation to the dust entrapped within focal atalectic areas (Schepers, 1955).

Control

Despite these drastic changes found when rare earth compounds are introduced into experimental animals, there appears to be small chance of worker illness at the present time. Exceptions are possible injuries to the cornea and thermal burns

122

from careless handling of mixtures of rare earths that are pyrophoric. Yttrium, an element usually included with the rare earths, is the only one assigned an exposure limit, 1 mg/m³, for steady exposure (NIOSH, 1978).

References

Graca JG, Garst EL, Lowry WE: Comparative toxicity of stable rare earth compounds. *Arch Ind Health* 1957;15:9–14.

Luckey TD, Venugopal B: *Metal Toxicity in Mammals: 1. Physiologic and Chemical Basis for Metal Toxicity.* New York, Plenum Press, 1977, p 174.

NIOSH: *NIOSH/OSHA Pocket Guide to Chemical Hazards.* Washington, DC, National Institute for Occupational Safety and Health, (NIOSH 78-210), 1978.

Schepers GWH: The biological action of rare earths: I. The experimental pulmonary histopathology produced by a blend having a relatively high oxide content. *Arch Ind Health* 1955;12:301–305.

26 • Selenium

Uses and Hazards

Selenium is a nonmetallic element, often referred to as a metalloid. It is widely distributed in nature, although nowhere in quantity, and it is recovered as a by-product in smelting and refining, especially of copper. Its occurrence and industrial and agricultural uses are summarized in a National Academy of Sciences monograph (1976).

Selenium has the remarkable property of increased electrical conductivity in the presence of light, for which reason it is used in the manufacture of photoelectric cells. Selenium is used for hardening and toughening of metals, for increasing resistance to abrasion of rubber hose and cable coverings, as a pigment in glass, paints, and ceramics, to improve the machineability of certain steels and copper-base alloys, as an antioxidant in lubricating oils, in rectifiers, television cameras, xerography, and in shampoos (Browning, 1969; Glover, 1970; Diskin et al., 1979). In refineries, workers may be exposed to selenium, which occurs as an impurity in sulfide ores of copper, gold, nickel, and silver. Rectifiers of all sizes, some very large, contain selenium, and a short circuit from overloading may result in harmful exposures. Sodium selenate has been used as an insecticide against aphids, especially in the commercial growing of carnations, by adding the chemical to the soil, a practice that presents a potential hazard since this compound is both stable and poisonous. Workers may be in danger in the production of chamber sulfuric acid from iron sulfide carrying selenium sulfide, and in the chemical production of hydrogen sulfide. Reclamation of materials that, unknown to those in charge of the work, contain selenium compounds is also a potential hazard. Disposal of selenium and its compounds is a real problem to industry. Dumping into public waterways is a public health matter unless great dilution is possible. Burning materials containing selenium produces an offensive odor so that this cannot be done in or near residential or other populated areas.

Toxic Effects of Industrial Exposure

The earliest report of chronic industrial selenium poisoning was published by Alice Hamilton in 1925. Symptoms occurred in workers in a copper refinery who had a strong odor of garlic in the breath and complaints of upper respiratory and gastrointestinal irritation. These characteristics of the "rose cold" are now thought to be secondary to the hepatic production and pulmonary excretion of dimethyl selenide (Diskin et al., 1979). Although the effects differ among the several selenium compounds, there are signs and symptoms common to all if the level of exposure is not controlled. Most common is the garlic odor of breath, sweat, and urine, of which the workers and their families are aware. Acute sore throats and coryza-like symptoms with lacrimation and metallic taste are frequently reported. Motley et al. (1937) reported acute sore throats in laboratory workers exposed to methyl selenide. Dudley (1938) stated that among men exposed to selenium in copper refining, workers were nervous, had garlic breath, gastrointestinal disturbances, and a striking pallor. Reports of porphyrinuria in cases of selenosis with skin lesions were interpreted by Halter (1938) as the effect of selenium in activating an individual's predisposition to porphyria. Scattered reports of weakness, apathy, depression, lack of power of concentration in workers chronically exposed to selenium compounds are hard to assess.

Occupational exposure may occur to elemental selenium, to selenium dioxide, to selenium oxychloride, and to hydrogen selenide (Cerwenka and Cooper, 1961). The fine dust of *metallic selenium,* which is sometimes considered to be nontoxic in poorly controlled exposures, collects in the workers' noses to produce catarrh, anosmia, and epistaxis. Clinton (1947) reported an acute exposure to selenium during reclaiming of aluminum that was covered with an unknown amount of selenium. A chemist recognized the clouds of pink vapors arising from the melting pots as selenium oxide and cleared the area of workers within two minutes. All of the exposed workers experienced sternal pain, cough, irritation of the mucous membranes of the eyes, nose and throat, and nausea, and some of the men vomited. No serious disability was detected, but there were no subsequent reports. Diskin et al. (1979) described the findings in a man who had worked in a selenium refinery for 50 years and who personally handled selenium and inhaled its fumes. He had red-orange hair and red fingernails from this exposure. Postmortem examination after death from acute myocardial infarction revealed numerous perivascular noncaseating granulomas throughout the lung that were interpreted to be a response to a blood-borne toxin, in this case, dimethyl selenide.

Pringle (1942) reported dermatitis and paronychia in workers chronically exposed to *selenium dioxide*. Finger, teeth, and hair may become stained red with the precipitation of minute amounts of amorphous selenium in the tissues. Amor and Pringle (1945) emphasized that selenium dioxide on the skin will readily produce burns, and absorption of selenium through the denuded surface may result in later toxic effects. Accidental contact with selenium dioxide inside a rubber glove can lead to a necrotizing skin lesion. Although *selenium oxychloride* ($SeOCl_2$) is known to be a severe vesicant (Dudley and Miller, 1941), occupational exposure has not been reported for it nor for organo-selenium compounds.

Hydrogen selenide (H_2Se) is a highly irritating gas with a bad odor and serious hazard to those exposed (Buchan, 1947). It has little industrial use, and exposure occurs by accident, especially in laboratories. It is formed when nascent hydrogen comes in contact with soluble selenium compounds or when selenium comes in contact with organic compounds at high temperatures (Cerwenka and Cooper, 1961). Besides garlic breath, it causes vertigo, nausea, vomiting, and, if the exposure is great enough, dyspnea, cyanosis, and pulmonary edema.

An unexpected clustering of cases of amyotrophic lateral sclerosis in male farmer-ranchers in a region where selenium poisoning is endemic in farm animals implicated seleniferous soils as a possible environmental factor in this disorder (Kilness and Hochberg, 1977).

Animal Studies

Considerable experimentation has been done because of the toxic effects of selenium compounds on animals, especially livestock grazing on seleniferous soils (Smith et al., 1940; Rosenfeld and Beath, 1964). Acute and chronic intoxication can be produced by ingestion, skin absorption, injection, and inhalation. Toxic selenium compounds are reduced after long-term exposure to the relatively harmless dimethyl selenide in the liver (Nakamuro et al., 1977). Exhalation and excretion of this compound is responsible for the garlic odor of breath and sweat. Short-term exposure to selenium compounds leads to the production of trimethyl-selenonium, which is excreted through the kidneys (Kiker and Burk, 1974). Hydrogen selenide gas produces a chemical pneumonitis in guinea pigs along with fatty changes in the liver and splenomegaly (Dudley, 1938).

Prevention and Treatment

Dudley in 1938 and Glover (1967) described a satisfactory method for the detection of selenium in the urine. Dudley found that male workers in copper refineries where selenium is encountered as an impurity had concentrations varying from a trace to 0.07 mg/L of urine. Glover (1967) reviewed the literature and his own experience with workers exposed to selenium and he urged control of selenium exposures, monitored by urine levels at the figure of 0.1 mg/L, a value consistent with the normal limits of 0.01 to 0.15 mg/L reported by Sterner and Lidfeldt (1941). The safe level in air is at present 0.2 mg/m³. Diskin et al. (1979) suggest that monitoring exhaled breath for dimethyl selenide may be a more effective screening procedure than measuring urinary levels of selenium.

HLH examined a number of selenium workers and found that the garlic odor of breath, sweat, and urine acts as a powerful control of overexposure enforced by the workers themselves or their families. However, in view of the considerable knowledge of the toxic effects of various soluble compounds and the vapor of this element, vague ill-health in workers exposed to selenium compounds should be studied and search made for involvement of the liver (Smith et al., 1940; Glover, 1967).

The use of British antilewisite (BAL) in human selenium poisoning is contraindicated (Belogorsky, 1949). In animal studies, BAL, while preventing liver damage, increased fatal renal injury. Ascorbic acid given daily in doses of 10 mg/kg has been reported to control the garlic odor in tellurium exposures (DeMeio, 1947) and may be similarly effective with selenium. Lemley and Merryman (1941) presented evidence that small doses of bromobenzine will hasten selenium excretion with resulting clinical improvement. Selenium-induced hepatitis should be treated as that of infectious etiology. Glover (1954) recommended the use of 10% sodium thiosulfate ointment or aqueous solution for burn or subungual contamination with selenium dioxide. The irritating dioxide is reduced by the thiosulfide to an inert selenium compound.

References

Amor AJ, Pringle P: A review of selenium as an industrial hazard. *Bull Hyg* 1945;20:239-241.

Belogorsky JB, Slaughter D: Administration of BAL in selenium poisoning. *Proc Soc Exp Biol Med* 1949;72:196.

Buchan RF: Industrial selenosis: Review of the literature, report of five cases and a general bibliography. *Occup Med* 1947;3:439-456.

Browning E: *Toxicity of Industrial Metals,* ed 2. New York, Appleton-Century-Crofts, 1969, pp 286-295.

Cerwenka EA, Cooper WC: Toxicology of selenium and tellurium and their compounds. *Arch Env Health* 1961;3:189-200.

Clinton M Jr: Selenium fume exposure. *J Ind Hyg Toxicol* 1947;29:225-226.

DeMeio RH: Tellurium: Effect of ascorbic acid on tellurium breath. *J Ind Hyg Toxicol* 1947; 29:393-395.

Diskin CJ, Tomasso CL, Alper JC, et al: Long-term selenium exposure. *Arch Intern Med* 1979; 139:824-826.

Dudley HC: Selenium as a potential industrial hazard. *Pub Health Rep* 1938;53:281-292.

Dudley HC, Miller JW: Toxicology of selenium: VI. Effect of subacute exposure to hydrogen selenide. *J Ind Hyg Toxicol* 1941;23: 470-477.

Glover JR: Some medical problems concerning selenium in industry. *Trans Assoc Ind Med Officers* 1954;4:94-96.

Glover JR: Selenium in human urine: A tentative maximum allowable concentration for industrial and rural populations. *Ann Occup Hyg* 1967;10:3-14.

Glover JR: Selenium and its industrial toxicology. *Ind Med Surg* 1970;39:50-54.

Halter K: Die Selenvergiftung unter besonderer Berück-ichtigung der dabei beobachtbaren Hautveränderungen in verbindung met sekundarer Porphyrie. *Arch Dermatol Syph* 1938;178:340-357, abstracted in *J Ind Hyg Toxicol* 1939;21:191.

Hamilton A: *Industrial Poisons in the United States.* New York, Macmillan, 1925.

Kiker KW, Burk RF: Production of urinary selenium metabolites in the rat following $^{75}SeO_3{}^{2-}$ administration. *Am J Physiol* 1974;227:643-646.

Kilness AW, Hochberg FH: Amyotrophic lateral sclerosis in a high selenium environment. *J Am Med Assoc* 1977;237:2843-2844.

Lemley RE, Merryman MP: Selenium poisoning in the human subject. *J Lancet* 1941;61:435-438.

Motley HL, Ellis MM, Ellis MD: Acute sore throats following exposure to selenium. *J Am Med Assoc* 1937;109:1718-1719.

Nakamuro K, Sayato Y, Ose Y: Studies on selenium-related compounds: VI. Biosynthesis of dimethyl selenide in rat liver after oral administration of sodium selenate. *Toxicol Appl Pharmacol* 1977;39:521-529.

National Academy of Sciences: *Selenium.* Washington, DC, 1976.

Pringle P: Occupational dermatitis following exposure to inorganic selenium compounds. *Br J Dermatol* 1942;54:54-58.

Rosenfeld I, Beath OA: *Selenium.* New York, Academic Press, 1964.

Smith MI, Lillie RD, Stohlman EF, et al: Studies in chronic selenosis. *National Inst Health Bull* No. 174, 1940.

Sterner JH, Lidfeldt V: Selenium content of "normal" urine. *J Pharmacol Exp Ther* 1941;73: 205-211.

27 • Silver

Uses

Silver is another of many formerly unimportant industrial substances that the requirements of the Second World War brought into greater prominence. Silver is used as a coating for steel in aviation bearings, in telephone and telegraph instruments, and for lining tanks and pipes in food processing. In addition to its older uses in the manufacture of silverware and jewelry, and in photography, silver is alloyed with a number of metals to increase strength and hardness or to give corrosion resistance. Such metals include copper, aluminum, lead, antimony, cadmium, and chrome-nickel steels. An important use of silver is in the manufacture of solders. So-named silver solder contains cadmium, a metal with great toxic potential. Fluxes containing fluoride are used with silver solder and present another hazard independent of silver or cadmium. Failure to realize that cadmium and fluoride are dangers in silver soldering has caused unrecognized pulmonary irritation. Intense exposures cause pulmonary edema, and repeated exposures may result in irreversible damage to lung function.

Reports of Worker Illness

Argyria, a bluish-black deposit of metallic silver in the skin, occurs in two forms. Localized argyria usually develops in those areas of the skin or other tissue that have been penetrated by fine particles of metallic silver (Weir, 1979). Generalized argyria may follow ingestion or inhalation of soluble silver compounds. Hill and Pillsbury (1939) described cases of localized and generalized argyria from occupational exposures that included silver nitrate production, silvering of glass beads, mirrors and Christmas ornaments, silver plating, and silver mining. The condition develops slowly, requiring from two to 25 years of ex-posure. Wigley and Deville (1944) described a typical case of argyria in a worker in the silver trade most of his life, chiefly in the production of silver nitrate crystals. This man had a gray to black pigmentation of the skin over all exposed surfaces, including the upper chest. Rosenman et al. (1979) studied 30 workers who had been exposed to both silver oxide and silver nitrate. Six individuals had argyria and 20 had ocular argyrosis. The clinical examinations generally supported the benign nature of occupational exposure to silver, although complaints of abdominal pain were associated with measurable blood silver levels. Both the abdominal distress and the history of nosebleeds may be attributable to exposure to corrosive substances at the plant. Argyria, local or generalized from prolonged application or ingestion of silver-containing medicaments, was common in the past and still occurs occasionally (Marshall and Schneider, 1977).

Two reports of respiratory tract argyrosis in silver workers are of some importance. Montaudon (1959), quoted by Browning (1969, p. 299), found plaques of pigmentation along the trachea and around the orifices of the smaller bronchi in a worker employed in silver nitrate manufacture. These observations were based on bronchoscopy. In the workers Montaudon studied there was no silver tattooing, as it is often called, of skin, eyes, or buccal mucosa but the nasal mucosa showed subepithelial silver deposition. The bronchial mucosa also had silver particles deposited in the basement membrane, but with much less phagocytosis than in the nasal mucosa, along with some squamous metaplasia. McLaughlin et al. (1945), describing metallic inhalation by silver finishers using iron oxide rouge, pointed out its benign character, although bilateral densities were discovered on chest x-ray. Failure to recognize the cause of such x-ray changes may result in unnecessary diagnostic studies or exclusion from employment.

Dermatologists and ophthalmologists have been fascinated with the biologic behavior of silver, which is converted to silver sulfide deposited in the elastic fibers of the corium to give dramatic grey-blue pigmentation. Argyrosis of the eyes, as silver deposits have been named, have been caused both by medication and by contact and inhalation of silver compounds in industry. Conjunctiva, cornea, and rarely the lens, have been reported as discolored, but this abnormality has not caused loss of vision. Moss et al. (1979), reporting the ophthalmic studies of the 30 silver workers studied by Rosenman (1979), confirmed the frequency of conjunctival and, to a lesser extent, corneal pigmentation. Ten workers complained of decreased night vision, but in seven of these individuals electrophysiologic and psychophysiologic studies demonstrated no functional deficits.

Animal Studies

Silver salts fed to animals have produced renal changes and vascular hypertension (Olcott, 1950). Large doses given by vein caused hemolysis and death due to generalized congestion and pulmonary edema. Smaller doses caused an anemia with consequent bone marrow hyperplasia. As might be expected, retention of silver is greatest in the reticulo-endothelial system (Shouse and Whipple, 1931). Silver is excreted almost entirely in the feces. Kehoe et al. (1940) showed that such excretion prevents silver storage.

Therapy and Control

Past efforts to encourage elimination of the silver have failed, and local treatment is of dubious benefit. Bessman and Doorenbos (1957), in disagreement with Luetscher (1948), claim that British antilewisite (BAL) is of value in trying to remove silver from the body.

The current (1977) safe level of exposure to silver and its soluble compounds is 0.01 mg/m³. This low figure is used to prevent generalized argyria since silver, once deposited in the body, is not excreted except in very small amounts. Weir (1979) has criticized this level because it does not distinguish between localized argyria from deposition of metallic silver *particles* and generalized argyria resulting from inhalation or ingestion of *soluble* silver compounds. He has suggested that

dusts from metallic silver (and copper) be regulated as nuisances at 10 mg/m³, a proposal that has elicited some controversy (Chien, 1979).

References

Bessmann SP, Doorenbos NJ: Chelation. *Ann Intern Med* 1957;47:1036–1041.

Browning E: *Toxicity of Industrial Metals,* ed 2. New York, Appleton-Century-Crofts, 1969, pp 296–301.

Chien PT: Metallic copper and silver dust hazards. *Am Ind Hyg Assoc J* 1979;40:747.

Hill WR, Pillsbury DM: *Argyria.* Baltimore, Williams and Wilkins, 1939.

Kehoe RA, Cholak J, Story RV: Manganese, lead, tin, aluminum, copper, and silver in normal biological materials. *J Nutr* 1940;20:85–98.

Luetscher JA Jr: Clinical application of British antilewisite. *Cincinnati J Med* 1948;29:491–501.

Marshall JP, Schneider RP: Systemic argyria secondary to topical silver nitrate. *Arch Dermatol* 1977;113:1077–1079.

McLaughlin AIG, Grout JLA, Barrie HJ, et al: Iron oxide dust and the lungs of silver finishers. *Lancet* 1945;1:337–341.

Moss AP, Sugar A, Hargett NA, et al: The ocular manifestations and functional effects of occupational argyrosis. *Arch Ophthalmol* 1979;97:906–908.

Olcott CT: Experimental argyrosis. *Arch Pathol* 1950;49:138–149.

Rosenman KD, Moss A, Kon S: Argyria: Clinical implications of exposure to silver nitrate and silver oxide. *J Occup Med* 1979;21:430–435.

Shouse SS, Whipple GH: Effects of intravenous injection of colloidal silver on hemopoietic system in dogs. *J Exp Med* 1931;53:413–420.

Weir FW: Health hazard from occupational exposure to metallic copper and silver dust. *Am Ind Hyg Assoc J* 1979;40:245–247.

Wigley JEM, Deville PM: Occupational argyria. *Proc R Soc Med* 1944;37:648–649.

28 • *Tellurium*

Industrial Uses

Production of tellurium is only one-fifth that of selenium, to which it is analagous chemically. Its chief source is as a by-product in the refining of bismuth. Since tellurium is encountered as an impurity in various minerals, the toxic effect of its compounds must be considered in the recovery of such elements as lead and copper. Tellurium has been used in rubber compounding to increase resistance to heat and aging and to enhance toughness of rubber hose and cable coverings. Alloys of tin, silver, and magnesium are improved by the addition of tellurium, which also has the property of hardening lead and improving its resistance to acids. Small amounts of tellurium are used in making chilled car wheels and chilled iron castings. Machinability of stainless steels and commercial bronze is increased by tellurium.

Toxic Effects of Exposure

Tellurium compounds can be absorbed by ingestion and by inhalation, and possibly also through the skin. They are excreted in exhaled air, sweat, urine, and feces. Less tellurium than selenium is needed to produce garlic breath, an observation made first in 1824 by Gmelin (Hunter, 1978, p. 470). Recent experience confirms the social problems this causes. An electronic company using tellurium sent workers for medical advice to HLH with the chief complaint that their wives refused to kiss them because of the garlic odor. Although Schroeder (1967) thought that the high concentration of tellurium in commercial garlic buds that he analyzed accounted for the characteristic odor of that plant, it is now known that the odors of garlic, chives, and onion are due to volatile compounds that contain sulfur (VanEtten and Wolff, 1973).

Earlier, Hofmeister (1894), cited in Browning (1969), believed that the characteristic odor of breath of tellurium workers was the result of methyl telluride formed by synthesis within the body. Shie and Deeds (1920) found that moderate exposure of the workers to fumes and dust for some weeks or months caused a dry mouth, a metallic taste and garlic odor, inhibition of sweat (selenium does not have this effect) with a scaling and itching skin, as well as anorexia, nausea, vomiting, and somnolence. These authors believed that the symptoms in workers they studied were due to hydrogen telluride. Mead and Gies (1901) examining men engaged in recovering pure lead, copper, and zinc by electrolysis, had found similar symptoms, of which drowsiness and apathy were the most striking.

In 1942, Steinberg et al. reported the medical studies of 62 men exposed in foundries where tellurium was added to molten iron, a mixture that produced dense white fumes of oxides of tellurium. Somnolence and garlic breath odor were the principal findings in these cases as well as in two reported by Blackadder and Manderson (1975) as a result of accidental inhalation of tellurium hexafluoride gas. Both of these patients developed bluish-black patches in the webs of the fingers and, to a lesser degree, in streaks on the neck and face. Recovery from all symptoms was complete, without treatment, within several weeks.

Animal Studies

The physiologic action of H_2Te in animals is that of a powerful hemolytic poison similar to hydrogen arsenide and hydrogen selenide. Webster (1946) confirmed this with *in vitro* studies of guinea pigs' blood. This effect has not been seen in humans. As in the case of selenium, elemental tellurium is far less toxic than the tellurites. De Meio (1946) found tellurite to be more toxic for rats than selenite or arsenite. The toxic effects arise while the body is reducing the tellurium compounds to the relatively harmless element tellurium and methyl telluride. Excretion takes place through the sweat, urine, and feces, which also have the garlic odor. Tellurium salts are converted into an insoluble form and excreted in the feces. De Meio's work with animals shows that tellurium compounds are soluble in tissue fluids and may be deposited in all tissues and concentrated in the kidney. Excretion of methyl telluride is slow.

Endotracheal administration of suspensions of metallic tellurium and tellurium dioxide particles produced a chronic inflammatory response in rat lungs but did not result in fibrosis (Geary et al., 1978). Blue-gray discoloration was found in the brain and testes.

Ingestion of tellurium by rats results in "black" brain from the localization of the dark tellurium particles in the lipofucsin granules in the cytoplasm of brain neurons (Duckett and White, 1974). Feeding of metallic tellurium to pregnant rats produces congenital communicating hydrocephalus in the offspring (Agnew and Curry, 1972), while a similar diet fed to weanling rats leads rapidly to paralysis caused by demyelination secondary to degeneration of Schwann cells, a process termed tellurium neuropathy (Lampert and Garrett, 1971).

Control and Treatment

The methods of prevention are similar to those described in the section on selenium. De Meio (1947) discovered that by reducing tellurite to elemental tellurium with administration of 10 mg ascorbic acid per kg body weight, the garlicky odor could be eliminated. Amdur (1947) gave BAL (British antilewisite) by a course of injections to three research metallurgists accidentally exposed to tellurium fumes, with resulting complete disappearance of their intensely garlic-smelling breath and sweat. The BAL was given 48 hours after the exposure, and 14 days passed before all trace of garlic odor disappeared. In 1958 Amdur published his animal studies warning that BAL used for tellurium poisoning could be nephrotoxic. There is no human experience to date to establish harmful complications of using BAL as therapy for tellurium poisoning.

In the United States and United Kingdom, the current level for safe use is 0.1 mg/m³ for tellurium and 0.2 for tellurium hexafluoride. In the USSR the maximum allowable concentration is 0.01 mg/m³.

References

Agnew WF, Curry E: Period of teratogenic vulnerability of rat embryo to induction of hydrocephalus by tellurium. *Experientia* 1972;28:1444–1445.

Amdur ML: Tellurium: Accidental exposure and treatment with BAL in oil. *Occup Med* 1947;3:386–391.

Amdur ML: Tellurium oxide, an animal study in acute toxicity. *Arch Ind Health* 1958;17:665–667.

Blackadder ES, Manderson MG: Occupational absorption of tellurium: A report of two cases. *Br J Ind Med* 1975;32:59–61.

Browning E: *Toxicity of Industrial Metals,* ed 2. New York, Appleton-Century-Crofts, 1969, pp 310–316.

De Meio RH: Tellurium: I. The toxicity of ingested elementary tellurium for rats and rat tissues. *J Ind Hyg Toxicol* 1946;28:229–232.

De Meio RH: Tellurium: Effect of ascorbic acid on tellurium breath. *J Ind Hyg Toxicol* 1947;29:393–395.

Duckett S, White R: Cerebral lipofucsinosis induced by tellurium: Electron dispersive x-ray spectrophotometry analysis. *Brain Res* 1974;73:205–214.

Geary DL Jr, Myers RC, Nachreiner DJ, et al: Tellurium and tellurium dioxide: Single endotracheal injection to rats. *Am Ind Hyg Assoc J* 1978;39:100–109.

Hunter D: *Diseases of Occupations,* ed 6. London, Hodder and Stoughton, 1978.

Lampert PW, Garrett RS: Mechanism of demyelination in tellurium neuropathy. *Lab Invest* 1971;25:380–388.

Mead LT, Gies WJ: Physiological and toxicological effects of tellurium compounds. *Am J Physiol* 1901;5:104–149.

Schroeder HA, Buckman J, Balassa JJ: Abnormal trace elements in man: Tellurium. *J Chron Dis* 1967;20:147–161.

Shie MD, Deeds FE: The importance of tellurium as a health hazard in industry. *Public Health Rep* 1920;35:939.

Steinberg HH, Massari SC, Miner AC, et al: Industrial exposure to tellurium: Atmospheric

130

studies and clinical evaluation. *J Ind Hyd Toxicol* 1942;24:183–192.

VanEtten CH, Wolff IA: Natural sulfur compounds, in *Toxicants Occurring in Natural Foods.*

Washington, DC, National Academy of Sciences, 1973.

Webster SH: Volatile hydrides of toxicological importance. *J Ind Hyg Toxicol* 1946;28:167–182.

29 • *Thallium*

Uses

The great majority of cases of thallium poisoning are not of industrial origin. Thallium as a rat exterminator has a grim history in its use for murder and suicide. Because thallium is absorbed through the skin, it has had wide use as a depilatory and for treatment of parasitic diseases of the hair follicles in children. If it is rightly given, it can be depended on to cause complete loss of hair in children on the 16th to the 18th day. Death has followed the rapid administration of thallium in amounts exceeding the therapeutic dose.

Industrial workers may be exposed to it in the extraction of thallium from ores, in the production of thallium compounds and in their use in making pigments and dyes, in making window glass, optical lenses and imitation precious jewelry, and in the production of luminous paint. While the quantities used are small, a number of uses have been found for the bromoiodide crystals of thallium because of the property of transmitting long wavelength radiation. Such crystals are used in lenses and optical systems prisms. Thallium compounds, because of sensitivity to long wavelength light, are to be found in place of selenium in photoelectric cells.

Toxic Effects

There is a large literature, both from Europe and the United States, on the subject of thallium poisoning (Heyroth, 1947; Prick et al., 1955). Acute cases have occurred in epidemic numbers, both from clinical use of thallium as a depilatory and as a result of eating food made of flour contaminated with a rodenticide containing thallium sulfate. Swelling of feet and legs, with pains in the joints suggesting acute articular rheumatism, colic, vomiting, sleeplessness, hyperesthesia and paresthesia of hands and feet, and mental confusion, as well as a striking loss of hair from the head and body, are most often reported. Cases of thallium poisoning have been mistaken for the Guillain-Barré syndrome in HLH's experience.

Hubler (1966) drew attention to chronic poisoning, often not recognized, causing mental abnormalities and hair loss. Industrial cases following work with thallium are milder in character with no report of fatalities, undoubtedly due to lower exposures than in nonoccupational poisonings. In 1927 Rube and Hendriks reported severe poisoning among men recovering thallium from the flue dust of sulfuric acid works (Hamilton and Hardy, 1949, p. 207). Six men developed joint pains, loss of appetite, fatigue, albuminuria, and loss of hair. In other reports industrial cases are described as showing epilation and severe cramp-like pains in the knees and calves (Heyroth, 1947; Prick et al., 1955; Sessions and Gorens, 1947; Glömme and Sjöström, 1955). There is a single case of iritis followed by optic atrophy in a worker severely exposed to thallium (Leschke, 1934). Sensory changes of fingers and toes, a mild polyneuritis, have been reported in workers manufacturing rodenticides. Several authors report lymphocytosis and eosinophilia accompanying mild symptoms that reverse with cessation of exposure (Meyer, 1928).

Animal Studies

Both acute and chronic thallium intoxication of experimental animals are reported in the literature (Browning, 1969; Heyroth, 1947). Acute poisoning is characterized by nervous system and gastrointestinal symptoms: restlessness, ataxia, chorea, athetosis, tremors, convulsions, dyspnea, and hemorrhagic diarrhea leading to death. Sensory nerve degeneration without motor nerve involve-

132

ment constitutes the chief neuropathy in thallium-poisoned cats (Kennedy and Cavanaugh, 1977). The chief feature of chronic poisoning in animals, as in man, is loss of hair, although lesions of bone, eyes, and skin have been reported.

Thallium poisoning in rats leads to depletion of important enzymes in the corpus striatum and an increased firing rate of the caudate neurons (Hasan et al., 1977). Thallium sulfate (0.6 mg/egg) applied to the chorioallantoic membranes of seven-day chick embryos induced achondroplasia (Hall, 1977) and the same compound fed to pregnant rats produced skeletal abnormalities in the fetuses (Gibson and Becker, 1970).

Therapy

British antilewisite (BAL) has proved ineffective in a few cases of thallium poisoning both in humans and in animal studies. HLH helped to care for three children poisoned by thallium with homicidal intent. In contrast with Moeschlin's report (1965), therapy with calcium sodium ethylenediaminetetraacetic acid (CaNa EDTA) and alternately with N-acetyl-D-penicillamine increased urinary excretion of thallium and apparently influenced the clinical course favorably. Moeschlin pointed out that, if thallium has not been absorbed from the gastrointestinal tract, insoluble compounds can be formed by using sodium iodide and hydrogen sulfide in a stabilized form. Paulson et al. (1972) reported successful treatment of thallium poisoning with dithizone and hemodialysis, although they point out that the latter is not necessary if renal function is intact. Rieders and Cordova (1965) showed that sodium diethyldithiocarbamate will hasten excretion of thallium. Bank et al. (1972) reported five patients with thallium intoxication, all of whom had neurologic symptoms. Treatment with oral KCl effectively released tissue thallium, but this maneuver aggravated symptoms by elevating plasma thallium.

Oral Prussian blue (potassium ferric hexacyanoferrate II) has been used successfully in treating human cases of thallium poisoning (Stevens et al., 1974), presumably by increasing the inflow of thallium ions into the gut. Constipation has to be treated to prevent recycled resorption of thallium from the bowel. No side effects of therapy were encountered with doses ranging from 88 to 416 mg/kg per day (Barbier, 1974).

Control

Considerable industrial experience supports the figure of 0.1 mg/m³ in air as safe for a 40-hour workweek. Since thallium persists in urine for a few weeks, its measurement may serve as a measure of exposure. Elkins (1959) pointed out that the physical properties of the thallium used in industry rather than low toxicity help to account for the few reported cases of occupational thallium poisoning.

References

Bank WJ, Pleasure DE, Suzuki K, et al: Thallium poisoning. *Arch Neurol* 1972;26:456-464.

Barbier F: Treatment of thallium poisoning. *Lancet* 1974;2:965.

Browning E: *Toxicity of Industrial Metals,* ed 2. New York, Appleton-Century-Crofts, 1969, pp 317-322.

Elkins HB: *The Chemistry of Industrial Toxicology,* ed 2. New York, John Wiley, 1959.

Gibson JE, Becker BA: Placental transfer, embryotoxicity, and teratogenicity of thallium sulfate in normal and potassium-deficient rats. *Toxicol Appl Pharmacol* 1970;16:120-132.

Glömme J, Sjöström B: Industrial thallium poisoning. *Svensk-Läkartidn* 1955;52:1436-1441, abstracted in *Arch Ind Health* 1956;13:513.

Hall BK: Thallium-induced achondroplasia in chicken embryos and the concept of critical periods during development. *Teratology* 1977;15:1-16.

Hamilton A, Hardy H: *Industrial Toxicology,* ed 2. New York, Paul B. Hoeber, Inc, 1969, pp 207-208.

Hasan M, Chandra SV, Dua PR, et al: Biochemical and electrophysiologic effects of thallium poisoning on the rat corpus striatum. *Toxicol Appl Pharmacol* 1977;41:353-359.

Heyroth FF: Thallium: A review and summary of medical literature. *Publ Health Rep* 1947; suppl 197.

Hubler WR: Hair loss as a symptom of chronic thallotoxicosis. *South Med J* 1966;59:436-442.

Kennedy P, Cavanaugh JB: Sensory neuropathy produced in the cat with thallous acetate. *Acta Neuropathol* 1977;39:81-87.

Leschke E: *Clinical Toxicology.* Baltimore, William Wood, 1934.

Meyer S: Changes in blood as reflecting industrial damage. *J Ind Hyg* 1928;10:29–55.

Moeschlin S: *Poisoning: Diagnosis and Treatment.* New York, Grune & Stratton, 1965.

Paulson G, Vergara G, Young J, et al: Thallium intoxication treated with dithizone and hemodialysis. *Arch Intern Med* 1972;129:100–103.

Prick JJG, Smitt WGS, Muller L: *Thallium Poisoning.* Amsterdam, Elsevier, 1955.

Rieders F, Cordova VF: Effect of diethyldithiocarbamate (Na DEDTC) on urinary thallium excretion in man. *The Pharmacologist* 1965;7:162.

Sessions HK, Gorens S: Health hazards in the industrial handling of thallium. *US Nav Med Bull* 1947;47:545–550.

Stevens W, van Peteghem C, Heyndrickx A, et al: Eleven cases of thallium intoxication treated with Prussian blue. *Int J Clin Pharmacol* 1974;10:1–22.

30 • Tin

Uses

Tin is obtained from ores such as tinstone and also from ores from which tungsten has been extracted. Tin is universally used as a plating or coating in containers for food and liquid because of its properties of corrosion resistance and the ease with which it can be soldered. Tin coatings are also used in electrical, radio, engineering, and automobile parts. Foil, collapsible tubing, and piping may be made with tin, and it is alloyed with zinc, nickel, lead, and copper. Modern pewter is made with tin, up to 90%, with tin replacing the lead used formerly. Organo-tin dialkyl compounds of high toxicity are used as stabilizers in the plastic and paint industries. Organo-tin compounds are used as pesticides, fungicides, molluscicides, anthelmintics in poultry, and for control of schistosomiasis.

Reports of Toxic Effects of Tin

Inorganic tin compounds were once used in bactericidal drugs. They proved ineffective and relatively nontoxic. However, an organic compound diethyltin di-iodide, named "Stalinon," used to treat osteomyelitis, skin infections, and anthrax, caused poisoning in 217 patients, 100 of whom died. The fatalities and residual symptoms were due to toxic effects of organic tin on the central nervous system (CNS). This severe CNS injury caused by organic tin compounds used as drugs has not been reported after industrial exposure. However, so toxic are these compounds that the potential hazard must not be forgotten. This subject was reviewed by Barnes and Stoner (1958) and by Lewis (1960).

Industrial workers who inhale dust or fumes of tin or tin oxide may develop stannosis, a benign dust disease (Oyanguren et al., 1958; Robertson et al., 1961). The chest x-ray changes, like those of siderosis, are dramatic and show dense bilateral nodular infiltrates. The discrete opacities are unusually dense because of the high radio-opacity of tin (atomic weight 119) compared with iron (atomic weight 56), a factor that should facilitate early diagnosis. The few autopsies done showed no fibrosis around tin deposits (Dundon and Hughes, 1950). Cases of stannosis were found in 121 of 215 smelters (Robertson and Whitaker, 1955). Stannosis has occurred in men working in tin processing and fettling, a cleaning operation.

Organic tin compounds present an entirely different and serious hazard, summarized by Browning (1969). Acute burns of skin and eyes from industrial exposure can be caused by tributyl and dibutyl tin compounds after brief contact (Lyle, 1958). Itching is the chief symptom. If vapor or liquid is spilled on the workman's clothes, he may develop patches of itching erythematous lesions of the skin of the abdomen, thigh, or groin. Such lesions disappear completely with control of skin contact. Gammeltoft (1978) studied two ship painters suspected of having dermatitis from antifouling paint containing tributyltinoxide (TBTO) and established that this compound is a primary irritant and not a sensitizing agent. Lacrimation and chemical conjunctivitis from accidental tin burns of the eye do not cause permanent damage.

Animal Studies

Barnes and co-workers (Barnes and Magee, 1958; Barnes and Stoner, 1958) found that the alkyl salts, chiefly the lower derivatives, produce central nervous system effects, such as cerebral edema. The dialkyl tin compounds, however, caused inflammation of the biliary ducts and, after repeated doses, necrosis of the liver in rats. Both acute and chronic exposure produced

134

changes in the animals similar to those seen in humans given organic tin as medication — paralysis, weight loss, encephalopathy. In animal studies, the survivors of trialkyl tin poisoning did not suffer permanent brain or spinal cord damage. Browning points out (Browning, 1969; Stoner et al., 1955) that this finding is in contrast to mercury alkyl compounds that do cause irreversible brain damage and demyelination of the spinal cord in exposed animals that survive.

Treatment and Control

Control of skin and eye exposure are obvious steps, or removal from work with tin, if lesions have appeared. If human poisoning with organic tin compounds should occur, therapy would be that for cerebral edema of any etiology. In the United states a limit of 2 mg/m³ is proposed for exposure to inorganic compounds of tin and 0.1 mg/m³ for organic compounds. This low figure is suggested because of the severe toxicity of some compounds to the central nervous system.

References

Barnes JM, Magee PN: The biliary and hepatic lesions produced experimentally by dibutyl tin salts. *J Pathol Bact* 1958;75:267–279.

Barnes JM, Stoner HB: Toxic properties of some dialkyl and trialkyl tin salts. *Br J Ind Med* 1958;15:15–22.

Browning E: *Toxicity of Industrial Metals,* ed 2. New York, Appleton-Century-Crofts, 1969, pp 323–330.

Dundon CC, Hughes JP: Stannic oxide pneumoconiosis. *Am J Roentgenol* 1950;63:797–812.

Gammeltoft M: Tributyltinoxide is not allergenic. *Contact Derm* 1978;4:238–239.

Lewis CE: The toxicology of organometallic compounds. *J Occup Med* 1960;2:183–187.

Lyle WH: Lesions of the skin in process workers caused by contact with butyl tin compounds. *Br J Ind Med* 1958;15:193–196.

Oyanguren H, Haddad R, Maass H: Stannosis: Benign pneumoconiosis owing to inhalation of tin dust and fume. I. Environmental and experimental studies. *Ind Med Surg* 1958;27:427–429.

Robertson AJ, Rivers D, Nagelschmidt G, et al: Stannosis: Benign pneumoconiosis due to tin dioxide. *Lancet* 1961;1:1089–1093.

Robertson AJ, Whitaker PH: Radiological changes of pneumoconiosis due to tin oxide. *J Fac Radiol* 1954–1955;6:224–233.

Stoner HB, Barnes JM, Duff JI: Studies on the toxicity of alkyl tin compounds. *Br J Pharmacol* 1955;10:16–25.

31 • *Titanium*

Uses

Titanium is abundant and widely distributed in the earth's crust. It has found many uses both in industry and medicine. Its best known use is in the manufacture of surgical appliances because of its lightness and tensile strength, which compare favorably with tantalum for the same use. Titanium salts have been used in cosmetics, for a variety of skin diseases, and as a protective cream to prevent flash burns. There are no reports of ill effects from this experience, an absence ascribable to the biological inertness of titanium. Titanium has a variety of industrial uses. The white oxide is used in paint manufacture as a substitute for lead and the chloride and tannate are used as mordants in the dye industry. Titanium is alloyed with a number of other metals, chiefly aluminum, tin, vanadium, and iron. Smaller amounts are used in the manufacture of welding rods, electrodes, lamp filaments, and x-ray tubes. Titanium salts are also used in the glass and ceramics industry. Titanium carbide is a component of "hard metal" made of cobalt-cemented carbides, which are widely used in cutting tools (see section on Cobalt). The military uses titanium chloride in smoke screens.

Industrial Exposures to Titanium

Chief titanium exposures in industry are to the metal, the dioxide, and chloride. It is well known that the powders of titanium are pyrophoric and its liquid form burns in air. Several explosions have been reported from careless handling of titanium. Published reports of the health of workers do not make clear whether or not a dust pneumoconiosis may follow exposure to titanium oxide inhalation (Browning, 1969). A single report of accidental exposure to hot liquid $TiCl_4$ described by Hermindinger and Klotz is reported by Browning. Not only did the accident cause skin burns, but the liberated fumes of titanic acid and oxychloride produced such damage to the mucous membranes that stenosis of larynx, trachea, and large bronchi developed. Such a sequence of events is not unique and can be caused by a wide variety of chemicals given the conditions of heating and exposure by explosion, release of the material under pressure, or accidental splashing. In this case formation of hydrochloric acid explains the irritant action.

Browning (1969) summarized some of the earlier European reports of absence of clinical effects from titanium dust exposures. However, in 1959, Moschinski et al. reported chest x-ray changes consistent with some degree of pulmonary fibrosis in three of 15 workers. HLH studied a case of chronic lung disease in a worker exposed to several metals including beryllium in whom titanium was found in lung biopsy.

Määtä and Arstila (1975) studied open lung biopsy samples, sputum specimens, and bronchial aspirations from three TiO_2 factory workers. They found that in the alveolar macrophages, the lysosomes contained significant amounts of electron-dense particles thought to be oxides of titanium. Smaller amounts of silicon, aluminum, and iron were also detected, a finding attributed to the coating of industrial TiO_2 with other elements such as silicon and aluminum since the late 1960s. Earlier, Elo et al. (1972) found deposition of TiO_2 in pulmonary interstitial tissue, where it was thought to behave as a mild irritant, and slight fibrosis in lung specimens from three titanium pigment workers. TiO_2 clearance by the lymphatic system was suggested by its presence in the pulmonary lymph nodes.

The generally nontoxic nature of titanium dust was confirmed by Uragoda and Pinto (1972) who found no significant difference in lung radiographs in ilmenite (iron titanium oxide) ore extraction workers in Ceylon from those of a control population. Similar results were reported by

Daum et al. (1977) who surveyed 207 workers in a plant producing TiO₂ from ilmenite where the exposures were to dusts of titanium ore, TiO₂, and to various oxides of sulfur. Clinically significant or symptomatic lung disease was infrequent except for airway obstruction in 47% of all workers (38% in nonsmokers) and undesirable irritation of the respiratory tract, none of which was thought to represent serious occupational lung disease. In a dissenting comment, Parkes (1977) emphasized the inertness of TiO₂ and the need to attribute the respiratory tract irritation to some other factor in the sulfuric acid extraction process.

Animal Studies

Many studies in animals by feeding, implantation in soft tissue, and exposure of bone to titanium plates have confirmed its low absorption by the gastrointestinal tract and its biological inertness. In her review of the subject, Browning (1969) reports that one Italian author (Lenzi, 1936) did produce lung fibrosis, which he called "titanicosis," in some animal species when he administered titanium oxide by inhalation. Stokinger (1963) recorded a 1956 Russian report of lung changes in animals exposed for five months to titanium combined with carbon. The changes were said to resemble silicosis, but such lesions were not found in animals exposed for several years to dust of hard metal, which contains titanium carbide as well as other metal carbides cemented with cobalt. Exposure of animals to titanium chloride produced severe reactions of respiratory distress at high levels and production of silicotic-like lesions at lower levels (8.4 ppm average) after repeated exposure (Stokinger, 1963).

Titanium phosphate is a new man-made fiber that has a potential utility as a reinforcing agent in a variety of applications and as a possible replacement for asbestos, since both are composed of bundles of submicronic fibers (Gross et al. 1977). Intratracheal and intraperitoneal administration to rats and hamsters by these authors induced no abdominal tumors and only a slight fibrogenic response in the lungs of these animals.

Control

Because of its chemical and biological properties, industrial titanium exposures are considered harmless. No exposure value has been established for the metallic dust. For titanium dioxide, which is considered an inert or nuisance dust, the TLV is 10 mg/m³. Attention to possible hydrochloric acid exposures due to hydrolysis of titanium chloride is mandatory. Because of its benign character, use of titanium in indoor paints as a substitute for lead should be, but is not, universal practice as a measure of protection against childhood lead poisoning.

References

Browning E: *Toxicity of Industrial Metals,* ed 2. New York, Appleton-Century-Crofts, 1969, pp 331–335.

Daum S, Anderson HA, Lilis R, et al: Pulmonary changes among titanium workers. *Proc R Soc Med* 1977;70:31–32.

Elo R, Määtä K, Uksila E, et al: Pulmonary deposits of titanium dioxide in man. *Arch Pathol* 1972;94:417–424.

Gross P, Kociba RJ, Sparschu GL, et al: The biologic response to titanium phosphate: A new synthetic mineral fiber. *Arch Pathol Lab Med* 1977;101:550–554.

Määtä K, Arstila AV: Pulmonary deposits of titanium dioxide in cytologic and lung biopsy specimens: Light and electron microscopic x-ray analysis. *Lab Invest* 1975;33:342–346.

Moschinski G, Jurisch A, Reinl W: Die Lungenveränderungen bei Sinterhartmetall Arbeitern. *Arch Gewerbepathol Gewerbehyg* 1959;697–721.

Parkes WR: Pulmonary changes among titanium workers. *Proc R Soc Med* 1977;70:289–290.

Stokinger HE: The metals (excluding lead), in Patty FA (ed): *Industrial Hygiene and Toxicology,* ed 2. New York, John Wiley, 1963.

Uragoda CG, Pinto MRM: An investigation into the health of workers in an ilmenite extracting plant. *Med J Aust* 1972;1:167–169.

32 • *Tungsten*

Tungsten dust exposures arise in the crushing and the milling of the ore, in preparing and in using powdered tungsten in "powder metallurgy," and in making cemented tungsten-carbide tool tips. Cemented tungsten-carbide, which contains titanium, cobalt, tungsten, and carbon, is of great hardness and therefore is widely used in making special tips for tools, and for high-speed steels that provide a sharp edge in lathe tools even when the tool becomes red hot. Electric-light and radio-tube filaments contain tungsten. Additional uses for tungsten are to be found in the textile industry, in making blue and green pigments known as the tungstates, and in electrodes prepared as a source of ultraviolet radiation.

It is only from the manufacture of cemented carbide cutting tools that reports of any illness associated with tungsten exposure arise. Cobalt is currently held responsible by some, but not all, students for the hard-metal pneumoconiosis arising in this industry, and the evidence and clinical findings are discussed under that heading.

Animal studies involving the dusts of tungsten and of tungsten carbide by investigators in the United States (Miller et al., 1953; Delahant, 1955) and in Sweden (Lundgren and Swensson, 1953) reached the same conclusion — namely, that without cobalt, tungsten causes no harmful biological reaction (Browning, 1969).

NIOSH recommended exposure standards are 5 mg W/m^3 for insoluble tungsten, 1 mg W/m^3 for soluble tungsten, 0.1 mg Co/m^3 for cemented tungsten carbide dust containing more than 2% Co, and 15 µg Ni/m^3 for such dust containing more than 0.3% Ni (NIOSH, 1977).

References

Browning E: *Toxicity of Industrial Metals,* ed 2. New York, Appleton-Century-Crofts, 1969, pp 336–339.

Delahant AB: An experimental study of the effects of rare metals on animal lungs. *Arch Ind Health* 1955;12:116–120.

Lundgren KD, Swensson A: Experimental investigations using method of Miller and Sayers on effect upon animals of cemented tungsten carbides, and powders used as raw material. *Acta Med Scand* 1953;145:20–27.

Miller CW, Davis MW, Goldman A, et al: Pneumoconiosis in the tungsten carbide tool industry. *Arch Ind Hyg Occup Med* 1963;8:453–465.

NIOSH: *Criteria for a Recommended Standard . . . .Occupational Exposure to Tungsten and Cemented Tungsten Carbide.* Washington, DC (NIOSH 77-127), 1977.

33 • *Vanadium*

Uses

Exposure to vanadium and its industrially useful compounds occurs in mining and processing of vanadium-bearing ore, in the manufacture of steel alloys, and in its use as a catalyst for many chemical reactions. Because most crude oils contain vanadium, workers cleaning oil-fired boilers or handling petroleum ash may be exposed to amounts of vanadium compounds associated with toxic effect. At least 90% of the world supply of vanadium goes into the hardening of steel because as little as 0.5% vanadium in ferrovanadium alloy will nearly double its tensile strength. As the pentoxide V_2O_5, vanadium is used as an accelerator or catalyst in such different processes as dye mordants, paint and varnish drying, and in the manufacturing of glass, ink, insecticides, sulfuric acid, and photographic chemicals.

Reports of Worker Illness

Experience with illness in industry has identified vanadium ore, the metal, and vanadium pentoxide as harmful. Breathing levels associated with toxic effect are reported from as little as 5 mg vanadium per cubic meter of air. Urinary levels correlated with illness ranged from 0.01 mg/L vanadium, so-called borderline exposure, up to 0.3 mg/L where exposure is excessive and engineering control is inadequate or lacking (Sjöberg, 1951; Vintinner et al., 1955). In evaluating reports of illness in workers found in the literature, it is important to understand that precise air sampling and urinary assay for vanadium are relatively recent practices. Early reports may be the result of gross overexposure. On the other hand, the vast literature on biological effects of vanadium, its discovery as a contaminant in urban air, and its value to industry require attention to all that can be learned of its potential for harm.

Dutton (1911) described vanadium poisoning as he had seen it in a plant where vanadium ore was ground and prepared for use in steel production. His patients suffered from anemia with evidence of destruction of red blood cells preceded by polycythemia. Loss of appetite, pallor, and emaciation followed. There were albumin, casts, and blood in the urine, and cough sometimes severe enough to cause hemoptysis. Nervous disorders and dimness of vision occurred. Vanadium was found in urine, feces, and saliva. This early picture of such severe disorders has never been confirmed. A Pennsylvania plant which one of the writers (AH) visited in 1919 worked on Peruvian ores by an aluminothermic process by which ferrovanadium was produced. The dusty processes here comprised the emptying of the ground ore from the sacks in which it was shipped. Most workers exposed to these operations complained of cough.

Symanski (1939), cited by Hamilton and Hardy (1949, p. 195), reviewed the literature and concluded that the pentoxide of vanadium is harmful to workers. In 19 exposed workers Symanski found conjunctivitis, cough, and profuse expectoration, sometimes with hemoptysis. The workers complained of chest pain, and a diagnosis of bronchitis was made on the basis of symptoms plus the presence of scattered râles. He saw no evidence of disturbance of gastrointestinal tract, kidneys, central nervous system, or blood-forming organs. Wyers (1946) reported his observations on over 50 workers in the vanadium industry seen over a period of nine years. He described the hazard of vanadium pentoxide that arose as dust mainly during the crushing of the vanadium oxide, and he presented 10 illustrative cases as evidence of vanadium dust disease of the chest and systemic intoxication. The chest x-ray changes included linear striations, reticulation after longer periods of exposure, and, finally, em-

139

physema. Chronic bronchitis, the long held characteristic in workers exposed to vanadium pentoxide, was a constant finding with paroxysmal cough and sputum as presenting symptoms and râles and rhonchi on physical examination. These findings disappeared in most cases in about 14 days if the worker changed his occupation. Wyers described a variety of findings, depending on the length of the exposure, that he considered as evidence of systemic intoxication: pallor of the skin, elevation of the blood pressure, palpitation on exertion, accentuation of the second pulmonic sound, and coarse tremors of the fingers and arms. In workers with dental caries and furred tongues, greenish black discoloration of the tongue was accompanied by a salty taste. Wyers suggested that this finding may be due to the reduction of vanadium pentoxide to trioxide and the formation of green salts by the ptyalin and acid-forming bacteria in the mouth. This finding also disappeared when exposure ceased.

Reports published since that of Wyers have appeared in the period from 1950 to 1962 from Peru (Vintinner et al., 1955), England (Williams, 1952; Browne, 1955), Australia (Thomas and Stiebris, 1956), Sweden (Sjöberg, 1955), and the United States (Zenz et al., 1962). The extensive literature on industrial vanadium poisoning is summarized by Browning (1969) and by NIOSH (1977). With few exceptions, the reports describe signs and symptoms of irritation of skin, mucous membranes of nose, throat, and respiratory tract. Itching papules or dry patches on exposed parts of the skin, conjunctivitis of all degrees of severity, nasal irritation including mild catarrh, epistaxis, chronic hyperplasia of the mucous membranes, and/or atrophic changes in the pharynx are recorded. Some, but not all, authors describe the greenish discoloration of the tongue. Most authors report reversal of signs and symptoms after varying periods of time if the worker is removed from vanadium exposure. Of special importance are reports of vanadium-induced bronchitis and, in a few instances, pneumonia. Tara et al., cited by Patty (1963, p. 1181), described four of 12 dockers bagging calcium vanadate who suffered cough, dyspnea, and hemoptysis after a day and a half of exposure. Sjöberg (1956) found that six vanadium workers out of 36 with wheezing and dyspnea had persistent evidence of bronchitis after eight years in spite of improved working conditions. Milder, but similar, symptoms of cough and wheezing are reported from open pit mining of vanadium in Peru and cleaning oil-fired burners in England and the United States. The fact that H_2SO_4 is present in the soot may aggravate the effect of vanadium on the respiratory tract.

Biological Effects and Animal Studies

Lewis (1959) studied vanadium workers in the Colorado Plateau and found no illness, but lowered plasma cholesterol values were detected. This action is known to students of the mechanism of the biological behavior of vanadium. An interesting observation was made by Mountain et al. (1955), based on the knowledge that vanadium alters sulfur metabolism in the body. They showed that the cystine content of the fingernails of vanadium workers is reduced by levels of vanadium exposure that caused no detectable harm. It has been suggested that this finding might be used to monitor vanadium exposures or to aid in diagnosis. Moeschlin (1965, p. 150) pointed out that a similar reduction in cystine content of fingernails is present in cirrhosis of the liver, rheumatoid arthritis, and some malignancies.

At the end of the 19th century, vanadium compounds were popular in the treatment of tuberculosis and diabetes, and were considered as therapy for syphilis. Animal experimentation with vanadium has been undertaken by many investigators to determine its nutritional significance (Schroeder et al., 1963) and its therapeutic possibilities. Fischer (1934) described a greenish coating containing vanadium covering the mucous membranes of the eyes, nose, and stomach of experimental animals. Daniel and Lillie (1938), working with rats, described pathologic changes due to vanadium chiefly in the gastrointestinal tract. They found no cumulative effect and stated that acute and chronic symptoms were similar. Wyers (1946), discussing the pathologic physiology of the signs and symptoms noted in his cases in the light of animal experimentation with vanadium compounds, considered the cause and effect relationship well established and, by so doing, confirmed Dutton's observations of 1911. Hudson (1964), in a useful monograph on the subject, has summarized the literature on the biological behavior of vanadium.

Control and Treatment

Since absorption of vanadium is chiefly by the respiratory tract, mechanical enclosure of many vanadium-using operations is required; if this is impractical, the worker must be provided with an airfed unit to ensure complete respiratory protection from vanadium pentoxide. The present air levels considered safe by United States authorities are 0.05 mg V/m^3 for vanadium compounds and 1.0 mg V/m^3 for metallic vanadium and vanadium carbide (NIOSH, 1977). Assay of nails for lowered cystine content in vanadium workers has been suggested as a biological monitor, but, like stippling of red blood cells caused by lead, this is a nonspecific effect. The chief excretion route of vanadium is the urine. Only a small percentage is absorbed by the gastrointestinal tract. Because urinary excretion of most absorbed vanadium is rapid, urinary assay is a reasonably accurate measure of exposure. The present urinary level in the United States thought to reflect a safe body burden is 0.5 mg/L.

Removal from exposure is the obvious first step. The only published specific therapy is the use of British antilewisite (BAL) reported by Sjöberg (1955) as successful in two human cases. Experimental animal studies by Mitchell and Floyd (1954) using high doses of BAL of 125 mg/kg given by vein provided more protection than did calcium sodium ethylenediaminetetraacetic acid (CaNa$_2$ EDTA).

References

Browne RC: Vanadium poisoning from gas turbines. *Br J Ind Med* 1955;12:57–59.

Browning E: *Toxicity of Industrial Metals,* ed 2. New York, Appleton-Century-Crofts, 1969, pp 340–347.

Daniel EP, Lillie RD: Experimental vanadium poisoning in the white rat. *Pub Health Rep* 1938; 53:765–777.

Dutton LF: Vanadiumism. *J Am Med Assoc* 1911;56:1648.

Fischer R: *Occupation and Health.* Geneva, International Labor Organization, 1934, vol 2, p 1177.

Hamilton A, Hardy HL: *Industrial Toxicology,* ed 2. New York, Paul B. Hoeber, 1949.

Hudson TGF: *Vanadium: Toxicology and Biological Significance.* New York, Elsevier, 1964.

Lewis CE: The biological actions of vanadium: I. Effects upon serum cholesterol levels in man. *Arch Ind Health* 1959;19:419–425.

Mitchell WG, Floyd EP: Ascorbic acid and ethylene diamine tetraacetate as antidotes in experimental vanadium poisoning. *Proc Soc Exp Biol Med* 1954;85:206–208.

Moeschlin S: *Poisoning: Diagnosis and Treatment.* New York, Grune & Stratton, 1965, p 150.

Mountain JT, Stockell FR, Stokinger HE: Studies in vanadium toxicology: III. Fingernail cystine as an early indicator of metabolic changes in vanadium workers. *Arch Ind Health* 1955; 12:494–502.

NIOSH: *Criteria for a Recommended Standard . . . .Occupational Exposure to Vanadium.* Washington, DC (NIOSH 77-222), 1977.

Patty FA: *Industrial Hygiene and Toxicology.* New York, Interscience, a division of John Wiley, 1963.

Schroeder HA, Balassa JJ, Tipton IH: Abnormal trace metals in man: Vanadium. *J Chron Dis* 1963;16:1047–1071.

Sjöberg SG: Health hazards in the production and handling of vanadium pentoxide. *Arch Ind Hyg Occup Med* 1951;3:631–646.

Sjöberg SG: Vanadium bronchitis from cleaning oil-fired boilers. *Arch Ind Health* 1955;12: 505–512.

Sjöberg SG: Follow-up investigation of workers at a vanadium factory. *Acta Med Scand* 1956; 154:381–386.

Thomas DLG, Stiebris K: Vanadium poisoning in industry. *Med J Aust* 1956;1:607–609.

Vintinner FJ, Vallenas R, Carlin CE, et al: Study of the health of workers employed in mining and processing of vanadium ore. *Arch Ind Health* 1955;12:635–642.

Williams N: Vanadium poisoning from cleaning oil-fired boilers. *Br J Ind Med* 1952;9:50–55.

Wyers H: Some toxic effects of vanadium pentoxide. *Br J Ind Med* 1946;3:177–182.

Zenz C, Bartlett JP, Thiede WH: Acute vanadium pentoxide intoxication. *Arch Environ Health* 1962;5:542–546.

34 • Zinc

Uses

Zinc has many industrial uses: as a coating on iron and steel; in the form of zinc sheet for building purposes; in the manufacture of bronze and brass; in alloys with copper, aluminum, and nickel; and in plating instead of cadmium (Browning, 1969). Zinc oxide is widely used as a white pigment in rubber formulations, photocopying processes, paints, and ceramics. It is also used in lacquers, varnishes, plastics, cosmetics, pharmaceuticals, glass, matches, and in dentistry (NIOSH, 1975). Since zinc is normal and necessary in human metabolism, there is less likelihood of occupational poisoning. Zinc is relatively nontoxic when compared with other trace elements in the body such as antimony, arsenic, cadmium, and lead (Prasad, 1978). When industrial poisoning does occur, it is almost always caused by inhalation of zinc oxide powder formed when zinc is elevated to temperatures above its melting point. Such exposures to zinc fumes occur in smelting, welding, and galvanizing processes, and in brass founding. These problems, including "zinc chills," are discussed in the chapter on Metal Fumes.

Worker Illness

Careful and detailed clinical and laboratory studies by Batchelor and his colleagues (1926) on 24 workmen exposed for from two to 35 years to dust, zinc oxide, zinc sulfide, or finely divided metallic zinc (poor in lead and cadmium) revealed no acute or chronic illness attributable to zinc. These authors concluded that "abnormal amounts of zinc may enter and leave the body for years without causing symptoms or evidence which can be detected clinically or by laboratory examinations of gastrointestinal, kidney, or other

damage." The great weight of evidence is against the existence of chronic industrial zinc poisoning, and the ill health of zinc workers when it exists can usually be traced to other causes.

The zinc salt that has given trouble in industry is the chloride, which is caustic, and which, because of the way it is used, causes an amount of disturbance disproportionate to its harmful nature. It is generally employed as a flux in soldering, and this process often causes spattering of droplets that may reach the eye or the skin of face and hands and produce painful burns. McCord and Kilker (1921) described a more severe form of zinc chloride burns in 17 men employed in using a mixture of tars, creosote, and zinc chloride for preserving wood. The injury spread in a fairly large area and resulted in detachment of the skin under which the tissues were white and bloodless with a cylinder of scar tissue in the center, the depth of which depended on the duration of the lesion. There was no infection and little or no swelling. Some lesions were exquisitely painful but others were painless. Gocher (1941) reported that, if men worked in uncontrolled levels of fumes or dust of zinc oxide, chromate, sulfate or chloride, they developed dermatitis, boils, conjunctivitis, and gastrointestinal disturbances. But these findings did not occur until exposure had lasted more than six months. There is evidence to show that the swallowing of a soluble zinc compound may cause chronic gastritis with vomiting (Hegsted et al., 1945). These upsets do not improve until the exposure to zinc in the air ceases.

During World War II it was discovered that a serious form of poisoning may result from the "smoke" deliberately produced by heating zinc chloride. Zinc chloride smoke was used in both World Wars, but in the first it was apparently not in sufficiently finely divided form to produce serious lung injury. During World War II the smoke was generated at a higher temperature, and the zinc chloride was volatilized to produce very finely divided particles. Evans (1945) reported a mass poisoning caused by such smoke generated at the mouth of a tunnel. Seventy men were exposed, and ten died. The symptoms pointed to damage of upper respiratory tract, followed in fatal cases by edema of the lungs. In those surviving, bronchopneumonia developed. Plugs of detached mucous membrane from the bronchi, trachea, larynx, and nose of those dying and in the sputum of survivors demonstrated the necrotizing action of the fumes. The concentration of zinc chloride in the air was estimated to be 0.2 lb/yd³ (86.4 gm/m³). Such a disaster can happen only as a result of an unusual accident, but it is good to know of the potential hazard.

Macaulay and Mant (1964) reported a fatal case of pulmonary edema after a short period of exposure to zinc chloride from a smoke bomb. The patient, a 19-year-old soldier, suffered vomiting, cough, and abdominal cramps immediately and, after 24 hours of remission, developed dyspnea, fever, and tachycardia, and he died 11 days after the accident. The left lung contained the equivalent of 92.9 mg of zinc. The pulmonary necrosis found at autopsy was attributed to inhalation of unhydrolyzed corrosive zinc chloride. Because this chemical is extremely hygroscopic, combination with the moisture of the lung produced damaging hydrochloric acid and zinc oxychloride. As Macaulay and Mant remarked, a number of similar accidents probably occur and are not recognized. Failure to understand the serious character of this exposure deprives the patient of therapy, which should include the use of oxygen, large doses of steroids, antibiotics and, above all, total bed rest from the moment of the accident.

Chronic zinc intoxication resulting from exposure to zinc chloride solutions was described by du Bray (1937) in a worker who was a feather renovator in a pillow factory. For four years, the employee had made up the solutions from the powder by hand but he had not followed the precaution of washing his hands immediately with a weak acid solution. The patient's complaints of fatigability, poor appetite, constipation, and pains in the long bones of the legs all subsided upon leaving employment. The portal of entry of zinc in this case was believed to be by absorption through the skin of the hands and forearms.

There are scattered reports cited by Moeschlin (1965, pp. 122–123) of harmful effects of other zinc compounds. Zinc chromate is said to cause occupational eczema, a finding also reported in 1945 by Hegsted et al. Zinc phosphide, used as vermin poison, produces the dangerous gas hydrogen phosphide and has been responsible for fatalities.

The single case reported by Noro and Uotila (1954) of fatal lung disease in a worker who inhaled zinc stearate used to prevent rubber from sticking may be important. The man worked at this job for 29 years and suffered gradually increasing dyspnea and productive cough. Small nodules radiating from the hilum and thickened pleura were visible in the chest x-ray. Increase in connective tissue and chronic inflammation with giant cell formation were found at autopsy. This case report is included because of the wide use of zinc stearate in place of talc or other powders to prevent adhesion in a number of operations in rubber and cable manufacture.

Treatment and Control

In the United States, treatment for harmful zinc effect has been symptomatic except for the vigorous therapy needed in cases of acute zinc-induced pneumonia. Chelation with sodium calciumedetate and hemodialysis were not successful in treating a patient suffering from acute intravenous zinc poisoning who had poor renal function (Brocks et al., 1977). Moeschlin (1965) recommended the use of British antilewisite (BAL).

For years the safe value of zinc oxide fume in industrial air was 15 mg/m³. Because of cases of "zinc chills" among those working at this concentration, the present recommendation is 5 mg/m³ determined as a time-weighted average (TWA) for exposure up to a 10-hour workday and a 40-hour workweek (NIOSH, 1975).

References

Batchelor RP, Fehnal JW, Thomson RM, et al: A clinical and laboratory investigation of the effect of metallic zinc, of zinc oxide and of zinc sulphide upon the health of workmen. *J Ind Hyg* 1926;8:322–363.

Brocks A, Reid H, Glazer G: Acute intravenous zinc poisoning. *Br Med J* 1977;1:1390–1391.

Browning E: *Toxicity of Industrial Metals,* ed 2. New York, Appleton-Century-Crofts, 1969, pp 348–355.

du Bray ES: Chronic zinc intoxication. *J Am Med Assoc* 1937;108:383–385.

144

Evans EH: Casualties following exposure to zinc chloride smoke. *Lancet* 1945;2:368–370.

Gocher TEP: Zinc poisoning. *Northwest Med* 1941;45:467–468.

Hegsted DM, McKibbin JM, Drinker CK: The biological, hygienic, and medical properties of zinc and zinc compounds. *Public Health Rep* 1945; (suppl 179) 1–44.

Macauley MB, Mant AK: Smoke-bomb poisoning: A fatal case following the inhalation of zinc chloride smoke. *J R Army Med Corps* 1964;110: 27–32.

McCord CP, Kilker CH: Zinc chlorid poisoning. *J Am Med Assoc* 1921;76:442–443.

Moeschlin S: *Poisoning: Diagnosis and Treatment*. New York, Grune & Stratton, 1965.

NIOSH: *Criteria for a Recommended Standard . . . .Occupational Exposure to Zinc Oxide*. Washington, DC. (NIOSH 76-104), 1975.

Noro L, Uotila U: *International Congress of Industrial Medicine*. Naples, 1954.

Prasad AS: *Trace Elements and Iron in Human Metabolism*. New York, Plenum Press, 1978, pp 251–346.

35 • *Zirconium*

Zirconium is used in the glass and ceramics industry as an opacifier and polishing powder. Among other uses are as a shielding material in nuclear reactors and as an alloy notably with silicon and manganese. Small amounts are used in flash bulbs and arc lamps, abrasives, ceramics, and paints. During the Second World War, and since, it has been used in tracer bullets and detonators (Browning, 1969).

While there are no reports of toxic effects from occupational exposure, accidents resulting from the explosion of zirconium are the greatest hazards in its industrial use. This danger results from the powder being highly reactive at low temperatures, with ready ignition by sparks. Zirconium fires cannot be put out by water because of the danger of explosion.

Zirconium compounds in technical use are insoluble for the most part, and perhaps this is the reason that there are at present no known cases of systemic poisoning (Fairhall, 1945). Reed (1956) studied 22 workers exposed to zirconium and found no associated illness. A single case with chest x-ray changes in this group proved to be chronic beryllium poisoning, subsequently verified at autopsy.

Of considerable interest are subcutaneous granulomata, thought to be due to hypersensitivity, that occur clinically and experimentally from the application of a deodorant containing an organic zirconium compound (Shelley and Hauley, 1958; Epstein et al., 1963). There are unpublished cases known to HLH of a similar reaction to zirconium salts used to prevent reaction to poison ivy. Telephone linesmen at one time used such a lotion provided by the company.

There are many studies of the biological behavior of zirconium and its salts in experimental animals, and they confirm the low order of zirconium toxicity (McClinton and Schubert, 1948). The experimental production of skin and lung lesions, principally granulomata, by zirconium continues to interest investigators (Leininger et al., 1977).

References

Browning E: *Toxicity of Industrial Metals,* ed 2. New York, Appleton-Century-Crofts, 1969, pp 356-360.

Epstein WL, Skahen JR, Krasnobrod H: The organized epithelioid cell granuloma: Differentiation of allergic (zirconium) from colloidal (silica) types. *Am J Pathol* 1963;43:391-405.

Fairhall LT: Inorganic industrial hazards. *Physiol Rev* 1945;25:182-202.

Leininger JR, Farrell RL, Johnson GR: Acute lung lesions due to zirconium and aluminum compounds in hamsters. *Arch Pathol Lab Med* 1977;101:545-549.

McClinton DT, Schubert J: Toxicity of some zirconium and thorium salts in rats. *J Pharmacol* 1948;94:1-6.

Reed CE: Effects on the lung of industrial exposure to zirconium dust. *Arch Ind Health* 1956; 13:578-581.

Shelley WB, Hauley HJ Jr: The allergic origin of zirconium deodorant granulomas. *Br J Dermatol* 1958;70:75-101.

36 • *Metal Fumes*

The term *metal fume fever* is used to cover recognized diseases that in the past had such titles as brass founders' ague, spelter shakes, metal shakes, and zinc chills. Such names were derived from knowledge that the symptoms are caused by fumes encountered in the founding of brass, the smelting of zinc, and in any operation giving rise to freshly generated metal fumes. It is an industrial disease that is as old as the metallurgy of brass and there are many descriptions of it in the early literature in England, France, and Germany. Attacks of intermittent fever among brass founders were described by Thackrah in 1832, who correctly attributed the malady to inhalation of zinc oxide fumes (Meiklejohn, 1957).

Metal fume fever may be caused by the freshly formed oxides of a number of metals that include antimony, arsenic, cadmium, cobalt, copper, iron, lead, magnesium, manganese, mercury, nickel, selenium, silver, tin, and zinc (Piscator, 1976), but it is the latter that is the principal offender (Drinker, 1922). Lehmann in 1910 (Hamilton and Hardy, 1949, p. 161) reporting experiments on himself and three others, observed that the course of metal fume fever did not resemble an intoxication by metallic compound but, rather, an infection by bacteria or the injection of foreign protein. A sudden chill and a rise of temperature followed inhalation; these effects subsided in a matter of hours and produced a temporary immunity that accounted for the term "Monday morning fever." His explanation was that brass poisoning is caused by the resorption of pyrogenic protein from alveolar lining cells released by the destructive action of the zinc oxide. Arnstein (Hamilton and Hardy, 1949, p. 161) contributed the further fact that brass fumes cause leukocytosis and that inhaled zinc can be recovered from the urine and feces. Lehmann was unable to explain why it was not possible to produce the same symptoms by inhalation of ordinary zinc oxide powder. This enigma was resolved by Drinker et al. (1927) who showed that freshly formed oxide particles, such as occur in fumes from heated zinc, are finely divided and not yet agglomerated and so pass easily through the air passages, just as they do through a glass tube. In a short time, however, the particles clump and will no longer pass with ease through a tube. This particle behavior is considered the reason that metal fume fever is never caused except by freshly formed fumes from heated metal.

Drinker et al. (1927) connected the temporary immunity, which is familiar to brass founders, with the leukocytosis, which is a defensive mechanism. If a man resumes work while he still has a high white cell count, there is no recurrence of chills and fever; but, if he waits over Sunday and the leukocytosis has subsided, he is likely to have a new attack. Kuh et al. (1946) believed that metal fume fever results from the absorption of endotoxins liberated in the lungs as a result of the killing of the microorganisms of the lower respiratory tract. The short-lived immunity that often follows an attack would then be due to the temporary sterilization of the tract and would be lost when microorganisms began to multiply again. Pernis et al. (1961) proposed that an endogenous pyrogen is produced by the direct effect of metal fumes on white blood cells to explain the clinical syndrome of metal fume fever. There have been no recent studies of this problem.

Clinical Syndrome

The symptoms of metal fume fever come on a few hours after exposure, very rarely in the foundry, more often after the worker has reached home. Chilling of the body is often the precipitating cause, and the cases are always much more numerous in winter, although this is partly engaged in rolling red-hot ingots of pure copper. Seven cases of "copper fever" were recorded after exposure to red oxide of copper (Cu_2O) that was being pulverized in a paint factory (Schiotz, 1948). In 1947 Friberg and Thrysin (Moeschlin, 1965, p. 124) described cases of copper fever in men who cleaned furnaces used in a chemical operation requiring finely divided copper as a catalyst. The syndrome they described began after a few hours of exposure with a sweetish taste in the mouth, burning of the eyes, and dryness of the throat — the well-known signs and symptoms of metal fume fever. In 13 out of 17 such cases the increased blood copper level reflected absorption of the metal fume.

Drinker (1927) found in experiments on himself that typical chills follow the inhalation of freshly precipitated magnesium oxide. Schiotz (1948) described cases of "iron fever" in four men engaged in electric welding of iron in a small and ill-ventilated space on a boat. In all of these, the symptoms were identical with those caused by zinc oxide. Schiotz proposed the term "metal fever" should be used rather than "metal fume fever" since some metal dusts as well as fumes may be the cause. Metal fever is probably an accurate title, but the term metal fume fever has been used so long it is likely to continue in use. While zinc, copper, iron, and magnesium in the form of freshly generated oxides are best documented as causing this syndrome, it is likely that most metals under the right circumstances will behave in a similar fashion.

Polymer fume fever, a syndrome very similar to metal fume fever, also occurs after exposures to pyrolysis products of fluorocarbon polymers, typically polytetrafluorethylene (PTFE) and fluorinated polyethylenepropylene (FEP) (Waritz, 1975; Arita and Soda, 1977). Two cases in a textile mill, aggravated by cigarette smoking, were reported by Wegman and Peters (1974).

References

Anseline P: Zinc-fume fever. *Med J Aust* 1972; 2:316-318.

Arita H, Soda R: Pyrolysis products of polytetrafluorethylene and polyfluorethelynepropylene with reference to inhalation toxicity. *Ann Occup Hyg* 1977;20:247-255.

Drinker P: Certain aspects of the problem of zinc toxicity. *J Ind Hyg* 1922;4:177-197.

Drinker P, Thomson RM, Finn JL: Metal fume fever. *J Ind Hyg* 1927;9:98-105.

Fishburn CW, Zenz C: Metal fume fever. *J Occup Med* 1969;11:142-144.

Hamilton A, Hardy H: *Industrial Toxicology,* ed 2. New York, Paul B. Hoeber, 1949.

Hammond JW: Metal fume fever in the crushed stone industry. *J Ind Hyg Toxicol* 1944;26: 117-119.

Kuh JR, Collen MF, Kuh C: Metal fume fever. *Permanente Found Med Bull* 1946;4:145-151.

Meiklejohn A: *The Life, Work and Times of Charles Turner Thackrah, Surgeon and Apothecary of Leeds (1795-1833).* Edinburgh, E & S Livingstone, 1957.

Moeschlin S: *Poisoning: Diagnosis and Treatment.* New York, Grune & Stratton, 1965.

NIOSH: *Criteria for a Recommended Standard . . . .Occupational Exposure to Zinc Oxide.* Washington, DC (NIOSH 76-104), 1975.

Papp JP: Metal fume fever. *Postgrad Med* 1968;43:160-163.

Pedley FG, Ward RV: Lead poisoning in brass and bronze foundries. *Can Med Assoc J* 1931;25: 299-303.

Pernis EC, Vigliani EC, Finulli M: Endogenous pyrogen in the pathogenesis of metal fume fever. *Proc 13th Intern Cong Occup Health,* 1961; p 770. (also in *Med lav* 1960;51:579-586).

Piscator M: Health hazards from inhalation of metal fumes. *Environ Res* 1976;11:268-270.

Rohrs LC: Metal fume fever from inhaling zinc oxide. *Arch Ind Health* 1957;16:42-47.

Schiotz EH: Metal fever produced by copper and iron. Abstracted in *J Ind Hyg Toxicol* 1948; 30:10.

Stokinger HE: The metals (excluding lead), ed 2, in Patty FA (ed): *Industrial Hygiene and Toxicology.* New York, John Wiley, 1963, vol 2.

Waritz RS: An industrial approach to evaluation of pyrolysis and combustion hazards. *Environ Health Pers* 1975;11:197-202.

Wegman DH, Peters JM: Polyfume fever and cigarette smoking. *Ann Intern Med* 1974;81: 55-57.

due to the better ventilation of the foundry in summer. Sometimes the attack comes on after the subject has undressed and gone to bed between chilly sheets. The actual chill is preceded by an unusual sweetish or metallic taste in the mouth, a feeling of dryness in the throat, cough and dyspnea, a sense of lassitude and malaise, sometimes nausea, rarely vomiting. The Russians have found that a warm bath taken at this stage may avert a chill. Fever and chills are followed by sweating and possibly prostration, but these pass off almost completely by morning and the sufferer usually goes back to work. The reported temperature rise varies from 38°C to 39°C and reaches maximum in 10 or 12 hours after the inhalation of the fumes. The leukocytosis persists longer. The "enzymes of injury," SGOT and SGPT, are reported to be normal but lactic dehydrogenase may be elevated (Anseline, 1972; Fishburn and Zenz, 1969). Chest radiographs are reported either to be normal (Rohrs, 1957; Papp, 1968) or to show an increase in bronchovascular markings in the acute phase (Anseline, 1972). In 1925 Gelman in Russia (Hamilton and Hardy, 1949, p. 162) reported relatively slight rise of temperature, but there was disturbance of liver function as shown by increased urobilin and hematoporphyrin in the urine and, in several cases, glycosuria. The liver was enlarged during the attack in a few cases.

Tanquerel (Drinker, 1922) and other authors have concluded that there is no such thing as chronic poisoning from brass. Any persistent illness was held to be due to lead, arsenic, and antimony. Many studies of brass workers show, however, that their general health is below the average for their economically similar group. There are scattered reports of ill-defined gastrointestinal disturbances associated with chronic exposure to zinc oxide fumes (NIOSH, 1975). The term "brass poisoning" is often used by workmen to refer to infected cuts and scratches that are more prevalent in workers with brass than in workers with iron and steel. Whether a cut is slower to heal when made by a sliver of brass than when made by sharp steel is doubtful.

In 1938, Pozzi (Hamilton and Hardy, 1949, p. 163) thought that alcoholism and malnutrition accounted for the severity of metal fume fever in arc welders. The explanation of more serious attacks in these men than in brass founders may be because arc welders are more often obliged to work in small, confined places and thus receive intense exposures to metal fume. Such exposures

may include the hazard of inhalation o nary irritants such as oxides of nitrogen

Because of the nonspecificity of suc logic changes as pulmonary fibrosis and forms of emphysema, it has been impo clearly associate repeated attacks of me with chronic pulmonary insufficiency. A lifetime with three or more bouts a weel syndrome, causing toxic effects on the cel the alveoli, must produce permanent, irre damage either alone or acting with cigarett ing, bacterial infection, or other in pulmonary insults.

In all cases of chronic illness in brass wo1 is wise to consider toxic lead effect. Bot and so-called railway bronze may contain a as 9% of lead that volatilizes with the zi1 causes typical plumbism (Pedley and 1931). Stokinger (1963) speculated that, sin per binds histamine to a protein (serum albu it may be that, as he puts it, "a local action inhalation) may become systemic (fume fe In view of the fact that other metal oxides metal fume fever, more investigation is rec to support this proposition.

Industrial Operations
Causing Metal Fume Fever

The great majority of cases of metal fume occur in brass foundries; the next most freq source is the smelting of zinc. Other source zinc oxide fumes give rise to a few cases o1 dustrial poisoning, but instances are repo from time to time from every industry in wl any metal is heated to the point of volatilizati Metal fume fever has occurred in the crush stone industry, where molten zinc is poured i1 the crushers to form a lining (Hammond, 194 During the cutting of the steel lining with an yacetylene torch, zinc fumes were produced th caused severe temporary illness after one to thi hours of exposure. The maximum fume conce tration of zinc was 580 mg/m^3 compared to 25 mg/m^3 for manganese and 2.0 mg/m^3 for lead, result supporting the diagnosis of metal fumes du to zinc.

Hamilton and Hardy (1949, p. 164) summa rized some of the older literature on metal fum fever from exposure to copper. Hanson in 191(reported "influenza-like" symptoms in 10 work men who were employed at an electric furnace where copper was raised to a very high tempera ture. In 1939 Koelsch described fever among men

SECTION THREE
CHEMICAL COMPOUNDS I

1 • *Introduction*

The industrially useful chemicals discussed in this Section are chiefly harmful to skin and mucous membranes. There are no unique symptoms and signs associated with occupational conjunctivitis, rhinitis, pharyngitis, bronchitis, and pneumonitis. The clue to correct diagnosis is to be found in the worker's job history (Hardy, 1960). Complicating factors are the nonspecific additional insults of cigarette smoking, urban air, and infection. The work of Green and Kass (1964) with animals demonstrates the influence of a series of events acting on the respiratory tract. Studies of Anderson and Ferris (1962) of the apparently overwhelming effect of smoking habits on the lungs of workers also inhaling potentially harmful chemicals illustrate the difficulties in identifying occupational chest disease if the exposure is long term at low levels that do not cause acute, easily recognized episodes. Additional problems for the physician are variations in tolerance of symptoms, inaccurate report of the work exposure, fear of loss of employment, and delay in settlement of a justified compensation claim.

There are certain patterns of response of the respiratory tract to occupational exposure to some chemicals that can be identified. Pulmonary edema follows high levels of exposure and is clinically obvious in from minutes to hours after exposure ceases, depending on the quantity inhaled and the victim's activity, as well described by Kleinfeld (1965). Failure to recognize the true etiology and treatment of symptoms with antibiotics instead of oxygen and steroids has led to unnecessary fatalities. After such an episode, the patient, with proper therapy, will recover completely. If he recovers after a stormy course, he may suffer permanent impairment of lung function (Conner et al., 1962). A less severe syndrome is caused by repeated, steady exposure at low levels to chemicals known to produce pulmonary edema at higher levels. It is wise to remember that steady exposure will lower the worker's threshold of awareness of irritation, such as the sense of smell. Such a worker tolerates symptoms such as cough and eye watering and will work in an atmosphere capable of damaging the respiratory tract. Progressive loss of lung function is influenced not only by occupational factors but also by smoking habits, urban air, infection, and aging (Brinkman et al., 1972; Skalpe, 1964).

References

Anderson DO, Ferris BG: Role of tobacco smoking in the causation of chronic respiratory disease. *N Engl J Med* 1962;267:787–794.

Brinkman GL, Block DL, Cress C: Effects of bronchitis and occupation on pulmonary ventilation over an 11-year period. *J Occup Med* 1972; 14:615–620.

Conner EH, DuBois AB, Comroe JH Jr: Acute chemical injury of the airway and lungs. Experience with six cases. *Anesthesiology* 1962;25: 538–547.

Green GM, Kass EH: Factors influencing the clearance of bacteria by the lung. *J Clin Invest* 1964;43:769–776.

Hardy HL: Toxic hazards: Pulmonary irritants. *N Engl J Med* 1960;263:813–814.

Kleinfeld M: Acute pulmonary edema of chemical origin. *Arch Environ Health* 1965;10: 942–946.

Skalpe IO: Long-term effects of sulphur dioxide exposure in pulp mills. *Br J Ind Med* 1964;21: 69–73.

2 • Alkalies

The alkalies that play an important part in industry are the hydroxides of sodium, potassium, and ammonium; anhydrous sodium carbonate (soda ash); calcium oxide (quicklime); calcium chloride; barium oxide and hydrate; the sulfides of sodium, calcium, and arsenic; and the alums. All have caustic properties of varying degrees but – while caustic soda and potash may cause fatal burns or blindness, and the fumes of concentrated ammonia may cause death from congestion and edema of the lungs – quicklime, the alums, and the sulfides will rarely be responsible for anything more severe than eye and skin irritation. A very severe skin reaction may follow exposure to calcium chloride dust. Contact with alkali ash may lead to an irritant dermatitis, especially when coupled with sweating and poor personal hygiene (Rycroft and Calnan, 1977).

Reference

Rycroft RJG, Calnan CD: Irritant dermatitis during the relining of a blast furnace. *Contact Derm* 1977;3:75–78.

Ammonia

Ammonia is defined as gaseous or liquified anhydrous ammonia and its aqueous solutions (NIOSH, 1974). It is used widely in the manufacture of fertilizers, nitric acid, plastic and synthetic fibers, and explosives. It is used in refrigeration plants, in petroleum refining, and as an important feedstock in the chemical manufacturing industry.

Acute industrial poisoning from ammonia usually results from the sudden accidental escape of the liquid or gas, frequently in connection with the installation or repair of refrigeration equipment or in the chemical and fertilizer industries.

The fact that ammonia is a gas makes it more dangerous than solid caustic potash or sodium. Ammonia gas is very irritating to the upper air passages and workers escape from the fumes as quickly as possible. If escape is delayed, the gas may be deeply inhaled with resulting congestion of the lungs, followed by edema. Fairbrother (1887) described an accident in a brewery where four men were installing a refrigerator. A large vat of ammonia broke, and the fluid ran over the floor and filled the room with vapors. During the three minutes before the men could be released, the exposure was so intense as to be fatal to one worker in 15 seconds and fatal to a second after two hours of delirium and cardiac and respiratory failure. The third man was conscious and could walk but developed marked dyspnea and died in five hours. The one man who survived for three months had repeated bouts of hemoptysis.

Kass et al. (1972) and Sabonya (1977) described bronchiectasis as a result of acute ammonia burns. Taplin et al. (1976) reported a case of acute inhalation of ammonia gas as a result of a loosened coupling from a tank of liquid fertilizer. Pulmonary edema was successfully treated with oxygen and positive end-expiratory pressure. Three weeks after the accident, the patient, a young adult male, appeared to be healthy except for shortness of breath on moderate exertion. Six months after the exposure, radionuclide lung-imaging studies revealed excessive deposition of the radioactive aerosol in the major airways with poor penetration to lung periphery, findings that are indicative of partial airway obstruction characteristic of the chronic bronchitic type of obstructive airway disease. Other cases of fatal and near-fatal ammonia gas poisoning have been reported by Slot (1938), Caplin (1941), Levy et al. (1964), White (1971) and Walton (1973).

Four individuals exposed to concentrated ammonia vapors when a truck carrying liquid ammonia fell from an overpass were studied by

Hatton et al. (1979). The finding of a significant increase in urinary excretion of hydroxylysine metabolites was interpreted as evidence of collagen breakdown in the airways and lung parenchyma. For this reason these authors recommend the measurement of these substances in the urine as a useful index to the severity of the pulmonary lesions resulting from the inhalation of ammonia and other noxious gases.

Severe injury may follow the splashing of ammonia into the eye. In one such case, which took place in the cooling room of an abattoir, the result was inflammation of the cornea and conjunctiva, followed by atrophy of the iris and opacity of the lens. The only way to prevent such distressing sequelae is to wash the eye immediately and thoroughly, for ammonia can be demonstrated in the anterior chamber within a few seconds of its introduction into the conjunctival sac. Thies (1929) reported a case of severe corneal and conjunctival ulcer that developed 10 days after ammonia water was splashed into the eye.

Chronic poisoning has been described in connection with prolonged exposure to ammonia fumes but here the data are scanty. Such exposures are encountered in stables, in refrigeration plants, in various chemical processes (such as diazo copying), and in the manufacture of latex cements. Subjects exposed to controlled concentrations of ammonia for six weeks developed a tolerance for the irritant effect of the fumes after three weeks (Ferguson et al., 1977). After acclimation, continuous exposure to 100 ppm in this study was easily tolerated with no observable adverse effects on health.

HLH cared for a man working in a walk-in refrigerator for milk who complained of chronic cough and increasing dyspnea on effort. Bilateral infiltrates were seen on chest x-ray, and lung function indices reflected both ventilatory and diffusion abnormalities. After three years away from ammonia exposure, this worker had persistent evidence of pulmonary damage. It is likely a number of such cases are not recognized and are classified as idiopathic pulmonary fibrosis.

Henderson and Haggard (1943) listed the physiological reactions to ammonia at various concentrations (Table 1).

The history of the changes in ammonia exposure standards is reviewed in the NIOSH criteria document (1974; see also *J Occup Med* 1976;20:200–204). There has been a reduction from 500 ppm proposed by Lehmann in 1886 to 100 ppm, which was adopted as the Threshold

Table 1

Ammonia Concentrations	ppm
Least detectable odor	53
Least amount causing immediate irritation to the eye	698
Least amount causing immediate irritation to the throat	408
Least amount causing coughing	1720
Maximum concentration allowable for prolonged exposure	100
Maximum concentration allowable for short exposure (½–1 hr)	300–500
Dangerous for even short exposure (½ hr)	2500–4500
Rapidly fatal for short exposure	5000–10,000

Limit Value (TLV) in 1948. The present federal standard for ammonia is an 8-hour TWA of 50 ppm (35 mg/m³).

References

Caplin M: Ammonia gas poisoning: Forty-seven cases in a London shelter. *Lancet* 1941;2:95–96.

Fairbrother HC: Poisoning from strong ammonia. *St. Louis Med Surg J* 1887;52:272.

Ferguson WS, Koch WC, Webster LB, et al: Human physiological response and adaptation to ammonia. *J Occup Med* 1977;19:319–326.

Hatton DV, Leach CS, Beaudet AL, et al: Collagen breakdown and ammonia inhalation. *Arch Environ Health* 1979;34:83–87.

Henderson Y, Haggard HW: *Noxious Gases.* New York, Reinhold, 1943.

Kass I, Zamel N, Dobry CA, et al: Bronchiectasis following ammonia burns of the respiratory tract. *Chest* 1972;62:282–285.

Levy DM, Divertie MB, Litzow TJ, et al: Ammonia burns of the face and respiratory tract. *J Am Med Assoc* 1964;190:873–876.

NIOSH: *Criteria for a Recommended Standard . . . .Occupational Exposure to Ammonia.* Washington, DC, National Institute for Occupational Safety and Health (NIOSH 74-136), 1974.

Sabonya R: Fatal anhydrous ammonia inhalation. *Human Pathol* 1977;8:293–299.

Slot GMS: Ammonia gas burns. Account of six cases. *Lancet* 1938;2:1356–1357.

Taplin GV, Chopra S, Yanda RJ, et al: Radionuclidic lung-imaging procedures in the assessment of injury due to ammonia inhalation. *Chest* 1976;69:582–586.

152

Thies O: Eye injuries in the chemical industry. Abstracted in *Bull Hyg* 1929;4:643.

Walton M: Industrial ammonia gassing. *Br J Ind Med* 1973;30:78–86.

White ES: A case of near fatal ammonia gas poisoning. *J Occup Med* 1971;13:549–550.

Cement

Cement is composed of 60% to 67% CaO, 17% to 25% SiO_2, 3% to 8% Al_2O_3, and smaller amounts of iron and magnesium oxides. Hydration of cement is slowly exothermic, but it is the alkalinity, not the heat, that is responsible for cement burns. These lesions typically develop in home "do-it-yourself" projects and more rarely in experienced cement workers (Vickers and Edwards, 1976; Hannuksela et al., 1976; Whiting, 1977; Flowers, 1978). Strong alkalies dissolve keratin, extract water from the tissue, and produce a soapy, slippery burn.

Sensitization dermatitis, particularly of the hands, is seen in some cement workers and has been attributed to the presence of hexavalent chromium that is present in many cements (Calnan, 1960). The addition of small amounts of iron sulfate to the cement reduces the chromium to the insoluble trivalent form and has been recommended to decrease the incidence of cement dermatitis (Fregert et al., 1979).

References

Calnan CD: Cement dermatitis. *J Occup Med* 1960;2:15–22.

Flowers MW: Burn hazard with cement. *Br Med J* 1978;1:1250.

Fregert S, Gruvberger B, Sandahl E: Reduction of chromate in cement by iron sulfate. *Contact Derm* 1979;5:39–52.

Hannuksela M, Suhonen R, Karvonen J: Caustic ulcers caused by cement. *Br J Dermatol* 1976;95:547–549.

Vickers HR, Edwards DH: Cement burns. *Contact Derm* 1976;2:73–78.

Whiting RK: Alkali burns caused by contact with cement. *Penn Med* 1977;80:48.

Sodium Hydroxide

Sodium hydroxide (also called caustic soda, soda lye, or white caustic) is now produced primarily by electrolysis of sodium chloride solution. It is used in a wide variety of manufacturing processes that include the production of rayon, mercerized cotton, soap, paper, aluminum, petroleum, and dyestuffs. Other uses involve metal cleaning, zinc extraction, tin plating, laundering, and bleaching (NIOSH, 1975).

Ramazzini in 1713 reported skin fissures in laundresses and washerwomen from occupational exposure to sodium hydroxide. Davidson (1927) demonstrated a delayed sense of irritation from concentrated sodium hydroxide applied to the skin of volunteers in contrast to the fairly rapid perception of acid similarly applied. The keratolytic effect of sodium hydroxide was demonstrated by a case reported by Morris (1952) where a concentrated solution dripped on the head of a worker repairing a clogged pipe: a scalp burn with local loss of hair occurred that was probably lessened by flushing with water even though that was delayed to the next day.

Burns of the eye have been the most severe effect of contact with sodium hydroxide solutions or dust. Hughes (1946a,b) summarized the sequence of events in severe alkali burns of the eye and he concluded that alkalinity and not a specific cation was responsible for the severity of the lesion. Since alkali penetrates through the cornea into the anterior chamber rapidly (within one to 10 minutes), immediate and copious irrigation with water is essential. The value of prompt treatment is illustrated by cases of sodium hydroxide splash burns of the eye reported by Dennis (1954) and Horwitz (1966).

Inhalation of sodium hydroxide has not been widely reported as a hazard although NIOSH in one of its investigations found symptoms of upper respiratory tract irritation among workers near an open vat in a chemical degreasing operation where the solvent containing NaOH was maintained at 93°C (200°F) by steam bubbling through it (NIOSH, 1975). In an epidemiologic study of 291 workers chronically exposed to caustic dusts for 30 years or more, Ott et al. (1977) found no significant increases in mortality in relation to duration or intensity of such exposure.

Interest in sodium hydroxide aerosols has developed in the nuclear reactor industry where leaks of molten sodium or of liquid sodium-potassium alloy (NaK) used as heat exchangers could produce aerosols from contact with water in the air. Cooper et al. (1979) pointed out that sodium hydroxide aerosols can quickly react with carbon dioxide to form aerosols of sodium carbonate that are much less alkaline and less hygroscopic. They pointed out the implications of this transformation in the setting of the current occupational exposure limit of 2 mg/m³. Potential skin burns with NaK may be prevented or retarded by prompt flooding with light mineral oil containing 1% to 2.5% stearic acid (Finkel and Lyons, 1958).

References

Cooper DW, Underhill DW, Ellenbecker MJ: A critique of the U.S. standard for industrial exposure to sodium hydroxide aerosols. *Am Ind Hyg Assoc J* 1979;40:365-371.

Davidson EC: The treatment of acid and alkali burns – An experimental study. *Ann Surg* 1927;85:481-489.

Dennis RH: A simple procedure for treatment of alkali burns of the eye. *J Maine Med Assoc* 1954;45:32-49.

Finkel AJ, Lyons WB: Sodium-potassium alloy. An experimental study of its hazards. *Arch Ind Health* 1958;17:624-633.

Horwitz ID: Management of alkali burns of cornea and conjunctiva. *Am J Ophthalmol* 1966; 61:340-341.

Hughes WF Jr: Alkali burns of the eye – I. Review of the literature and summary of present knowledge. *Arch Ophthalmol* 1946a;92:423-449.

Hughes WF Jr: Alkali burns of the eye – II. Clinical and pathologic course. *Arch Ophthalmol* 1946b;93:189-214.

Morris GE: Chemical alopecia. *Arch Ind Hyg Occup Med* 1952;6:530-531.

NIOSH: *Criteria for a Recommended Standard . . . .Occupational Exposure to Sodium Hydroxide.* Washington, DC, National Institute for Occupational Safety and Health (NIOSH 76-105), 1975.

Ott MG, Gordon HL, Schneider EJ: Mortality among employees chronically exposed to caustic dust. *J Occup Med* 1977;19:813-816.

3 • Carbon Dioxide

Sources and Uses

Carbon dioxide (CO_2) is one of the gases found in mines, in natural gas wells, in silos, and in holds of industrial fishing ships. It is produced from carbonaceous material that is easily oxidized and takes up the oxygen from the air. "Black damp" consists of 87% nitrogen and 13% CO_2. Miners test for this gas by lowering a candle into a shaft, for the candle will go out if the air has less than 17% oxygen. Schultzik (Hamilton and Hardy, 1949, p. 246) called attention to the fact that not all kinds of flames can be used for this test. He found that, while most flames are extinguished by 10% CO_2, acetylene does not go out until 26% to 31% is reached. Candles or petroleum lamps should be used, and it is wise to use mice in addition to the flame test.

Carbon dioxide is widely used in industry and research laboratories. It is usually stored in cylinders and tanks under pressure but can also be stored at low temperatures in solid form ("dry ice") that is mainly used as a refrigerant and as a chilling agent. Gaseous CO_2 is used in the textile, leather, and paint industries, and in the manufacture of drugs. Due to its relative inertness it is used in fire extinguishers and as an aerosol propellant, as a pressure medium in food preservation, in welding, and in purging pipelines and tanks. It is widely involved in the manufacture of carbonated drinks. CO_2 is generated as a by-product in synthetic ammonia production, in lime-kiln operations, in the manufacture of methanol and ethylene oxide, and in fermentation (NIOSH, 1976).

Physiological Action

The most important physiological effect of carbon dioxide is to stimulate the respiratory center. At concentrations of 5%, the stimulation is pronounced. The use of CO_2 for the resuscitation of gas victims and for bringing on respiration in newborn babies shows that as much as 30% may be tolerated for some time provided the oxygen supply is adequate. Haldane (Hamilton and Hardy, 1949, p. 247) believed that the symptoms caused by breathing carbon dioxide are chiefly due to oxygen deprivation and begin when the latter has fallen to 12%; the symptoms (headache, rapid breathing) become severe when oxygen reaches 8%. Unconsciousness and death do not occur until the oxygen is down to 5% — unless the victim makes strenuous exertions, in which case death may come while there is still 8% oxygen.

In addition to its effects on the respiratory center, carbon dioxide in appropriate concentrations can produce headache, somnolence, mental confusion, hyporeflexia, lassitude, and eventually more severe neurological disturbances such as tremors, flaccid paralysis, unconsciousness, and death (Johnston, 1959). Respiratory acclimatization to 3% carbon dioxide has been demonstrated by several investigators (Schaefer, 1963). Schaefer (1961) pointed out that while the health of submarine personnel exposed continually to 3% CO_2 was only slightly affected if the oxygen content of the air was maintained at normal levels, more recent studies in the U.S. Navy established the need to keep CO_2 concentrations below 1% for conditions of continuous prolonged exposure. Impairment of performance was noted during prolonged exposure to 3% carbon dioxide even when the oxygen concentration was 21%. Prolonged exposure to 1.5% CO_2 resulted in respiratory acidosis that was not compensated until after the 24th day (Schaefer et al., 1963).

Studies of British coal miners, engaged as part-time rescue workers, demonstrated that they are unlikely to tolerate inspired CO_2 concentrations greater than 3%; higher concentrations of 4% and 5% produced breathlessness and headaches (Love et al., 1979).

Toxic Effects On Man

One source of CO_2 poisoning in industry is fermentation. Troisi (1957) reported deaths from entering silos containing green fodder. Another illustrative case was reported by Lillevik and Geddes (1943). A man was asphyxiated by a 10-minute exposure to carbon dioxide in a grain elevator where 4700 bushels of flaxseed had been stored for 58 days. The man was rescued at once and given prompt treatment with oxygen inhalation, but he died in 48 hours. The air just over the flaxseed bin had 1.8% oxygen and 11.1% CO_2; that within the flaxseed contained 0.4% oxygen and 12.6% CO_2. Bacteria and saprophytic fungi were held responsible for the abnormally high respiratory activity of the flaxseed.

Residues in brewery vats have caused fatal poisoning in this country and England; making compressed yeast caused six cases of poisoning in a German factory as reported by Brezina (Hamilton and Hardy, 1949, p. 247). Carbon dioxide may also be a danger in beet-sugar production, since the juice of the beets is treated with lime and the calcium saccharate is precipitated by CO_2. Schultzik (Hamilton and Hardy, 1949, p. 247) reported a case involving the death of a workman who had entered a vessel in a beet-sugar factory. From the factory inspection service of South Africa, there is a report concerning a case of fatal CO_2 asphyxia in a laborer who, contrary to orders, climbed into a wine vat to gauge the depth of the wine, was overcome by the fumes, and died before he could be lifted out. Four cases occurred in England from the vapors arising from a pit filled with powdered coal.

Sevel and Freedman (1967) described cerebral and retinal degeneration in a patient who was in a coma for 11 months after asphyxiation in a wellhead chamber during the dismantling of an artesian well in central London. Earlier, they had described neurological and ocular changes in two patients who survived CO_2 asphyxia in a similar incident (Freedman and Sevel, 1966). Specifically, they reported headache, photophobia, abnormalities of eye movements, constriction of peripheral visual fields, enlargement of blind spots, deficient dark adaptation, and personality changes, largely depression and irritability.

Carbon dioxide poisoning has been reported aboard ships. Dalgaard et al. (1972) reviewed the literature dealing with cases of unconsciousness and deaths in holds of industrial fishing ships containing trash fish and fish meal. High CO_2 levels (up to 22%) and low O_2 concentrations were incriminated although H_2S may also have been involved. Earlier, Williams (1958) had described a fatal incident aboard a ship with a cargo of onions and crude brown sugar. The two dead men had cyanosis of the oral mucosa and nail beds and markedly congested conjunctivae. Ill persons who survived had headache, giddiness, tinnitus, and weakness, signs and symptoms considered to be consistent with CO_2 poisoning. Another incident involved the wrecked liner *Celtic,* which lay for a year at the entrance to Cork Harbor, fastened to the rocks so that it could not be floated off, and the cargo had to be removed. While engaged in this work in one of the holds, 19 men were overcome by poisonous fumes and four of them died. The nature of the fumes was not definitely ascertained, but the symptoms were not those of carbon monoxide poisoning. Since the fumes were apparently generated by rotting apples, it was decided that the gas was carbon dioxide.

Similar accidents have been reported when dry ice has been used in high quantities as a refrigerant. Chronic poisoning is improbable under most conditions. Prolonged exposure to excessive concentrations is most likely in sealed quarters such as submarines and space crafts. Gibbons (1977) reviewed reports of actual or potential CO_2 poisoning from use of carbon dioxide fire extinguishers and significant loads of dry ice aboard civil and military airplanes. He concluded that the use of dry ice aboard pressurized aircraft could have serious consequences although small amounts of dry ice in unpressurized planes were probably safe. Similar hazards could be associated with the use of CO_2 fire extinguishers aboard planes. Dry ice or carbon dioxide snow may cause injury to the skin when it is improperly handled.

Tolerance Limits

The present tolerance limit of 0.5% for CO_2 would appear to provide a good margin of safety for an 8-hour daily exposure, providing normal amounts of oxygen are inhaled. NIOSH (1976) has recommended a limit of 1% by volume determined as a TWA concentration for up to a 10-hour work shift in a 40-hour workweek, with a ceiling concentration of 3% by volume for a sampling period not to exceed 10 minutes. For higher concentrations of CO_2, respiratory protection is satisfactory only with a self-contained type of respirator or a hose mask with a blower. Adequate ventilation of suspect areas is essential.

References

Dalgaard JB, Deneker F, Fallentin B, et al: Fatal poisoning and other health hazards connected with industrial fishing. *Br J Ind Med* 1972; 29:307–316.

Freedman A, Sevel D: The cerebro-ocular effects of carbon dioxide poisoning. *Arch Ophthalmol* 1966;76:59–65.

Gibbons HL: Carbon dioxide hazards in general aviation. *Aviation Space Environ Med* 1977;48:261–263.

Hamilton A, Hardy HL: *Industrial Toxicology,* ed 2. New York, Paul B. Hoeber, 1949.

Johnston RF: The syndrome of carbon dioxide intoxication: Its etiology, diagnosis, and treatment. *Univ Mich Med Bull* 1959;25:280–292.

Lillevik HA, Geddes WF: Investigation of a death by asphyxiation in a grain-elevator bin containing flaxseed. *Cereal Chem* 1943;20:318–328.

Love RG, Muir DCF, Sweetland KF, et al: Tolerance and ventilatory response to inhaled CO_2 during exercise and with inspiratory resistive loading. *Ann Occup Hyg* 1979;22:43–53.

NIOSH: *Criteria for a Recommended Standard . . . .Occupational Exposure to Carbon Dioxide.* Washington, DC, National Institute of Occupational Safety and Health (NIOSH 76-194), 1976.

Schaefer KE: A concept of triple tolerance limits based on chronic carbon dioxide toxicity studies. *Aerospace Med* 1961;32:197–204.

Schaefer KE: Acclimatization to low concentrations of carbon dioxide. *Ind Med Surg* 1963;32:11–13.

Schaefer KE, Hastings BJ, Carey CR, et al: Respiratory acclimatization to carbon dioxide. *J Appl Physiol* 1963;18:1071–1078.

Sevel D, Freedman A: Cerebro-retinal degeneration due to carbon dioxide poisoning. *Br J Ophthalmol* 1967;51:475–482.

Troisi FM: Delayed death caused by gassing in a silo containing green forage. *Br J Ind Med* 1957; 14:56–58.

Williams HI: Carbon dioxide poisoning. Report of eight cases with two deaths. *Br Med J* 1958;2:1012–1014.

4 • Carbon Monoxide

Sources of Exposure

Carbon monoxide (CO) is a toxic gas that is odorless, colorless, and tasteless, and is slightly less dense than air. It is the oldest of the industrial poisons, for it must have attacked the first men who used heat to break stone for implements or who burned wood with little air to make charcoal. It is still encountered often in industry, since it is formed whenever there is incomplete combustion of oxygen.

Carbon monoxide is produced in nature in amounts estimated to be as much as ten times that from man-made sources (Spedding, 1974). Oxidation of methane is the largest source of CO in the atmosphere and may reach 3×10^9 metric tons of CO annually in the northern hemisphere alone (WHO, 1979). About 220×10^6 metric tons per year are released from the oceans, a large part of which originates in the float cells of kelp (Chapman and Tocher, 1966), and to some extent from pneumatophores of deep-sea coelenterates (Pickwell, 1970). Other natural sources include forest and grass fires, volcanos, marsh gases, electrical storms, and the destruction of chlorophyll in autumn. Carbon monoxide is also produced endogenously from the normal catabolism of hemoglobin at a rate of 42 ml per hour in normal males at rest (Coburn et al., 1963).

Man-made carbon monoxide results from the incomplete combustion of carbonaceous substances. The most important source is the gasoline (spark ignition) engine, which accounts for 60% of the annual total CO emission (Lawther, 1975; Stewart, 1976). Another 20% comes from stationary sources such as space and water heaters, furnaces, and from industrial processes, coal mine explosions, and solid waste disposal procedures. CO plays a necessary part in the production of steel since it is used in the reduction process to take up oxygen. Gases that are used for illumination and for heat and power contain varying amounts of CO, and the gases that result from the explosion of coal dust, from the detonation of blasting charges, and from the partial burning of such charges are also more or less rich in carbon monoxide.

Natural gas in this country does not contain carbon monoxide, but, unless it is burned with a sufficient supply of oxygen, the vapors that form may be very rich in CO. For this reason, water heaters are a common source of carbon monoxide. When a flame touches a surface cooler than the ignition temperature of the gaseous portion of the flame, carbon monoxide will be formed, especially since the temperature of the water-filled coils cannot rise appreciably above the boiling point of water. If these heaters are not properly vented, the room atmosphere readily becomes contaminated. Gas and coal space heaters are also frequent sources of carbon monoxide unless properly vented.

Additional sources of carbon monoxide are the manufacture of synthetic methanol and other organic compounds from carbon monoxide, industrial and residential fires, carbide manufacture, distillation of coal or wood, operations near furnaces and ovens, pyrolysis and oxidation of lubricants in air compressors, operation of snow melting machines, and testing of internal combustion engines. Although tobacco smoking contributes negligible amounts of CO to the air, cigarette smokers are the most heavily exposed nonindustrial portion of the population and this exposure obviously affects industrial workers as well.

The most common hazard, of course, is automobile exhaust in garages. Goldsmith et al. (1963) stated that the average motor vehicle exhaust at that time contained 3.5% carbon monoxide, and they found that in Los Angeles alone motor vehicles emitted 9000 tons of CO per day or 3.4 million tons per year. It has been estimated that 60 million tons were released in 1953 into the United States atmosphere, a value that rose to 100 million tons annually by 1970 (US EPA, 1973).

Prolonged exposure to carbon monoxide can occur in garage work, especially in poorly ventilated places. An investigation of 1308 garages and repair shops was made by the New York State Department of Labor in 1920. These shops employed 5960 men, most of whom were quite ignorant of the dangerous properties of the gas from the exhaust, although they knew that now and then a man would be "knocked out." The investigators found that 113 cases of asphyxia had occurred in two years, and they also found 150 persons suffering from headaches that they attributed to the air in the garages. Chovin (1967) reported average carbon monoxide levels as high as 172 mg/m³ (150 ppm) and 205 mg/m³ (179 ppm) in a Paris police garage in early mornings and early evenings.

Complaints of malaise from traffic policemen have led to the testing the air of streets where traffic is heavy. In the air of New York City streets, Henderson and Haggard (1943) found 0.01% CO. In Philadelphia, Wilson et al. (1926) demonstrated CO in the blood of 14 traffic policemen, in six of whom the amount ranged from 20% to 30%. When, however, during an oil importation crisis, the only traffic in central London was diesel powered (which produces very little CO in the exhaust), carbon monoxide concentrations fell almost to zero (Lawther et al., 1962). Generally, CO concentrations in street air fall away rapidly with distance because of dispersion by wind and vehicle-produced turbulence (Lawther, 1975).

Apart from emissions from industrial and other processes as sources of carbon monoxide, the use of CO-containing gases for heat or power is widespread, and there is consequently ample opportunity in industry for contamination of the air of workrooms with this gas. Outside of garages, the amount found in the air is usually small, and it is difficult to state, as a result of occupational experience, at just what point such contamination begins to constitute a danger to health. It is a common experience among printers, pressers in tailor shops, bakers, cooks, laundry workers, lead molders, felt hat finishers, and painters who use open charcoal burners to heat cold rooms that the air from gas and charcoal burners causes dull headache and inability to do prolonged mental work efficiently or to do skilled work well. These workers complain of a feeling of fatigue and lack of energy, and sometimes of anorexia. The installation of exhaust ventilation is followed by a distinct feeling of improved well being and increased energy. In France, where charcoal is much used for cooking, CO fumes apparently cause trouble fairly often, for the French write of the "folie des cuisiniers."

Another source of carbon monoxide is the metabolism of absorbed methylene chloride (dichloromethane, CH_2Cl_2), which is a principal ingredient of most paint removers (Stewart and Hake, 1976). Barrowcliff and Knell (1979) reported a case of serious cerebral deterioration in a middle-aged man who had used methylene chloride as a solvent for three years in a road material laboratory. They suggested the possibility of both the immediate risk of anoxia due to carboxyhemoglobinemia and the long-term hazard of chronic CO toxicity affecting the brain. Rodkey and Collison (1977) concluded from their studies with rats that methylene chloride acts as a direct substrate for the metabolic formation of CO.

Absorption and Excretion

Carbon monoxide is absorbed through the lungs and combines reversibly with hemoglobin and to a lesser extent with myoglobin, cytochrome oxidase, and other compounds with iron-containing porphyrin. The relation between equilibrium concentrations of oxygen (O_2) and carbon monoxide (CO) in inspired air and oxyhemoglobin (HbO_2) and carboxyhemoglobin (COHb) is expressed by Haldane's first law in the following equation:

$$\frac{COHb}{HbO_2} = M \times \frac{P_{CO}}{P_{O_2}}$$

where M is an affinity constant (208 to 235 at 37°C) and P_{CO} and P_{O_2} are the partial pressures of CO and O_2, respectively (Lawther, 1975). This relationship is affected by the concentration of COHb before exposure, normally about 0.5% to 0.8% from endogenous breakdown of hemoglobin plus that produced by the inhalation of tobacco smoke. COHb also dissociates in accordance with this equation, a process that is accelerated by increased concentration of oxygen in inspired air and increased pulmonary ventilation by exercise. Without these measures, appreciable levels of COHb have a half-life of about 4.5 hours. Under conditions of cessation of exposure, excretion of carbon monoxide begins rapidly but becomes slower with time and with lowered levels of carboxyhemoglobin. Hyperbaric oxygen will accelerate the lowering of high levels of carboxyhemoglobin (Pace et al., 1950; Smith et al., 1962; Sluijter, 1967).

Peterson and Stewart (1970) exposed healthy volunteers to different concentrations of CO for periods of 0.5 to 24 hours. They derived an empirical relationship for blood COHb levels as a function of ambient CO concentration and exposure time:

$$\log_{10} y = 0.85753 \log_{10} x + 0.62995 \log_{10} t - 2.29519$$

where y = percent COHb, x = ppm CO, and t = time in minutes. This formulation has been criticized as being basically a static model that would not reflect true situations when averaging periods longer than 15 minutes are used. More sophisticated equations have been proposed but they are generally beyond the needs of occupational toxicology. In any case, because of shifts of COHb from smoking, varying exposure levels, and variable physical activity, it is considered preferable to measure COHb concentrations in blood rather than CO concentrations in air.

Sayers and Yant (1935) stated that men may be exposed all day to small amounts of carbon monoxide while at rest and not experience any effects; however, on the way home, in the open air, they may suffer severe symptoms, even to unconsciousness. Elimination is supposedly very rapid but, according to these authors, it takes some hours for excessive carbon monoxide to leave the blood unless oxygen and carbon dioxide inhalations are administered to hasten elimination. In their experiments with human subjects it took from 10 to 11 hours to reduce a 35% saturation to 5%.

Apthorp and his colleagues (1958) carried out an interesting experiment on four normal subjects who, during steady exercise, were given pure carbon monoxide in sufficient amounts to raise their blood CO to levels between 30% to 50% saturation. The rate of elimination of CO was compared during the breathing of oxygen with that of breathing carbogen (5% CO_2 in oxygen). The addition of CO_2 led to an increase in the rate of elimination of carbon monoxide because of the increase in minute-volume that it produced. Apthorp et al. estimated that doubling the minute-volume led to a 30% increase in the rate of CO excretion.

Action of Carbon Monoxide

The action of carbon monoxide is favored by heat, humidity, and muscular exertion (Sayers and Yant, 1935). Young men are more susceptible than older men in industrial experience, probably because they breathe more deeply, although there is among coal miners a strong belief that the older men have acquired a degree of "immunity." Men with chronic bronchitis or asthma handle CO poorly and the course of CO poisoning is unfavorably influenced by alcoholism, obesity, and chronic heart disease. Chronic vascular disease increases the damage by CO to the basal ganglia (Hill and Semerak, 1918).

The asphyxia brought about by CO is caused by the affinity of hemoglobin for this gas, which is 240 times as great as its affinity for oxygen, and the resulting carboxyhemoglobin is much more stable than oxyhemoglobin. The asphyxia, however, differs from that caused by suffocation. Haldane showed that the presence of COHb in the blood interferes with the dissociation of the remaining oxyhemoglobin, so that a person with an anemia of 50% is better able to utilize the oxygen in his blood than one with a CO saturation of 50%. A third effect is that reduced oxyhemoglobin acts as a catalyst in the liberation of carbon dioxide; therefore, if there is a loss of oxyhemoglobin by its conversion to COHb, the removal of CO_2 may be hindered (von Oettingen, 1944).

Haldane (1930) reported that breathing 1.0% CO produces a carbon monoxide saturation of the blood up to 50% in 15 minutes and up to 80% in 23 minutes; but if a man is exerting himself, 50% saturation may be reached in five minutes. At just what level of COHb saturation death will occur is not known, for the blood loses carbon monoxide rapidly when the victim is removed to fresh air. A high degree of saturation may not be fatal provided treatment is instituted promptly.

It is inaccurate, but unfortunately convenient, to use the term "carbon monoxide poisoning" or to include carbon monoxide among the poisonous gases. It is physiologically inert except for one property — it drives oxygen out of the red cells of the blood and thus deprives the body of its normal supply of oxygen. In the strictest sense, it is an asphyxiant and the damage that it produces can be traced to oxygen starvation. Erythrocytes once freed from carbon monoxide are ready to function normally. Nerve cells will live in an atmosphere of carbon monoxide (Haggard, 1922). Lhermitte and Ajuriaguerra (1946), however, believed that there is a toxic factor in carbon monoxide "poisoning," in addition to the anoxic effect, that affects the neuroglia and vascular network of the central nervous system, with specific involvement of the basilar region and the white fibers of the centrum semiovale.

Lewey and Drabkin (1944) noted in their experiments on dogs that the electrocardiographic and morphologic changes in the heart in carbon monoxide poisoning closely resemble those observed in anoxia produced by other causes, such as exposure to oxygen-poor air. On the other hand, certain differences have been noted between simple oxygen deprivation and carbon monoxide poisoning. Klebs (Hamilton and Hardy, 1949, p. 226) found no pleural hemorrhages associated with the latter while they were present in victims of asphyxia. C. K. Drinker (1938) stated that in asphyxia the respiratory symptoms appear first and the nervous symptoms later, while in CO poisoning this order is reversed. Haldane agreed and said that there is less dyspnea in carbon monoxide asphyxia than in mountain sickness, but that there is a greater tendency to loss of consciousness. Lewey suggested that the difference may depend on the course of the case — a slow asphyxiation producing changes typical of anoxia, while one that is sudden and/or violent results in a different picture.

Clinically, there is a wide difference between a sudden, rapid, and excessive exposure to carbon monoxide and one that is less great but more prolonged. This difference is shown by the complete recovery of victims in an incident of severe sudden exposure to carbon monoxide that had escaped from a blast furnace. If, however, the inhalation of carbon monoxide proceeds slowly and if the victim lives for some time in an atmosphere of carbon monoxide, there may be cell destruction from the prolonged anoxemia. This consequence is seen in the victims of coal mine explosions or fires and in those overcome by the exhaust gases from motor engines, who recover consciousness but are left with transient or permanent psychoses, paralyses, cardiac disturbances, impaired vision, and similar problems.

The sequelae of intense exposures are usually abnormalities of cerebral or spinal function, and the anatomic changes are found chiefly in the nervous system. Those cases that present striking sequelae are important from the medical and medicolegal point of view, but it must not be forgotten that they are exceptional and that the vast majority of patients who recover from the acute effects do so completely (Forbes, 1921). Engel (1925), who had 12 years' experience in a large steel works, saw some 1200 cases among blast furnace men but noted no sequelae in the central nervous system or the lungs. In the experience of the senior authors of this book, lasting damage from acute exposure is rare in view of the number of men who have been so affected.

Fire fighters have unusual intermittent exposures to carbon monoxide from smoke inhalation. Sammons and Coleman (1974) concluded from their studies of 36 fire fighters that the nonsmokers sampled randomly achieved the maximum allowable COHb saturation under NIOSH guidelines (5.0%) and that as a group fire fighters exhibited changes in the enzymes of injury that suggested myocardial damage. Loke et al. (1976) found a significant increase in mean COHb levels in 16 fire fighters studied after three building fires, and they suggested that fire fighters avoid cigarette smoking after a fire in order to prevent further increases in COHb levels. The need for rapid estimations of these levels after each exposure was stressed by Stewart et al. (1976), and they described an electrochemical breath analysis instrument that permitted such determinations in the field by the fire fighters themselves.

Increased COHb levels regardless of smoking habits were noted by Radford and Levine (1976) in their study of Baltimore fire fighters. They also found that *intermittent* use of self-contained compressed air breathing apparatus offered no advantage over non-use and that *continuous* use of this equipment was required for adequate protection. Griggs (1977) found that while such equipment provided full protection, its use was associated with significantly increased heart rates. He emphasized the point that in fighting fires the exertion levels and, hence, the ventilation rates may be so great that even in low or moderate concentrations of carbon monoxide the COHb can rise to dangerous levels within minutes. The seriousness of this hazard in burning buildings was also pointed out by Barnard and Weber (1979) in their investigations of 25 fires in Los Angeles.

Concentration Necessary to Produce Symptoms

Table 2 is based on the work of Haldane (1930), Henderson and Haggard (1943), and Sayers and Yant (1935). The work of McFarland and his colleagues (1944) on the effects of CO and altitude on the visual thresholds of aviators had shown that CO anoxia produces a loss of visual efficiency at an ambient concentration much lower than had been supposed. Indeed, the amount is so small that even the effect of smoking a few cigarettes and inhaling the smoke was enough to bring the COHb level up to a point where visual sensitivity was impaired. In industrial work, such an impairment may make accurate work impossible and may be the cause of accidents. Horvath et al. (1971) subjected volunteers for two hours to concentrations that approximated the mean (26 ppm) and the peak (111 ppm) levels that raised the average COHb concentration to 6.6%. The 111-ppm level of carbon monoxide resulted in definite impairment of visual vigilance in urban traffic driving.

Table 2
Concentration of CO Necessary
to Produce Symptoms

Concentration in Air		
Percent	*ppm*	*Effects*
0.02	200	Possibly headache, mild frontal in 2 to 3 hours
0.04	400	Headache, frontal, and nausea after 1 to 2 hours; occipital after 2½ to 3½ hours
0.08	800	Headache, dizziness and nausea in ¾ hour, collapse and possibly unconciousness in 2 hours
0.16	1600	Headache, dizziness and nausea in 20 minutes; collapse, unconsciousness, possibly death in 2 hours
0.32	3200	Headache and dizziness in 5 to 10 minutes, unconsciousness and danger of death in 30 minutes
0.64	6400	Headache and dizziness in 1 to 2 minutes, unconsciousness and danger of death in 10 to 15 minutes
1.28	12,800	Immediate effect; unconsciousness and danger of death in 1 to 3 minutes

Drinker (1938) stated that, when an individual is exercising or working, the safety constant must be reduced to one-third or less. Ebersole (1960) reported that submariners exposed to 50 ppm of carbon monoxide for many days complained of headaches. However, there were no complaints when the level was dropped to 40 ppm and exposure lasted 60 days. Haldane (1930) put the COHb level necessary to produce symptoms at 20%. Stern (1964) felt that when the blood carbon monoxide reaches 10%, signs of borderline effects are first seen. He also believed that if the air concentration is 50 ppm or less the blood level will remain below 10%. Schulte (1964) corroborated these findings when he exposed young healthy men to 44 ppm for long periods without any deleterious effects. He felt that 50 ppm should be the limit for any exposure over four hours.

It is important to remember that other gases may be mixed with carbon monoxide and complicate the clinical picture. Thus, in coal mines there may be nitrous fumes from explosions and sulfur dioxide from sulfur in the coal. In factory fires these same gases may be formed along with hydrogen chloride, and there may also be acrolein from burning oil or fat.

Toxic Effects: Blood

Since carbon monoxide, like oxygen, is reversibly bound by hemoglobin, it is consequently in competition with oxygen for binding sites on the hemoglobin molecule. As noted above, the equilibrium constant, M, expresses the relative affinity of hemoglobin for CO and O_2, and ranges in man from 185 to 238 (Douglas et al., 1912). In the presence of COHb the oxyhemoglobin dissociation curve is "shifted to the left" so that CO not only diminishes the total amount of available oxygen by direct replacement in the alveolar air but it also alters the binding of oxygen to hemoglobin so that it is held more tenaciously and is released at lower oxygen tensions. Since myoglobin may act as a reservoir for oxygen within the muscle fibers, it too can combine with CO to form carboxymyoglobin, although the affinity constant, M, is much lower in this case, approximately 40 (Rossi-Fanelli and Antonini, 1958). This value may be higher for cardiac muscle so that when blood COHb is 10%, 30% of the cardiac myoglobin may be saturated with CO.

The blood cell count in carbon monoxide asphyxia is usually reported to be normal, although a polycythemia has been found in both acute and chronic poisoning. This has been regarded as a compensatory effort to make up for the red cells that are incapacitated by COHb. Barcroft and his colleagues (1925), working on the anoxemia of mountain sickness, observed that the blood in the spleen contained less carbon monoxide than did the circulating blood. Contraction of the spleen, they believed, sends out fresh red cells to meet the demand for oxygen transport. According to deBoer and Carroll (1924), the

162

spleen contracts when there is as little as 8% COHb in the blood. Theoretically, then, polycythemia should be a frequent finding in CO poisoning, but as a matter of fact, it is decidedly rare. If it does occur, it is only at an early stage and it is transient. Brieger's (1944) study of dogs exposed to 96 ppm of carbon monoxide for 11 weeks showed a significant rise in the red cell count in the first weeks, but then it dropped to the original level or below. Brieger believed that the increase in red cell count was due to marrow activity, not to contraction of the spleen, for he found increased numbers of reticulocytes and some normoblasts. Nor did he believe that the polycythemia indicated an acclimatization to carbon monoxide, for the dogs suffered from the usual circulatory and nervous disturbances, and characteristic anatomic changes were found.

Toxic Effects:
Cardiovascular System

Haggard, experimenting with dogs, saw no direct toxic action of CO on the heart and Drinker's studies of fatal poisoning in men gave the same results. In extreme asphyxia the most characteristic effect was heart block. In young, vigorous men there is often low blood pressure and a dilated heart, and sometimes auricular fibrillation. Sandall (1922), in clinical studies, found no abnormality in the heart in 85% of the cases in which tachycardia had been a definite sign.

There is, however, some difference of opinion on this matter. According to British writers, cardiac symptoms are not at all unusual immediately after severe exposure, and they may be persistent or even permanent, findings pointing to myocarditis as a sequel. Palpitation, breathlessness on exertion, and precordial pain are fairly common complaints in CO poisoning. Carbon monoxide asphyxia may exacerbate preexisting disease of the coronary arteries. Neubuerger and Clark (1945) described a nonindustrial case of subacute carbon monoxide poisoning with cerebral changes and multiple myocardial necroses. A 19-year-old girl was found comatose in a camp cottage with a dead companion. Both had been exposed to what was judged to be a low concentration of carbon monoxide for 18 hours at a room temperature of 90°F (32°C). The girl who was found comatose lived for 18 days. The main findings at autopsy were widespread degenerative changes in the white

substance of the brain, areas of hemorrhage and atalectasis in the lungs, and numerous foci of myocardial necrosis. This case is illustrative of the damage wrought by long-continued exposure to a low concentration of carbon monoxide.

Liebman (Hamilton and Hardy, 1949, p. 233) seems to have been the first, in 1919, to describe myocardial necrosis in carbon monoxide poisoning. In the following year Herzog reported that in 14 out of 16 cases he had found necrosis and fatty dystrophy in the papillary muscle of the mitral valve, in the apex of the heart and in the left ventricle wall. Kroetz (1936) described a case of angina pectoris that followed acute exposure to carbon monoxide in a locomotive engineer whose freight train was stalled for some time in a tunnel. Ehrich et al. (1944) quote Klebs as having been the first, in 1865, to note pathologic lesions in the heart, hemorrhages in the pericardium extending to the tips of the papillary muscles. Colvin (1928) and Kroetz (1936) both found changes in the electrocardiogram. In their experiments on dogs, Ehrich and his colleagues (1944) found that, if the concentration of COHb reached 75% or over (even if for only 15 minutes), pathologic changes such as hemorrhage and necrosis would occur in the myocardium.

Beck and Suter (1938) were impressed with the frequency with which cardiac symptoms appeared in 136 patients "where illness could unquestionably be attributed to frequent and prolonged exposure to carbon monoxide gas." The symptoms were in most instances functional, but in some they were organic. In only one of their patients whose histories are given in full was the poisoning of occupational origin. This patient was a toll bridge executive who worked seven hours daily in an office where approximately 18,000 automobiles stopped daily to pay toll and thereby pollute the air with exhaust gases. A blood test made while the man was on duty showed a CO saturation of 27%, and tests on five other employees gave values from 5.0% to 30.75%. The patient eventually developed symptoms of congestive heart failure, with dyspnea, palpitations, precordial anginal pains, and extrasystoles, as well as electrocardiographic indications of auricular fibrillation. Removal from that atmosphere cleared up the patient's symptoms. Beck and Suter also suggest carbon monoxide as a causative agent in producing myocardial disease as an explanation of the seasonal incidence of coronary thrombosis, to which Wood and Hedley (1935) had called attention. These authors had reported 95 cases observed in Philadelphia during autumn and winter and only 14 in spring and summer. They attributed these findings to the increased combustion of CO-producing fuel for motor power and heating and to improper ventilation during the cold months that rendered more people susceptible to cardiovascular diseases.

Cohen and colleagues (1969), studying 36 hospital admissions for myocardial infarction in the Los Angeles area, discovered a direct relationship between ambient carbon monoxide and myocardial infarction mortality rates, a finding that confirmed reports and opinions over the past 50 years. In a review of carbon monoxide and coronary artery disease, Goldsmith and Aronow (1975) concluded that "the most vulnerable target organ for low level carbon monoxide exposure appears to be the heart." They found convincing evidence for the effect of CO on aggravation of angina pectoris (after exposure to 50 ppm for 90 minutes), aggravation of intermittent claudication (after exposure to 50 ppm for 120 minutes), and alterations of the ECG in normal subjects (after exposure to 100 ppm for four hours). They also found suggestive evidence for production or worsening of arteriosclerosis to be associated with CO in smokers, and for impairment of survival of patients with acute myocardial infarction. In a later review, Aronow (1979) collected evidence of carboxyhemoglobin interfering with myocardial oxygen delivery, aggravating myocardial ischemia, reducing the threshold for ventricular fibrillation during an episode of myocardial ischemia, and increasing platelet stickiness and hence thrombotic tendency. He also found experimental data that implicated carbon monoxide in the pathogenesis of cardiovascular disease by tobacco smoking or by heavy occupational exposure.

Davies and Smith (1980) stated that P wave changes are an early indication of the adverse effect of CO on myocardial conducting tissues, since they found such changes in six of 15 subjects at 7.1% COHb and in three of 16 at 2.4% COHb. They concluded that the P wave abnormalities that they found were due to a specific toxic effect of CO on the normal atrial pacemaking or conducting tissue activity.

Siggard-Anderson and his co-workers (1968) exposed eight young nonsmokers to carbon monoxide inhalations five times daily for eight days. This exposure regimen resulted in an increase in vascular permeability with variable reductions in plasma volume, and, of greater significance, reduced oxygen tension in the tissues. Kjeldsen (1969) examined 1000 workers not exposed occupationally to carbon monoxide and he discovered that the 59 workers with evidence of arteriosclerosis had significantly higher COHb levels than their nonarteriosclerotic counterparts.

Theodore et al. (1971) found that the prominent effect of chronic exposure in animals was marked erythrocytosis, which they felt was an adaptation to chronic tissue hypoxia induced by carbon monoxide. Eckardt and his colleagues (1972), on the other hand, found from their work on monkeys that elevated carboxyhemoglobin levels did not lead to compensatory increases in hematocrit, hemoglobin, or erythrocyte determinations, or to cardiac fibrosis or brain pathology.

Astrup et al. (1967) exposed rabbits to carbon monoxide for eight weeks and found that the uptake of cholesterol in the intima of blood vessels was considerably enhanced. Histologically, the changes in the vessel walls were indistinguishable from those caused spontaneously. In a more recent reevaluation of the relationship between CO and/or nicotine to arteriosclerosis and cardiovascular disease, Astrup and Kjeldsen (1979) pointed out that CO exposure leads to degenerative changes and partial necrosis of myofibrils that are similar to changes after hypoxia. However, the previously reported effects of CO on arterial intimal changes have not been confirmed, and they view these structural alterations as produced primarily by nicotine and secondarily by CO so that CO-induced changes in cholesterol metabolism enhance the accumulation of cholesterol in smokers' arteries.

Toxic Effects:
Central Nervous System

Marked hyperemia of the cerebral vessels seems to be the first effect of CO-induced anoxemia. Forbes et al. (1924) repeatedly showed in animal experiments that a rise in intracranial blood pressure occurs under the influence of carbon monoxide, a rise that they attributed to the increased congestion and edema. The elevation of pressure was accompanied by dilation of the veins about the optic disc, a finding also seen in man at the height of headache produced experimentally. Dempsey et al. (1976) reported the case of a comatose young adult with a hospital admission COHb level of 51%. In addition to the presence of intermittent decerebrate posturing with opisthotonus, ophthalmoscopy revealed bilateral venous engorgement, normal optic discs, and peripapillary hemorrhages in the nerve fiber layer.

Glaister and Logan (1914) saw many cases with cerebrovascular accidents after severe carbon monoxide poisoning. Small hemorrhages into the substance of the cerebrum were a common finding at autopsy, as were hemorrhages into the meninges. In fact, hemorrhage may occur in practically every organ and tissue as a result of the high blood pressure and of the dilatation and weakening of vessel walls. The greater vulnerability of alcoholics to carbon monoxide asphyxia has been attributed to preexisting vascular disease, and the same explanation has been given for the severity of lesions in the middle aged and elderly as compared with the youthful (Hill and Semerak, 1918).

Chiodi and his colleagues (1941) found depression of the respiratory center in severe carbon monoxide poisoning and an increase of the cardiac output by as much as one-half when COHb saturation was 30% to 50%. Degeneration and necrosis of the cells varied in intensity according to the adequacy or inadequacy of the blood supply, and were typically most marked in the lenticular nucleus of the corpus striatum, particularly the pallidal region, as first described by Klebs in 1865 and confirmed by many others (e.g., LaPresle and Fardeau, 1967). The exaggeration of this process in the globus pallidus is explained by the poor blood supply, the end arteries here making a sharp bend backward, or by the ease with which thrombosis occurs in the long, thin pallidal vessels that are devoid of vasa vasorum. Other foci of degeneration may be found scattered widely throughout the cerebrum (Wilson and Winkelman, 1925; LaPresle and Fardeau, 1967), and their varied localization accounts for the wide variety of symptoms that have been described in severe carbon monoxide asphyxia. Strecker (1927) found a diffuse infiltration of the cerebral white matter with proliferation of glial elements and endothelial cells.

Hearing loss has been reported from acute carbon monoxide poisoning. Baker and Lilly (1977) described this effect in a young woman who recovered from severe poisoning but who showed a persistent U-shaped audiogram. They believed that acute CO asphyxia involves vestibular function more often than hearing, the loss of which they thought resulted from hypoxia of the cochlea, eighth nerve, and brain stem nuclei. Makashima

et al. (1977) studied CO poisoning in guinea pigs and concluded that loss of auditory threshold sensitivity was most prominent at the auditory cortex and the inferior colliculus, with no loss at the cochlea. These findings were interpreted to demonstrate the relative vulnerability of the central auditory pathway to carbon monoxide compared to the end organ.

Blindness — complete or incomplete, transient or permanent — is a rare accompaniment or sequel of carbon monoxide asphyxia. Usually, when it is present, it is a part of the symptom complex that includes marked involvement of the central nervous system. The cases are not numerous, but there are enough to demonstrate that oxygen starvation that results from the prolonged action of CO may be sufficient to cause degeneration of the cortical centers, the optic thalamus, or the optic nerve.

Neuroretinitis with subsequent optic atrophy was described by Wilmer (1921) whose patient was a workman who used a gasoline torch in a closed room. He had an attack of faintness, dizziness, nausea, and headache that soon subsided but two days later he experienced transient blurring of vision. Two months later he did the same work and again two days later developed blurring of vision that did not clear up. Two months later he was found to have contracted visual fields, defective color sense, and atrophy of the optic nerve. Thompson (1922) attributed to carbon monoxide the amblyopia of a garage worker whose vision was lost on the temporal side of the left eye and in the right eye was reduced to counting fingers. Fejer's (1924) patient recovered consciousness after severe asphyxia, with partial sight, but suffered complete loss of vision on the third day, followed by gradual recovery. In an industrial case described by Beck (1936), transient loss of sight in both eyes was accompanied by symptoms suggestive of multiple sclerosis, but all cleared in 20 days. Francois (1942) reported a case of homonymous hemianopsia that followed carbon monoxide exposure, and found two additional cases in the literature. Ramsey (1973) found no effect on depth perception, visual discrimination for brightness, or flicker fusion discrimination at COHb concentrations of 7.6% and 11.2%, although reaction time to a visual stimulus was reduced significantly in both test groups.

Beard and Wertheim (1967) noted a definite behavior impairment in young adults that followed inhalation of carbon monoxide: a deterioration of performance occurred after 90 minutes at 50 ppm of CO, and at proportionately shorter times after 250 ppm. These results could not be confirmed by Stewart et al. (1970). In a study involving 49 healthy adult men, Schulte (1963) found that psychomotor abilities were sensitive to CO in the blood, although reaction time, static steadiness, and muscle persistence were not altered by COHb concentrations less than 20%. However, he found that tests of cognitive ability involving choice discrimination showed impairment at COHb levels below 5%. Horvath et al. (1971) found impaired visual vigilance when subjects breathed 111 ppm CO, which raised the mean COHb level to 6.6%.

Lawther (1975) pointed out that many studies designed to detect deterioration of perception, judgment, behavior, and performance of skilled tasks at low concentrations of COHb suffer from failure to use double-blind techniques. He emphasized the difficulties inherent when small effects are sought that can also be produced by anxiety, drugs, foods, and stimulants, and he concluded that "there is slender evidence that COHb concentrations of less than 3% can impair perception and performance."

Several authors have stressed the incidence of neuropsychiatric sequelae of acute CO poisoning and the need for prolonged administration of oxygen to prevent them. Smith and Brandon (1970) reviewed 206 cases in Newcastle-upon-Tyne and found that in about 20% recovery was complicated by prolonged delirium. Irritability, restlessness, and depression were also present in 20% of the cases. Three men developed permanent dementia, and spastic hemiplegia occurred in two older patients. In a follow-up study three years later (1973), they found deterioration of personality in 33% and impairment of memory in 43% of the 63 patients available for evaluation. Gross neuropsychiatric damage was directly attributable to the CO poisoning in eight patients. Remick and Miles (1977) reported organic brain damage with parietal lobe signs in a young woman who attempted suicide with a combination of barbiturate overdosage and CO poisoning. Ginsburg and Romano (1976) described severe neurologic and psychiatric sequelae in another suicide attempt with CO, and their review of the literature revealed that 15% to 40% of survivors of CO poisoning develop neuropsychiatric symptoms. These writers emphasized the need for adequate evaluation of COHb, presence of depressants, arterial gases for acidosis, and electrocardiographic status. Treatment should include oxygen, prefer-

ably hyperbaric, avoidance of tranquilizers that decrease REM (rapid eye movement) sleep, possible use of dexamethasone or mannitol to treat central nervous system edema, and bed rest for two to four weeks to avoid delayed onset of undesirable neuropsychiatric complications.

Clinical Syndromes

The diagnosis of *acute carbon monoxide poisoning* depends on the history of exposure; the appearance of the victim (marked pink color of cheeks and lips, red blotches on various parts of the skin); the symptoms (as of alcoholic intoxication if consciousness is still maintained, with dull, fixed eyes); the evidences of anoxemia, exaggerated by exertion; and the detection of carbon monoxide in the blood or in the air of the place in which the victim was overcome. It can be seen then that the effects of carbon monoxide on the worker depend not only on the carbon monoxide content in the blood but on many other factors such as the work effect, duration of exposure, the partial pressure of the oxygen breathed, the temperature, the general health of the worker and the degree and capacity of inurement to exposure.

The symptoms of acute poisoning may come on without warning since the gas is odorless, tasteless, and quite nonirritating. The odor of "escaped gas" is due to other volatile compounds. But usually some warning of danger is given unless the amount of carbon monoxide is very great. Such a warning is usually a subjective symptom pointing to involvement of the central nervous system, which is the part of the body most vulnerable to the attack of carbon monoxide. It may be a sense of pressure in the head or a bandlike constriction or throbbing, a feeling of weakness in the knees, mental confusion, headache, roaring in the ears, nausea, perhaps vomiting. These constitute the first stage.

The second stage is characterized by increasing weakness and confusion. The headache, dizziness, and inability to think clearly, to decide and act with energy, increase and render the victim peculiarly helpless, so that even if escape is possible he may perish. A person may become not only indifferent to the danger, but even soothed to drowsiness, to a condition like drunkenness. As the action of the anoxemia spreads to the spinal cord, the legs feel heavy, as if the knees were giving way. If rescue does not come in time, consciousness is lost, with vomiting and involuntary evacuations, sometimes with localized or general muscular contractions. Some speak of stiffness of the jaws like lockjaw. General convulsions, however, are not usual in industrial cases even of the severe type.

Atypical forms may occur: sudden apoplectiform seizures without subjective warning symptoms; severe dyspnea or cardiac symptoms that come on at the outset and lead to death, or appear with the return to consciousness. In this class also belong those relapsing forms in which, after a varying period of apparent recovery, there is a reappearance of the symptoms, sometimes severer than in the initial attack.

Pulmonary edema is a common feature of acute gassing, and death is often due to pneumonia. In some cases it is aspiration pneumonia because the patient has vomited before recovering consciousness. The pneumonia comes on early when it is of this etiology. Pulmonary edema is found in the victims whose death is rapid, edema with foci of inflammation in those surviving some 36 hours, and pneumonia in those who live several days. Or a pneumonia may develop some weeks after the accident. It is said to follow a very rapid course with high fever.

Recovery from severe exposure depends on several factors. If the rescue from the poisoned atmosphere is delayed, and if there is preexisting disease — especially disease of the blood vessels or the respiratory tract — recovery is unlikely. Moreover, the elimination of carbon monoxide from the blood does not always halt the changes that have been set up in such cells as those of the central nervous system, which may proceed to profound degeneration with late and progressive symptoms of mental impairment, motor and sensory involvement, loss of vision, cardiac disturbances, or hemorrhage from a sudden rise in blood pressure.

In those cases of severe asphyxia in which recovery is incomplete for some time after the accident or possibly where normal health is never regained, the symptoms are usually mental. In a typical case of severe exposure, if death does not occur, consciousness is regained and a stage of excitement, even delirium, comes on, followed by depression, apathy, indifference to the surroundings, and inability to remember anything about the accident. An intense headache usually goes with this stage. Rarely, however, do these symptoms persist for more than two or three days.

The great majority of victims of carbon monox-ide asphyxia recover without any lasting symptoms, but there are exceptional cases in which structural damage has occurred, usually as a result of slow and prolonged asphyxia. Since this damage involves the basal ganglia especially, and more rarely the cortex and peripheral nerves, the clinical picture may be one of great variety. It has been known for many years that mental disorders may follow severe carbon monoxide poisoning, and instances have been described after exposure in garages (Hitchcock, 1918; O'Malley, 1912). Haldane considered loss of memory and lack of judgment as definite symptoms of carbon monoxide asphyxia, both while the victim is under its influence and after recovery.

Symptoms of brain involvement may come on some time after the accident, in the form either of an apoplectic seizure or of an increasing psychosis. Epileptoid convulsions may be a symptom, not of the early stage, but of recovery. Attacks of headache and dizziness may persist for many weeks after recovery from severe symptoms.

Chronic carbon monoxide poisoning is not accepted as a clinical entity by all. Some explain chronic effects as being due to a slow accumulation of day by day damage that results in pathologic change. In cases of chronic carbon monoxide overexposure such as may be seen in industry, there are few objective signs that can help the physician make the diagnosis unless an abnormal level of COHb can be detected in the blood. However, if this test is made after the patient has left the supposedly contaminated environment for fresh air, the COHb value may be below its maximum because carbon monoxide begins to leave the blood rapidly. But studies have shown that this disappearance is not as rapid as has been supposed. Sayers and Yant (1935) showed that without administration of oxygen it takes from nine to 11 hours to lower a saturation of 35% to 5%. Gilbert and Glaser (1959) showed that when a person has been overcome by carbon monoxide and is removed to an atmosphere of pure air, 50% of the CO in the blood will be removed in three hours.

Beck (1936) called chronic carbon monoxide poisoning "a neglected clinical problem." In his examination of 279 persons whose living conditions involved continual exposure to carbon monoxide, he found evidence suggestive of chronic poisoning in 137, and he stated that most of the symptoms were those of uncomplicated anoxemia but that other findings suggested organic lesions of the central nervous system. Neuromuscular and joint pains, spasms of the voluntary and involuntary muscles, nausea and vomiting, and increase of red cells and of hemoglobin were reported. Duvoir and Gaultier (1946) tried to establish a picture of chronic carbon monoxide poisoning free from the multiplicity of somewhat dubious symptoms that have been attributed to this form of intoxication. In addition to an increase in carboxyhemoglobin, three symptoms are characteristic: asthenia (both muscular and mental), severe headache (not strictly localized), and vertigo and syncope (especially the former). Sumari (1946) found neurological changes in 60 of 71 individuals with chronic coalgas poisoning in Finland.

On the other hand, Rossiter (1942) denied the possibility of injury by small, repeated doses of carbon monoxide, since all damage by this gas results from anoxemia and low concentrations of COHb cannot produce anoxemia. Sievers et al. (1942) made a significant report on the effect of working for 13 years in the Holland Tunnel. The study covered 156 traffic officers working in an atmosphere that averaged 70 ppm of carbon monoxide. There was no sign of impairment of health that would suggest occupational disease; the response to standard neurological tests was good and there was a low incidence of tremors. Blood analysis showed carboxyhemoglobin higher in smokers, averaging 4.1% in light smokers, and 5.4% in those smoking at least 20 cigarettes daily. Nonsmokers averaged 1.7% COHb. Cohen and his colleagues (1971) studied carbon monoxide uptake in federal inspectors at a United States–Mexico border station and found that there was a definite and significant increase in COHb among the inspectors. They also showed concern for the drivers waiting in line to be inspected and raised the question of whether an increase in carboxyhemoglobin in these drivers might lead to more highway accidents.

Well-informed observers and research workers both here and abroad differ on the question as to whether chronic carbon monoxide poisoning exists (Grüt, 1949; Cooper, 1966). One important factor is the role that cigarette smoking plays in chronic poisoning. Another factor involves CO produced endogenously by the breakdown of hemoglobin, and what effect this might have. These and other problems are discussed in recent reviews (Coburn, 1970; National Academy of Sciences, 1977; WHO, 1979).

Control

For many years, the threshold limit value (TLV) for carbon monoxide was set at 100 ppm for eight hours and 400 ppm for not over one hour. During the Second World War, Lewey and Drabkin (1944) questioned whether this figure might be too high and whether working in atmospheres lower in CO might be sufficient to cause changes that, in the case of aviators or men handling complicated machinery, might result in serious accidents. Since it now seems well established that psychomotor performance can be impaired after a 2% to 3% increase in COHb levels, standards of 40 ppm for one hour and 15 ppm for eight hours (as proposed by the Ontario Air Pollution Act of 1967) would seem to be the maximum compatible with safe operation of aircraft.

The American Conference of Governmental Industrial Hygienists (1971) recommended 50 ppm (55 mg/m³) as a TLV for carbon monoxide, a value that is now adopted in the United States. It stated that the apparent success of 100 ppm was due to inurement and accumulation of individuals of low degree of susceptibility. It further recommended that when heavy labor, high temperatures, or high altitude (5000 to 8000 feet; 1525 to 2440 meters) are involved, this figure be reduced to 25 ppm. As has become fairly customary, the USSR and Czechoslovakia recommend lower values; the former uses a TLV of 18 ppm and the latter 30 ppm.

NIOSH (1972) proposed standards that would prevent acute carbon monoxide poisoning, protect employees from harmful myocardial changes associated with COHb levels above 5%, and protect employees from adverse behavioral manifestations that result from exposures to low levels of CO. To this end, NIOSH proposed a concentration limit of 35 ppm determined as a time-weighted average for an eight-hour workday, and a ceiling concentration of 200 ppm.

References

American Conference of Governmental Industrial Hygienists (ACGIH): *Documentation of the Threshold Limit Values,* ed 3. Cincinnati, Ohio, 1971.

Apthorp GH, Bates DV, Marshall R, et al: Effect of acute carbon monoxide poisoning on work capacity: Influence of 5% CO_2 on rate of recovery. *Br Med J* 1958;2:476–478.

Aronow WS: Effect of carbon monoxide on cardiovascular disease. *Prevent Med* 1979;8:271–278.

Astrup P, Kjeldsen K, Wanstrup J: Enhancing influence of carbon monoxide on the development of atherosclerosis in cholesterol fed rabbits. *J Athero Res* 1967;7:343–354.

Astrup P, Kjeldsen K: Model studies linking carbon monoxide and/or nicotine to arteriosclerosis and cardiovascular disease. *Prevent Med* 1979;8:295–302.

Baker SR, Lilly DJ: Hearing loss from acute carbon monoxide intoxication. *Ann Otol Rhinol Laryngol* 1977;86:323–328.

Barcroft J, Murray CS, Orchovats D, et al: Influence of the spleen in carbon monoxide poisoning. *J Physiol* 1925;60:79–84.

Barnard RJ, Weber JS: Carbon monoxide: A hazard to fire fighters. *Arch Environ Health* 1979;34:255–257.

Barrowcliff DF, Knell AJ: Cerebral damage due to endogenous chronic carbon monoxide poisoning caused by exposure to methylene chloride. *J Soc Occup Med* 1979;29:12–14.

Beard RR, Wertheim GA: Behavioral impairment associated with small doses of carbon monoxide. *Am J Public Health* 1967;57:2012. 2022.

Beck HG: Slow carbon monoxide asphyxiation. *J Am Med Assoc* 1936;107:1025–1029.

Beck HG, Suter GM: Role of carbon monoxide in the causation of myocardial disease. *J Am Med Assoc* 1938;110:1982–1986.

Brieger H: Carbon monoxide polycythemia. *J Ind Hyg Toxicol* 1944;26:321–327.

Chapman DJ, Tocher RD: Occurrence and production of carbon monoxide in some brown algae. *Can J Bot* 1966;44:1438–1442.

Chiodi H, Dill DB, Consolazio F, et al: Respiratory and circulatory response to acute carbon monoxide poisoning. *Am J Physiol* 1941;134:683–693.

Chovin P: Carbon monoxide: Analysis of exhaust gas investigations in Paris. *Environ Res* 1967;1:198–216.

Coburn RF (ed): Biological effects of carbon monoxide. *Ann NY Acad Sci* 1970;174:1–430.

Coburn RF, Blakemore WS, Forster RE: Endogenous carbon monoxide production in man. *J Clin Invest* 1963;42:1172–1178.

Cohen SI, Deane M, Goldsmith JR: Carbon monoxide and survival from myocardial infarction. *Arch Environ Health* 1969;19:510–517.

Cohen SI, Dorion G, Goldsmith JR, et al: Carbon monoxide uptake by inspectors at the U.S.-Mexico border station. *Arch Environ Health* 1971;22:47–54.

Colvin LT: Electrocardiographic changes in a case of severe carbon monoxide poisoning. *Am Heart J* 1928;3:484–488.

Cooper AG: *Carbon Monoxide, a Bibliography with Abstracts.* Publ Hlth Service Publ No. 1053, Washington, DC, 1966.

Davies DM, Smith DJ: Electrocardiographic changes in healthy men during continuous low-level carbon monoxide exposure. *Environ Res* 1980;21:197–206.

de Boer S, Carroll DC: Mechanism of spleen reaction to general CO poisoning. *J Physiol* 1924;59:312–332.

Dempsey LC, O'Donnell JJ, Hoff JT: Carbon monoxide retinopathy. *Am J Ophthalmol* 1976;82:692–693.

Douglas CG, Haldane JS, Haldane JBS: The laws of combination of haemoglobin with carbon monoxide and oxygen. *J Physiol* 1912;44:275–305.

Drinker CK: *Carbon Monoxide Asphyxia.* New York, Oxford University Press, 1938.

Duvoir M, Gaultier M: Etude étiologique, clinique et chimique de 40 cas d'oxycarbonisme chronique professionnel. *Arch d mal profess* 1946;7:449–452, abstracted in *J Ind Hyg Toxicol* 1947;27:119.

Ebersole JH: The new dimensions of submarine medicine. *N Engl J Med* 1960;262:599–610.

Eckardt RE, MacFarland HN, Alarie YCE, et al: The biologic effect from long-term exposure of primates to carbon monoxide. *Arch Environ Health* 1972;25:381–387.

Ehrich WE, Bellet S, Lewey FH: Cardiac changes from CO poisoning. *Am J Med Sci* 1944;208:511–523.

Engel RC: Observations in blast furnace gassing. *J Ind Hyg* 1925;7:122–123.

Fejer G: Blindness caused by inhalation of coal gases: Recovery. *Am J Ophthalmol* 1924;7:522–523.

Forbes HS: A survey of carbon monoxide poisoning in American steel works, metal mines and coal mines. *J Ind Hyg* 1921;3:11–15.

Forbes HS, Cobb S, Freemont-Smith F: Central edema and headache following carbon monoxide asphyxia. *Arch Neurol Psychiatry* 1924;11:264–281.

Francois J: Hémianopsie homonyme par intoxication oxycarbonée aiquë. *Ophthalmologica* 1942;103:143–149, abstracted in *J Ind Hyg Toxicol* 1942;103:142.

Gilbert GJ, Glaser GH: Neurologic manifestations of chronic carbon monoxide poisoning. *N Engl J Med* 1959;261:1217–1220.

Ginsburg R, Romano J: Carbon monoxide encephalopathy: Need for appropriate treatment. *Am J Psychiatry* 1976;133:317–320.

Glaister J, Logan DD: *Gas Poisoning in Mining and Other Industries.* New York, W. Wood, 1914.

Goldsmith JR, Aronow WS: Carbon monoxide and coronary heart disease: A review. *Environ Res* 1975;10:236–248.

Goldsmith JR, Terzaghi J, Hackney JD: Evaluations of fluctuating carbon monoxide exposures. *Arch Environ Health* 1963;7:647–663.

Griggs TR: The role of exertion as a determinant of carboxyhemoglobin accumulation in firefighters. *J Occup Med* 1977;19:759–761.

Grüt A: *Chronic Carbon Monoxide Poisoning.* Copenhagen, Mundsgaard, 1949.

Haggard HW: Studies in carbon monoxide asphyxia: The growth of the neuroblast in the presence of carbon monoxide. *Am J Physiol* 1922;60:244–249.

Haldane JS: Carbon monoxide poisoning. *Br Med J* 1930;2:16–17.

Hamilton A, Hardy HL: *Industrial Toxicology,* ed 2. New York, Paul B. Hoeber, 1949.

Henderson Y, Haggard HW: *Noxious Gases,* ed 2. New York, Reinhold, 1943.

Hill E, Semerak CB: Changes in the brain in gas (carbon monoxid) poisoning. *J Am Med Assoc* 1918;71:644–648.

Hitchcock CW: Carbon monoxid poisoning: Its nervous and mental symptoms. *J Am Med Assoc* 1918;71:257–260.

Horvath SM, Dahms TE, O'Hanlon JF: Carbon monoxide and human vigilance. *Arch Environ Health* 1971;23:343–347.

Kjeldsen K: *Smoking and Atherosclerosis.* Copenhagen, Mundsgaard, 1969.

Kroetz C: Angina pectoris nach Rauchgasvergiftung. *Med Klin* 1936;32:1521–1524, abstracted in *J Ind Hyg Toxicol* 1937;19:36.

LaPresle J, Fardeau M: The central nervous system and carbon monoxide poisoning: II. Anatomical study of brain lesions following intoxication with carbon monoxide (22 cases). *Prog Brain Res* 1967;24:31–74.

Lawther PJ: Carbon monoxide. *Br Med Bull* 1975;31:256–260.

Lawther PJ, Commins BT, Henderson M: Carbon monoxide in town air. An interim report. *Ann Occup Hyg* 1962;5:241–248.

Lewey FH, Drabkin DL: Experimental chronic carbon monoxide poisoning of dogs. *Am J Med Sci* 1944;208:502–511.

Lhermitte J, de Ajuriaguerra DE: Les lesions du système nerveux central provoquées par l'intoxication par l'oxyde de carbon. *Semaine de hôp Paris* 1946;22:1945–1948, abstracted in *J Ind Hyg Toxicol* 1947;29:73.

Loke J, Farmer WC, Matthay RA, et al: Carboxyhemoglobin levels in fire fighters. *Lung* 1976;154:35–39.

Makishima K, Keene WM, Vernose GV, et al: Hearing loss of a central type secondary to carbon monoxide poisoning. *Trans Am Acad Ophthalmol Otolaryngol* 1977;84:452–457.

McFarland RA, Roughton FJW: Halperin MH, et al: The effects of carbon monoxide and altitude on visual thresholds. *J Aviat Med* 1944;15:381–394.

National Academy of Sciences: *Carbon Monoxide.* Washington, DC, 1977.

Neubuerger KT, Clarke ER: Subacute carbon monoxide poisoning with cerebral myelinopathy and multiple myocardial necroses. *Rocky Mt J Med* 1945;42:29–35, with correction 42:196.

NIOSH: *Criteria for a Recommended Standard . . . .Occupational Exposure to Carbon Monoxide.* Washington, DC, National Institute for Occupational Safety and Health (NIOSH 73-11000), 1972.

O'Malley M: Carbon monoxid poisoning with acute symptoms, relapse with psychotic symptoms, and complete recovery. *J Am Med Assoc* 1912;59:1540–1541.

Pace N, Strajman E, Walker EL: Acceleration of carbon monoxide elimination in man by high pressure oxygen. *Science* 1950;111:652–654.

Pickwell GV: The physiology of carbon monoxide production by deep-sea coelenterates: Causes and consequences. *Ann NY Acad Sci* 1970;174:102–115.

Peterson JE, Stewart RD: Absorption and elimination of carbon monoxide by inactive young men. *Arch Environ Health* 1970;21:165–171.

Radford EP, Levine MS: Occupational exposures to carbon monoxide in Baltimore firefighters. *J Occup Med* 1976;18:628–632.

Ramsey JM: Effects of single exposures of carbon monoxide on sensory and psychomotor response. *Am Ind Hyg Assoc J* 1973;34:212–216.

Remick RA, Miles JE: Carbon monoxide poisoning: Neurologic and psychiatric sequelae. *Calif Med Assoc J* 1977;117:654–657.

Rodkey FL, Collison HA: Biological oxidation

of (^{14}C) methylene chloride to carbon monoxide and carbon dioxide by the rat. *Toxicol Appl Pharmacol* 1977;40:33–38.

Rossi-Fanelli A, Antonini E: Studies on the oxygen and carbon monoxide equilibria of human myoglobin. *Arch Biochem Biophys* 1958;77:478–492.

Rossiter FS: Carbon monoxide. *Ind Med* 1942;11:586–589.

Sammons JH, Coleman RL: Firefighters' occupational exposure to carbon monoxide. *J Occup Med* 1974;16:543–546.

Sandall TE: The later effects of gas poisoning. *Lancet* 1922;2:857–859.

Sayers RR, Yant WP: Dangers of and treatment for carbon monoxide poisoning. *U.S. Bureau of Mines Rep* No. 2476, 1935.

Schulte JH: Effects of mild carbon monoxide intoxication. *Arch Environ Health* 1963;7:524–530.

Schulte JH: Sealed environments in relation to health and disease. *Arch Environ Health* 1964;8:438–452.

Sievers RF, Edwards TI, Murray AL, et al: Effects of exposure to known concentrations of carbon monoxide. A study of traffic officers stationed at the Holland Tunnel for 13 years. *J Am Med Assoc* 1942;118:585–588.

Siggard-Anderson J, Petersen FB, Hansen TI, et al: Plasma volume and vascular permeability during hypoxia and carbon monoxide exposure. *Scand J Clin Lab Invest* 1968;22(suppl 103):39–48.

Sluijter ME: The treatment of carbon monoxide poisoning by administration of oxygen at high atmospheric pressure. *Prog Brain Res* 1967;24:123–182.

Smith G, Ledingham IMcA, Sharp GR, et al: Treatment of coal-gas poisoning with oxygen at 2 atmospheres pressure. *Lancet* 1962;1:816–818.

Smith JS, Brandon S: Acute carbon monoxide poisoning – 3 years experience in a defined population. *Postgrad Med J* 1970;46:65–70.

Smith JS, Brandon S: Morbidity from acute carbon monoxide poisoning at three-year follow-up. *Br Med J* 1973;1:318–321.

Spedding DJ: *Air Pollution.* Oxford, Clarendon Press. 1974.

Stern AC: Summary of existing air pollution standards. *J Air Poll Control Assoc* 1964;14:5–15.

Stewart RD: The effect of carbon monoxide on humans. *J Occup Med* 1976;18:304–309.

Stewart RD, Hake CL: Paint-remover hazard. *J Am Med Assoc* 1976;235:398–401.

Stewart RD, Peterson JE, Baretta ED, et al: Experimental human exposure to carbon monoxide. *Arch Environ Health* 1970;21:154–164.

Stewart RD, Stewart RS, Stamm W, et al: Rapid estimation of carboxyhemoglobin level in fire fighters. *J Am Med Assoc* 1976;235:390–392.

Strecker EA: Mental sequelae of carbon monoxide poisoning with reports of autopsy in two cases. *Arch Neurol Psychiatry* 1927;17:552–554.

Sumari P: Clinical observations in chronic carbon monoxide (generator gas) intoxication: Preliminary report. *Nord Med* 1946;30:943–945.

Theodore J, O'Donnell RD, Back KC: Toxicological evaluation of carbon monoxide in humans and other mammalian species. *J Occup Med* 1971;13:242–255.

Thompson HM: Chronic carbon monoxid amblyopia. *Colorado Med* 1922;19:145–147.

von Oettingen WF: Carbon monoxide: Its hazards and the mechanism of its action. *Public Health Bull* No. 290, Washington, DC, 1944.

US EPA: The national air monitoring program: Air quality and emission trends. *Annual Report,* Environmental Protection Agency, 1973, vol 1.

WHO: *Environmental Health Criteria 13: Carbon Monoxide.* Geneva, World Health Organization, 1979.

Wilmer WH: Effects of carbon monoxide on the eye. *Am J Ophthalmol* 1921;4:73–90.

Wilson ED, Gates I, Owens HR, et al: Street risk of carbon monoxide poisoning. *J Am Med Assoc* 1926;87:319–320.

Wilson G, Winkelman NW: An unusual cortical change in carbon monoxide poisoning. *Arch Neurol Psychiatry* 1925;13:191–196.

Wood FC, Hedley OF: The seasonal incidence of acute coronary occlusion in Philadelphia. *Med Clin North Am* 1935;19:151–157.

5 • Cyanides

Sources of Hazard

Exposure to *hydrogen cyanide* (HCN, prussic acid) occurs most often in connection with the fumigation of ships, workshops, and dwellings, but this gas is also encountered in fumigation intended to kill agricultural pests, in chemical laboratories, in blast-furnace gas, in the manufacture of illuminating gas, and in the gas from burning nitrocellulose. Industrial processes that carry with them some danger of hydrogen cyanide or cyanogen exposure include the preparation and the decomposition of cyanides, the synthesis of acrylonitrile, the preparation of resin monomers, and the extraction of phosphoric acid from bones. The presence of HCN in various industrial gases results from an incomplete combustion of nitrogen-containing organic compounds, and its presence is often not suspected until some accident occurs. Nut meats, beans, peas, and seeds are fumigated in vacuum chambers with HCN, and partial sterilization of soil is accomplished with this poisonous gas. Curiously, certain plants produce HCN as a side reaction in their protein metabolism with occasional accidental poisoning to agricultural workers and animals.

Sodium and *potassium cyanide* (NaCN, KCN) are used in metallurgy for the extraction of gold and silver from ores. The greatest use, however, for these salts is in electroplating and case-hardening of steel and iron. Cyanide salts are also used for cleaning and coating silver, in silver polishes, and in photography. The manufacture of cyanide compounds must be considered a source of danger.

Cyanogen chloride (CNCl) resembles the other cyanides in its action, but, according to Reed (1920), it is more irritating to the air passages and to the skin. It is used as a pesticide.

Calcium cyanamide ($CaCN_2$), an intermediate in the production of nitric acid and more commonly used as a fertilizer, is severely irritating to the skin and has, in addition, a vasodepressant effect. The vasodepressant effect appears when some other agent such as alcohol — and in one curious case report, paregoric — is also taken. There is a flushing of the skin, a rapid pulse, fall in blood pressure, sweating, pressure in the head or headache, dyspnea, and sometimes syncope.

Biological Effects

HCN is a rapidly acting poison. Its behavior in the body is the result of inactivation of the respiratory enzyme, cytochrome oxidase, by formation of a cyanide complex by CN^- reacting with trivalent iron in cytochrome oxidase, an action shared by all the soluble inorganic cyanide salts. This mechanism of CN ion action prevents the uptake of oxygen by the tissues with resulting cytotoxic hypoxia. The blood itself, saturated with oxygen, remains arterial in color after it reaches the venous circulation to produce the characteristic cherry-color appearance of the victim of acute cyanide poisoning. In low concentration in the human body the CN ion stimulates respiration. Chemical warfare studies demonstrated that electrocardiographic changes follow the intravenous introduction of the CN ion into human volunteers (Wexler et al., 1947).

Since the cyanide ion is absorbed by all tissues, it is important to remember that HCN can be absorbed through human skin (Walton and Witherspoon, 1925; Drinker, 1932; Fairley et al., 1934). This fact means that a gas mask is not sufficient protection against dangerous concentrations of HCN in the air, and it also explains the occurrence of symptoms of poisoning in individuals who have put on clothing from which the fumigating gas had not yet been removed. When the ambient concentration of HCN is high, the cyanide is absorbed through the lungs and transported throughout the body so rapidly that the skin as a mode of entry does not have time to play a significant part in the poisoning. Part of the absorbed cyanide is exhaled unchanged. The greater part is changed by tissue sulfur transferase (rhodanese) to the relatively nontoxic thiocyanate radical (SCN^-) that is distributed unaltered to all body fluids and remains extracellular (Goodman and Gilman, 1975, p. 904). Since this transformation is limited by the endogenous supply of thiosulfate, the toxicity of the cyanide ion depends upon the fact that the rate of conversion to the less harmful thiocyanate cannot be swift enough in any but minute doses to prevent the direct asphyxial action on the tissue cells. Thiocyanate is excreted for the most part by the kidney, but at an irregular rate and can be detected in the urine and blood serum of human beings (Baumann et al., 1934). The ingestion of certain cyanogenetic foodstuffs, notably members of the cabbage family, and the use of tobacco result in amounts of thiocyanate in the urine above the usual range of daily excretion considered to be from 0.5 to 3.0 mg.

The ability of the body to convert the cyanide ion into thiocyanate may account for the many industrial exposures to cyanides without apparent ill effect. At the workroom air level of 10 ppm or under, the ability of the body to convert cyanide to thiocyanate is, in most cases, capable of preventing cyanide intoxication.

The United States Public Health Service (Hamilton and Hardy, 1949, p. 250) has shown that 500 ppm of air can be breathed by a man for one minute without injury, 375 ppm for a minute and a half, and 250 ppm for two minutes. Based on these findings, a rule was established that an experienced man may be allowed to enter a room that has been fumigated if the air contains no more than 100 ppm. The signs and symptoms of acute poisoning appear rapidly after ingestion or inhalation of toxic levels of cyanide, and they include giddiness, vertigo, hyperpnea, headache, palpitation, cyanosis, coma, apnea, asphyxial convulsions, and death (Wolfsie and Shaffer, 1959). Acute poisoning from cyanides does occur from time to time in industry, but it is rare. Johnstone (1948) reported accidental poisoning by cyanide dust in three men spraying insecticide — one was found dead, the other two unconscious. One fatality was reported from Germany (Hamilton, 1925, pp. 345–347) where a woman carried a jar of potassium cyanide down a flight of stairs to the galvano-plating room and on the way inhaled enough fumes to cause her death.

Many cases of fatal poisoning occurred during the First World War because of the extensive use of hydrocyanic acid for the destruction of vermin, for which purpose it continues to be used. HCN fumes are formed by combining dilute sulfuric acid and sodium cyanide. Since the gas is evolved immediately, the disinfectors are instructed to drop the package of sodium cyanide (paper and all) into the acid and run. After the building doors are closed, they must be sealed and warning signs must be placed outside. The action of the gas is complete in two hours, but usually the building is vacated overnight. The doors and windows must be opened from the outside; when this is impossible, an oxygen-supplied respirator must be used. From half an hour to two hours' ventilation is long enough for the disappearance of the gas, but the apparatus in which it has been generated must be removed with great care.

The following cases from European experience are summarized from those cited in Hamilton and Hardy (1949, pp. 251–256). Lambert's case was in an Italian disinfector who was found unconscious in a room filled with this gas. The immediate symptoms were stertorous breathing, flushed skin, red and engorged veins, contracted pupils, and rigid muscles. Later there was free sweating and muscular twitching. The man lived 16 days with fever, sweating, tremors, and rigidity of the muscles, occasional convulsions, ataxia, and aphasia. A fatal incident was described by Koelsch in 1920 in which two men carried a receptacle in which HCN gas had been produced. As they lifted it, an unchanged portion of sodium cyanide was brought into contact with the acid; the fumes that developed poisoned the workman who was carrying the rear handles of the apparatus. He died in a short time. Fühner told of 100 soldiers who put on deloused clothing too soon, before sufficient airing had occurred. All were poisoned — 10 lost consciousness, but none suffered any permanent effect. Fühner told also of an accident in Essen in some Krupp workmen's barracks that had been treated with the gas and then imperfectly aired. Ten men died from the fumes, and five became comatose but revived. The same investigator described a syndrome in men spraying trees with HCN that he considered a mild form of acute poisoning. The symptoms were sudden faintness, weakness, and trembling of the muscles, followed by a splitting headache. The warning signs are itching of the throat and nose, burning and reddening of the eyes, then a metallic taste in the mouth and burning of the tongue, and finally pressure in the head and a feeling of apprehension. In milder poisoning, such as occurs among fumigators, the symptoms are those of moderate oxygen starvation, as seen in mountain climbers. In some cases these symptoms appear in factory workers every day and then pass off when the workers leave work and go out into the open air. A report from Connecticut told of an accident involving eight workers who were overcome by HCN vapors when a new employee put cyanide eggs into a solution of sulfuric acid. These reports bring out the fact that acute cyanide poisoning in industry is accidental in origin, and occurs through ignorance or deliberate disregard of precautionary instruction.

Chronic Occupational Cyanide Exposure

Dermatitis is a familiar occurrence in workers, such as electroplaters, who are chronically exposed to cyanide solutions. The effect is thought to be due to the fact that the solution is strongly irritating and in some individuals causes severe itching. Cyanide rash is described as consisting usually of pruritic papules and vesicles. Occasionally, a blotchy eruption of the face may follow low-level exposure to HCN vapors and solutions of cyanide salts. According to Braddock and Tingle (1930) the so-called cyanide rash among American gold miners is to be attributed rather to the caustic action of quicklime than to the cyanides.

Although Parmenter (1926) questioned whether chronic cyanide poisoning existed, there are numerous reports that controvert this view. Barsky (1937) reported that a group of men engaged in plating with alkaline cyanide solutions of copper, bronze, and nickel suffered from upper respiratory tract irritation. He reported on 18 workers who complained in varying degrees of persistent running nose, nasal obstruction, and bleeding. Examination showed congestion of the nasal mucosa with sloughs of various sizes on the septal wall and on the middle and inferior turbinates. In three cases the sloughs went on to perforation. Barsky noted that no chromic acid was used in the plating process used by these workers. Also, he was able to report that improvement in ventilation of the cyanide baths resulted in complete cessation of signs and symptoms. There are other reports of irritation of the nasal passages among workers in a plant where plating was done

with a copper cyanide solution and in which the air concentration averaged 5 ppm of cyanide, and where the workers had to wear respirators to control the symptoms.

Martin in 1888 reported the case of a 21-year-old servant who applied a silver coating containing the double cyanide of potassium and silver to antiques. As she continued at this work, and the subsequent polishing, she experienced great weakness, severe abdominal pain, vomiting, headache, and ataxia. Merzbach in 1899 described the case of a worker in a printing shop who placed copper plates in a solution of cyanide salts and then passed a galvanic current through the solution, which released hydrogen cyanide as a gas. After a year, severe gastrointestinal symptoms and disturbance of the whole nervous system, including the intellect, resulted in complete disability and death within two years of cessation of cyanide exposure. Collins and Martland (1908) reported a disease of the primary motor neurons resembling the clinical picture of acute anterior poliomyelitis that was the result of poisoning by potassium cyanide. The patient was a 60-year-old hotel worker who polished silver by dropping it into a potassium cyanide solution and then drying it. He had severe pruritis and brownish-red pigmentation of the forearms. Severe vertigo and signs of meningitis were followed by loss of power in legs and arms. Improvement came slowly after six months. Parmenter (1926) described a photographic worker who suffered from numbness, weakness, vertigo, nausea, tachycardia, headache, flushing of the face, and gastric distress while working over a sink containing potassium cyanide and ferrous sulfate.

Two of the three cases reported by Smith (1932) qualify as examples of chronic cyanide poisoning. In one case, the worker had been a gold plater for 20 years, 10 of which he had spent in a small shop with insufficient ventilation. He was first bothered with a rash on his arms, hands, and face. Coincidentally, he had spells of nausea and vomiting. After a prevacation rush of business, he was seized with violent abdominal pain and convulsions that recurred with renewed exposure to the potassium cyanide solution. He gave up work, incapacitated by weakness, weight loss, headache, vertigo, muscular cramps, and recurring abdominal pain and vomiting. The second worker had been employed as a case hardener for 15 years. Weight loss and muscle weakness involving the arms and legs developed to such a degree that he had to give up work. Ullmann (Hardy et al.,

1950), investigating the cause of general malaise and headaches in several girls employed in a shoe store in Germany, found a considerable quantity of cyanide in a fluid shoe cleaner.

Hardy et al. (1950) reported on a worker who, after 15 years in the case hardening industry, had an attack of mental confusion, motor aphasia, and slurred speech. He recovered, and, after 15 years of good health working as a truck driver, he returned to cyanide exposure, whereupon his symptoms returned. His complaints of coughing and sneezing recalled the fact that one of the actions of the thiocyanate radical is iodide-like, and causes mucous membrane reactions, such as coryza. While cyanide exposure continued, this patient complained of muscular tremors and gastrointestinal symptoms that increased in severity until vomiting and abdominal cramps (in addition to the weakness and headache already mentioned) were almost completely disabling. Two years after the renewed cyanide exposure, the worker, then age 59, had a left hemiplegia from which he recovered in three weeks. Wald et al. (1939) reported such episodes in hypertensive patients being treated with thiocyanate as a result of relative hypotension that caused vascular insufficiency.

El Ghawabi et al. (1975) investigated the effects of chronic cyanide exposure in the electroplating sections of three factories in Egypt that employed 36 workers. Cyanide concentrations ranged from 4.2 to 12.4 ppm and a linear regression line was established for urinary excretion of thiocyanates and ppm of CN in workplace air. The exposed workers had significantly higher hemoglobin values and lymphocyte counts compared with the unexposed controls, and 78% also had punctate basophilia. Cyanmethemoglobin was detected only in the exposed group, 20 of whom had variable thyroid enlargements, presumably from the thiocyanate formed from the cyanide in the blood. Symptoms noted with greatest frequency included headache, weakness, changes in taste and smell, giddiness, throat irritation, vomiting, and effort dyspnea.

Levine and Radford (1978) studied a group of 479 Baltimore fire fighters and found that they were exposed to HCN levels that were sufficient to raise their mean serum thiocyanate levels above that of controls. This elevation occurred independently of tobacco smoking and of the use of supplied air respiratory equipment.

A patient with chronic cyanide poisoning was brought to the Massachusetts General Hospital for study. It was found that he had signs of thyrotoxicosis including nervousness, lid lag, and tremor of the extended hands and fingers. The thyroid gland was enlarged two to three times its normal size with a small nodule in the left lobe, and auricular fibrillation was present. The blood pressure ranged between 140 to 175 systolic and 75 to 100 diastolic. The thyroid gland was removed and pathologic examination showed a fetal adenoma superimposed on the picture of underlying goiter. After surgery and removal from exposure to HCN solution, the man was well and worked daily (Hardy et al., 1950). A number of carefully studied cases of goiter following thiocyanate therapy for hypertension have been reported. In all reported cases of thiocyanate-therapy goiter, the goiter decreased in size when the thiocyanate was withdrawn or when thyroid was administered. It has been suggested that continued exposure to cyanide in industry, even at low levels, can produce thiocyanate-induced changes in the thyroid gland.

Treatment and Control

In the early 1930s methylene blue was used to treat cyanide poisoning because of its capacity to compete with cytochrome oxidase for CN^- ions (Geiger, 1933; Wendel, 1933). However, its lack of efficiency stimulated a search for a better antidote that led to the use of nitrites and thiosulfate (Chen et al., 1944). The following reactions provide an understanding of the mechanisms that are involved:

$$\text{Cytochrome oxidase} + CN^- \rightleftharpoons$$
$$\text{Cytochrome oxidase cyanide}$$
$$NaNO_2 + \text{hemoglobin} \rightarrow \text{Methemoglobin}$$
$$\text{Methemoglobin} + CN^- \rightarrow \text{Cyanmethemoglobin}$$
$$Na_2S_2O_3 + NaCN + O \rightarrow NaSCN + Na_2SO_4$$

Formation of methemoglobin, which competes for CN^- because its iron is trivalent, drives the first equation to the left, restores the function of the cytochrome oxidase, and leads to the formation of cyanmethemoglobin, which has a low toxicity. Cyanide is detoxified by conversion to thiocyanate, and the extent of this reaction is enhanced by the combined use of nitrite and thiosulfate (Chen and Rose, 1952). Continued or repeated treatment may be required because of liberation of cyanide ions from cyanmethemoglobin and from thiocyanate.

In practice, emergency treatment is started by breaking pearls of amyl nitrite, one at a time, in a handkerchief over the patient's nose for 15 to 30 seconds. Immediately thereafter 10 ml of 3% sodium nitrite (300 mg) are given intravenously over a period of 2 to 4 minutes. With the needle left in place, this injection is followed by an infusion of 50 ml of a 25% solution of sodium thiosulfate (12.5 g) given slowly over the next 10 minutes. Injections of both sodium nitrite and sodium thiosulfate should be repeated in full doses if toxic signs persist or reappear. Physicians in industrial clinics, clinical laboratories, emergency rooms, and ambulances who elect this form of treatment should see to it that these settings are fully supplied with nitrites and thiosulfate, together with an exact outline for their immediate use in handling acute cyanide poisoning. Cyanide antidote kits are available commercially that have a long shelf life, over 17 years according to Chen and Rose (1952) and over 14 years in another report (Hirsch, 1964).

Recently, this method of treatment of cyanide poisoning has been challenged on the basis of unproven efficacy and intrinsic toxicity of sodium nitrite (Graham et al., 1977). Alternative treatments have been proposed that utilize either dicobalt edetate to chelate cyanide or hydroxocobalamin (vitamin B_{12a}), which reverses cyanide toxicity by combining with cyanide to form cyanocobalamin (vitamin B_{12}). Successful use of dicobalt edetate by Bain and Knowles (1967), Thomas and Brooks (1970), and Hillman et al. (1974) have led to recommendation of its use instead of the nitrite/thiosulfate regimen, since it reacts with CN^- to form cobalticyanide $(CO(CN)_6^{3-})$ and monocobalt edetate, both of which are excreted in the urine within 24 hours. Dicobalt edetate is commercially available in Britain and France in 20 ml-ampules that contain 350 mg of the compound in 20% glucose. Nagler et al. (1978) used this method to treat three cases of cyanide poisoning in an electroplating factory and concluded that this chelating agent should be reserved for severely poisoned cases because of the ominous side effects that included nausea, vomiting, profuse diaphoresis, crushing retrosternal pain, cardiac arrhythmias, and facial and palpebral edema. Milder cases in their view should be treated with nitrite/thiosulfate. Graham et al. also noted that dicobalt edetate may also lead to loss of calcium and magnesium ions and to intense purgation.

Hydroxocobalamin is said to be free from toxic effects and has been used with success in treating acute cyanide poisoning in man (Yacoub et al., 1974). Evans (1964) found that the use of thiosulfate enhanced the effect, and Graham et al. (1977) recommended intravenous hydroxocobalamin along with thiosulfate as the treatment of choice. The use of supportive therapy, especially the administration of oxygen, was stressed by Graham et al. who successfully treated a case of massive cyanide poisoning by these methods alone.

The handling of industrial chronic cyanide poisoning must properly be one of prevention by use of ventilating equipment and protective clothing, with the awareness that skin absorption, ingestion, and inhalation are routes of entry. After development of chronic symptoms, the worker should be made to change his work.

The current permissible limit for HCN and cyanide salts in the United States is 5 mg/m³ air, expressed as CN (4.7 ppm), determined during a 10-minute sampling period (NIOSH, 1976).

References

Bain JTB, Knowles EL: Successful treatment of cyanide poisoning. *Br Med J* 1967;2:763.

Barsky MH: Ulcerations of the nasal membranes and perforation of the septum in a copperplating factory — Unusual and sudden incidence. *NY State J Med* 1937;37:1031–1034.

Baumann EJ, Sprinson DB, Metzger N: The estimation of thiocyanate in urine. *J Biol Chem* 1934;105:269–277.

Braddock WH, Tingle GR: So-called cyanide rash in gold mine mill workers. *J Ind Hyg* 1930;12:259–264.

Chen KK, Rose CL: Nitrite and thiosulfate therapy in cyanide poisoning. *J Am Med Assoc* 1952;149:113–119.

Chen KK, Rose CL, Clowes GHA: The modern treatment of cyanide poisoning. *J Indiana Med Assoc* 1944;37:344–350.

Collins J, Martland HS: Disease of primary motor neurons causing clinical picture of acute anterior poliomyelitis: The result of poisoning by cyanide of potassium — A clinical and experimental contribution to toxic effects of cyanide of potassium upon the peripheral motor neurons. *J Nerve Ment Dis* 1908;35:417–426.

Drinker P: Hydrocyanic gas poisoning by absorption through skin. *J Ind Hyg Toxicol* 1932; 14:1–2.

El Ghawabi SH, Gaafar MA, El-Saharti AA, et al: Chronic cyanide exposure: A clinical, radioisotope, and laboratory study. *Br J Ind Med* 1975; 32:215–219.

Evans CL: Cobalt compounds as antidotes for hydrocyanic acid. *Br J Pharmacol* 1964;23:455–475.

Fairley A, Linton EC, Ward FE: The absorption of hydrocyanic acid vapors through the skin. *J Hyg* 1934;34:283–294.

Geiger JC: Cyanide poisoning in San Francisco. *J Am Med Assoc* 1932;99:1944–1945.

Geiger JC: Methylene blue solutions in potassium cyanide poisoning. *J Am Med Assoc* 1933; 101:269.

Goodman LS, Gilman AG: *The Pharmacological Basis of Therapeutics,* ed 5. New York, Macmillan, 1975.

Graham DL, Laman D, Theodore J, et al: Acute cyanide poisoning complicated by lactic acidosis and pulmonary edema. *Arch Intern Med* 1977;137:1051–1055.

Hamilton A: *Industrial Poisons in the United States.* New York, Macmillan, 1925.

Hamilton A, Hardy HL: *Industrial Toxicology,* ed 2. New York, Paul B. Hoeber, 1949.

Hardy HL, Jeffries WM, Wasserman MM, et al: Thiocyanate effect following industrial cyanide exposure. *N Engl J Med* 1950;242:968–972.

Hillman B, Bardhan KD, Bain JTB: The use of dicobalt edetate (Kelocyanor) in cyanide poisoning. *Postgrad Med J* 1974;50:171–174.

Hirsch FG: Cyanide poisoning. *Arch Environ Health* 1964;8:622–624.

Johnstone RT: *Occupational Medicine and Industrial Hygiene.* St. Louis, CV Mosby, 1948.

Levine MS, Radford EP: Occupational exposure to cyanide in Baltimore fire fighters. *J Occup Med* 1978;20:53–56.

Nagler J, Provoost RA, Parizel G: Hydrogen cyanide poisoning: Treatment with cobalt EDTA. *J Occup Med* 1978;20:414–416.

NIOSH: *Criteria for a Recommended Standard . . . .Occupational Exposure to Hydrogen Cyanide and Cyanide Salts.* Washington, DC, National Institute for Occupational Safety and Health (NIOSH 77-108), 1976.

Parmenter DC: Mild cyanide poisoning. *J Ind Hyg* 1926;8:280–282.

Reed CI: Chronic poisoning from cyanogen chloride. *J Ind Hyg* 1920;2:140–143.

Smith AR: Cyanide poisoning. *NY State Dept Labor Ind Bull* 1932;11:169–170.

Thomas TA, Brooks NW: Accidental cyanide poisoning. *Anesthesia* 1970;25:110–114.

Wald MH, Lindberg HA, Barker MH: The toxic manifestations of the thiocyanates. *J Am Med Assoc* 1939;112:1120–1124.

Walton DC, Witherspoon MG: Skin absorption of certain gases. *J Pharmacol Exp Ther* 1925; 26:315–324.

Wendel WB: Methylene blue and cyanide poisoning. *J Am Med Assoc* 1933;100:1054–1055.

Wexler J, Whittenberg JL, Dumke PR: The effect of cyanide on the electrocardiogram of man. *Am Heart J* 1947;34:163–173.

Wolfsie JH, Shaffer CB: Hydrogen cyanide: Hazards, toxicology, prevention and management of poisoning. *J Occup Med* 1959;1:281–288.

Yacoub J, Faure J, Morena H, et al: Acute cyanide poisoning. Current data on the metabolism of cyanide and treatment with hydroxocobalamine [French]. *Eur J Tox* 1974; 71:22–29.

6 • Halogens

Chlorine

Chlorine is produced industrially by the electrolysis of sodium chloride (fused or in brine) in diaphragm cells or in mercury cells, and by the chemical oxidation of chlorides. Chlorine is used as a bleach in the production of pulp and paper, and is important in the manufacture of plastics and resins. It is also used in textile and household bleaches, refrigerants, cosmetics, pharmaceuticals, beneficiation of ores, metal extraction, and automobile antifreezes. Chlorinated solvents and chlorinated pesticides also utilize this halogen. NIOSH (1976) lists over 50 occupations that have a potential exposure to chlorine.

Chlorine is a highly reactive, noninflammable, yellowish-green gas with a strong, pungent, irritating odor. The military services in this country and abroad were obliged to study carefully the question of the chronic effects of chlorine and phosgene in connection with the many claims of permanent disability from these gases that were used in chemical warfare in the First World War. Gilchrist and Matz (1933) studied 838 U.S. veterans who had a history of exposure to chlorine gas in order to ascertain the long-term sequelae. Of the 96 men who were examined clinically and radiographically, only nine showed definite residual effects attributable to the gassing. These conditions included reactivated pulmonary tuberculosis, chronic bronchitis, and emphysema.

Knowledge of the effects of acute chlorine poisoning has largely come from accidents involving leaking chlorine cylinders. Dixon and Drew (1968) reported a fatality due to inhalation of chlorine and called attention to the confusion of opinions in the literature regarding the development of pulmonary edema after acute exposures to chlorine.

An accidental mass poisoning with chlorine gas occurred when a leaking cylinder containing 100 lb (about 45 kg) of chlorine was inadvertently placed over the ventilator grating of a busy Brooklyn subway station so that 1000 persons were exposed to the gas (Chasis et al., 1947). Of these, 208 were admitted to eight hospitals and 33 were observed for one to two weeks. All 33 had tracheobronchitis and 23 had some degree of pulmonary edema. Pneumonia developed in 14, but only three had a severe form. The exposed persons who did not require hospitalization complained of burning of the eyes and nose, lacrimation, and rhinorrhea; respiratory distress, nausea, and vomiting were generally absent. However, those who were hospitalized had early symptoms of burning of the eyes with lacrimation (65%), burning of the nose and throat with salivation, rhinorrhea, and hoarseness (37%), cough, choking sensation, substernal burning, pain and constriction (96%), nausea (40%), vomiting (25%), and headache and dizziness (18%). All of the immediate symptoms subsided within 24 hours, except for cough, substernal pain, and respiratory distress, which persisted for up to two weeks.

Kowitz et al. (1967) reported an incident in which 150 longshoremen were accidentally exposed when the main valve of a cylinder of liquid chlorine was ruptured. Fifty-nine of these workers were studied over a three-year period after the accident. Eleven, who were heavily exposed, showed evidence of alveocapillary injury and gradually developed increasing airway resistance. Lung function studies of the 59 workers who were followed showed that the chlorine exposure produced decreased vital capacity, decreased diffusing capacity, and increased elastic work of breathing.

Beach et al. (1969) studied seven chemical workers who were exposed to chlorine gas in separate accidents. The usual symptoms of cough, dyspnea, and chest pains started within 10 minutes of exposure and lasted two to eight days.

Congestion, consolidation, and nodulation were seen on chest x-rays, and pulmonary edema was present in a severe case. Hypoxemia was corrected by oxygen therapy, and this treatment had to be continued for four days in the one severe case. All recovered completely.

Kaufman and Burkons (1971) were able to study 18 persons accidentally exposed to chlorine as early as 24 to 48 hours after exposure and serially over the ensuing 14 months. Pulmonary function studies showed a pattern of airway obstruction and hypoxemia that cleared entirely within three months in most cases but that persisted in some workers for 12 to 14 months. Similar absence of long-term sequelae from exposure to chlorine gas was reported by Weill and his colleagues (1969) who found no significant permanent lung damage in 12 persons studied for up to seven years after acute, heavy accidental exposure. Chester et al. (1969) studied 139 workers in a chlorine gas plant exposed to an average air concentration less than 1 ppm. Of these, 55 had accidental additional exposures that required oxygen therapy. The immediate effect of these exposures was an obstructive ventilatory deficit that cleared rapidly.

The relation of symptoms and signs to level of chlorine exposure are summarized in Table 3, adapted from the National Academy of Sciences monograph (1976, p. 123).

Chronic exposure to low levels of chlorine also seems to be without lasting effects. Patil et al. (1970) studied 600 diaphragm cell workers in 25 North American chlorine manufacturing plants whose time-weighted average exposure ranged from 0.006 to 1.42 ppm, most of whom were exposed to less than 1 ppm. There were no statistically significant correlations between exposure and signs, symptoms, or abnormal chest x-rays, ECGs, or pulmonary function tests.

The effects of chlorine on the mucous membranes was once attributed to the formation of hydrochloric acid and later to the toxic effects of nascent oxygen released by the oxidative action of the gas (Kramer, 1967). This effect of nascent oxygen has more recently been explained to be the result of a complex series of reactions in which unstable oxidizing agents (e.g., hypochlorous acid, perchloric acid) produce damage by forming stable hydrates of organic chlorine (Chester et al. 1977).

Postmortem changes after fatal massive exposures to chlorine include destruction of mucous membranes lining the bronchi and bronchioles,

Table 3
Chlorine Exposure Thresholds and Limits

Cl_2 Concentration ppm	Effect or Limit
.03–3.5	Range of reported odor thresholds
1	TLV, OSHA time-weighted average (TWA); permissible level, 8-hour workday
1–3	Slight irritation; work possible without interruption
3	Permissible level for 15 minutes; 60-minute emergency exposure limit (EEL)
3–6	Stinging or burning of eyes, nose, throat; lacrimation, sneezing, coughing; bloody nose or blood-tinged sputum
4	Suggested 30-minute EEL
5	Severe irritation of eyes, nose, respiratory tract, intolerable after a few minutes; suggested 15-minute EEL
7	Suggested 5-minute EEL
14–21	Dangerous for 30 to 60 minutes
35–50	Lethal in 60 to 90 minutes

Adapted from Table 5-10, National Academy of Sciences (1976).

focal and confluent areas of edema in the alveoli, patchy superimposed pneumonia, hyaline membrane formation, multiple recent fibrinocellular thromboses of the pulmonary vessels, and ulcerative tracheobronchitis (Adelson and Kaufman, 1971). Some of the pulmonary damage was attributed to the use of high pressure oxygen in treatment.

Treatment of acute chlorine gas inhalation includes intermittent positive pressure oxygen, use of nebulized bronchodilators, and administration of mild sedatives and a cough medication containing codeine (Noe, 1963; Kramer, 1967). Chester et al. (1977) suggested the possible beneficial effects of intramuscular and oral corticosteroid therapy. Hedges and Morrissey (1979) suggested additional measures.

Although the permissible exposure limit for many years has been 1 ppm (3 mg/m³) as a time-weighted average, NIOSH (1976) recommended a ceiling airborne concentration of 0.5 ppm for any 15-minute sampling period. In 1979, OSHA changed the occupational exposure limit for chlorine to a ceiling limit of 1 ppm rather than as a time-weighted average.

Hydrogen Chloride

Acute poisoning from hydrochloric acid fumes practically never occurs in industry, but occasionally a claim is made for compensation by men who draw steel wire and breathe some of the hydrochloric acid from the baths through which the wire passes. The hydrogen evolved in this process rises as tiny bubbles, each with a film of dilute hydrochloric acid.

Anhydrous HCl is highly hygroscopic and its affinity for water makes chronic exposures to the anhydrous form unlikely. Hydrogen chloride exposures, then, are almost always to hydrochloric acid aerosols, which affect the conjunctivae and the mucous membranes of the nose, mouth, and respiratory tract (National Academy of Sciences, 1976). The effects of exposure to HCl are summarized in Table 4, adapted from that report (p. 142).

Table 4
Effects of Exposure to HCl Vapor

HCl Concentration ppm	Effects or Comments
.067–.134	Threshold for odor detection and change in respiratory pattern
5	No organic damage
10	Irritation; work undisturbed
10–50	Work difficult but possible
35	Throat irritation after short exposure
50–100	Intolerable; work impossible
1000–2000	Brief exposures dangerous; laryngospasm
1300–2000	Lethal after a few minutes

Adapted from Table 5-23, National Academy of Sciences (1976).

Patil et al. (1970), in their study of workers in chlorine manufacturing plants referred to above, noted that complaints of tooth decay in the medical histories were not corroborated by physical examination. On the other hand, ten Bruggen Cate (1968) did report industrial dental erosion among workers exposed to hydrochloric and sulfuric acids, and he presented a classification of the severity of this problem. Apart from tooth erosion, no significant abnormalities have been reported from chronic exposures to low levels of gaseous hydrogen chloride (Toyama et al., 1962).

However, thermal degradation of polyvinyl chloride by fires results in the formation of at least 75 toxic compounds, the chief of which is the massive evolution of HCl gas. This hazard constitutes a serious problem for fire fighters and is thought to be the cause of death in the case reported by Dyer and Esch (1976).

The ceiling limit for anhydrous HCl exposure in industry is 5 ppm (7 mg/m³) (NIOSH/OSHA, 1978).

References

Adelson L, Kaufman J: Fatal chlorine poisoning: Report of two cases with clinicopathologic correlation. *Am J Clin Pathol* 1971;56:430–442.

Beach FXM, Jones ES, Scarrow GD: Respiratory effects of chlorine gas. *Br J Ind Med* 1969;26:231–236.

ten Bruggen Cate HJ: Dental erosion in industry. *Br J Ind Med* 1968;25:249–266.

Chasis H, Zapp JA, Bannon JH, et al: Chlorine accident in Brooklyn. *Occup Med* 1947;4:152–176.

Chester EH, Gillespie DG, Krause FD: The prevalence of chronic obstructive pulmonary disease in chlorine gas workers. *Am Rev Resp Dis* 1969;99:365–373.

Chester EH, Kaimal PJ, Payne CB Jr, et al: Pulmonary injury following exposure to chlorine gas. Possible beneficial effects of steroid treatment. *Chest* 1977;72:247–250.

Dixon WM, Drew D: Fatal chlorine poisoning. *J Occup Med* 1968;10:249–251.

Dyer RF, Esch VH: Polyvinyl chloride toxicity in fires: Hydrogen chloride toxicity in fire fighters. *J Am Med Assoc* 1976;235:393–397.

Gilchrist HL, Matz PB: The residual effect of warfare gases. The use of chlorine gas, with report of cases. *Med Bull Vet Admin* 1933;9:229–270.

Hedges JR, Morrissey WL: Acute chlorine gas exposure. *JACEP* 1979;8:59–63.

Kaufman J, Burkons D: Clinical, roentgenologic, and physiologic effects of acute chlorine exposure. *Arch Environ Health* 1971;23:29–34.

Kowitz TA, Reba RC, Parker RT, et al: Effects of chlorine gas upon respiratory function. *Arch Environ Health* 1967;14:545–558.

Kramer CG: Chlorine. *J Occup Med* 1967;9:193–196.

National Academy of Sciences: *Chlorine and Hydrogen Chloride.* Washington, DC, 1976.

NIOSH: *Criteria for a Recommended Standard*

180

. . . .*Occupational Exposure to Chlorine.*
Washington, DC, National Institute for Occupational Safety and Health (NIOSH 76-170), 1976.

NIOSH/OSHA: *Pocket Guide to Chemical Hazards.* Washington, DC, National Institute for Occupational Safety and Health (NIOSH 78-210), 1978.

Noe JT: Therapy for chlorine gas inhalation. *Ind Med Surg* 1963;32:411–414.

Patil LRS, Smith RG, Vorwald AJ, et al: The health of diaphragm cell workers exposed to chlorine. *Am Ind Hyg Assoc J* 1970;31:678–686.

Toyama T, Kondo T, Nakamura K: Environments in acid aerosol producing workplaces and maximum flow rate of workers. *Jap J Ind Health* 1962;4:15–22.

Weill H, George R, Schwarz M, et al: Late evaluation of pulmonary function after acute exposure to chlorine gas. *Am Rev Resp Dis* 1969; 99:374–379.

Phosgene

Phosgene (carbonyl chloride, carbon oxychloride, $COCl_2$), well-known as a deadly war gas, is of minor importance in industry as far as its use is concerned, but the cases of poisoning that occur from time to time are so startling as to claim attention that is out of proportion to their frequency. Phosgene is used in peacetime as an intermediate in the production of aniline dyes. It is also encountered as a thermal decomposition product of chlorinated hydrocarbons, such as carbon tetrachloride and trichloroethylene.

Cases of poisoning were first documented in this country during the First World War in the production of phosgene for chemical warfare and for the dye industry. Phosgene is not an irritating gas, and it has an odor like hay at low concentrations and a pungent smell at high concentrations. It hydrolyzes in the presence of water to form HCl. Since there is no protective respiratory reflex, deep inspiration of the gas may occur, whereupon HCl is liberated in the lower respiratory tract and causes congestion and edema. If this is not quickly fatal, lobular pneumonia may develop with abscess formation. Winternitz (1920) emphasized that phosgene caused damage to the smaller bronchioles and, by destruction of the natural defenses, allowed rapid invasion of the lower respiratory tract by pathogens.

The famous Hamburg cases of 1928 were caused by the explosion of a tank of phosgene, and pathologic effects were found all through the respiratory tract, with degeneration in the nerves as later sequelae (Hegler, 1928). An unusual case of phosgene poisoning occurred when a laborer in an English chemical works removed the cap from a cylinder of phosgene and received a blast of the gas that made him cough and vomit. He returned to work after 20 minutes, and three hours later he bicycled home feeling quite well, ate supper, and went for a walk. An hour later, he developed cough and severe dyspnea, typical of phosgene poisoning, that responded to oxygen and rest (Hamilton and Hardy, 1949, p. 35). The effect of exercise in activating chemically initiated pulmonary edema is well illustrated by this case.

The treatment is that of pulmonary edema of chemical etiology: oxygen, antibiotics, and steroids. The present permissible exposure limit in air in the United States is 0.1 ppm (0.4 mg/m³) of phosgene. NIOSH (1976) proposed that occupational exposures to phosgene be no greater than 0.1 ppm determined as a time-weighted average for a 10-hour workday, 40-hour workweek, with a ceiling value of 0.2 ppm for any 15-minute period.

References

Hamilton A, Hardy HL: *Industrial Toxicology,* ed 2. New York, Paul B. Hoeber, 1949.

Hegler C: Uber eine Massenvergiftung durch Phosgengas in Hamburg; klinische Beobachtungen. *Deutsche med Wchnschr* 1928;54:1551–1553.

NIOSH: *Criteria for a Recommended Standard . . . .Occupational Exposure to Phosgene.* Washington, DC, National Institute for Occupational Safety and Health (NIOSH 77-137), 1976.

Winternitz MC: *Collected Studies on the Pathology of War Gas Poisoning.* New Haven, Yale University Press, 1920.

Fluorine and Its Compounds

Hydrogen fluoride (HF) and its compounds are important in industry. Hydrogen fluoride is used in the processing of cryolite in the aluminum industry, in steel production, in the manufacture of fluorocarbons, as a catalyst in alkylation processes, and in electroplating (NIOSH, 1976). The acid is used in glass etching and clouding of electric bulbs, but sand-blasting has replaced it in the manufacture of ordinary ground glass. Cut glass may be finished by polishing with "putty powder," consisting of oxides of lead and tin, but cheap cut glass is finished with hydrofluoric acid. This acid is also used in pickling steel, especially wire, in removing enamel from defective enamel ware, in treating textiles, in cleaning sandstone and marble, and it may be added to laundry mixtures in place of oxalic acid, as may also the fluorides, especially sodium silicofluoride. Anhydrous hydrofluoric acid is used in the production of high-octane aviation fuel.

Other sources of industrial fluorine exposure are the use of fluorine compounds in insecticidal sprays for fruits and vegetables and the mining and conversion of phosphate rock to superphosphate to be used as fertilizer. The fluorine content of phosphate rock is about 4%, and this source of fluorine is expected to increase as the supply of fluorspar dwindles (NIOSH, 1975). During the conversion to superphosphate, about 25% of the fluorine present is volatilized and is lost to the atmosphere. Fluorides are used in the smelting of many metals and in the production of glass, enamel, and brick as well as in electroplating. Still other uses of the acid or its compounds include removing molding sand from castings and rust from steel and iron, bleaching of cane for seats, disinfecting hides (silicofluorides), and poison for rats and roaches. Fluorides are used in many public water supplies to prevent tooth decay. NIOSH (1975) estimates that in the United States 350,000 workers in 92 occupations have potential exposures to inorganic fluorides, and NIOSH (1976) similarly tabulates 57 occupations involving 22,000 workers with potential exposures to HF.

Acute exposures to HF or F_2 can produce skin, eye, and respiratory tract injuries. Acute and chronic conjunctivitis and eczema of the eyelids have been reported. Gaseous F_2 reacts violently with the skin to produce thermal burns, while solutions of HF produce painful chemical burns (Stokinger, 1949). HF fumes have been found to produce irritation of the eyes and nose at levels of 26 mg/m^3 and serious respiratory irritation at 50 mg/m^3 (Machle et al., 1934). High levels of HF can lead to fatal damage to the respiratory tract as shown in the two cases described by Greendyke and Hodge (1964). Kleinfeld (1965) also reported a fatal case with acute hemorrhagic pulmonary edema and severe tracheobronchitis in a chemist who was accidentally exposed to HF.

The severity of hydrofluoric acid burns of the skin depends on the concentration of the acid and the duration of exposure. HF acts on the skin in three ways: dehydration, low pH, and the specific toxic effect of the fluoride ion, which involves inactivation of calcium ions in the tissues. HF burns are characterized by white necrosis and excruciating pain, the onset of which may be delayed after contact with less concentrated solutions. Successful treatment has traditionally involved initial copious irrigation with water and then soaks with iced saturated solutions of $MgSO_4$, followed by subcutaneous infiltration of 10% calcium gluconate to complex the fluoride ion in the tissues. This treatment, which usually leads to very rapid relief of pain and remarkably rapid healing (Finkel, 1973; Shewmake and Anderson, 1979), has been modified in recent years by use of high molecular weight quaternary ammonium compounds (benzethonium or benzalkonium) soaks in place of the $MgSO_4$ (Dibbell et al., 1970).

Worker illness from exposure to fluorides has been reported from the aluminum production and the phosphate rock-processing industries (Hodge and Smith, 1977). In the former, severe industrial fluorosis was first reported by Møller and Gudjonsson (1932) who examined 78 workers engaged in crushing and refining of cryolite, a double fluoride of sodium and aluminum. They called attention to changes in the skeleton noted on x-rays of 30 workers that showed increased bone density of the spine and pelvis, calcification of ligaments, and hyperostoses. Roholm (1937) confirmed and expanded these findings. Exposures had been estimated by Møller and Gudjonsson to range from 20 to 80 mg F taken into the body daily for 10 to 20 years. Brun, Buchwald and Roholm (1941) estimated that the air concentrations had ranged from 15 to 20 mg F/m^3.

Hodge and Smith (1977) pointed out that the industrial fluorosis of crippling severity reported by the Danish investigators has since been seen in only a few isolated workmen, and that the exposures that led to these changes exceeded any known condition in the United States where ventilation and industrial hygiene practices have largely averted this problem. Kaltreider et al. (1972) did note that some degree of skeletal fluorosis developed in aluminum potroom workers after 10 years of exposure, and that after 15 years of such exposure moderate to severe osteosclerosis of the dorsal spine occurred, with some degree of limitation of mobility. However, these changes were not disabling nor was there any evidence of systemic intoxication. Exposure levels here ranged from 2.4 to 6 mg F/m^3 and urine fluoride varied from 8.7 to 9.8 mg F/L.

Fluorides given to experimental animals in toxic amounts can produce kidney damage. But the exposures to cryolite workers under very dusty conditions were not accompanied by albuminuria or glycosuria, according to Roholm (1937). Kaltrieder et al. (1972) similarly detected no excess albuminuria nor did Dinman et al. (1976), who studied the results of over 16,000 urinalyses for protein and found no correlation between urinary fluoride concentrations and the presence of albuminuria.

The possibility of chronic fluoride poisoning exists, however, as evidenced by the case reports of Burke et al. (1973), in which systemic disease resulted from an extensive HF burn, and of Waldbott and Lee (1978) and White (1980).

No osteosclerosis develops when TWA air fluoride concentrations remain below 2.5 mg/m³ (Hodge and Smith, 1977). The United States permissible limit for hydrogen fluoride exposure is 3 ppm (2 mg/m³), for fluorine 0.1 ppm (0.2 mg/m³), and for fluoride dust 2.5 mg/m³. An average daily urinary output of less than 5 mg/L of fluorine provides an index of safe working levels for long-term exposures.

Boron Trifluoride

Boron trifluoride is a highly reactive compound that is used primarily as a catalyst in chemical reactions. It is a colorless gas that fumes in moist air and has a pungent odor. Although it is very irritating to the skin and the respiratory tract so that contact and inhalation should be avoided, its toxicity has not been adequately studied (NIOSH, 1976). The permissible exposure limit is 1 ppm (3 mg/m³).

Bromine and Iodine

The two halogens, bromine and iodine, are similar to chlorine in biological effect. Iodine is more toxic than bromine, and both are more toxic than chlorine. They are skin, eye, and lung irritants, and the permissible exposure levels for safety at work are low: bromine 1 ppm (0.7 mg/m³) and iodine 0.1 ppm (0.1 mg/m³) (NIOSH/OSHA, 1978).

References

Burn GC, Buchwald H, Roholm K: Die Fluorausscheidung im Harn bei chronischer Fluorvergiftung von Kryolitharbeitern. *Acta Med Scand* 1941;106:261–273.

Burke WJ, Hoegg UR, Phillips RE: Systemic fluoride poisoning resulting from a fluoride skin burn. *J Occup Med* 1973;15:39–41.

Dibbell DG, Iverson RE, Jones W, et al: Hydrofluoric acid burns of the hand. *J Bone Joint Surg* 1970;52A:931–936.

Dinman BD, Backenstose DL, Carter RP, et al: Prevention of bony fluorosis in aluminum smelter workers. A five-year study of fluoride absorption and excretion–Pt. 3. *J Occup Med* 1976;18:17–20.

Finkel AJ: Treatment of hydrogen fluoride injuries. *Adv Fluorine Chem* 1973;7:199–203.

Greendyke RM, Hodge HC: Accidental death due to hydrofluoric acid. *J Forensic Sci* 1964;9:383–390.

Hodge HC, Smith FA: Occupational fluoride exposure. *J Occup Med* 1977;19:12–39.

Kaltreider NL, Elder MJ, Cralley LV, et al: Health survey of aluminum workers with special reference to fluoride exposure. *J Occup Med* 1972;14:531–541.

Kleinfeld M: Acute pulmonary edema of chemical origin. *Arch Environ Health* 1965;10:942–946.

Machle W, Thamann F, Kitzmiller K, et al: The effects of the inhalation of hydrogen fluoride. I. The response following exposure to high concentrations. *J Ind Hyg* 1934;16:129–145.

Møller PF, Gudjonsson SV: Massive fluorosis of bones and ligaments. *Acta Radiol* 1932;13:269–294.

NIOSH: *Criteria for a Recommended Standard . . . .Occupational Exposure to Inorganic Fluorides.* Washington, DC, National Institute of Occupational Safety and Health (NIOSH 76-103), 1975.

NIOSH: *Criteria for a Recommended Standard . . . .Occupational Exposure to Hydrogen Fluoride.* Washington, DC, National Institute for Occupational Safety and Health (NIOSH 76-143), 1976.

NIOSH: *Criteria for a Recommended Standard . . . .Occupational Exposure to Boron Trifluoride.* Washington, DC, National Institute for Occupational Safety and Health (NIOSH 77-122), 1976.

NIOSH/OSHA: *Pocket Guide to Chemical*

Hazards. Washington, DC, National Institute for Occupational Safety and Health (NIOSH 78-210), 1978.

Roholm K: *Fluorine Intoxication. A Clinical-Hygiene Study with a Review of the Literature and Some Experimental Investigations.* London, H.K. Lewis, 1937.

Shewmake SW, Anderson BG: Hydrofluoric acid burns. *Arch Dermatol* 1979;115:593–596.

Stokinger HE: Toxicity following inhalation of fluorine and hydrogen fluoride, in Voegtlin C, Hodge HC (eds): *Pharmacology and Toxicology of Uranium Compounds.* New York, McGraw-Hill, 1949.

Waldbott GL, Lee JR: Toxicity from repeated low-grade exposure to hydrogen fluoride — Case report. *Clin Toxicol* 1978;13:391–402.

White DA: Hydrofluoric acid — A chronic poisoning effect. *J Soc Occup Med* 1980;30: 12–14.

7 • Nitrogen Compounds

Nitric acid must be considered in connection with the various oxides of nitrogen, which make up what were once commonly called "nitrous fumes," because exposure of nitric acid to the air at once liberates such compounds. Nitric acid is the second most important industrial acid with about 75% used in the production of ammonium nitrate fertilizer and about 15% in the manufacture of explosives (NIOSH, 1976a).

Contact of nitric acid with organic matter, such as wood shavings and sawdust, produces an evolution of nitrogen oxides, and such contact is an essential part of many important industrial processes. Firemen may be exposed to these compounds as a result of burning materials such as bed mattresses. All of the commonly used explosives, with the exception of gunpowder, are nitrated products and are made by the action of nitric acid on cellulose, glycerine, phenol, benzol, toluol, and similar substances. Nitrocellulose is the basis, not only for smokeless powder, but also for lacquers, photographic film, and celluloid. Nitrobenzol and nitrophenols are used in the production of dyes and drugs as well as of explosives. Metal etching and photoengraving both use nitric acid, and in dilute form it is used for cleaning ("bright dipping") copper and brass.

Nitric acid can injure tissues on direct contact because of its corrosive properties. The familiar yellow burn of skin from concentrated nitric acid, the xanthoproteic reaction, is the result of the formation of denatured colored proteins. When splashed onto the eye, concentrated nitric acid produces immediate opacification of the cornea, and, when severe, this accident may result in blindness, symblepharon, and shrinkage of the eyeball (Grant, 1974). The progression of ocular changes in a chemist who was splashed with hot nitric acid was described by McAdams and Krop (1955). Exposure to nitric acid vapor and mists sometimes causes dental erosion but not as often as sulfuric or hydrochloric acids (ten Bruggen Cate, 1968).

The inhalation effects of nitric acid cannot be separated from those of the oxides of nitrogen since they invariably occur together. The oxides of nitrogen, principally nitrogen dioxide (NO_2) and nitric oxide (NO), are formed when nitric acid reacts with reducing agents as well as by combustion of nitrogen-containing materials. Nitric oxide produced in welding arcs or flames is oxidized in air to nitrogen dioxide. Apart from welding and other flame operations, such as glassblowing, nitrogen oxides are produced by fuel combustion, by catalytic oxidation of ammonia in the production of nitric acid, by underground blasting operations, in the decomposition of agricultural silage, and by ice arena resurfacing machines (NIOSH, 1976b). Acute exposure to high concentrations of nitrogen dioxide is an occupational hazard of welders, miners, chemists, fire fighters, silo-fillers, and those employed in the manufacture of nitric acid (National Academy of Sciences, 1977).

The shocking accident at the Cleveland Clinic in 1929 brought the hazard of nitric oxide into general prominence when the combustion of nitrocellulose x-ray films caused the deaths of 97 persons (Nichols, 1930). Industrial physicians, especially those with experience in the war industries, knew of this hazard (McAdams, 1955). The United States Navy reported nine serious cases of poisoning among 23 men who were exposed to gases from burning blasting gelatin (Charleroy, 1945). The lack of warning symptoms was emphasized and also the fact that the prodromal symptoms of cough, headache, and sensations of fullness in the head and chest are exactly the same for those suffering the slightest effects as for those who will later show a sudden circulatory collapse.

The usual course of overexposure is one of delayed symptoms, coming on from one to 24 hours after inhalation and beginning with dyspnea, which increases as acute pulmonary congestion is followed by edema. Cyanosis may also develop. If the victim has not breathed deeply while exposed, he may recover with oxygen therapy and prompt use of steroids. Unfortunately, it is usual that he will have breathed deeply, for the instinctive reaction to the offending gas is to hold the breath as long as possible and then take a few deep gasping respirations. In such cases death may follow within 36 hours because of pulmonary edema. The relation between acute exposure levels of NO_2 and clinical effects is summarized in Table 5, taken from the National Academy of Sciences monograph (1977).

Table 5
Clinical Effects Resulting From Acute
Exposure to High Nitrogen Dioxide Levels

NO_2 Concentration		Clinical Effect	Time Between Exposure and Termination of Effect
ppm	mg/m³		
500	940	Acute pulmonary edema; fatal	Within 48 hours
300	564	Bronchopneumonia; fatal	2–10 days
150	282	Bronchiolitis fibrosa obliterans; fatal	3–5 weeks
50	94	Bronchiolitis, focal pneumonitis; recovery	6–8 weeks
25	47	Bronchitis, bronchopneumonia; recovery	6–8 weeks

From Table 10-19, National Academy of Sciences (1977).

Experimental studies with healthy, young, adult male volunteers exposed to 1 or 2 ppm NO_2 for 2.5 to 3 hours demonstrated small transitory reductions in hemoglobin and hematocrit levels, and changes in acetylcholinesterase and other blood enzyme levels (Posin et al., 1978).

Victims of acute exposure to high levels of oxides of nitrogen fall into three classes: 1) those who die almost immediately after very heavy exposure, a rare occurrence caused by a serious accident; 2) those with delayed symptoms who develop edema of the lungs within 48 hours, the form most often seen in industry; and 3) those who recover apparently from the immediate effects but fall victims to chronic chest disease of varying severity, probably depending on the dose received, intercurrent infection, previous chemical injury to the lungs, or smoking habits. There are probably a far larger number of cases belonging to this third class than has been recognized in American industry.

Several authors have classified the clinical types that follow inhalation of nitrogen oxides. Milne (1969) wrote of a biphasic pattern marked by initial pulmonary edema. If this episode is survived, a second one follows after an interval of some days of seemingly good health. Becklake et al. (1957) classified cases in this way:

Type 1: Acute pulmonary edema, developing after a latent period of up to 30 hours, frequently fatal, but followed by complete recovery if the initial episode is survived.

Type 2: Exposure and acute symptoms followed by a latent period and apparent improvement sometimes lasting up to a month. Thereafter, progressive development of unremitting dyspnea with severe cough and frank cyanosis, and typical roentgenographic findings of irregular soft mottling throughout both lungs that clear quickly if the patient recovers.

Type 3: Development of a pneumonia of chemical origin (a category that implies gradual deterioration).

Transient lung infiltrates seen on x-ray are noted in all reports (Camiel and Berkan, 1944). Lung function of no single pattern is recorded but the general opinion is that the lesion is damage of the small bronchioles. The end picture is altered by therapy as well as by the original chemical injury (Ramirez-R and Dowell, 1971).

Silo-filler's disease, affecting those who work with silage, is believed to be due to oxides of nitrogen emitted by the anaerobic fermentation of potassium nitrate that is especially high in young plants. When freshly stored the hay or corn becomes elevated in temperature due to the fermentation process, which releases the various nitrogen compounds including the harmful dioxide (Scott and Hunt, 1973). Lowry and Schuman (1956) described four cases, two of whom died one month after exposure to irritating gases from corn silage, and two of whom were probably saved by steroid therapy. Nitrogen dioxide, as shown by experience with silo-filler's disease, produces an early pulmonary edema that is followed by bronchiolitis fibrosa obliterans. Ramirez-R and Dowell (1971) concluded from their study of the literature that persistent lung malfunction after exposure to silage gas is uncommon in those patients who recover from the initial toxic pulmonary edema and bronchiolitis.

In addition to the action on the lungs, necropsy studies in cases of nitrogen oxide poisoning show that there may be intense congestion in the gastrointestinal tract, sometimes with hemorrhage, and congestion of the meninges, or even of the cerebrum, with punctate hemorrhages. The changes in the blood are striking: the venous blood is thick and tarry, and coagulates rapidly. Formation of methemoglobin occurs when nitric oxide is present in the offending gas. Destruction of erythrocytes has been described after oxides of nitrogen poisoning, and lesions in the liver and kidneys have been reported, including jaundice, with increase of bile pigments in blood and urine (Doremus and McNally, 1923). Most common, however, as a sequel of nitrogen oxides poisoning are various forms of pulmonary disease that vary according to the length of time that elapses between exposure and death.

Experience with welders working in confined spaces and underground miners has impressed HLH with the fact that nitrogen oxides inhaled over a period of time without acute episodes can cause lung damage. Further, an acute nitrogen oxide pneumonitis can result in measurably decreased lung function. If the original acute episode is promptly treated with bed rest, adequate oxygen, antibiotics, and steroids, the course of reaction will be favorably altered.

The current standard for the tolerable limit for workers is set at 2 ppm (5 mg/m^3) for nitric acid, 25 ppm (30 mg/m^3) for nitric oxide, and 5 ppm (9 mg/m^3) for nitrogen dioxide. NIOSH (1976b) has recommended a ceiling concentration of 1 ppm (1.8 mg/m^3) for nitrogen dioxide, determined by a 15-minute sample, while it concurs with the current ceilings for HNO$_3$ and NO (NIOSH, 1976a).

References

Becklake MR, Goldman HI, Bosman AR, et al: The long-term effects of exposure to nitrous fumes. *Am Rev Tubercul* 1957;76:398–409.

ten Bruggen Cate HJ: Dental erosion in industry. *Br J Ind Med* 1968;25:249–266.

Camiel MR, Berkan HS: Inhalation pneumonia from nitric fumes. *Radiology* 1944;42:175–182.

Charleroy DK: Nitrous and nitric gas casualties. *US Naval Med Bull* 1945;44:435–437.

Doremus CA, McNally WD: Gaseous poisons, in Haines WS, Webster RW (eds): *Legal Medicine and Toxicology*, ed 2. Philadelphia, WB Saunders, 1923, vol 2.

Grant WM: *Toxicology of the Eye,* ed 2. Springfield IL, Charles C Thomas, 1974.

Lowry T, Schuman LM: "Silo-filler's disease" — A syndrome caused by nitrogen dioxide. *J Am Med Assoc* 1956;162:153–160.

McAdams AJ Jr: Bronchiolitis obliterans. *Am J Med* 1955;19:314–322.

McAdams AJ Jr: Krop S: Injury and death from red fuming nitric acid. *J Am Med Assoc* 1955;158:1022–1024.

Milne JEH: Nitrogen dioxide inhalation and bronchiolitis obliterans. *J Occup Med* 1969;11: 538–547.

National Academy of Sciences: *Nitrogen Oxides.* Washington, DC, 1977.

Nichols, BH: The clinical effects of the inhalation of nitrogen dioxide. *Am J Roentgentol* 1930; 23:516–520.

NIOSH: *Criteria for a Recommended Standard . . . . Occupational Exposure to Nitric Acid.* Washington, DC, National Institute for Occupational Safety and Health (NIOSH 76-141), 1976a.

NIOSH: *Criteria for a Recommended Standard . . . . Occupational Exposure to Oxides of Nitrogen (Nitrogen Dioxide and Nitric Oxide).* Washington, DC, National Institute for Occupational Safety and Health (NIOSH 76-149), 1976b.

Posin C, Clark K, Jones MP, et al: Nitrogen dioxide inhalation and human blood biochemistry. *Arch Environ Health* 1978;33:318–324.

Ramirez-R J, Dowell AR: Silo-filler's disease: Nitrogen dioxide-induced lung injury. Long-term follow-up and review of the literature. *Ann Intern Med* 1971;74:569–576.

Scott EG, Hunt WB Jr: Silo filler's disease. *Chest* 1973;63:701–706.

8 • Oxygen and Ozone

Oxygen

Prolonged breathing of oxygen at partial pressures greater than that in normal air leads to toxic effects that involve the lungs, central nervous system, and eyes (Clark and Lambertsen, 1971). Inhalation of 100% oxygen at 1 atm results, after several days, in disruption of capillary endothelium and type I alveolar cells, edema of the lung interstitium, and deposition of fibrin over the alveolar lining. This exudative reaction is replaced by proliferation of interstitial fibers and alveolar type II cells (Senior et al., 1971). Breathing oxygen at pressures above 2 atm results in central nervous system dysfunction with convulsions, retinal damage, paralysis, and death. This hazard is not encountered occupationally except in divers and in rescue brigades in tunnels and mines (Young, 1971), and possibly to hyperbaric chamber personnel. Oxygen toxicity has also been reviewed by Winter and Smith (1972) and by Frank and Massaro (1979). In general, no significant pulmonary impairment has been found from prolonged breathing of oxygen at partial pressures of 0.5 atm or less (Clark and Lambertsen, 1971).

References

Clark JM, Lambertsen CJ: Pulmonary oxygen toxicity: A review. *Pharmacol Rev* 1971;23:37–133.

Frank L, Massaro D: The lung and oxygen toxicity. *Arch Intern Med* 1979;139:347–350.

Senior RM, Wessler S, Avioli LV: Pulmonary oxygen toxicity. *J Am Med Assoc* 1971;217:1373–1377.

Winter PM, Smith G. The toxicity of oxygen. *Anesthesiology* 1972;37:210–241.

Young JM: Acute oxygen toxicity in working man, in Lambertsen CJ (ed): *Underwater Physiology*. New York, Academic Press, 1971, pp 67–76.

———

Ozone

Ozone (O_3) is a gas with a characteristic pungent odor that is detectable in dilutions of less than 0.1 ppm in air. It is a powerful oxidizing agent and it attacks most metals as well as many organic compounds (Stokinger, 1954). Apart from the stratosphere, where it is produced by the action of ultraviolet light on oxygen, it is produced in industry in electric arc welding shielded by inert gases such as argon and helium (Kleinfeld et al., 1957). Other sources include room air ozonizers, office photocopying machines, fumigation chambers, ozonizers for treatment of sewage and for water purification, high voltage electrical equipment, and ultraviolet ray quartz lamps (Jaffe, 1968).

Since ozone is a powerful oxidant, it can injure mucous membranes with resultant eye irritation and pulmonary tract damage. Edematous thickening of the alveolar walls results in decreased diffusing capacity even at exposures as low as 0.6 to 0.8 ppm (Young et al., 1964). At higher concentrations (2 ppm), a two-hour experimental exposure in an outdoor fumigation chamber resulted in throat and mouth dryness, decreased mental ability, chest pains, cough, and fatigue that persisted for two weeks (Griswold et al., 1957). In another study, Hazucha et al. (1973) found that breathing 0.37 ppm ozone for two hours with intermittent exercise significantly lowered all of the maximal expiratory tests, and they attributed the changes to decreased lung elastic recoil, increased airway resistance, and small airway obstruction. Golden et al. (1978) found that a two-hour exposure to 0.6 ppm produced bronchial hyperirritability, probably by damaging airway epithelium and sensitizing bronchial irritant receptors.

Kleinfeld et al. (1957) described severe pulmonary symptoms (edema, bronchopneumonia)

188

along with persistent headache, fatigue, and exertional dyspnea in three workers exposed to ozone while engaged in inert-gas shielded metal arc welding. Fabbri et al. (1979) examined 31 workers (27 men, 4 women) in a plastic bag factory who were exposed to ozone levels of 0.1 to 0.92 mg/m³ during extrusion, printing, and sealing operations for about two years. They concluded that chronic exposure to these levels of ozone below 0.5 ppm caused impairment of small airways only in smokers.

Human experience, both clinical and experimental, has established the extreme toxicity of ozone and that it can cause acute and chronic disease manifested as bronchitis and bronchiolitis (Stokinger, 1954, 1965; Jaffe, 1967, 1968; Nasr, 1971). The photochemical action of sunshine on automobile exhaust fumes containing hydrocarbons produces ozone in Los Angeles-type smog (Jaffe, 1967). As much as 0.06 ppm of ozone has been measured in Los Angeles smog, with associated smarting of the eyes and irritation of nose and throat.

The permissible exposure limit in the United States is 0.1 ppm (0.2 mg/m³) (NIOSH, 1978).

References

Fabbri L, Mapp C, Rossi A, et al: Pulmonary changes due to low-level occupational exposure to ozone. *Med lavoro* 1979;4:307–312.

Golden JA, Nadel JA, Boushey HA: Bronchial hyperirritability in healthy subjects after exposure to ozone. *Am Rev Resp Dis* 1978;118:287–294.

Griswold SS, Chambers LA, Motley HL: Report of a case of exposure to high ozone concentrations for two hours. *Arch Ind Health* 1957; 15:108–110.

Hazucha M, Silverman F, Parent C, et al: Pulmonary function in man after short-term exposure to ozone. *Arch Environ Health* 1973;27: 183–188.

Jaffe LS: Photochemical air pollutants and their effects on man and animals. I. General characteristics and community concentrations. *Arch Environ Health* 1967;15:782–791.

Jaffe LS: Photochemical air pollutants and their effects on man and animals. II. Adverse effects. *Arch Environ Health* 1968;16:241–255.

Kleinfeld M, Giel C, Tabershaw IR: Health hazards associated with inert-gas shielded metal arc welding. *Arch Ind Health* 1957;15:27–31.

Nasr ANM: Ozone poisoning in man: clinical manifestations and differential diagnosis — A review. *Clin Toxicology* 1971;4:461–466.

NIOSH: *NIOSH/OSHA Pocket Guide to Chemical Hazards.* Washington, DC, National Institute for Occupational Safety and Health (NIOSH 78-210), 1978.

Stokinger H: Ozone toxicity. A review of the literature through 1953. *Arch Ind Hyg Occup Med* 1954;9:366–383.

Stokinger H: Ozone toxicology. A review of research and industrial experience: 1954–1964. *Arch Environ Health* 1965;10:719–731.

Young WA, Shaw DG, Bates DV: Effect of low concentrations of ozone on pulmonary function. *J Appl Physiol* 1964;19:765–768.

9 • Sulfur Compounds

Hydrogen Sulfide

Sources of poisoning Hydrogen sulfide (H_2S), also known as sulfur hydride, is a powerful asphyxiant that has little use in industry but is formed in the course of certain industrial processes where elemental sulfur or its compounds come into contact with organic chemicals at high temperatures. It is also found in nature and it is produced by the decay of organic substances containing sulfur (e.g., industrial waste water and sewage). Industrial poisoning from this gas, therefore, is almost always the result of an accident and it is a leading cause of sudden death in the workplace (NIOSH, 1977).

Wherever sulfur is deposited, pockets of hydrogen sulfide may be encountered. Thus, it has been known to collect in pools of water in coal mines formed by the decomposition of iron pyrites and to rise when the water is disturbed; sometimes it is liberated by the blasting of coal. Edington (1938) found it in a lead mine where there was stagnant water with sulfur deposits. It is recognized as a danger in gypsum and sulfur mines. An unusual source of H_2S gas was discovered in the course of digging through limestone during the construction of a sewer main in Florida (Robinson et al., 1942). Underground streams of water were charged with the gas, and men working in shallow holes complained of dyspnea, lassitude, nausea, smarting and burning of the eyes, and lacrimation. One man who reached a depth of 4.9 meters (16 feet) lost consciousness, but he was quickly rescued and he recovered.

Hydrogen sulfide is also present in natural gas from some fields. At the present time the greatest source of danger from H_2S poisoning in the United States is in the production and refining of high-sulfur petroleum from some of the oil fields of Mexico, Wyoming, and western Texas. It was the refining of light Mexican oils that first called the attention of the petroleum industry to this poisonous gas. Shortly thereafter, the discovery of oil in western Texas brought the danger into much greater prominence. Hydrogen sulfide in toxic quantities was found in solution in the crude oil, and exposure to H_2S in the petroleum industry became a major occupational hazard (Yant, 1930; NIOSH, 1977). The gas begins to pass off into the air as soon as it reaches the surface, and this process is greatly accelerated by the heat of refining. There is, therefore, great risk of exposure at many points in the refining of "sour crude." This problem is also present in Canada in the fossil fuel-rich province of Alberta where Burnett et al. (1977) collected 221 cases of exposure to H_2S in the five years from 1969 to 1973. Of these, 92% occurred in the oil, gas, and petrochemical industries.

The decay of organic matter gives rise to H_2S in sewers and waste waters from industrial plants where animal products are handled. Thus, there have been accidental poisonings from H_2S in tanneries, glue factories, fur-dressing and felt-making plants, abattoirs, fertilizer cookers, beet-sugar factories, and liquid manure tanks. An accident in Lowell, Massachusetts, resulted in the poisoning of five men who were sent to repair a street sewer that also drained waste from a tannery. Four of them died—three, as is so often the case, in a vain attempt to save the first victim. The danger of H_2S formation is ever present in tanneries because of the methods used in preparing and tanning hides. First, all hair is removed by coating the hair side of the hide with a depilatory paste composed primarily of sodium sulfide. After the hair is removed the hide is then "chrome" tanned with a liquor that is basically sodium chromate that has been treated with sulfuric acid. It is imperative that there be separate sewerage lines for the dehairing and tanning processes. If these two effluents are mixed, H_2S is readily formed. Five

189

deaths in a Maine factory resulted from the accidental discharge of sulfuric acid from a delivery truck into a sulfide vat (Maloof, in a personal communication to HLH, 1971).

Hydrogen sulfide is formed in certain industrial processes such as the production of sulfur dyes (brown, black, and blue), in the production of carbon disulfide, and in heating rubber containing sulfur compounds in the process of vulcanizing. An accidental poisoning described by Nau et al. (1944) resulted from the pouring of water on hot dross that contained antimony, arsenic, and sulfur. Gaseous hydrides of all three were formed.

A source of hydrogen sulfide poisoning, mild in character but fairly troublesome, is in the making of rayon by the viscose process. The method calls for the use of sodium hydrate, followed by carbon disulfide, by which reaction sodium trithiocarbonate (Na_2CS_3) is formed; this compound decomposes, especially in the spinning bath of warm dilute sulfuric acid, into sodium carbonate and hydrogen sulfide. It is in the spinning room that these fumes are given off, and reports from all industrial countries show that the irritation from the gas is a troublesome feature of rayon manufacture.

Hydrogen sulfide is used in many chemical procedures. Carelessness, ignorance of the risk, and faulty cylinders result in dangerous exposures to chemical workers, students, and research workers in ill-equipped laboratories. The practice of graduate students working alone at night has resulted in near fatal accidents caused by the inhalation of hydrogen sulfide.

Toxic action and therapy   Because the sulfide is detoxified so rapidly in the body, complete recovery may take place if the victim is moved quickly enough from continuing exposure to hydrogen sulfide. Artificial respiration and oxygen inhalation should be used in all cases because the intensity of hydrogen sulfide exposure is seldom known. Such measures may allow unexpected recovery and perhaps prevent pulmonary edema.

Hydrogen sulfide, according to Yant (1930), is about as toxic as hydrogen cyanide, and its action is as rapid. Death may result from respiratory failure, sometimes within a few seconds, depending on the dose received in an acute exposure, as a result of central respiratory paralysis accelerated by toxic action on the carotid body (Yant, 1930; Heymans and Neil, 1958). Smith and Gosselin (1979) have documented the similarities between acute cyanide and sulfide poisoning, particularly the fact that both are reversible inhibitors of cytochrome oxidase. They suggested that treatment of cyanosis in H_2S poisoning consist of induction of methemoglobinemia by intravenous sodium nitrite (10 ml of a 3% solution) over two to four minutes, but that the use of sodium thiosulfate be omitted. This procedure should be supplemented by oxygen inhalation therapy. Presumably, the methemoglobin thus formed would trap the free sulfide and spare the cytochrome oxidase.

Burnett et al. (1977) questioned whether this procedure can be effective once the cytochrome oxidase system has been poisoned, and they cited the lack of benefit of nitrite therapy in the few cases in their series that had received it. They also suggested that the availability of this antidote might distract physicians and other rescuers from providing needed respiratory and cardiovascular support for the victims. Nevertheless, effective use of nitrite therapy was reported by Stine et al. (1976) in a case of accidental H_2S poisoning from exposure to acid sulfide waste.

Hydrogen sulfide is not only an asphyxiating gas, but it has a decidedly irritating action that becomes noticeable in the milder forms of poisoning when it is not masked by the severer symptoms of asphyxia. In lower concentrations (50 to 500 ppm) its action may be primarily as a respiratory irritant. Exposure to concentrations of 250 to 600 ppm may result in pulmonary edema and bronchopneumonia. The mildest forms of poisoning are characterized by irritation of the conjunctivae with photophobia and sometimes a severe conjunctivitis with keratitis. The latter is usually of brief duration and may last several days but leaves no permanent injury to the cornea. The appearance of colored rings around lights and increased photophobia may be warning signs.

Table 6 (Gafafer, 1964) indicates the responses that one might expect at various concentrations, although physiologic responses to different levels of exposure may vary greatly among individuals. Of greatest importance is the paralysis of the sense of smell at 150 ppm, so that the victim may be unaware of his danger.

Reports of occupational illness   It is usually held that chronic poisoning by H_2S in industrial workers is characterized by conjunctivitis, headache, attacks of dizziness, digestive disturbances, diarrhea, and loss of weight. The skin is said to have a tendency to furunculosis. Haggard (1924) wrote of local irritation to the air passages,

Table 6

ppm	Responses
0.2	Detectable odor
10	Threshold limit value for daily 8-hour exposure
150	Olfactory nerve paralysis
250	Prolonged exposure may cause pulmonary edema
500	Systemic symptoms may occur in one-half to one hour
1000	Rapid collapse—respiratory collapse imminent
5000	Immediate death

From Gafafer (1964).

but Aves (1929) stated that Texas oil workers rarely suffer from respiratory infections. From early French writings one learns of the "plomb des fosses," the colic and diarrhea from which Paris sewer workers suffered, with the colic resembling that of plumbism.

Larsen (Hamilton and Hardy, 1949, p. 265) gave the histories of 50 tunnel workers in Denmark who had attacks of acute keratitis with severe pain, photophobia, and corneal vesicles that broke within 24 hours. These effects occurred after exposure to H_2S liberated from the decaying organic matter on the floor of the sea and from anaerobic decomposition. Aves (1929) described much more serious eye problems in Texas workers, where in some cases the reaction was severe, with swelling of the lids so great as to evert both upper and lower lids. However, corneal ulcers rarely developed and recovery was fairly rapid. The other mucous membranes did not seem to suffer.

While earlier authorities stated that conjunctivitis began to appear at a concentration of 100 to 150 ppm, Barthelemy (1939), who had supervised the spinners in a large rayon factory for some years, stated that the gas should be kept down to 20 ppm by volume if inflammation of the eyes is to be prevented. He described the injury to the eyes produced by H_2S as consisting of intense photophobia, blepharospasm, excessive lacrimation, intense congestion, pain, blurred vision, and a hazy and sometimes blistered cornea. Nevertheless, the acute symptoms usually subside quickly with treatment and removal from the offending exposure, but severe cases may result in lasting damage if corneal ulcers occur with scarring. More recently a number of reported eye effects at 20 ppm or less indicate that a tolerance level of less than that value is required.

Beasley (1963) described three cases of delayed eye irritation consisting of gritty sensation, blurred and hazy vision, rainbow rings around lights, blepharospasm, and retro-orbital pain. These complaints were attributed to the H_2S in the gas plant where exposure took place, and not to the ammonia and steam that were also present. Brown (1969) reported that a foreman in a rubber factory developed transient "blue vision" for one day after exposure to H_2S. Poda (1966), in compiling the effects of H_2S exposure in a heavy water plant, found that eye irritation was relatively uncommon in plants where a working level of 10 ppm was used. More common findings were cough, nausea, headache, nervousness, and insomnia, all thought to be due to hydrogen sulfide. Workers that had consumed alcohol in the 24 hours before exposure appeared to be affected at lower concentrations of H_2S.

Neurological sequelae might be expected when acute poisoning with H_2S results in unconsciousness, but frequently recovery is practically complete (Kaipainen, 1954; Kemper, 1966). During the unconscious stage there may be convulsions, spasticity, and abnormal or absent deep reflexes. McCabe and Clayton (1952) reported lasting neurological changes in four of 320 survivors of an air pollution incident in Mexico: two had acoustic neuritis, one had dysarthria, and one had aggravated epilepsy. Burnett et al. (1977) reported no permanent neurological after-effects in survivors in their series of cases. Matsuo et al. (1979) suggested that the severe cerebral hypoxia from systemic hypotension in massive H_2S poisoning leads, in fatal cases, to focal brain lesions.

Control The currently accepted ceiling concentration for H_2S is 10 ppm (approximately 15 mg/m³) for up to a 10-hour work shift in a 40-hour workweek (NIOSH, 1977). Russia and Czechoslovakia have a 7 ppm limit. Repeated or long-term exposures tolerated in spite of symptoms may cause loss of the sense of smell, a serious matter since subsequent acute exposures leading to pulmonary edema may occur with the worker unaware of the risk.

References

Aves, CM: Hydrogen sulphide poisoning in Texas. *Texas State J Med* 1929;24:761–766.

Barthelemy HL: Ten years' experience with industrial hygiene in connection with manufacture of viscose rayon. *J Ind Hyg Toxicol* 1939;21:141–151.

Beasley RWR: The eye and hydrogen sulfide. *Br J Ind Med* 1963;20:32-34.

Brown KE: Some toxicology problems in a rubber industry. *Med J Aust* 1969;1:534-538.

Burnett WW, King EG, Grace M, et al: Hydrogen sulfide poisoning: Review of 5 years' experience. *Can Med Assoc J* 1977;117:1277-1280.

Edington JW: Sulphuretted hydrogen production by bacteria in a lead mine. *J Hyg* 1938;38:683-687.

Gafafer, WM (ed): *Occupational Diseases: A Guide to Their Recognition,* Washington, DC, US Government Printing Office, 1964.

Haggard HW: Action of irritant gases on the respiratory tract. *J Ind Hyg* 1924;5:390-398.

Hamilton A, Hardy HL: *Industrial Toxicology,* ed 2. New York, Paul B. Hoeber, 1949.

Heymans C, Neil E: *Reflexogenic Areas of the Cardiovascular System.* Boston, Little Brown, 1958.

Kaipainen WJ: Hydrogen sulfide intoxication: Rapidly transient changes in the electrocardiogram suggestive of myocardial infarction. *Ann Med Intern Fenniae* 1954;43:97-101.

Kemper, FD: A near-fatal case of hydrogen sulfide poisoning. *Can Med Assoc J* 1966;94:1130-1131.

Matsuo F, Cummins JW, Anderson RE: Neurological sequelae of massive hydrogen sulfide inhalation. *Arch Neurol* 1979;36:451-452.

McCabe LC, Clayton GD: Air pollution by hydrogen sulfide in Poza Rica, Mexico. *Arch Ind Hyg Occup Med* 1952;6:199-213.

Nau CA, Anderson W, Cone RE: Arsine, stibine and hydrogen sulphide; Accidental industrial poisoning by a mixture. *Ind Med* 1944;13:308-310.

NIOSH: *Criteria for a Recommended Standard . . . . Occupational Exposure to Hydrogen Sulfide.* Washington, DC, National Institute for Occupational Safety and Health (NIOSH 77-158), 1977.

Poda GA: Hydrogen sulfide can be handled safely. *Arch Environ Health* 1966;12:795-800.

Robinson LF, Camp MN, Chamberlain EC: A source of industrial hazard from hydrogen sulphide gas. *South Med J* 1942;25:621-623.

Smith RP, Gosselin RE: Hydrogen sulfide poisoning. *J Occup Med* 1979;21:93-97.

Stine RJ, Slosberg B, Beacham BE: Hydrogen sulfide intoxication. A case report and discussion of treatment. *Ann Intern Med* 1976;85:756-758.

Yant WP: Hydrogen sulphide in industry; Occurrence, effects, and treatment. *Am J Pub Health* 1930;20:598-608.

Sulfur Dioxide

Sulfur dioxide is used in the manufacture of sodium sulfite and of sulfuric acid, and in many other chemical processes. Other uses include refrigeration, bleaching, fumigation, and as an antioxidant in magnesium processing. It is generated as a by-product of paper manufacturing, petroleum refining, and of combustion of fossil fuels that contain sulfur as an impurity (NIOSH, 1974). Large quantities of sulfur dioxide are produced in the smelting of sulfide ores of lead, iron, zinc, and copper. So-called contact acid is made by the use of a catalyzer to produce this oxidation, the sulfur dioxide passing over platinized asbestos or iron or vanadium oxide. Sulfuric acid produced from sulfide ores is almost sure to be contaminated with as much as 1% of arsenic or selenium. Such impurities are very troublesome, for they cannot be removed by scrubbing but must be driven out by heat, a process that may result in the formation of the higher toxic gaseous compounds of arsenic or selenium.

Sulfur dioxide is almost irrespirable to those unaccustomed to it, but men who have worked in a fairly heavily contaminated atmosphere acquired a decided degree of tolerance. The gas causes a violent cough reflex that acts as a defense against a dangerous amount, provided the workers can escape quickly. In fatal cases, when death has come on rapidly, the postmortem changes are those of asphyxia. When the symptoms do not appear for several hours and death is delayed, the changes are those that follow inhalation of any irritant gas.

The following history of an unusual accident that happened in an American plant describes acute sulfur dioxide effect. Thirteen men were unloading sulfur from the hold of a ship when the bucket or chain struck a spark and ignited the sulfur dust in the air and the flames spread to the fine powder on the ceiling and walls, so that the air was filled with sulfur dioxide fumes. All were "knocked out" at once, but those nearest the hatchway climbed out and gave the alarm. Rescue was impossible until gas masks were procured and 15 minutes had elapsed before the last man was rescued. The victims suffered inflammation of the eyes, nausea, vomiting, pain in abdomen, sore throat, and later bronchitis. One worker seemed to be recovering, but then developed pneumonia and died on the tenth day. All but two of the remaining men were back at work in three weeks. The two who did not return at that time ran a low-grade fever and complained of weakness for some weeks. Such reports, incomplete as they are, support the conclusion that edema, destruction of protective ciliated epithelium, and invasion of the lung by bacteria are consequences of acute sulfur dioxide poisoning. Prompt use of oxygen, steroids, bronchodilators, and antibiotics may prove to be not only lifesaving but also may prevent irreversible damage.

Cases of unconsciousness and death from asphyxia were reported among commercial shrimp fisherman where a 1.25% sodium bisulfite solution was used as a dip to prevent "black spot" discoloration of the catch (Ford et al., 1978). Exposure to high concentrations of sulfur dioxide was suggested in this incident by the absence of methemoglobin and the findings of sulfhemoglobin levels of 6% and 12% in the postmortem blood of two fatal cases.

Charan et al. (1979) described an accident in a paper mill in which five persons were acutely exposed to very high concentrations of SO_2. Two men died with five minutes of rescue and were found to have extensive sloughing of the mucosa of the large and small airways as well as hemorrhagic alveolar edema. The three survivors had irritation and soreness of the eyes, nose, and throat, tightness of the chest, and severe dyspnea. Chest roentgenograms were normal despite diffuse râles and bronchi; no pulmonary edema was evident. One man developed severe airway obstruction that did not respond to bronchodilators; one man developed asymptomatic mild obstructive and restrictive disease, and the third had normal pulmonary function tests.

The question of chronic poisoning from sulfur dioxide is relatively more important than that of acute poisoning, which is rare and is usually due to an accident. Haggard (1924) said that there is no true tolerance to this gas. In contrast, Kehoe et al. (1932) studied the effect of prolonged exposure to sulfur dioxide on 100 workmen exposed to this gas in the course of their employment. Forty-seven had from four to 12 years' exposure, the severity of which fluctuated through a wide range. They found a significantly higher incidence of chronic nasopharyngitis, alteration in sense of smell and taste, and dyspnea on exertion. The workers in this group suffered upper respiratory tract infections that lasted three times as long as such infections among the control group. This report confirms a relationship between chronic illness and the frequency of heavy exposure to the fumes of sulfur dioxide.

Pulmonary function was tested in 113 copper smelter workers by Smith et al. (1977). Exposure to 1.0 to 2.5 ppm (2.6 to 6.5 mg/m³) sulfur dioxide was associated with excessive loss of 1-sec forced expiratory volume and an increase in respiratory symptoms. Those workers with impaired $FEV_{1.0}$ on initial measurements showed even greater losses of pulmonary function related to SO_2 exposure. In another study of men in an open pit copper mine and its associated smelter, Archer and Gillam (1978) found significant reduction of forced vital capacity (FVC) and $FEV_{1.0}$ to be associated with chronic exposure to SO_2 in a TWA range of 1 to 6 mg/m³ (0.4 to 3 ppm), and they suggested that the current occupational standard, which is based on acute effects, needs to be reconsidered. The situation is not clear, however, since Lebowitz et al. (1979) in a study of another copper smelter concluded that their investigation could not demonstrate consistent effects of SO_2 or dust exposure on pulmonary function. Fairchild et al. (1972) found in their animal experiments that influenza-infected mice exposed to sulfur dioxide developed more pneumonia than virus-controlled mice. They felt the increase in pneumonia was due to the sulfur dioxide concentration that induced low-grade inflammatory changes in the lungs.

The current literature dealing with chronic chest disease in England and the United States correlated with levels of sulfur dioxide in urban air is vast. (See, for example, the symposium on sulfur oxides and related particulates, *Bull NY Acad Med,* December 1978;54[11]). Amdur (1969) concluded that sulfur dioxide, not alone, but with fine particles of fly ash plus moisture, causes pulmonary damage by penetration to the lower respiratory tract where conversion to sulfuric acid takes place.

The occupational exposure standard recommended by NIOSH (1974) for exposure to sulfur dioxide states that such exposure should not exceed 2 ppm of air (5 mg/m³) determined as a TWA for up to a 10-hour workday, 40-hour workweek.

References

Amdur MO: Toxicologic appraisal of particulate matter, oxides of sulfur, and sulfuric acid.

J Air Pollution Control Assoc 1969;19:638–644.

Archer VE, Gillam JD: Chronic sulfur dioxide exposure in a smelter: II. Indices of chest disease. *J Occup Med* 1978;20:88–95.

Charan NB, Myers CG, Lakshminarayan S, et al: Pulmonary injuries associated with acute sulfur dioxide inhalation. *Am Rev Resp Dis* 1979;119:555–560.

Fairchild GA, Roan J, McCarrol J: Atmospheric pollutants and the pathogenesis of viral respiratory infection. *Arch Environ Health* 1972;25:174–182.

Ford R, Shkor J, Akman WV, et al: Deaths from asphyxia among fishermen. *Morb Mort Weekly Rep* 1978;27:309–315.

Haggard HW: Action of irritant gases on the respiratory tract. *J Ind Hyg* 1924;5:390–398.

Kehoe RA, Machle WF, Kitzmiller K, et al: On effects of prolonged exposure to sulphur dioxide. *J Ind Hyg* 1932;14:159–173.

Lebowitz MD, Burton A, Kaltenborn W: Pulmonary function in smelter workers. *J Occup Med* 1979;21:255–259.

NIOSH: *Criteria for a Recommended Standard . . . . Occupational Exposure to Sulfur Dioxide.* Washington DC, National Institute for Occupational Safety and Health (NIOSH 74-111), 1974.

Smith TJ, Peters JM, Reading JC, et al: Pulmonary impairment from chronic exposure to sulfur dioxide in a smelter. *Am Rev Resp Dis* 1977;116:31–39.

Sulfuric Acid

Sulfuric acid is one of the most widely used compounds in industry. Enormous quantities are used in the refining of petroleum, in the production of artificial fertilizers, in pickling steel and iron, in manufacture of halogen acids and of organic sulfonates used in detergents and lubricants, in dehydration procedures, and in the charging of storage batteries (NIOSH, 1974).

Concentrated sulfuric acid has a corrosive action on living tissues because of its very strong affinity to water so that it produces charring rather than acid burns. In contrast, dilute sulfuric acid injures skin and mucous membranes because of its acidity. Oleum (fuming sulfuric acid) is a solution of sulfuric anhydride (sulfur trioxide) in anhydrous sulfuric acid. Sulfuric acid mist is an aerosol whose particle sizes depend upon hygroscopic addition of water.

Two types of sulfuric acid injuries are encountered: (1) primary irritant effects on skin, eyes and other mucous membranes, and respiratory tract and (2) corrosion of teeth. Splash injuries to the eyes are serious because of the danger of permanent damage to the cornea. Skin burns, especially of the face, may lead to cosmetic problems. Exposure to fuming sulfuric acid led, in the case reported by Goldman and Hill (1953), to severe burns of the face and body, and to immediate respiratory distress that required oxygen therapy for 10 days; 18 months after the accident the patient had disabling pulmonary fibrosis, residual bronchiectasis, and pulmonary emphysema.

Inhalation of sulfuric acid mist leads, at low concentrations (0.35 to 5 mg/m^3), to reflex changes resulting in shallower and more rapid breathing (Amdur et al., 1952). Exposures to higher concentrations produced lacrimation, rhinorrhea, râles and increased airway resistance in healthy male volunteers, two of whom developed chronic bronchitic symptoms (Sim and Pattle, 1957). Bronchitis was found in excess in men occupationally exposed to high concentrations of sulfuric acid mist in an electric accumulator factory (Williams, 1970). In this study, absence of lower respiratory tract disease was attributed to the large mist particle size. However, sulfuric acid can reach the finer bronchioles and alveoli when the usual defenses of the respiratory tract are rendered inoperative. An unusual incident studied by HLH occurred when four diesel engineers were simultaneously exposed to sulfuric acid and cyanide and became unconscious. All developed persistent dyspnea and hypoxemia that were still present four years later.

Erosion of teeth occurs in workers exposed to sulfuric acid mist in the storage battery industry (Malcolm and Paul, 1961). The incisors are principally affected, with canines to a lesser extent and with no involvement of the premolars and molars. Progressive destruction of the tooth crown occurs on the labial surface and the painless erosion ceases when lip level is reached. These findings were confirmed by ten Bruggen Cate (1968) in his study of dental erosion in industry where workers are exposed to a variety of acids.

The recommended occupational exposure limit for sulfuric acid mist is 1.0 mg/m^3 for a TWA exposure for up to a 10-hour workday, 40-hour workweek (NIOSH, 1974).

References

Amdur MO, Silverman L, Drinker P: Inhalation of sulfuric acid mists by human subjects. *Arch Ind Hyg Occup Med* 1952;6:305–313.

ten Bruggen Cate HJ: Dental erosion in industry. *Br J Ind Med* 1968;25:249–266.

Goldman A, Hill WT: Chronic bronchopulmonary disease due to inhalation of sulfuric acid fumes. *Arch Ind Hyg Occup Med* 1953;8:205–211.

Malcolm D, Paul E: Erosion of teeth due to sulphuric acid in the battery industry. *Br J Ind Med* 1961;18:63–69.

NIOSH: *Criteria for a Recommended Standard .... Occupational Exposure to Sulfuric Acid.* Washington, DC, National Institute for Occupational Safety and Health (NIOSH 74-128), 1974.

Sim VM, Pattle RE: Effect of possible smog irritants on human subjects. *J Am Med Assoc* 1957; 165:1908–1913.

Williams MK: Sickness absence and ventilatory capacity of workers exposed to sulphuric acid mist. *Br J Ind Med* 1970;27:61–66.

Sulfate Dusts

Sodium sulfate beds are mined for use in the Kraft paper and other industries. Kelada and Euinton (1978) studied 119 workers from five Canadian mines who were exposed to sodium sulfate dusts during crushing, melting, evaporating, drying, loading, and bagging operations of this salt. No abnormalities in pulmonary function, serum electrolytes, or other aspects of health were encountered, even though 42 workers had more than 10 years' exposure. Nevertheless, epidemiologic studies in the United States have shown an excess risk of asthmatic attacks in the general population to be correlated with elevated levels of suspended sulfates in the air (French, 1975).

References

French J: Effects of suspended sulfates on human health. *Environ Health Pers* 1975;10: 35–37.

Kelada F, Euinton LE: Health effects of long-term exposure to sodium sulfate dust. *J Occup Med* 1978;20:812–814.

SECTION FOUR
CHEMICAL COMPOUNDS II

1 • *Aliphatic Hydrocarbons*

The aliphatic series of hydrocarbons includes the saturated (paraffin, methane, or alkane) and the unsaturated (olefin, ethylene, or alkene) compounds, which are derived almost exclusively from petroleum or petroleum processing.

Saturated Aliphatic Hydrocarbons

The saturated aliphatic series is comprised of gases (methane, ethane, propane, and butanes), liquids from pentanes (C_5) through C_{16} compounds, and longer chain solids. The compounds in this series are used as fuels, solvents, and lubricants, most commonly in mixtures. The first two members of the series, methane and ethane, have no known toxicologic properties and exert an effect simply as oxygen-displacing asphyxiants. Methane, the principal constituent of natural gas, is widely used as a domestic fuel. As such, it is biologically inert and is markedly different from the toxic carbon monoxide-containing manufactured gases, water gas and producer gas, that were in common use prior to the cross-country transportation of natural gas from petroleum-producing fields to commercial markets. However, the concept of toxic domestic fuel gas remains sufficiently prominent in American thinking to result in a number of suicide attempts each year by persons who "take gas." The usual consequence of this attempt is an explosion rather than an intoxication, since the lower limit of flammability for methane is approximately 5%. In mines methane may be known as marsh gas or fire damp, and is the principal cause of explosions in coal mines. Methane may become a simple asphyxiant in poorly ventilated pockets in coal mines into which the gas may rise because of its low density.

From time to time one notes clinical reports in the medical literature that refer to a "gas leak syndrome" (Sherman and Harris, 1968). The usual history includes an upper respiratory infection or other mild illness that requires a patient to be confined in a room that has a gas heater. Complaints of headache, weakness, myalgia, ataxia, and light-headedness or fainting appear to be associated with the confinement and unrelated to the primary illness. Medical examination is usually noncontributory, and there is no evidence that leaking natural gas has produced these clinical complaints. It is more than likely that whatever symptoms are related to the heating system are in fact related to faulty flues, so that there is leakage of carbon monoxide. Insufficient supply of air to replace that consumed by the heating system may result in negative pressure that in turn causes back drafts from the flues.

In general, the saturated hydrocarbons from propane (C_3) through the octanes (C_8) show increasingly strong narcotic properties. Heavier members of the series become insufficiently volatile to produce narcotizing concentrations in air unless heat is applied or vapor-saturated atmospheres are encountered in tanks or other confined spaces. The margin between narcosis and lethal depression of vital centers is too narrow to permit these compounds to be used as surgical anesthetics. Narcotic effects may be accompanied by exhilaration, dizziness, and headache. There may also be a loss of appetite, nausea, a persisting taste of gasoline, confusion, inability to do fine work, and loss of consciousness in extreme cases. Removal from exposure usually results in a rapid clearing of symptoms, although there may be a transient exacerbation upon coming into the open air.

In addition to the narcotic properties of *n*-hexane, this compound has been shown to be responsible for the polyneuropathy of shoe and leather workers in Japan and Italy (Sobue et al., 1968; Inoue et al., 1970; Cianchetti et al., 1976;

Buiatti et al., 1978) and furniture finishers in the United States (Herskowitz et al., 1971). Subjective symptoms associated with this exposure included muscle spasms, pelvic girdle and leg weakness and pain, and arm paresthesias. Lowered nerve conduction velocity and demonstrable damage to distal nerve axons ("dying-back" neuropathy) also have been reported (Scala, 1976; Schaumberg and Spencer, 1976). Moderate neuropathy from n-hexane exposure can be completely reversed with reduction of worker exposure (Paulson and Waylonis, 1976). Perbellini et al. (1981) have suggested that assay of urine for excretion of hexane metabolites may be used for monitoring occupational exposure to this compound and its isomers.

The unbranched hydrocarbons such as n-heptane and n-hexane are metabolized to alcohols, which are further degraded to carbon monoxide or conjugated to glucuronic acid (Toftgård and Gustafsson, 1980). The 2,5-hexanedione formed from n-hexane has been implicated as responsible for the neurotoxic effects of n-hexane and methyl-n-butyl ketone. This neurotoxicity has been verified in studies with rats that were given hexanol-2, a metabolic precursor of 2,5-hexanedione, intraperitoneally for eight months (Perbellini et al., 1978). Takeuchi et al. (1980) showed that n-hexane is much more toxic to rat peripheral nerve than is either n-pentane or n-heptane.

The vapors of compounds from pentane through octane are increasingly irritating to mucous membranes, although none of these compounds is actually a strong irritant. The liquids, as fat solvents, extract sebum from the skin to leave a dry irritated surface prone to cracking and bacterial infection. The likelihood of exposure to individual members of this series is very small; most commonly exposures are to mixtures that may be variously termed petroleum ether, benzine (not benzene), petroleum naphtha, gasoline, mineral spirits, Stoddard solvent, and varsol. Higher boiling mixtures appear as kerosine or jet fuels, and as diesel oils; heavier yet are the lubricating oils. Such mixtures may contain various branched and cyclic compounds such as benzene that have important toxicologic properties of much greater significance than those of the quantitatively predominant aliphatics. The composition of these mixtures will reflect the origin of the petroleum, molecular modifications effected at the refineries, seasonal fuel adjustments, and the addition of highly dissimilar materials such as antioxidants, anti-knock compounds, corrosion inhibitors, combustion improvers, and dyes.

From the practical point of view, and in the absence of benzene, the manifestations of exposure to vapors of these hydrocarbon mixes are those typical of exposure to heptane or octane: giddiness, vertigo, headache, and anesthetic stupor. In massive acute exposures, such as may be experienced upon entry into gasoline storage tanks, rapid central nervous system depression may occur with sudden collapse, deep coma, and death. There may be convulsions indicative of brain irritation or apneic anoxia. Full recovery without sequelae may occur but cerebral microhemorrhages or focal postinflammatory scarring may result in epileptiform seizures months after the acute episode. Irritation of the upper and lower respiratory tract and visceral damage also have been described (Machle, 1941).

From time to time cases are reported of sudden death in persons who have inhaled vapors of volatile liquids such as gasoline. Usually this exposure is not in the line of work but reflects an attempt to obtain an exhilarating or similar psychopharmacologic experience. It appears that these deaths are due to fatal cardiac arrhythmias in which endogenous releases of epinephrine are implicated (Reinhardt et al., 1971). There is no convincing evidence that prolonged exposures to vapors of aliphatic compounds in the case of gasoline station attendants can cause harmful effects. Yet, careful studies of aircraft factory workers heavily exposed to jet fuel vapors have demonstrated slightly reduced peripheral nerve conduction velocities and a tendency to higher peripheral vibration perception thresholds, along with repeated acute symptoms such as dizziness, chest pressure, palpitations, nausea, and headache (Knave et al., 1976). Further investigations have revealed psychiatric symptoms, such as anxiety and depression, and neurasthenic complaints in the exposed workers (Knave et al., 1978).

These solvent mixes are all primary irritants and defatting agents when applied to the skin. Carcinoma of the skin that has followed prolonged topical exposure to cutting oils almost certainly represents a reaction to specific carcinogenic polycyclic aromatic compounds and not to the aliphatic materials that are the predominant constituents (Bingham et al., 1980).

In industrial situations, kerosine and lubricating oils are insufficiently volatile to cause respiratory tract damage. These substances can enter the lungs by aspiration that follows ingestion and spontaneous or induced vomiting. Gerarde (1963) showed experimentally that the ingestion of these mixtures is not especially injurious in the absence of vomiting. When vomiting does occur, however, hydrocarbon mixtures of low viscosity (e.g., gasoline) are readily aspirated into the lungs and in such cases there may be rapid death from cardiac arrest, asphyxia, or respiratory paralysis. Rapid systemic absorption may lead to central nervous system disturbances such as convulsions, depression, or coma. The aspiration of lesser amounts or of somewhat heavier molecular weight compounds (C_{10} to C_{15}), such as kerosine, results in a slower progression of events, marked by chemical pneumonitis with prominent endothelial damage, pulmonary hemorrhage and edema, and complicating bacterial pneumonia. Thus, when hydrocarbons have been ingested, accidentally or deliberately, the prevention of aspiration is of the utmost importance. The advisability of gastric lavage is a debatable point (Press, 1962), but the best current practice seems to indicate this procedure if precautions, such as intratracheal intubation, are taken.

Heavier and more viscous materials, such as mineral oil and motor oil are not readily aspirated. The pulmonary reaction to these high-viscosity hydrocarbons is one of lipoid pneumonia, a chronic localized tissue response that has been observed in persons using mineral oil-based nose drops over the course of several years.

Occasionally, one reads of acute oliguric renal failure from topical exposures such as washing hair (Barrientos et al., 1977) or hands (Crisp et al., 1979) with diesel oil. Similar nephrotoxic effects were reported by Reidenberg et al. (1964) as a result of inhalation of diesel oil vapors in a truck cab. Chronic glomerulonephritis and Goodpasture's syndrome have also been reported to follow exposure to petroleum fuels (Beirne and Brennan, 1972; Zimmerman et al., 1975).

Lubricating oils Lubricating oils are based upon aliphatic hydrocarbon molecules containing 17 or more carbon atoms. Such oils are complex mixtures that contain small amounts of aromatic and polycyclic substances and a broad variety of dissimilar materials known collectively as "additives." The functions of these additives are multiple: they may inhibit corrosion or oxidation, preserve film integrity, alter viscosity, suppress bacterial growth, or act as detergents. Some of these materials have biological properties that may cause lubricating oils to have toxic effects in excess of those of simple aliphatic compounds. Skin reactions to these petroleum oil additives are described in treatises on occupational dermatology. These problems are not common, however, and they primarily affect those individuals who have developed a high degree of hypersensitivity.

Cutting oils Cutting fluids are applied to metal-cutting tools to facilitate and accelerate machining operations, to cool cutting surfaces, and to carry metal chips away from work surfaces. It is believed that cutting fluids are the most common cause of industrial dermatitis and, as such, represent a major cause of disability, lost work time, and work restriction. The problem is exacerbated by the fact that large volumes of fluid may be used at each machine, that the compressed air used in chip removal may spatter fluids over the operator and his clothing, and that sharp metal chips imbedded in rags and clothing or on the skin cause small lacerations that impair skin resistance to irritating compounds and infection.

Cutting fluids are for the most part dissimilar in composition to the lubricating oils. Cutting fluids can be classified into three categories: 1) insoluble oils, 2) soluble fluids, and 3) synthetic fluids. Insoluble oils are based upon petroleum oils to which are added various animal or vegetable fats, oils, and waxes. These oils are commonly recirculated for long periods, with metal chips removed by filtration, and are used chiefly in heavy machining operations, such as the cutting of engine blocks. Soluble fluids or oils are based upon an emulsion of oils and water, and are milky in appearance. The chemical or synthetic fluids are mostly water with small amounts of wetting agents. Various materials may be added to the basic fluid, regardless of type, to provide or improve specific desirable properties. These additives include germicides such as formalin, mercurials, or phenolic compounds; emulsifiers such as soaps and sulfonates; corrosion inhibitors such as borates, dichromates, or amines; and extreme pressure compounds of sulfur, chlorine, or phosphorus. The oil-water emulsions tend to become rancid, but they are good coolants, economical, and noncombustible.

The prevalence of cutting fluid dermatitis is related to the hygienic status of the working place and the worker. Poor machine enclosure, the use of degraded and contaminated fluid, inadequate washing facilities for personnel, and an insufficient supply of clean clothes and protective garments contribute to the problem. Machinists who are prone to acne and seborrhea or who are hirsute are relatively susceptible to blockage of hair follicles by insoluble oils and the consequent folliculitis. Individuals with a previously unresolved skin problem or who have a dry, atrophic skin are vulnerable to soluble fluids, especially those that are clearly alkaline or that contain wetting agents.

The usual cutaneous response to oil-based materials is an oil folliculitis that arises as a result of chemical irritation and mechanical plugging of the follicular canals. Onset of the problem usually occurs soon after the first exposure and is marked by acute reactions starting on the dorsal surfaces of the hands and fingers, the extensor surfaces of the forearms and thighs, and the abdomen (i.e., those surfaces that are in contact with oil or oil-soaked clothing). Comedones and perifollicular papules and pustules ("oil boils") develop. Secondary infections may occur, but the bacteria in the oil are rarely primary skin pathogens and are rarely the single cause of the folliculitis. Melanosis may appear later. Clinical manifestations clear rapidly with the termination of exposure and do not resolve if the exposure is continued. Exposure is controlled through proper machine design to prevent spattering, clean clothing, protective garments, and careful attention to handwashing and other aspects of personal hygiene.

Since emulsion and synthetic fluids are potent defatting agents, the skin reaction to them may include maceration, dryness and "chapping," reddening, and vesiculation. Bacterial growths in the fluid do not appear to be directly injurious to workers, but rancid fluids and products of bacterial action can lead to skin disorders. As is the case with insoluble oils, both treatment and prevention are based on the control of exposure. Corticosteroid creams may be used as an adjunct in the treatment. The value of "barrier" creams and other protective gels is not unanimously accepted, but they do offer modest usefulness in certain situations, and have been shown to reduce ultrastructural and cytoarchitectural changes in human epidermis after applications of acetone and kerosine (Lupulescu and Birmingham, 1976).

Individual additives in cutting fluids can be a cause of either primary irritative or hypersensitive dermatitis. Detergents, soaps, and wetting agents defat the skin, and alkaline materials damage the keratin of the upper, protective skin layers. Ulcerative and erythematous lesions on the genitals and buttocks have been reported for workers wearing coveralls that had been dry-cleaned with Stoddard solvent, a mixture of petroleum distillates (Nethercott et al., 1980). Formalin in germicides is a sensitizer. Additives containing sulfur and chlorine are direct irritants, although so-called chloracne is not associated with cutting fluids. Nickel or chromates derived from metals being cut can be a source of allergic dermatitis. Harsh abrasive soaps and solvents, such as gasoline and kerosine, may contribute to chemical and traumatic dermatitis, since these cleaning materials are common in machine shops. While grime and grease can certainly be removed from the skin with these substances, it is safer to utilize less injurious cleansers available commercially.

Certain petroleum oils have carcinogenic constituents; this is especially the case with shale oils, which are currently extracted and used outside the United States (Kahn, 1979; Weaver and Gibson, 1979). Since American potential supplies of oil shale tars constitute 94% of the known world resources, these substances may present toxic problems in this country in the future. There are no good data that would establish the prevalence of skin cancers among machinists in this country, but scrotal and other skin cancers have been reported among British cotton mule spinners prior to 1953 (International Agency for Research on Cancer, 1973) and more recently among toolsetters and machine operators in the British Midlands (Waldron and Waterhouse, 1976). Reports from other European countries have recently been summarized by Bingham et al. (1980). Knowledge of occupational malignancies of the skin has a long and important history that dates back to 1775 when Pott identified scrotal cancer in English chimney sweeps.

Exposures to mist sprays of insoluble oils used as coolants, cutting fluids, and lubricants in machine operations are usually not harmful to the respiratory tract (Ely et al., 1970; Goldstein et al., 1970; Pasternack and Ehrlich, 1972), although worker discomfort occurs at oil mist levels above 5 mg/m^3 (Hendricks et al., 1962). Mineral oil droplets less than 5μ in diameter may be inhaled and result in fibrotic nodules, paraffinomas, or in lipoid pneumonitis (Waldron, 1977). Decoufle (1976) could find no evidence that machinists exposed to cutting-oil mists had any unusual mortality from respiratory tract cancer.

Unsaturated Aliphatic Compounds

In general, the unsaturated aliphatic hydrocarbons lack biological properties that are important to occupational medicine. These compounds are for the most part products of the petrochemical industry and are formed in the cracking and dehydrogenation of petroleum fractions. Ethylene and propylene are anesthetics at high concentrations and have been used in surgical procedures. The butylenes, butadiene, and isoprene (C_5) have similar properties. Acetylene is also an anesthetic material with no known injurious effects upon man. When acetylene is prepared from the addition of water to calcium carbide, phosphine (PH_3) may be generated from phosphides in the impure carbide. Hence, phosphine, the toxicity of which is discussed in the chapter on phosphorus, may be a significant contaminant of commercial grades of acetylene. The wide range of flammability of this gas and its tendency to form explosive acetylides with metals warrant special attention.

Inhalation toxicity studies of 1,3-butadiene on rats failed to demonstrate any adverse effects with a variety of exposure concentrations, except for moderately increased salivation at the higher levels (Crouch et al., 1979).

Exposure Limits

The permissible exposure limits for occupational exposure range from 1000 ppm for propane and pentane to 500 ppm for hexane, heptane, octane, and petroleum distillates. These values are roughly equivalent to 1800 to 3000 mg/m^3, depending on the molecular weights of the compounds. For mineral oil mist the permissible limit is much lower and has been set at 5 mg/m^3. The butadiene permissible limit is 1000 ppm (= 2200 mg/m^3). NIOSH has recommended much lower limits for the C_5 to C_8 aliphatics, with values ranging from 75 to 120 ppm (NIOSH/OSHA, 1978).

References

Barrientos A, Ortuño MT, Morales JM, et al: Acute renal failure after use of diesel oil as shampoo. *Arch Intern Med* 1977;137:1217.

Beirne GJ, Brennan JT: Glomerulonephritis associated with hydrocarbon solvents: Mediated by antiglomerular basement membrane antibody. *Arch Environ Health* 1972;25:365–369.

Bingham E. Trosset RP, Warshawsky D: Carcinogenic potential of petroleum hydrocarbons. *J Environ Pathol Toxicol* 1980;3:483–563.

Buiatti E, Cecchini S, Ronchi O, et al: Relationship between clinical and electromyographic findings and exposure to solvents, in shoe and leather workers. *Br J Indust Med* 1978;35:168–173.

Cianchetti C, Abbritti G, Perticoni G, et al: Toxic polyneuropathy of shoe-industry workers. *J Neurol Neurosurg Psychiatry* 1976;39:1151–1161.

Crisp AJ, Bhalla AK, Hoffbrand BI: Acute tubular necrosis after exposure to diesel oil. *Br Med J* 1979;2:177.

Crouch CN, Pullinger DH, Gaunt IF: Inhalation toxicity studies with 1,3-butadiene: 2. 3 month toxicity study in rats. *Am Ind Hyg Asoc J* 1979;40:796–802.

Decoufle P: Cancer mortality among workers exposed to cutting oil mist. *Ann NY Acad Sci* 1976;271:94–101.

Ely TS, Pedley SF, Hearne FT, et al: A study of mortality, symptoms and respiratory function in humans occupationally exposed to oil mist. *J Occup Med* 1970;12:253–261.

Gerarde HW: Toxicological studies on hydrocarbons: IX. The aspiration hazard and toxicity of hydrocarbons and hydrocarbon mixtures. *Arch Environ Health* 1963;6:329–341.

Goldstein DH, Benoit JN, Tyroler HA: An epidemiological study of oil mist exposure. *Arch Environ Health* 1970;21:600–603.

Hendricks NV, Collins GH, Dooley AE, et al: A review of exposures to oil mist. *Arch Environ Health* 1962;4:139–145.

Herskowitz A, Ishii N, Schaumberg H: n-Hexane neuropathy. A syndrome occurring as a result of industrial exposure. *N Engl J Med* 1971;285:82–85.

Inoue T, Takeuchi Y, Takeuchi S, et al: A health survey on vinyl sandal manufacturers with high incidence of n-hexane intoxication. *Jap J Ind Health* 1970;12:73–84.

International Agency for Research on Cancer: *Monographs on the Evaluation of Carcinogenic Risk of Chemicals to Man. Vol 3. Certain Polycyclic Aromatic Hydrocarbons and Heterocyclic Compounds.* Lyon, France, IARC, 1973.

Kahn H: Toxicity of shale oil chemical products: A review. *Scand J Work Environ Health* 1979;5:1–9.

Knave B, Persson HE, Goldberg JM, et al: Long-term exposure to jet fuel. An investigation

202

on occupationally exposed workers with special reference to the nervous system. *Scand J Work Environ Health* 1976;3:152–164.

Knave B, Olson BA, Elofsson, et al: Long-term exposure to jet fuel. A cross-sectional epidemiologic investigation on occupationally exposed industrial workers with special reference to the nervous system. *Scand J Work Environ Health* 1978;4:19–45.

Lupulescu AP, Birmingham DJ: Effect of protective agent against lipid-solvent-induced damages. Ultrastructural and scanning electron microscopical study of human epidermis. *Arch Environ Health* 1976;31:33–36.

Machle W: Gasoline intoxication. *J Am Med Assoc* 1941;117:1965–1971.

Nethercott JR, Pierce JM, Likwornick G, et al: Genital ulceration due to Stoddard solvent. *J Occup Med* 1980;22:549–552.

NIOSH/OSHA: *Pocket Guide to Chemical Hazards.* Washington, DC, National Institute for Occupational Safety and Health (NIOSH 78-210), 1978.

Pasternack B, Ehrlich L: Occupational exposure to an oil mist atmosphere. A 12-year mortality study. *Arch Environ Health* 1972;25:286–294.

Paulson GW, Waylonis GW: Polyneuropathy due to *n*-hexane. *Arch Intern Med* 1976;136:880–882.

Perbellini L, De Grandis D, Semenzato F, et al: An experimental study on the neurotoxicity of *n*-hexane metabolites: Hexanol-1 and hexanol-2. *Toxicol Appl Pharmacol* 1978;46:421–427.

Perbellini L, Brugnone F, Faggionato G: Urinary excretion of the metabolites of *n*-hexane and its isomers during occupational exposure. *Br J Indust Med* 1981;38:20–26.

Press E: Cooperative kerosine poisoning study: Evaluation of gastric lavage and other factors in the treatment of accidental ingestion of petroleum distillate products. *Pediatrics* 1962;29:649–674.

Reidenberg MM, Powers DV, Sevy RW, et al: Acute renal failure due to nephrotoxins. *Am J Med Sci* 1964;247:25–29.

Reinhardt CF, Azar A, Maxfield ME, et al: Cardiac arrhythmias and aerosol "sniffing." *Arch Environ Health* 1971;22:265–279.

Scala RA: Hydrocarbon neuropathy. *Ann Occup Hyg* 1976;19:293–299.

Schaumberg HH, Spencer PS: Degeneration in central and peripheral nervous systems produced by pure *n*-hexane: An experimental study. *Brain* 1976;99:183–192.

Sherman BR, Harris EH: Gas leak syndrome.

Pediatrics 1968;42:710–711.

Sobue I, Yamamura Y, Ando K, et al: n-hexane polyneuropathy. Outbreak among vinyl sandal manufacturers. *Clin Neurol* 1968;8:393–403.

Takeuchi Y, Ono Y, Hisanaga N, et al: A comparative study on the neurotoxicity of n-pentane, n-hexane, and n-heptane in the rat. *Br J Ind Med* 1980;37:241–247.

Toftgård R, Gustafsson J-Å: Biotransformation of organic solvents. A review. *Scand J Work Environ Health* 1980;6:1–18.

Waldron HA: Health care of people at work. Exposure to oil mist in industry. *J Soc Occup Med* 1977;27:45–49.

Waldron HA, Waterhouse JAH: Mineral-oil cancers. *Lancet* 1976;1:805.

Weaver NK, Gibson RL: The U.S. oil shale industry: A health perspective. *Am Ind Hyg Assoc J* 1979;40:460–467.

Zimmerman SW, Groehler K, Beirne GJ: Hydrocarbon exposure and chronic glomerulonephritis. *Lancet* 1975;2:199–201.

2 • Alcohols and Glycols

Alcohols and glycols do not usually present serious hazards in the industrial setting. Although specific compounds, such as methanol and ethylene glycol, are involved in epidemics or in isolated instances of intoxication, the observed illness is almost invariably the result of intentional oral consumption of these compounds. Industrial exposures to alcohol and glycol vapors rarely produce symptoms of systemic intoxication, and the toxicity that is observed is usually related to irritation of the conjunctivae and the mucous membranes of the upper airway. In most industrial situations only the low molecular weight alcohols are sufficiently volatile to yield significant air concentrations. The alcohols and glycols have narcotic properties but these are much less prominent than those associated with the solvent hydrocarbons or halogenated hydrocarbons.

Alcohols

Methanol Methanol (CH_3OH, methyl alcohol, wood alcohol, carbinol) is used extensively as a solvent for lacquers, paints, varnishes, cements, inks, dyes, plastics, and various industrial coatings. Large quantities are used in the production of formaldehyde and other chemical derivatives such as acetic acid, methyl halides and terephthalate, methyl methacrylate, and methylamines (NIOSH, 1976). Most of the methanol produced in the United States is now prepared synthetically by the reduction of carbon monoxide with hydrogen rather than by the former method of distillation of wood. Methanol is also used as a gasoline additive, a component of lacquer thinners, in antifreeze preparations of the "nonpermanent" type, and in canned heating preparations of jellied alcohol. It is also used in duplicating fluid, in paint removers, and as a cleaning agent. Crude wood alcohol contains substances such as acetone, methyl ethyl ketone, methyl acetate, and furfural that contribute to a disagreeable odor and taste (McNally, 1937). Proposed new uses for methanol are primarily in various forms of energy generation (Posner, 1975).

Toxic effects The literature of the early 1900s does describe cases of systemic intoxication by the inhalation of methanol in various varnishing operations or similar situations in which large quantities were evaporated into an enclosed space (see, for example, De Schweinitz, 1901; Jelliffe, 1905). While the possibility of ingestion cannot be excluded definitely in every report, it is probable that some of these exposures were, in fact, only by inhalation. The levels of such exposures, however, must have been extremely high, for there is ample evidence today from the photographic film industry that repeated exposures to air levels well in excess of the threshold limit value of 200 ppm do not cause significant discomfort or illness. Scherberger et al. (1958) found that the average minimum identifiable odor level for methanol was 1500 ppm (roughly 2000 mg/m³).

The onset of symptoms may follow ingestion by a period of less than an hour or may be delayed for up to 30 hours; a latent period of 12 to 18 hours is common. In the usual case of methanol poisoning by ingestion the initial symptoms may include those suggestive of ethanol intoxication: headache, weakness, vertigo, visual disturbances, and coma (Tyson, 1912; Røe, 1946; Røe, 1955; Bennett et al., 1953). There may be nausea, vomiting, and abdominal or lumbar pain. Onset symptoms of occupational exposure to methanol vapor have included paresthesias, numbness, and shooting pains in the hands and forearms (Jelliffe, 1905). The symptoms are associated with metabolic acidosis, as a result of the accumulation of acid metabolites in the body. The severity of the symptoms is believed to be proportional to the intensity of the acidosis. Coma, seizures, and prolonged acidosis are signs of poor prognosis (Naraqi et al., 1979).

Visual disturbances, the most striking and often the most damaging aspect of methanol intoxication, may develop early (Benton and Calhoun, 1953). Blurring of vision, occasionally with changes in color perception and scotomata, and constriction of visual fields, may develop suddenly with little warning. The loss of acuity may involve a gray mist sensation, and there may be pain or tenderness of the eyes or photophobia. The initial impairment of vision may be transitory, but improvement in vision may be followed by complete and permanent blindness. Clinical observations suggest that if there is no improvement within six days the prognosis is very poor. The eye in methanol poisoning may have dilated and unreactive pupils. Visual loss is associated with hyperemia of the optic disc, and blurring of the disc margins, indicative of retinal edema, can also be seen. When severe, such blurring warns of at least some degree of permanent loss of vision. Atrophy of the disc is observed in some 30 to 60 days. Computerized tomography scanning of the skull can be helpful in the diagnosis by demonstrating symmetrical areas of low attenuation in the putamens (Aquilonius et al., 1978; McLean et al., 1980).

Pathologic changes noted in fatal cases of methanol ingestion were primarily edema, hyperemia, and necrosis of the stomach, intestines, brain, and retinas (Menne, 1938). Survivors of severe methanol poisoning may show mild dementia and a Parkinson-like extrapyramidal syndrome (Guggenheim et al., 1971; McLean et al., 1980).

The physiological explanation for the vulnerability of the eye in methanol intoxication lies in the very high relative oxygen consumption of the retina and the impairment of retinal metabolism by formaldehyde, the normal metabolite of methanol, or perhaps, as has recently been suggested, by accumulation of formate in the blood (Martin-Amat et al., 1978).

Therapy Since the metabolic acidosis and eye injury of methanol poisoning are related to the metabolites of methanol rather than to the alcohol itself, the treatment of methanol intoxication is based upon attempts to impair the metabolism of this compound so that it may be excreted unchanged in the urine. Methanol oxidation to formaldehyde is catalyzed by alcohol dehydrogenase, a zinc metalloenzyme that oxidizes other alcohols as well (Li and Vallee, 1969). Ethanol can compete with methanol for active sites of this enzyme, and in fact the enzyme has a greater affinity for the former than the latter. Consequently, the therapeutic administration of ethanol permits it to be preferentially oxidized and diminishes the production of methanol metabolites. Røe (1955) believes that sufficient ethanol must be administered to produce a blood level of at least 0.1%. Control of acidosis is essential in methanol poisoning and the use of intravenous bicarbonate has frequently been lifesaving. More recently the value of hemodialysis or peritoneal dialysis has been emphasized (Cowen, 1964; Keyvan-Larijarni and Tannenberg, 1974). The availability of one or other form of dialysis and of rapid determinations of blood methanol levels and acid-base balance has dramatically improved the prognosis of methanol intoxication.

References

Aquilonius S-M, Askmark H, Enoksson P, et al: Computerized tomography in severe methanol intoxication. *Br Med J* 1978;2:929–930.

Bennett IL Jr, Cary FH, Mitchell GL Jr, et al: Acute methyl alcohol poisoning: A review based on experiences in an outbreak of 323 cases. *Medicine* 1953; 32:431–463.

Benton CD Jr, Calhoun FP Jr: The ocular effects of methyl alcohol poisoning: Report of a catastrophe involving 320 persons. *Am J Ophthalmol* 1953;36:1677–1685.

Cowen DL: Extracorporeal dialysis in methanol poisoning. *Ann Intern Med* 1964;61:134–135.

De Schweinitz GE: A case of methyl-alcohol amaurosis, the pathway of entrance of the poison being the lungs and the cutaneous surface. *Ophthalmic Rec* 1901; 10:289–296.

Guggenheim MA, Couch JR, Weinberg W: Motor dysfunction as a permanent complication of methanol ingestion. *Arch Neurol* 1971;24: 550–554.

Jelliffe SE: Multiple neuritis in wood alcohol poisoning. *Med News (NY)* 1905;86:387–390.

Keyvan-Larijarni H, Tannenberg AM: Methanol intoxication. Comparison of peritoneal dialysis and hemodialysis treatment. *Arch Intern Med* 1974;134:293–296.

Li T-K, Vallee BL: Alcohol dehydrogenase and ethanol metabolism. *Surg Clin North Am* 1969; 49:577–582.

Martin-Amat G, McMartin KE, Hayreh SS, et

al: Methanol poisoning: Ocular toxicity produced by formate. *Toxicol Appl Pharmacol* 1978;45:201-208.

McLean DR, Jacobs H, Mielke BW: Methanol poisoning: A clinical and pathological study. *Ann Neurol* 1980;8:161-167.

McNally WD: *Toxicology*. Chicago, Industrial Medicine, 1937, pp 613-631.

Menne FR: Acute methyl alcohol poisoning. A report of twenty-two instances with postmortem examinations. *Arch Pathol* 1938;26:77-92.

Naraqi S, Dethiefs RF, Slobodniuk RA, et al: An outbreak of acute methyl alcohol intoxication. *Aust NZ J Med* 1979;9:65-68.

NIOSH: *Criteria for a Recommended Standard . . . . Occupational Exposure to Methyl Alcohol*. Washington, DC, National Institute for Occupational Safety and Health (NIOSH 76-148), 1976.

Posner HS: Biohazards of methanol in proposed new uses. *J Toxicol Environ Health* 1975;1:153-171.

Røe O: Methanol poisoning: Its clinical course, pathogenesis and treatment. *Acta Med Scand* 1946;Suppl 182:1-253.

Røe O: The metabolism and toxicity of methanol. *Pharmacol Rev* 1955;7:399-412.

Scherberger RF, Happ GP, Miller FA, et al: A dynamic apparatus for preparing air-vapor mixtures of known concentrations. *Am Ind Hyg Assoc J* 1958;19:494-498.

Tyson HH: Amblyopia from inhalation of methyl alcohol. *Arch Ophthalmol (NY)* 1912;41:459-471.

Ethanol   Ethanol (C_2H_5OH, ethyl alcohol, grain alcohol) that is used in industry is synthesized almost entirely by hydration of ethylene. Ethanol is used as a starting material for the synthesis of a wide variety of organic compounds used in industry. Beverage alcohol is derived from the fermentation of carbohydrates, and the supply for this purpose is not augmented by synthetic ethanol.

While the problems of ethanol intoxication associated with beverage ingestion are well-known, industrial exposures to ethanol vapors are of no practical importance, although Browning (1965) suggested that such exposure on a chronic basis may irritate the mucous membranes as well as produce headache, inebriation, and somnolence. Lester and Greenberg (1951) computed the absorption via the respiratory tract that would

be necessary to cause any continuous increase in blood ethanol levels. They concluded that a workman exposed to 1000 ppm would have to breathe at a rate of 65 L/min. Since a ventilation rate of 30 L/min is associated with hard work, the hazard of systemic effects from airborne ethanol is unlikely. At air concentrations of 5000 to 10,000 ppm there may be mild transient coughing or eye irritation. Concentrations of 20,000 ppm are intolerable. Workers sometimes drink ethanol, on hand for manufacturing or other non-beverage purposes, a practice that thereby adds to the total dose absorbed and increases susceptibility to accidents.

Ethanol absorption, regardless of the route of administration, may produce very undesirable effects in workers taking disulfiram, or exposed occupationally to this compound or to thiuram. Contact dermatitis from ethanol occurs rarely (van Ketel and Tan-Lim, 1975), but reports have not mentioned occupational exposure.

References

Browning E: *Toxicity and Metabolism of Industrial Solvents*. New York, Elsevier, 1965, pp 324-331.

Lester D, Greenberg LA: The inhalation of ethyl alcohol by man: Industrial hygiene and medicolegal aspects. *Q J Study Alcohol* 1951;12:167-178.

van Ketel WG, Tan-Lim KN: Contact dermatitis from ethanol. *Contact Derm* 1975;1:7-10.

Propanols and butanols   The propanols, propyl and isopropyl alcohol, have no current toxicological importance in industry. When ingested they have toxic properties that resemble ethanol but they are more injurious, perhaps because they are converted to metabolites more slowly. A rare instance of sensitivity to isopropyl alcohol was encountered in a cosmetic patch testing program (Ludwig and Hausen, 1977).

Of the four isomeric forms of butanol, n-butyl alcohol is of industrial importance and has been studied most intensively (Tabershaw et al., 1944; Sterner et al., 1949). No systemic effects have been noted with exposures below 100 ppm. Eye irritation, with corneal inflammation, burning sensation, lacrimation, photophobia, and blurred vision, was seen when the air concentration was 200 ppm or more. Dermatitis of hands and fingers was reported by Tabershaw et al. (1944) but could be prevented by protective ointments. The apparently specific formation of minute vacuoles of the cornea has been observed in workers coating raincoats with material containing this solvent (Cogan and Grant, 1945). The other butyl alcohols have similar irritative properties.

References

Cogan DG, Grant WM: An unusual type of keratitis associated with exposure to n-butyl alcohol (butanol). *Arch Ophthalmol* 1945;33: 106–109.

Ludwig E, Hausen BM: Sensitivity to isopropyl alcohol. *Contact Derm* 1977;3:240–244.

Tabershaw IR, Fahy JP, Skinner JB: Industrial exposure to butanol. *J Ind Hyg Toxicol* 1944;26: 328–330.

Sterner JH, Crouch HC, Brockmyre HF, et al: A ten-year study of butyl alcohol exposure. *Am Ind Hyg Assoc Q* 1949;10:53–59.

Pentanols The pentanols (pentyl or amyl alcohol, "fusel oil") are irritating as well as narcotic, and have produced illnesses, some fatal, upon ingestion. The toxicological significance in industry of these alcohols and their heavier homologues is small, but Browning (1965) has collected a number of case reports implicating amyl alcohol in industrial exposures that produced neurological and gastrointestinal symptoms.

Reference

Browning E: *Toxicity and Metabolism of Industrial Solvents*. New York, Elsevier, 1965, pp 356–367.

Allyl alcohol Allyl alcohol ($H_2C=CH-CH_2-OH$) is a pungent chemical intermediate with potent irritant properties. Absorption through the skin leads to deep muscle pain, presumably due to spasm. Lacrimation, retrobulbar pain, photophobia, and blurring of vision may result from exposure to vapors, and corneal injury has been described (Dunlap et al., 1958; Torkelson et al., 1959). Allyl alcohol and many of its esters are hepatic toxins that cause periportal necrosis and other liver injury (Kodama and Hine,

1958; Taylor et al., 1964), perhaps as a result of oxidation of allyl alcohol to acrolein ($H_2C=CH-CHO$) (Reid, 1972). When allyl alcohol is used in an open system, exhaust ventilation is essential, and clean-up of spills requires the use of personal protective equipment.

References

Dunlap MK, Kodama JK, Wellington JS, et al: The toxicity of allyl alcohol. *Arch Ind Health* 1958;18:303–311.

Kodama JK, Hine CH: Pharmacodynamic aspects of allyl alcohol toxicity. *J Pharmacol Exp Ther* 1958;124:97–107.

Reid WD: Mechanism of allyl alcohol-induced hepatic necrosis. *Experientia* 1972;28:1058–1061.

Taylor JM, Jenner PM, Jones WI: A comparison of the toxicity of some allyl, propenyl, and propyl compounds in the rat. *Toxicol Appl Pharmacol* 1964;6:378–387.

Torkelson TR, Wolf MA, Oyen F, et al: Vapor toxicity of allyl alcohol as determined on laboratory animals. *Am Ind Hyg Assoc J* 1959;20:224–229.

Ethylene chlorohydrin Ethylene chlorohydrin (CH_2Cl-CH_2-OH; 2-chloroethyl alcohol) is an extremely toxic compound used for its special solvent properties and as a chemical intermediate. It readily penetrates the skin and most rubber gloves. The mechanism of toxicity is not fully understood, but apparently its metabolite, chloroacetic acid, acts as an inhibitor in the tricarboxylic acid cycle. The central nervous system is especially susceptible with muscle incoordination and convulsions resulting from exposure (Middleton, 1930; Goldblatt and Chiesman, 1944; Bush et al., 1949).

References

Bush AF, Abrams HK, Brown HV: Fatality and illness caused by ethylene chlorhydrin in an agricultural operation. *J Ind Hyg Toxicol* 1949;31:352–358.

Goldblatt MW, Chiesman WE: Toxic effects of ethylene chlorhydrin (clinical). *Br J Ind Med* 1944;1:207–213.

Middleton EL: Fatal case of poisoning by ethylene chlorhydrin. *J Ind Hyg* 1930;12:265.

Glycols

Glycols are dihydroxyalcohols that are usually formed by adding two hydroxyl groups to the double bonds in alkene compounds. Glycols and their derivatives have a variety of uses such as antifreeze agents, dye solvents, vehicles for pharmaceuticals, cosmetics and food extracts, hygroscopic agents in textiles and tobacco, and plasticizers.

Ethylene glycol Ethylene glycol (1,2-ethanediol) is the basic constituent of "permanent" antifreeze and many hydraulic fluids. It has a low vapor pressure, and significant air concentrations are not achieved unless the compound is heated or sprayed as a mist. Respiratory exposures or topical application to the skin are not considered to be toxic, although Troisi (1950) reported nystagmus and attacks of loss of consciousness among women working in an electrolytic condenser factory that utilized ethylene glycol mixtures at 105°C. Intoxication does occur when ethylene glycol is taken by mouth, and an estimated 50 fatalities annually in the United States result from the ingestion of this compound by mistake or as a substitute for beverage ethanol. Recent case reports of such instances have been provided by Moriarty and McDonald (1974), Parry and Wallach (1974), Lavelle (1977), and Peterson et al. (1981).

In most cases the initial symptoms are similar to those of ethanol intoxication, but there may be significant nausea and vomiting, and abdominal pain. Severe intoxication progresses to include ataxia, prostration, cyanosis, stupor, convulsions, and coma, frequently ending in death (Winek et al., 1978). The mean lethal dose for an adult has been estimated to be about 100 ml (Milles, 1946). The cause of death in these cases is either central nervous system depression or renal failure related to the formation of glycollic and oxalic acids, the normal metabolites of the glycol. Renal disease is marked by albuminuria and oliguria, and by calcium oxalate crystals in the urinary sediment that may take many forms (Godolphin et al., 1980). Clinical experience suggests that large doses of ethylene glycol lead to death from relatively prompt central nervous system depression, while somewhat smaller and repeated doses, insufficient to cause this depression, result in renal insufficiency.

The metabolic basis of ethylene poisoning is related to the oxidation of this compound to oxalic acid by alcohol dehydrogenase. Since impairment of this metabolic pathway has therapeutic value, administration of ethanol has been used to compete with glycol for active enzyme sites (Li and Vallee, 1969). Human alcohol dehydrogenase has an affinity for ethanol that is 30 to 40 times that for ethylene glycol. That ethanol administration leads to increased urinary excretion of unchanged glycol and reduction in oxalate production has been shown in monkeys and in a number of human patients. Dialysis is also of value for the removal of ethylene glycol. Supportive measures often require vigorous treatment with sodium bicarbonate or sodium lactate to control severe and persistent acidosis as well as gastric lavage with potassium permanganate (1:5000), and early diuretic therapy.

Diethylene glycol Diethylene glycol (2,2'-oxydiethanol; polyglycol) is a similar compound but with little industrial hazard. From the toxicological point of view it is significant mainly in that over 100 deaths occurred in the United States in the late 1930s as a result of the ingestion of an elixir of sulfanilamide in a 72% diethylene glycol vehicle (Geiling and Cannon, 1938). Fatal cases showed progressive renal failure with death in less than eight days after onset of anuria.

Other glycols Other glycols, such as propylene glycol (1,2-propanediol) and the polyethylene glycols, have not been found to be of toxicological importance in industry (AIHA, 1980). Their low vapor pressure makes inhalation unlikely and skin irritation is minimal although some workers have experienced mild eye irritation. Occasional allergic contact reactions to polyethylene glycol have been reported (Fisher, 1978). Metabolites do not include oxalates, formic acid, or formaldehyde, but ingestion of propylene glycol in sufficient amounts may lead to lactic acidosis (Cate and Hedrick, 1980).

Alkyl derivatives of ethylene and diethylene glycols The principal alkyl derivatives of ethylene glycol are the monoethyl ether (Cellosolve), the monomethyl ether (methyl Cellosolve), and the butyl ether (butyl Cellosolve). They are important solvents for industrial coatings, cellulose, and inks. The three compounds are considered to have similar harmful properties with toxicity increasing in this order (Browning, 1965). All can be absorbed through the skin, lungs, or gastrointestinal tract. The monomethyl compound is converted in the body to methanol and ethylene glycol, which in turn are metabolized to formic and oxalic acids, respectively. Acute poisoning usually affects the central nervous system and the kidneys. With less intense and more prolonged exposure, involvement of the hematopoietic system is also seen. Macrocytic anemia with a predominance of immature leukocytes, and which resolves on cessation of exposure, has been reported especially after exposure to methyl Cellosolve. The hemolytic anemia that occurs in experimental animals exposed to butyl Cellosolve (Carpenter et al., 1956) has not been reported in man. While the Cellosolves are all irritating to the skin and mucous membranes, the central nervous system may be the important target since methyl Cellosolve produces hind-limb paresis, glial cell damage, and demyelination in rats (Savolainen, 1980). In humans, the effects of these glycol derivatives upon the central nervous system include headache, drowsiness, weakness, slurred speech, recrudescent stuttering, staggering gait, tremor, and blurred vision (Zavon, 1963). Changes in personality are often noted first by the family of the affected individual. These changes are such that the patient, in the absence of an accurate occupational exposure history, may be treated for schizophrenia or narcolepsy.

In acute poisoning with the ethylene glycol monoalkyl ethers, there is frequently evidence of renal injury: albuminuria and hematuria. The clinical nature of this renal disorder is not well established but it is not related to oxalates.

A similar series of monoalkyl ethers of diethylene glycol form the series of solvents known in industry as Carbitols. Diethylene glycol monoethyl ether (Carbitol), diethylene glycol monomethyl ether (methyl Carbitol), and diethylene glycol monobutyl ether (butyl Carbitol) have not been associated with industrial intoxication (Browning, 1965).

References

AIHA: Workplace environmental exposure level guide: Polyethylene glycols. *Am Ind Hyg Assoc J* 1980;41:A55–A57.

Browning E: *Toxicity and Metabolism of Industrial Solvents*. New York, Elsevier, 1965, pp 594–690.

Carpenter CP, Pozzani UC, Weil CS, et al: The toxicity of butyl cellosolve solvent. *Arch Ind Health* 1956;14:114–131.

Cate JC IV, Hedrick R: Propylene glycol intoxication and lactic acidosis. *N Engl J Med* 1980; 303:1237.

Fisher AA: Immediate and delayed allergic contact reactions to polyethylene glycol. *Contact Derm* 1978;4:135–138.

Geiling EHK, Cannon PR: Pathological effects of elixir of sulfanilamide (diethylene glycol) poisoning, clinical and experimental correlation: Final report. *J Am Med Assoc* 1938;111:919–926.

Godolphin W, Meagher EP, Frohlich J, et al: Case 38-1979: Ethylene glycol poisoning. *N Engl J Med* 1980;302:465–466.

Lavelle KJ: Ethylene glycol poisoning. *J Ind State Med Assoc* 1977;70:249–252.

Li T-K, Vallee BL: Alcohol dehydrogenase and ethanol metabolism. *Surg Clin North Am* 1969; 49:577–582.

Milles G: Ethylene glycol poisoning with suggestions for its treatment as oxalate poisoning. *Arch Pathol* 1946;41:631–638.

Moriarty RW, McDonald RH Jr: The spectrum of ethylene glycol poisoning. *Clin Toxicol* 1974;7: 583–596.

Parry MF, Wallach R: Ethylene glycol poisoning. *Am J Med* 1974;57:143–150.

Peterson CD, Collins AJ, Himes JM, et al: Ethylene glycol poisoning. Pharmacokinetics during therapy with ethanol and hemodialysis. *N Engl J Med* 1981;304:21–23.

Savolainen H: Glial cell toxicity of ethyleneglycol monomethylether vapor. *Environ Res* 1980;22:423–430.

Troisi FM: Chronic intoxication by ethylene glycol vapour. *Br J Ind Med* 1950;7:65–69.

Winek CL, Shingleton DP, Shanor SP: Ethylene and diethylene toxicity. *Clin Toxicol* 1978;13:297–324.

Zavon MR: Methyl cellosolve intoxication. *Am Ind Hyg Assoc J* 1963;24:36–41.

3 • *Aldehydes and Ketones*

Of the aldehydes and ketones, which together comprise the group known as carbonyl compounds, only a few are of significance in occupational toxicology. Some are important as industrial solvents and others as intermediates in chemical processes and in the manufacture of plastics. Some are irritants of the eyes, skin, and mucous membranes but reports of other occupational injury are rare, perhaps because, as Browning (1965) suggests, their metabolism is too rapid to produce the cumulative effects needed for systemic toxicity. Industrial limits of exposure are based primarily on air levels that do not produce irritation or an unpleasant sensory response.

Aldehydes

Formaldehyde Formaldehyde ($H_2C = O$; methanal) is a component of urea-formaldehyde and melamine-formaldehyde based amino resins that are typically used for electrical switch housings, knobs, molded dinnerware, adhesives, plywood glues, coatings, and industrial laminates. Formaldehyde is used as a disinfectant and fumigant, as a wood preservative, in the production of rosaniline and indigo dyes, in the manufacture of paper and rubber, in the modification of natural and synthetic textile fibers, and in cosmetics and deodorants. It is a gas that boils at $-21°C$; formalin is an aqueous solution that contains 40% formaldehyde by volume. The threshold for recognition of formaldehyde odor varies between 0.1 and 1.0 ppm, which is close to the limit that produces minimal irritant effects on the eyes and airway (Loomis, 1979). Such symptoms have been seen among embalming room employees in funeral homes (Kerfoot and Mooney, 1975). Higher air levels cause severe burning sensations, coughing, conjunctivitis, and lacrimation. Deep lung irritation in man has not been observed, but long-term exposure to phenol-formaldehyde resin vapors may result in chronic airway obstruction (Schoenberg and Mitchell, 1975; Gamble et al., 1976). Pulmonary hypersensitivity in the form of asthmatic bronchitis occasionally develops in exposed workers (Hendrick and Lane, 1977; NIOSH, 1976).

Formaldehyde is a potent skin irritant and sensitizer. Eczematous reactions have been observed in textile and leather workers (Schorr et al., 1974, Foussereau et al., 1976; Helander, 1977), in handlers of formaldehyde resins (Markusen et al., 1943; Glass, 1961), and even in a shampoo packer (Ancona-Alayon et al., 1976). Other instances have been collected by Browning (1965) and Fisher (1976). Hexamethylenetetramine, called "hexa," used as a stabilizer in amino resin systems to prevent premature hardening, decomposes to formaldehyde and is a possible source of irritating and sensitizing cutaneous reactions.

Squamous cell carcinomas of the rat nasal cavity have been produced by inhalation exposure to 15 ppm formaldehyde vapor, although lower levels of exposure did not lead to similar results (Swenberg et al., 1980). In this connection, a preliminary survey of physician deaths in Denmark for the period 1943 to 1976 failed to reveal any nasal cavity malignancies among pathologists or anatomists (Jensen, 1980).

The permissible exposure limit for formaldehyde is 3 ppm, although NIOSH (1976) has recommended a more stringent limit of 1 ppm (1.2 mg/m³).

Other aldehydes Acetaldehyde (CH_3CHO; ethanal) has industrial uses as a solvent and as an intermediate in chemical manufacture. While it is a narcotic and an irritant, especially at air levels above the permissible exposure limit of 200 ppm, it is usually handled in closed systems because of its explosive properties. No occupational injury has been reported (Browning, 1965).

210

The higher aliphatic aldehydes, propion alde-hyde, butyraldehyde, and methylal, have no in-dustrial toxicological importance nor have paraldehyde or furfural.

References

Ancona-Alayon A, Jiminez-Castilla JL, Gomez-Alvarez EM: Dermatitis from epoxy resin and formaldehyde in shampoo packers. *Contact Derm* 1976;2:356.

Browning E: *Toxicity and Metabolism of Industrial Solvents.* New York, Elsevier, 1965, pp. 463–492.

Fisher AA: Formaldehyde: Some recent experiences. *Cutis* 1976;17:665–686.

Foussereau J, Cavelier C, Selig D: Occupational eczema from para-tertiary-butylphenol formaldehyde resins: A review of the sensitizing resins. *Contact Derm* 1976;2:254–258.

Gamble JF, McMichael AJ, Williams T, et al: Respiratory function and symptoms: An environmental-epidemiological study of rubber workers exposed to a phenol-formaldehyde-type resin. *Am Ind Hyg Assoc J* 1976;37:499–513.

Glass WI: Outbreak of formaldehyde dermatitis. *N Z Med J* 1961;60:423–427.

Hendrick DJ, Lane DJ: Occupational formalin asthma. *Br J Ind Med* 1977;34:11–18.

Helander I: Contact urticaria from leather containing formaldehyde. *Arch Dermatol* 1977;113:1443.

Jensen OM: Cancer risk from formaldehyde. *Lancet* 1980;2:480–481.

Kerfoot EJ, Mooney TF Jr: Formaldehyde and paraformaldehyde study in funeral homes. *Am Ind Hyg Assoc J* 1975;36:533–537.

Loomis TA: Formaldehyde toxicity. *Arch Pathol Lab Med* 1979;103:321–324.

Markusen KE, Mancuso TF, Soet JS: Dermatitis due to the formaldehyde resins. *Ind Med Surg* 1943;12:383–386.

NIOSH: *Criteria for a Recommended Standard . . . . Occupational Exposure to Formaldehyde.* Washington, DC, National Institute for Occupational Safety and Health (NIOSH 77-126), 1976.

NIOSH: Health Hazard Evaluation Report #70-146-670, 1980. Also in *Morb Mort Weekly Rep* 1980; 29:395–401.

Schoenberg JB, Mitchell CA: Airway disease caused by phenolic (phenol-formaldehyde) resin exposure. *Arch Environ Health* 1975;30:574–577.

Schorr WF, Keran E, Plotka E: Formaldehyde allergy. The quantitative analysis of American clothing for free formaldehyde and its relevance in clinical practice. *Arch Dermatol* 1974;110:73–76.

Swenberg JA, Kerns WD, Mitchell RI, et al: Induction of squamous cell carcinomas of the rat nasal cavity by inhalation exposure to formaldehyde vapor. *Cancer Res* 1980;40:3398–3402.

Ketones

Ketones are widely used as solvents, as raw materials in chemical manufacture, and as components of coatings and adhesives. They are not highly toxic except for certain halogenated or unsaturated compounds. The ketones can be irritating to the eyes and mucous membranes, and at high concentrations they may be narcotic. They are not readily metabolized and some may, to a large extent, be eliminated unchanged in expired air (Browning, 1965).

Acetone Acetone $((CH_3)_2C = 0$; dimethyl ketone; propanone) is the simplest of the aliphatic ketones. It is used as a solvent for fats, oils, lacquers, varnishes, resins, acetylene, and cellulose derivatives. Inhaled acetone is readily absorbed from the lungs but it is largely excreted unchanged. Small amounts are slowly oxidized to carbon dioxide (Price and Rittenberg, 1950), perhaps by way of conversion to pyruvate in the liver (Sakami and Lafaye, 1951).

Extensive industrial experience with acetone along with careful industrial hygiene and occupational medical studies on hundreds of workers exposed to air levels of 1000 to 2000 ppm for many years have confirmed the relative safety of this compound (Haggard et al., 1944; Raleigh and McGee, 1972). Cases of acute inhalation intoxication, collected by Browning (1965), developed gastric distress and vomiting, fainting and collapse, and loss of consciousness, but no fatality occurred. Reports of symptoms from chronic occupational exposure are rare but, when they occur, they include headache, vertigo, sensation of heat, throat irritation, and cough. Eye, nose, and throat irritation has occurred in a majority of subjects studied at 500 ppm, while the highest satisfactory concentration for an eight-hour exposure was judged to be 200 ppm (Nelson et al., 1943).

Nonoccupational acetone intoxication has occurred from the application of plaster casts that used acetone as a setting agent. Inhalation of vapor as well as penetration through the skin may have been involved in these cases (Chatterton and Elliott, 1946; Harris and Jackson, 1952; Renshaw and Mitchell, 1956).

The permissible exposure limit for acetone has been 1000 ppm (2400 mg/m³), a level deemed to be safe by Raleigh and McGee (1972), but NIOSH (1978) has recommended lowering this level to 250 ppm (590 mg/m³). A similar reduction had been recommended by Vigliani and Zurlo (1955), who suggested 500 ppm (1186 mg/m³).

Methyl ethyl ketone Methyl ethyl ketone (CH₃COCH₂CH₃; butanone; MEK) resembles acetone in odor and physical properties but it is much more irritating to the eyes and upper airway. It is used as a solvent for gums, resins, and nitrocellulose, frequently in mixtures with alcohol, acetone, and other ketones. It is also used in artificial leather and synthetic rubber manufacture, in lacquers and varnishes, in lubricating oils, and in synthetic surface coatings (Browning, 1965; NIOSH, 1978).

Reports of injury from occupational exposure have been rare except for dermatoses. Toxic effects on the eye have been noted twice (Smyth, 1956; Berg, 1971), the optic nerve injury perhaps having resulted from methanol as a metabolite. While MEK is known to enhance the toxicity of methyl n-butyl ketone, it has also been incriminated as the cause of polyneuropathy in shoe factory workers (Dyro, 1978).

The recommended permissible exposure limit for methyl ethyl ketone is 200 ppm (590 mg/m³) (NIOSH, 1978).

Methyl n-butyl ketone Methyl n-butyl ketone (CH₃CO(CH₂)₃CH₃; 2-hexanone; MBK) also resembles acetone but has an odor somewhat more pungent than MEK. It is a solvent for lacquers, nitrocellulose, resins, fats, and waxes. It is readily absorbed from lungs, gastrointestinal tract, and skin in man and dogs, and it is not eliminated unchanged in breath or urine but is broken down to CO₂, 2,5-hexanedione, and other metabolites (DiVincenzo et al., 1978).

In 1974 methyl n-butyl ketone was found to be responsible for an outbreak of polyneuropathy in a plant that produced plastic-coated and color-printed fabrics (Mendell et al., 1974; Billmaier et al., 1974). Distal muscle weakness and sensory deficits were noted along with electromyographic

abnormalities, but most of these improved after the use of MBK was eliminated (Allen et al., 1975). Exposure of rats to 2,5-hexanedione, the principal metabolite of MBK, produced a clinical peripheral neuropathy in these animals that was characterized by both peripheral and central nervous system "dying-back" degeneration with giant axonal swellings filled with neurofilaments (Spencer and Schaumburg, 1975). These pathological changes have also been seen in workers exposed to acrylamide (Davenport et al., 1976) and in persons sniffing glue containing n-hexane (Korobkin et al., 1975). Both MBK and n-hexane are converted in the body to similar metabolites, 2,5-hexanediol and 2,5-hexanedione, both of which are neurotoxic (Krasavage et al., 1980). These investigators also found that these metabolites produced atrophy of the rat testicular germinal epithelium, a property shared with other neurotoxins.

Peripheral neuropathy attributable to MBK has also been reported among spray painters working on the gates of two Ohio River dams (Mallov, 1976). Potentiation of MBK peripheral neurotoxicity by methyl ethyl ketone (MEK) has been shown in experimental animals (Saida et al., 1976; Abdel-Rahman et al., 1976).

Although the current exposure limit for MBK is 100 ppm (410 mg/m³), NIOSH (1978) has recommended a much more stringent value of 1 ppm (4 mg/m³).

Methyl n-amyl ketone Methyl n-amyl ketone (CH₃CO(CH₂)₄CH₃; 2-heptanone; MAK) is used as a solvent for synthetic resin finishes and lacquer thinners. It has a fruity odor and occurs naturally in oil of cloves and Ceylon cinnamon oil. Many fewer workers are exposed to it than to the other common ketone solvents. It is irritating to the mucous membranes of experimental animals and is strongly narcotic at high concentrations, but no reports of adverse occupational effects have emerged. Recent studies with rats and monkeys have shown that MAK does not possess the neurotoxic properties of MBK (Johnson et al., 1978).

Other ketones Methyl propyl ketone (ethyl acetone; 2-pentanone) is used as a solvent, but very few workers are exposed to this compound. It is sufficiently irritating to the eyes and nose that its odor serves as a warning and reduces the toxic hazard. No injuries from industrial exposure have been reported.

Methyl isobutyl ketone ($CH_3COCH_2CH(CH_3)_2$; 4-methyl-2-pentanone; hexone; MiBK) is also used as a solvent for lacquers, but it has a strong odor that limits its use. It shares the irritant and narcotic properties of the other ketones. Adverse effects of exposure to this compound have rarely been reported, but AuBuchon et al. (1979) described a sensorimotor polyneuropathy in a spray painter that differed from that induced by exposure to MBK. The young man had burning paresthesias and decreased muscle strength of the hands and feet that gradually resolved. Electromyography suggested a demyelinating bilateral distal polyneuropathy that was confirmed by sural nerve biopsy. The permissible exposure limit for MiBK is 100 ppm (410 mg/m^3); NIOSH (1978) has recommended lowering this to half of the current value.

Cyclohexanone, mesityl oxide, and isophorone have irritant and narcotic effects but are not of industrial toxicological importance. Ethyl n-butyl ketone (EBK) has been found to lack neurotoxicity for rats, apparently because its metabolite, 2,5-heptanedione, which is neurotoxic, is present in low serum concentrations after EBK exposure (Katz et al., 1980).

References

Abel-Rahman MS, Hetland LB, Couri D: Toxicity and metabolism of methyl n-butyl ketone. Am Ind Hyg Assoc J 1976; 37:95–102.

Allen N, Mendell JR, Billmaier DJ, et al: Toxic polyneuropathy due to methyl n-butyl ketone. Arch Neurol 1975;32:209–218.

AuBuchon J, Robins HI, Viseskul C: Peripheral neuropathy after exposure to methylisobutyl ketone in paint spray. Lancet 1979;2:363–364.

Berg EF: Retrobulbar neuritis. A case report of presumed solvent toxicity. Ann Ophthalmol 1971; 3:1351–1353.

Billmaier D, Yee HT, Allen N: Peripheral neuropathy in a coated fabrics plant. J Occup Med 1974;16:665–671.

Browning E: Toxicity and Metabolism of Industrial Solvents. New York, Elsevier, 1965, pp 412–462.

Chatterton CC, Elliott RB: Acute acetone poisoning from leg casts of a synthetic plaster substitute. J Am Med Assoc 1946;130:1222–1223.

Davenport JG, Farrell DF, Sumi SM: 'Giant axonal neuropathy' caused by industrial chemicals:

Neurofilamentous axonal masses in man. Neurology 1976;26:919–923.

DiVincenzo GD, Hamilton ML, Kaplan CJ, et al: Studies on the respiratory uptake and excretion and the skin absorption of methyl n-butyl ketone in humans and dogs. Toxicol Appl Pharmacol 1978;44:593–604.

Dyro FM: Methyl ethyl ketone polyneuropathy in shoe factory workers. Clin Toxicol 1978;13:371–376.

Haggard HW, Greenberg LA, Turner JM: The physiological principles governing the action of acetone together with determination of toxicity. J Ind Hyg Toxicol 1944;26:133–151.

Harris LC, Jackson RH: Acute acetone poisoning caused by setting fluid for immobilizing casts. Br Med J 1952;2:1024–1026.

Johnson BL, Setzer JV, Lewis TR, et al: An electrodiagnostic study of the neurotoxicity of methyl n-amyl ketone. Am Ind Hyg Assoc J 1978;39:866–872.

Katz GV, O'Donoghue JL, DiVincenzo GD, et al: Comparative neurotoxicity and metabolism of ethyl n-butyl ketone and methyl n-butyl ketone in rats. Toxicol Appl Pharmacol 1980;52:153–158.

Korobkin R, Asbury AK, Summer AJ, et al: Glue-sniffing neuropathy. Arch Neurol 1975;32:158–162.

Krasavage WJ, O'Donoghue JL, DiVincenzo GD, et al: The relative neurotoxicity of methyl n-butyl ketone, n-hexane and their metabolites. Toxicol Appl Pharmacol 1980; 52:433–441.

Mallov JS: MBK neuropathy among spray painters. J Am Med Assoc 1976; 235:1455–1457.

Mendell JR, Saida K, Ganansia MF, et al: Toxic polyneuropathy produced by methyl n-butyl ketone. Science 1974; 185:787–789.

Nelson KW, Ege JF Jr, Ross M, et al: Sensory response to certain industrial solvent vapors. J Ind Hyg Toxicol 1943;25:282–285.

NIOSH: Criteria for a Recommended Standard . . . . Occupational Exposure to Ketones. Washington, DC, National Institute for Occupational Safety and Health (NIOSH 78-173), 1978.

Price TD, Rittenberg D: The metabolism of acetone: Gross aspects of catabolism and excretion. J Biol Chem 1950;185:449–459.

Raleigh RL, McGee WA: Effects of short, high-concentration exposures to acetone as determined by observation in the work area. J Occup Med 1972;14:607–610.

Renshaw PK, Mitchell RM: Acetone poisoning following the application of a lightweight cast. Br Med J 1956;1:615.

Saida K, Mendell JR, Weiss HS: Peripheral nerve changes induced by methyl n-butyl ketone and potentiation by methyl ethyl ketone. *J Neuropathol Exp Neurol* 1976;35:207–225.

Sakami W, Lafaye JM: The metabolism of acetone in the intact rat. *J. Biol Chem* 1951;193: 199–203.

Smyth HF Jr: Improved communication — Hygienic standards for daily inhalation. *Am Ind Hyg Assoc Q* 1956;17:129–185.

Spencer PS, Schaumburg HH: Experimental neuropathy produced by 2,5-hexanedione — a major metabolite of the neurotoxic industrial solvent methyl n-butyl ketone. *J Neurol Neurosurg Psychiatry* 1975;38:771–775.

Vigliani EC, Zurlo N: Erfahrungen der Clinica del Lavoro mit einigen maximalen Arbeitsplatzkonzentrationen (MAK) von Industriegiften. *Arch Gewerbepathol Gewerbehyg* 1955;13: 528–534.

4 • *Ethers and Epoxides*

Several classes of ethers have occupational toxicological importance. Many have narcotic and solvent properties or are used as chemical intermediates in organic syntheses. Epoxides are ethers that contain the three-membered oxirane ring, and are found in insecticides, plasticizers, resins, rubber and paint stabilizers, lubricants, detergents, emulsifiers, and waxes.

Diethyl Ether

Diethyl ether (C_2H_5-O-C_2H_5; ethyl ether; sulfuric ether) is the well-known anesthetic that may be dangerous in laboratory and industrial work because it forms explosive peroxides on standing in air. In addition to its use in surgery, it is employed as a solvent for fats, oils, waxes, gums, resins, alkaloids, and in the manufacture of cellulose acetate rayon and dyes (Browning, 1965). It is rapidly absorbed when inhaled and is quickly transferred by the blood to the central nervous system and other fatty tissues. Haggard (1924) showed that about 87% is expired unchanged while only 1% to 2% is excreted in the urine.

During the First World War diethyl ether was used extensively in the production of gun cotton and smokeless powder in mixtures with ethyl alcohol. Hamilton and Minot (1920) studied persons engaged in this work and found high job turnover among the men, who had complaints of apathy, drowsiness, depression, anorexia, constipation, and loss of weight. Many of the young women, who replaced most of the men during 1917 to 1918, had "ether jags" with excitement, singing, weeping, nausea, constipation, loss of weight, dizziness, confusion, drowsiness, and loss of consciousness. Some also developed an itching eruption on the face. An interesting feature of this study was the finding of marked polycythemia among the young women but not among the men.

Apart from this industrial experience, which was paralleled in Britain, reports of occupational toxicity have been rare. Browning (1965) cited a case of acute mania and uremic convulsions in a man working in perfume manufacture where ether was used as an extracting agent. Addiction to ether sniffing has also been described (Bartholomew, 1962).

The permissible exposure limit for diethyl ether has been set at 400 ppm (1200 mg/m^3).

References

Bartholomew AA: Two cases of ether addiction/habituation. *Med J Aust* 1962;49:550–553.

Browning E: *Toxicity and Metabolism of Industrial Solvents.* New York, Elsevier, 1965, pp 493–521.

Haggard HW: The absorption, distribution and elimination of ethyl ether. *J Biol Chem* 1924;59:737–802.

Hamilton A, Minot GR: Ether poisoning in the manufacture of smokeless powder. *J Ind Hyg* 1920;2:41–49.

Halo Ethers

Two chloromethyl ethers are of toxicologic importance: chloromethyl methyl ether (CMME) and bis-chloromethyl ether (BCME), the latter contaminating commercial grades of the former to the extent of 1% to 8%. CMME has been used for over 30 years as a cross-linking agent in the manufacture of ion-exchange resins. Both CMME and BCME are biologically active alkylating agents that are carcinogenic for mucosa, skin, and respiratory tract. Laskin et al. (1971) found rather high incidence levels of bronchogenic carcinomas and neuroepitheliomas in rats exposed to as little as 0.1 ppm of BCME. Epidemiological studies in industry, both retrospective and prospective, have correlated exposure to CMME/BCME with induction of small-cell ("oat cell") carcinomas of the lung (Thiess et al., 1973; Figueroa et al., 1973; Weiss and Figueroa, 1976; DeFonso and Kelton, 1976; Pasternack et al., 1977). The evidence from industry of the potent carcinogenicity of BCME and the fact that airborne levels of this compound are detectable when formaldehyde and hydrochloric acid react would suggest that histology technicians who carry out procedures in which this reaction may occur should be protected by suitable ventilation.

References

DeFonso LR, Kelton SC Jr: Lung cancer following exposure to chloromethyl methyl ether. An epidemiological study. *Arch Environ Health* 1976;31:125–130.

Figueroa WG, Raszkowski R, Weiss W: Lung cancer in chloromethyl methyl ether workers. *N Engl J Med* 1973;288:1096–1097.

Laskin S, Kuschner M, Drew RT, et al: Tumors of the respiratory tract induced by inhalation of bis (chloromethyl) ether. *Arch Environ Health* 1971;23:135–136.

Pasternack BS, Shore RE, Albert RE: Occupational exposure to chloromethyl ethers. A retrospective cohort mortality study (1948–1972). *J Occup Med* 1977;19:741–746.

Thiess AM, Hey W, Zeller H: Zur Toxicologie von Dichlordimethyläther-Verdacht auf kanzeroge Wirkung auch beim Menschen. *Zbl Arbeitsmed* 1973;23:97–102.

Weiss W, Figueroa WG: The characteristics of lung cancer due to chloromethyl ethers. *J Occup Med* 1976;18:623–627.

Ethylene Oxide

Ethylene oxide (CH_2CH_2O; dimethyl oxide; oxirane; EtO) is the simplest of the epoxides and is an effective and widely used sterilant for drugs and medical supplies. It is also an intermediate in the production of ethylene glycol, surface active agents, and other bulk chemical compounds. Significant ethylene oxide residues have been found after its use in sterilizing foods, cosmetics, and medical devices (Charlesworth, 1976). Concern over its safety has stemmed from numerous demonstrations of its mutagenicity in a variety of plant and invertebrate systems (Wolman, 1979), but its mutagenic potential for mammals has now been established in male rat germinal cells (Embree et al., 1977).

Ethylene oxide toxicity reported for man has largely been matters of irritation of skin, mucous membranes, and conjunctivae (Sexton and Henson, 1949; Hanifin, 1971; Bird et al., 1974; Taylor, 1977). Gross et al. (1979) have collected a number of earlier reports detailing acute neurological symptoms that included nausea and vomiting, headache, disorientation, and decreased levels of consciousness. Their own study was of four workers exposed to leaks from a large ethylene oxide sterilizer. Acute encephalopathy occurred in one man and peripheral neuropathy was noted in the other three. Nerve conduction velocities were abnormal and were consistent with an axonal degenerative neuropathy. Conduction abnormalities improved in the patient who was removed from exposure, but they persisted in two of the men who continued to work at a lower level of exposure.

Concern over ethylene oxide carcinogenicity has been intensified since the reports of Hogstedt and his colleagues (1979), who noted three cases of leukemia, where only 0.2 cases would have been expected, in a relatively small group of Swedish factory workers exposed to ethylene oxide and methyl formate in equal proportions for sterilizing hospital equipment. The time-weighted average ethylene oxide exposure concentration was 20 ± 10 ppm. Hogstedt et al. (1979) also conducted a cohort study of mortality and cancer incidence in ethylene oxide production workers for the period from 1961 through 1977. Here they found a significant excess of mortality and cancer incidence that included leukemia, and gastrointestinal and urogenital tract malignancies, as well as an increase in diseases of the circulatory system.

The United States permissible exposure limit of 50 ppm (90 mg/m^3) exceeds that in Sweden where the threshold limit value was lowered to 10 ppm as an eight-hour time-weighted average concentration, partly as a result of the reports of Hogstedt and his group. NIOSH has recommended a re-examination of the 50 ppm limit because of a recently concluded two-year inhalation study with male rats that resulted in peritoneal mesotheliomas arising from testis mesothelium after exposures to 33 and 100 ppm (NIOSH, 1981).

References

Bird L, Fisher AA, Price E: Ethylene oxide burns. *Arch Dermatol* 1974;110:924–925.

Charlesworth FA: Ethylene oxide residues in sterilized medical devices. *Food Cosmetic Toxicol* 1976;14:61.

Embree JW, Lyon JP, Hine CH: The mutagenic potential of ethylene oxide using the dominant-lethal assay in rats. *Toxicol Appl Pharmacol* 1977;40:261–267.

Gross JA, Haas ML, Swift TR: Ethylene oxide neurotoxicity: Report of four cases and review of the literature. *Neurology* 1979;29:978–983.

Hanifin JM: Ethylene oxide dermatitis. *J Am Med Assoc* 1971;217:213.

Hogstedt C, Malmqvist N, Wadman B: Leukemia in workers exposed to ethylene oxide. *J Am Med Assoc* 1979;241:1132–1133.

Hogstedt C, Rohlen O, Berndtsson BS, et al: A cohort study of mortality and cancer incidence in ethylene oxide production workers. *Br J Ind Med* 1979;36:276–280.

NIOSH: Ethylene oxide (EtO): Evidence of carcinogenicity. *NIOSH Current Intelligence Bulletin 35,* Washington, DC, National Institute for Occupational Safety and Health (NIOSH 81-103), May 22, 1981.

Sexton RJ, Henson EV: Dermatological injuries by ethylene oxide. *J Ind Hyg Toxicol* 1949;31:297–300.

Taylor JS: Dermatologic hazards from ethylene oxide. *Cutis* 1977;19:189–192.

Wolman SR: Mutational consequences of exposure to ethylene oxide. *J Environ Pathol Toxicol* 1979;2:1289–1303.

Dioxane

Dioxane (diethylene dioxide; diethylene ether; $C_4H_8O_2$), a valuable solvent for industrial coatings and a dehydrating agent in the preparation of histological slides, can be inhaled in amounts sufficient to cause systemic intoxication. Although irritation of the eyes, nose, and throat are noted at dioxane concentrations above 200 ppm, its warning properties are poor (Browning, 1965). Consequently, injury may be delayed hours after termination of an exposure that had erroneously been considered to be negligible. Dioxane can also be absorbed through the skin (Fairley et al., 1934). Acute exposures, such as of technicians in a histology laboratory, may lead to headache, nausea, vomiting, and irritation of the eyes. Five fatalities were reported as a result of acute exposure in a cellulose acetate "silk" manufacturing plant (Barber, 1934). While the quantitative aspects of the exposure were unclear, postmortem studies in these cases demonstrated prominent renal and hepatic injury, and the cause of death was considered to be hemorrhagic nephritis.

Exposure of workers to dioxane at low concentrations (1 to 2 ppm) results in its rapid metabolism to β-hydroxyethoxyacetic acid (HEAA), which is excreted in the urine (Young et al., 1976). When volunteers were exposed to 50 ppm dioxane vapor for six hours, the rapid conversion to HEAA prevented accumulation of dioxane within the body (Young et al., 1977). Animal experiments have confirmed the nephrotoxicity and hepatotoxicity of dioxane, and there is some evidence for hepatocarcinogenicity of dioxane administered to rats and mice (summarized in NIOSH, 1977).

Because dioxane penetrates skin rapidly and because there is some suggestion of carcinogenicity, NIOSH has recommended that occupational exposure not exceed airborne concentrations greater than 1 ppm (3.6 mg/m^3) based on a 30-minute sampling period although the current OSHA upper limit is 100 ppm and the ACGIH adopted value (1979) was 50 ppm.

References

Barber H: Haemorrhagic nephritis and necrosis of the liver from dioxan poisoning. *Guys Hosp Rep* 1934;84:267–280.

Browning E: *Toxicity and Metabolism of Industrial Solvents,* New York, Elsevier, 1965, pp 722–727.

Fairley A, Linton EC, Ford-Moore AH: The toxicity to animals of 1:4 dioxan. *J Hyg* 1934;34:486–501.

NIOSH: *Criteria for a Recommended Standard . . . . Occupational Exposure to Dioxane.* Washington, DC, National Institute of Occupational Safety and Health (NIOSH 77-226), 1977.

Young JD, Braun WH, Gehring PJ, et al: 1,4-dioxane and β-hydroxyethoxyacetic acid excretion in urine of humans exposed to dioxane vapors. *Toxicol Appl Pharmacol* 1976;38:643–646.

Young JD, Braun WH, Rampy LW: Pharmacokinetics of 1,4-dioxane in humans. *J Toxicol Environ Health* 1977;3:507–520.

Glycidyl Ethers

These compounds are characterized by having a 2,3-epoxypropyl group and an ether linkage to another organic group. While a large number of mono- and di-glycidyl ethers are theoretically possible, only a few are in use in industry. The ones that are currently utilized include allyl glycidyl ether (AGE), *n*-butyl glycidyl ether (BGE), *o*-cresyl glycidyl ether (CGE), diglycidyl ether (DGE), isopropyl glycidyl ether (IGE), phenyl glycidyl ether (PGE), resorcinol diglycidyl ether, 1,4-butanediol diglycidyl ether, and certain other alkyl or aliphatic glycidyl ethers (NIOSH, 1978).

The principal use of the glycidyl ethers is as reactive diluents in epoxy resin systems in which the epoxide groups form cross-linkages. Workers handling uncured resins in processes such as tooling and molding, manufacture of adhesives, and application of protective coatings may be exposed to vapors and mists that contain glycidyl ethers.

Dermatitis has been reported from exposure to AGE and PGE with the latter causing more severe manifestations, such as blister formation and second-degree burns, that were more persistent and less responsive to treatment (Hine et al., 1956). The sensitizing properties of BGE have been investigated by Lea et al. (1958) and Kligman (1966). Both studies showed that the sensitizing capacities as well as the irritative effects of BGE are dose dependent. Moreover, Fregert and Rorsman (1964) found that cross-sensitization may occur among AGE, BGE, and PGE. Inhalation exposure of rats to heated PGE has resulted in alopecia with a perifollicular inflammation and atrophy of the hair follicles (Lee et al., 1977), a finding that has not yet been reported for man.

Systemic effects from occupational exposure to glycidyl ethers have not been reported except for an accident described by Wallace (1979) in which two men were exposed to a BGE spill, the vapors of which they inhaled. On admission to the hospital both men complained of cough, vomiting, ataxia, and headache; ten days later they still had gastrointestinal irritation manifested by anorexia, nausea and vomiting, and hematemesis that persisted for several weeks along with severe headaches. Irritation of the respiratory track was mild and brief by comparison.

References

Fregert S, Rorsman H: Allergens in epoxy resins. *Acta Allergol* 1964;19:296–299.

Hine CH, Kodama JK, Wellington JS, et al: The toxicology of glycidol and some glycidyl ethers. *Arch Ind Health* 1956;14:250–264.

Kligman AM: The identification of contact allergens by human assay. III. The maximization test – A procedure for screening and rating contact sensitizers. *J Invest Dermatol* 1966;47: 393–409.

Lea VA Jr, Block WB, Cornish HH: The irritating and sensitizing capacity of epoxy resins. *Arch Dermatol* 1958;78:304–308.

Lee KP, Terill JB, Henry NW III: Alopecia induced by inhalation exposure to phenyl glycidyl ether. *J Toxicol Environ Health* 1977;3:859–869.

NIOSH: *Criteria for a Recommended Standard . . . . Occupational Exposure to Glycidyl Ethers.* Washington, DC, National Institute for Occupational Safety and Health (NIOSH 78-166), 1978.

Wallace E: Effects of n-butyl glycidyl ether exposure. *J Soc Occup Med* 1979;29:142–143.

Other Ethers and Epoxides

Isopropyl ether $((CH_3)_2CHO(CH_3)_2$; diisopropyl ether; 2-isopropoxypropane) has important industrial uses as a solvent and as a fuel. It also has anesthetic properties, but it is unsuitable for surgery because of its unpleasant odor, its depressant action, and its narrow margin of safety (Browning, 1965). Its potential hazard to workmen who use lacquers and varnishes containing it while in confined and unventilated areas was pointed out by Jackson (1933).

Dimethyl ether $(CH_3OCH_3$; methyl ether, methyl oxide; methoxymethane) is used as a refrigerant, solvent, aerosol propellant, methylating agent, and catalyst and stabilizer in polymerization. No adverse occupational effects have been reported, but 500 ppm appears to be a justifiable permissible exposure limit since the no-effect level for man is in the region of 50,000 ppm (AIHA, 1980).

Propylene oxide, which resembles chlorhydrin chemically, has been reported to produce contact dermatitis in an electron microscope technician (van Ketel, 1979).

218

References

AIHA: Workplace environmental exposure level guide: Dimethyl ether. *Am Ind Hyg Assoc J* 1980;41:A45–A46.

Browning E: *Toxicity and Metabolism of Industrial Solvents.* New York, Elsevier, 1965, pp 502–505.

Jackson DE: The pharmacological action of isopropyl ether. *J Pharmacol Exp Ther* 1933;48:278–279.

van Ketel WG: Contact dermatitis from propylene oxide. *Contact Derm* 1979;5:191–192.

5 • Esters

Esters are formed when an organic grouping, simple or complex, replaces an acidic hydrogen atom in an organic or inorganic acid. They are used extensively in the plastics industry, either as resins or as plasticizers, and as solvents for lacquers. Esters of inorganic acids may have prominent corrosive or pharmacological properties, and indeed this group may be considered to include the clearly toxic organophosphate insecticides. Although there are notable exceptions, esters of organic acids are generally of low toxicity. Nonspecific irritative effects are commonly associated with the presence of a double bond in these esters that, if saturated, would be essentially harmless. Conjunctivitis and upper airway symptoms may occur and pulmonary edema is possible in cases of massive overexposure. These irritating unsaturated esters include the acrylates, methacrylates, crotonates, and various vinyl and allyl esters.

With the exception of certain phosphate esters used as plasticizers, those esters used as resins and plasticizers are essentially physiologically inert in the industrial environment. This group includes the succinate, adipate, azelate, sebacate, citrate, and phthalate plasticizers. Phthalate ester toxicity has been especially investigated, and while these compounds do have biological activity of interest, they do not appear to be hazardous at ordinary levels of exposure (Daniel, 1978; Lawrence, 1978; Thomas et al., 1978). Chronic inhalation of phthalic ester vapors for a period of six to 10 years by workers engaged in plastics manufacture did result in neurological effects that included toxic polyneuritis and increased excitability of vestibular and olfactory receptors (Milkov et al., 1973).

With most of the esters listed above, minor degrees of epithelial irritation may follow highly unusual or intentionally created exposure conditions in which vapors of heated material are inhaled or in which skin exposures are prolonged. Even then, observed manifestations may be due to impurities, decomposition products, or physical aspects of the exposure situation. Reports of sensitizing reactions are rare and do not always suggest unequivocal etiologies. Inhalation of dusts has produced no specific pulmonary reactions.

Aliphatic Esters

The aliphatic esters are used as solvents for lacquer, cellulose, and drying oils. Ethyl acetate, butyl acetates, and propyl acetates have narcotic properties that are less prominent than those associated with the chlorinated hydrocarbons. Ethyl, methyl, and butyl formates also have narcotic and irritating properties. The ester solvents are powerful defatting agents when applied to the skin and produce a nonspecific drying, cracking, and an increased susceptibility to infection. Sensitization is rarely if ever encountered, except perhaps with vinyl acetate. Solvent ester vapors are generally irritating to the conjunctivae and mucous membranes of the upper airway, but they leave no residual effects. There have been rare reports in the literature of visceral injury, bone marrow effects, and nervous symptoms, the latter more often after methyl acetate exposure (Browning, 1965). Careful consideration of all exposure and diagnostic data in these cases almost always suggests that the esters mentioned were not necessarily responsible for the reported observations, particularly when they occurred in mixtures with other compounds, some of which may have been contaminants. As a group, the ester lacquer solvents have relatively insignificant toxic properties.

Halogenated Acid Esters

A small number of halogenated acid esters are potent lacrimators and vesicants and have the potential capacity for producing pulmonary edema. Compounds in this category are important organic intermediates and include ethyl chloroformate, ethyl chloroacetate, and related bromo- and iodo-compounds. Several of these materials have been used as chemical warfare agents. There is no evidence that they produce chronic disease, but fatalities have occurred from acute pulmonary edema. The highly hazardous character of these compounds appears to be related to the high reactivity of the halogen atom and not to the fact that they are esters.

Alkyl Esters of Sulfuric Acid

Alkyl esters of sulfuric acid, primarily dimethyl and diethyl sulfate, are important alkylating agents in industrial organic syntheses. These are intensely irritating substances, producing inflammation of the eyes, vesication of the skin, and pulmonary edema. Dimethyl sulfate was used in World War I as an irritant and vesicant, and it is extremely hazardous because of its lack of warning properties and the delayed deep lung reaction. Two cases, reported by Littler and McConnell (1955), are typical of those that occur. In one incident a young chemist splashed dimethyl sulfate on his skin and clothing but immediately flooded the contaminated areas with water, diluted sodium hydroxide, and ammonia. Although there were no immediate symptoms, bronchospasm, râles, tachycardia, and marked swelling of the eyes occurred about four hours later. Thirteen hours after exposure, large blisters appeared on the penis, scrotum, and thigh. Severe cough developed with sputum containing chunks of necrotic tracheal mucosa. Subcutaneous emphysema indicated perforation of the trachea. The second man, probably exposed only to vapors of dimethyl sulfate, developed pulmonary edema 12 hours after exposure, as well as swelling of the face and hands, disturbance of visual fields, and analgesia, which has been reported in others. Both men recovered without residual effects except for some skin scarring. Cases of this sort were often fatal before antibiotics became available for control of skin and lung infection. These cases illustrate the potent toxic properties of dimethyl sulfate vapor, the latent period between exposure and illness, and the serious complications that may ensue. There have also been indications that this compound may have carcinogenic properties. The permissible exposure limit for dimethyl sulfate is 1 ppm (5 mg/m^3) although the American Conference of Governmental Industrial Hygienists has set 0.1 ppm as its TLV.

Clinical manifestations due to methylchlorosulfonate, ethylchlorosulfonate, and methyl-p-toluene sulfonate are similar to those associated with dimethyl sulfate, and similar precautions are warranted. Contaminated areas should be entered only by trained personnel with impervious clothing and air-supplied respirators. Contact of these compounds with the skin or eyes is an indication for rapid and prolonged irrigation with large volumes of water. Decontamination of floors and equipment may be accomplished by flushing with dilute alkali or ammonia.

Phosphate Esters

Specific phosphate esters comprise a major category of organic insecticides with important associated occupational medical implications. Other phosphate and phosphite esters, lacking significant insecticidal properties, are widely used as plasticizers and as gasoline additives. Included in this group are tri-o-cresyl phosphate, triphenyl phosphate, tri-2-ethylhexyl phosphate, and 2-ethylhexyl diphenyl phosphate. As plasticizers, these compounds offer the additional property of flame retardancy and are widely used in vinyl and cellulose formulations. Triphenyl phosphite is a color stabilizer in alkyl resins and is an additive to epoxy plastics. Many phosphate esters used as plasticizers, such as tricresyl phosphate (TCP), may be added to gasoline to control pre-ignition.

While some of these plasticizer and fuel-additive phosphate esters do have weak cholinesterase-inhibiting properties, clinical effects associated with disturbances of transsynaptic transmission are not important. Of great significance, however, is the fact that some of these compounds induce delayed neurological effects marked by destruction of axons and demyelination in peripheral nerves and spinal cord. Experimentally one can demonstrate that certain cholinesterase-inhibiting insecticides are also delayed neurotoxins; however, this effect can usually be shown only when the animal is protected from prompt lethal cholinergic effects with prophylactic atropine and oximes. There does not appear to be a correlation, positive or negative, between cholinesterase inhibition and delayed neurotoxicity.

Tri-o-cresyl phosphate (TOCP) and phosphite

and triphenyl phosphate and phosphite are delayed neurotoxins lacking potent anticholinesterase properties. There are other phosphorus esters in this category, and more will undoubtedly be developed. Health officers responsible for the surveillance of workers handling phosphorus esters should insist upon accurate information describing the presence or absence of associated acute or delayed neurotoxic properties. Since there are species differences in susceptibility to delayed neurotoxic effects, toxicologic data must be evaluated critically, and information derived exclusively from rodents should be regarded as suggestive but insufficient.

Although cases of delayed neurotoxicity as a result of industrial exposures to several aryl phosphates have been reported, the vast majority of cases has followed ingestion of food or drinks that had been previously contaminated with tricresyl phosphate esters of the ortho isomer. This problem has been briefly alluded to in the chapter on aromatic hydrocarbons. The United States epidemic occurred in 1930 during Prohibition and produced as many as 15,000 cases of permanent paralysis, often slight, and a small number of deaths. The epidemic of paralytic disease was due to the ingestion of Jamaica ginger extract ("jake") that had become contaminated with tri-o-cresyl phosphate. "Jake" was an alcoholic preparation sold as a flavoring, but was used as a substitute for conventional alcoholic beverages, especially by heavy drinkers and homeless male drifters (Kiely and Rich, 1932). There are various theories, none proved, giving explanations for the distribution of the contamination in communities across the country.

Similar paralytic disease has followed the ingestion of this ester as an abortifacient, in several cooking oil epidemics, and in illegal alcoholic beverages. A recent epidemic occurred in Morocco in 1959 and involved 10,000 people who used olive oil adulterated with jet engine lubricating oil containing TOCP (Albertini et al., 1968). Of these, some 10% to 15% remained permanently crippled and unable to resume previous employment.

In each of these episodes, the clinical picture has been consistent. There may be a prompt transient gastrointestinal disturbance with nausea, vomiting, and diarrhea lasting a few hours to a few days. The onset of neurological disease is delayed for three days to a month and is marked by sharp, cramping pains in the legs, numbness and tingling in the feet, and, subsequently, leg weakness and foot drop. The upper extremities may become involved days later. The effects are symmetrical, the cranial nerves are rarely involved, and persistent sensory manifestations are variable. Flaccid paralysis is associated with wasting of the calf muscles and the small muscles of the hands. Upper motor neuron effects, which may develop over the course of months and bring spasticity, suggest an unfavorable prognosis as far as complete recovery is concerned. In milder cases, recovery appears to be complete, but residual effects are often demonstrable by careful neurologic examination. Many cases of apparent full recovery may, to a large extent, be examples of effective adaptation to permanent motor loss.

Hexamethylphosphoramide, $((CH_3)_2N)_3P:O$, is a relatively new solvent that is used in small quantities in organic and organo-metallic reactions. It has also been proposed as an insect chemosterilant. While no cases of human toxicity have been reported, it is a skin irritant for experimental animals and inhalation by rats frequently results in fatal pneumonia (Zapp, 1975), perhaps by enhancing murine respiratory mycoplasmosis (Overcash et al., 1976). Of greatest interest and importance is its induction of squamous cell carcinomas of the nasal cavity of rats after eight months' daily exposure to 0.4 and 4.0 ppm.

Nitrate Esters

Nitrate esters are derived from nitric acid and alcohols. Their most common use has been in military and mining explosives, and industrial experience with aliphatic nitrates has been primarily in the explosives industry, which has produced glyceryl trinitrate (nitrogylcerin) and ethylene glycol dinitrate for many years. The former compound, also known as trinitropropanetriol, is the active component of dynamite and is used as a coronary vasodilator in clinical medicine. Ethylene glycol dinitrate (dinitroethanediol), more volatile than the original glyceryl nitrate of the early dynamites, is added to the latter substance to increase the stability of the product and to lower its freezing point for low-temperature mining operations. In preparing dynamite these nitrates are absorbed in a "dope" of oxidizing salts and various inert fillers such as wood fibers or cornstarch. Small amounts of other nitrogen-containing compounds, such as dinitrotoluene, may be added. Both glyceryl trinitrate and ethylene glycol dinitrate pass readily through the skin (Hogstedt and Ståhl, 1980) and are sufficiently volatile to produce symptoms in a short period. The effects of absorption are observed in explosive makers, dynamite packagers, miners, and workers handling cordite (a smokeless powder composed of nitroglycerin, guncotton, mineral jelly, and acetone).

The principal biological properties of these nitrate esters are their ability to cause vasodilatation and to oxidize heme to the ferric state to produce methemoglobinemia. Vasodilatation is associated with hypotension, intense throbbing headache, dizziness, flushing, palpitation, and, less frequently, nausea, vomiting, or abdominal distress. The interval between exposure and the onset of symptoms and the duration of the "nitrate effect" varies with individual compounds. Glyceryl trinitrate typically produces a prompt response of brief duration; other agents are slower in producing effects. There is also variability in the ability of various nitrates to produce methemoglobin: ethylene glycol dinitrate is very active, glyceryl nitrate is less so, and ethyl nitrate is weakly active.

Most nitrates produce Heinz bodies, small round erythrocyte inclusions commonly associated with methemoglobin and a history of exposure to organic and inorganic nitrates, and aromatic nitro- and amino-compounds (Harley and Mauer, 1961). Red cells containing Heinz bodies have relatively short life spans and appear to be preferentially sequestered by the spleen. Their persistence in the peripheral blood usually outlasts the associated methemoglobinemia.

The "powder" headache characteristic of exposure to glyceryl trinitrate and ethylene glycol dinitrate usually begins as a feeling of warmth or fullness in the head and develops into a throbbing sensation that progresses from the forehead to the occiput or back of the neck. Although there is wide variability between individuals, most powder workers develop a tolerance to the effects of these nitrates and have no symptoms as long as exposure is maintained. The tolerance may be lost over a weekend or holiday, in which case the return to work is marked by a return of symptoms. There are many reports of workers who carried small pieces of dynamite in their hatbands or who placed pieces around their homes so as to maintain exposure and tolerance. Such reports also describe, however, the violent headaches experienced by persons who enter these homes as visitors and thereby become exposed to an acute dose of nitrate ester. The throbbing headaches have been attributed to dilatation of intracerebral blood vessels, and can be minimized or prevented by pretreatment with oral vasopressors such as amphetamine sulfate or prostigmine bromide (Schwartz, 1946).

More intense exposure has led to hypotension, confusion, and methemoglobinemia. The concurrent absorption of alcohol has been noted on many occasions to intensify the confusion, and frankly maniacal episodes have been reported.

There is evidence that the cardiovascular effects induced by glyceryl trinitrate and ethylene glycol dinitrate may be associated with sudden death in explosives workers—often on Monday mornings, on return from a holiday or weekend (Carmichael and Lieben, 1963; Lund et al., 1968). The clinical diagnosis has been acute myocardial infarction, often, but not always, with little evidence of antecedent coronary artery disease or of coronary occlusion. Critical review of the literature suggests that some three fourths of the sudden deaths in these workers occurred after one or two days' absence from exposure. It may be that coronary artery vasospasm follows the vasodilatation of acute re-exposure without tolerance or that vasodilatation and a drop in blood pressure causes insufficient return of blood to the right heart and cardiovascular collapse. These views are favored in the literature when no anatomical explanation for death is found at postmortem examination. It is of interest in this connection that dynamite workers do not differ from nonexposed "controls" with respect to numbers of ectopic beats or to mean QT-time during the abstinence phase (Hogstedt et al., 1980). An additional view is that chronic exposure to vasodilating drugs may impair the nutrient arterioles in the walls of the coronary arteries to cause the deposition of hyaline connective tissue, a process for which there is some experimental evidence. Nevertheless, the explanation for the epidemiological observations is not yet clearly established, although dynamite workers have been shown to have an excess mortality from coronary heart disease and cerebrovascular disease (Hogstedt and Axelson, 1977; Hogstedt and Andersson, 1979).

The permissible exposure limit for nitroglycerin and for ethylene glycol dinitrate is 0.2 ppm (1 mg/m³) but NIOSH (1978) recommended that this be reduced to 0.02 ppm (0.1 mg/m³) for either or a mixture of these compounds.

Pentaerythritol Tetranitrate

Pentaerythritol tetranitrate is used as a detonator or booster, or can be combined with trinitrotoluene. The nitrate effects of PETN are much less apparent than those associated with the use of nitroglycerin or ethylene glycol dinitrate, although there may be a contact dermatitis.

Alkyl Nitrites

The alkyl nitrous acid esters, such as amyl, butyl, and isobutyl nitrite, produce vasodilatation, tachycardia, and hypotension that may lead to collapse and shock. A throbbing headache and rapid flushing of the face are characteristic, along with vertigo, cyanosis, confusion, weakness, and yellow vision. Tolerance is developed with repeated exposure. Methemoglobinemia may occur and when it does it aggravates the oxygen deprivation in tissues produced by the hypotension (Haley, 1980). For the most part, the effects of alkyl nitrates and nitrites are similar.

Aliphatic Nitro Compounds

Aliphatic nitro compounds that are not esters do not produce nitrate effects but they can induce methemoglobinemia. Dyspnea, cough, and dizziness in workers handling crude TNT has been attributed to tetranitromethane, an impurity with prominent irritating properties (Sievers et al., 1947). Other aliphatic nitro compounds are also irritants.

2-Nitropropane is one of the nitroparaffins that have come into use as solvents for coatings, waxes, resins, gums, dyes, printing inks, and adhesives. Fatalities have occurred from occupational exposure and the downhill course ending in hepatic failure has been characterized by nausea, vomiting, diarrhea, gastrointestinal bleeding, headache, dyspnea, ataxia, and chest and abdominal pain. Liver failure was due to hepatocyte destruction (Hine et al., 1978). OSHA and NIOSH have recently issued a Health Hazard Alert on this compound because as a confirmed carcinogen in laboratory rats it is presumed to be potentially carcinogenic for man (OSHA/NIOSH, 1980).

The chlorinated aliphatic nitro compounds can be extremely irritating, and trichloronitromethane (chloropicrin), which has been used as a military lacrimator, produces coughing, nausea, vomiting, and pulmonary edema.

References

Albertini A, Gross D, Zinn UM: *Triaryl-phosphate Poisoning in Morocco 1959; Experiences and Findings.* Stuttgart, Georg Thieme, 1968.

Browning E: *Toxicity and Metabolism of Industrial Solvents.* New York, Elsevier, 1965, pp 522–593.

Carmichael P, Lieben J: Sudden death in explosives workers. *Arch Environ Health* 1963; 7:424–439.

Daniel JW: Toxicity and metabolism of phthalate esters. *Clin Toxicol* 1978;13:257–268.

Haley TJ: Review of the physiological effects of amyl, butyl, and isobutyl nitrites. *Clin Toxicol* 1980;16:317–329.

Harley JD, Mauer AM: Studies on the formation of Heinz bodies: II. The nature and significance of Heinz bodies. *Blood* 1961;17:418–433.

Hine CH, Pasi A, Stephens BG: Fatalities following exposure to 2-nitropropane. *J Occup Med* 1978;20:333–337.

Hogstedt C, Andersson K: A cohort study on mortality among dynamite workers. *J Occup Med* 1979;21:553–556.

Hogstedt C, Axelson O: Nitroglycerine-nitroglycol exposure and the mortality in cardio-cerebrovascular diseases among dynamite workers. *J Occup Med* 1977;19:675–678.

Hogstedt C, Söderholm B, Bodin L: 48-hour ambulatory electrocardiography in dynamite workers and controls. *Br J Ind Med* 1980; 37:299–306.

Hogstedt C, Ståhl R: Skin absorption and protective gloves in dynamite work. *Am Ind Hyg Assoc J* 1980;41:367–372.

Kiely CE, Rich ML: An epidemic of motor neuritis in Cincinnati, Ohio, due to drinking adulterated Jamaica ginger; history, symptomatology, and clinical report. *Publ Health Rep* 1932;47:2039–2063.

Lawrence WH: Phthalate esters: The question of safety. *Clin Toxicol* 1978;13:89–139.

Littler TR, McConnell RB: Dimethyl sulphate poisoning. *Br J Ind Med* 1955;12:54–56.

Lund RP, Häggendal J, Johnsson G: Withdrawal symptoms in workers exposed to nitroglycerine. *Br J Ind Med* 1968;25:136–138.

Milkov LE, Aldyreva MV, Popova TB, et al: Health status of workers exposed to phthalate plasticizers in the manufacture of artificial leather and films based on PVC resins. *Environ Health Persp* 1973;3:175–178.

NIOSH: *Criteria for a Recommended Standard .... Occupational Exposure to Nitroglycerin and Ethylene Glycol Dinitrate.* Washington, DC, National Institute for Occupational Safety and Health (NIOSH 78-167), 1978.

OSHA/NIOSH: *Health Hazard Alert: 2-Nitropropane.* (NIOSH 80-142), 1980. (Also published in *Am Ind Hyg Assoc J* 41:A18–A24, 1980).

Overcash RG, Lindsey JR, Cassell GH, et al: Enhancement of natural and experimental respiratory mycoplasmosis in rats by hexamethylphosphoramide. *Am J Pathol* 1976;82:171–189.

Schwartz AM: Cause, relief, and prevention of headaches arising from contact with dynalite. *N Engl J Med* 1946;235:541–544.

Sievers RF, Rushing E, Gay H, et al: Toxic effects of tetranitromethane: Contaminant in crude TNT. *Publ Health Rep* 1947;62:1048–1061.

Thomas JA, Darby TD, Wallin RF, et al: A review of the biological effects of di-(2-ethylhexyl) phthalate. *J Toxicol Appl Pharmacol* 1978; 45:1–27.

Zapp JA Jr: Inhalation toxicity of hexamethylphosphoramide. *Am Ind Hyg Assoc J* 1975;36: 916.

6 • Chlorinated Hydrocarbons

Simple chlorinated hydrocarbons have a widespread and essential role in the chemical industry and in a variety of manufacturing operations of great economic significance. The simple chlorohydrocarbons are widely used because of their excellent solvent properties for oils, fats, waxes, and various organic molecules, their relatively low cost, and the noninflammable characteristics associated with most of them. Accordingly, they are valuable extractants, dry cleaning agents, surface degreasing compounds, and vehicles for paints, varnishes, and other industrial coatings. Some chlorohydrocarbons are constituents of paint removers and many are intermediates in chemical syntheses.

Chlorohydrocarbon Solvents

Although the number of solvent chlorohydrocarbon compounds is large, about a dozen of them are of industrial significance and, as such, are of potential occupational medical importance. Three of the four chloromethanes and seven of

the nine chloroethanes are liquid solvents. Methyl chloride and ethyl chloride are gases at room temperature and hexachloroethane is a solid. Familiarity with the nomenclature of these compounds will help avoid possible confusion when the several common or technical names are used. Not all of the compounds listed in Table 7 are widely used.

Many of the members of this series of compounds are extremely volatile, a property that permits a hazardous exposure to occur more rapidly than might be anticipated by the inexperienced worker.

While many such compounds are of relatively low chemical toxicity, the rate at which a hazardous atmospheric concentration may be achieved can be very rapid, especially when the application of heat may further increase the air levels. Consequently, a relatively high threshold limit value (TLV) may be misinterpreted as a low hazard rating. As with many categories of industrial solvents, mixtures of compounds are the rule, although the material may be sold under a single chemical or common name. While this practice

Table 7
Chlorohydrocarbon Solvents

Common Name	Chemical Name	Formula
Methylene chloride	Dichloromethane	CH_2Cl_2
Chloroform	Trichloromethane	$CHCl_3$
Carbon tetrachloride	Tetrachloromethane	CCl_4
Ethylene dichloride	1,2-Dichloroethane	$ClCH_2CH_2Cl$
Ethylidene dichloride	1,1-Dichloroethane	Cl_2CHCH_3
Vinyl trichloride	1,1,2-Trichloroethane	$ClCH_2CHCl_2$
Methyl chloroform	1,1,1-Trichloroethane	CH_3CCl_3
Acetylene tetrachloride	1,1,2,2-Tetrachloroethane	$Cl_2CHCHCl_2$
Vinylidene chloride	1,1-Dichloroethene	$CH_2 = CCl_2$
Acetylene dichloride ⎫ Dichloroethylene ⎭	⎰ 1,2-Dichloroethene (cis and trans)	$ClCH = CHCl$
Acetylene trichloride ⎫ Trichloroethylene ⎭	Trichloroethene	$ClCH = CCl_2$
Perchloroethylene	Tetrachloroethene	$Cl_2C = CCl_2$

225

may be of no particular health significance because of a similarity of the effects associated with the specific compounds, there are several molecules of clearly greater toxicity. Establishing the purity of a solvent is therefore an essential prerequisite in the investigation of working conditions or possible etiological factors in disease.

Chlorohydrocarbons may be thermally decomposed (cracked) at high temperatures to yield, among others, hydrogen chloride and phosgene gases. The former is a highly irritant toxic gas that, because of its irritant effects upon the mucous membranes of the eyes and upper airway, has excellent warning properties that tend to limit exposure. Phosgene, on the other hand, is the classical insidious deep lung irritant without significant sensory effects to warn of its presence. When chlorohydrocarbon vapors are thermally cracked in open flames or arcs associated with furnaces, boilers, or welding operations, sufficient phosgene may be generated to create a hazard of far greater magnitude than that associated with the airborne solvent vapors alone. The amount of phosgene produced varies with the compound being cracked and the conditions of heating, moisture, and hot ferrous surfaces that are involved. While phosgene poisoning from this type of exposure has not been common, it is obviously important to isolate heating and welding operations from chlorohydrocarbon vapors. The temperatures of burning cigarettes are high enough to decompose these vapors, but there is no evidence that smoking has ever produced phosgene or phosgene poisoning. In situations where exhaust gases from furnaces may contain cracked solvent products including hydrogen chloride, special attention should be paid to the duct work since it is unusually susceptible to corrosion with consequent leaks and release of carbon monoxide into the work space.

Compounds of the chlorohydrocarbon group are most commonly absorbed through the lungs, although absorption from the gastrointestinal tract does occur in cases of ingestion. For the most part, chlorinated hydrocarbons that enter the body through the lungs leave unchanged by the same route. Those compounds that are metabolized may have degradation products that appear in the urine. Stewart and his colleagues (1961a,b) developed techniques that permit the retrieval of solvent vapors from the exhaled air of exposed workers as well as analyses of these vapors to characterize various quantitative and qualitative aspects of the exposures. They have

been able to demonstrate, for example, the continuing exhalation of tetrachloroethylene vapors more than 350 hours after the conclusion of exposure. Chlorohydrocarbons that are actively metabolized, of course, disappear from the breath much more rapidly, e.g., trichloroethylene. In cases of suspected exposure to these materials, the breath collection and analysis technique permits the identification of solvents and the construction of breath excretion curves that can be used to estimate the quantity of material absorbed.

Absorption through the skin occurs but it is not of practical industrial significance except possibly in the case of carbon tetrachloride, which may penetrate the skin in toxic amounts.

While the chlorohydrocarbons as a group share several biological properties, other effects are associated with only certain members of the series. Intercompound variability has been most clearly examined in situations in which the liver is the target organ. Plaa and his colleagues (1958) evaluated hepatotoxicity in mice by assessing the impairment of barbiturate detoxification after exposure to members of the chlorinated hydrocarbon series. More recently, hepatic damage has been evaluated in mice by determination of the serum enzymes of injury (e.g., serum glutamic pyruvic transaminase, SGPT) levels after exposure (Gehring, 1968). These experimental studies are in general agreement with each other and with clinical evidence that has accumulated over the years from cases of human overexposure. In order of decreasing hepatotoxicity are: tetrachlorethane, carbon tetrachloride, 1,1,2-trichloroethane, chloroform, perchloroethylene, trichloroethylene, methylene dichloride, and 1,1,1,-trichloroethane. Acute liver injury produced by these chlorinated aliphatic compounds usually consists of centrizonal necrosis and steatosis (Zimmerman, 1978).

Ability to depress the central nervous system is a characteristic property of all members of this series. Such effects may lead through the several stages of clinical anesthesia ultimately to death from respiratory paralysis. This property is well-known, for indeed chloroform and trichloroethylene have been used as surgical anesthetics. While there are differences in anesthetic potency among the chlorohydrocarbons, the generally observed phenomena in many are typical of the group and include dizziness, confusion, drowsiness, nausea and vomiting, and occasionally abdominal pain. Visual disturbances may also occur. Deep anesthesia may lead to death from respiratory depression or circulatory failure. Actual anesthesia is not commonly encountered in industry unless the worker enters tanks or confined places, or there is spillage, gross misuse of materials, or intentional inhalation of vapors to produce euphoria or a "jag." It is not uncommon, however, for complaints of vague nonspecific psychological or psychophysiological reactions to be associated with exposures to chlorohydrocarbons. Headache, fatigue, irritability, impaired memory, anorexia, and nausea are typical symptoms. Whether or not there is a specific pharmacodynamic explanation for these complaints has not been established and would have to be evaluated for each case in terms of specific compounds and degree of exposure.

There have been several reports over the years of sudden death in apparently healthy individuals who had been exposed to chlorohydrocarbons of relatively low toxicity. Autopsies in such cases have failed to reveal a cause of death and point perhaps to the possibility of transient ventricular fibrillation. There is experimental evidence that chlorohydrocarbons can sensitize the myocardium to the effects of endogenous epinephrine (Reinhardt et al., 1971; Aviado and Belej, 1974).

The vapors of the chlorohydrocarbons are not especially irritating to the mucous membranes of the eyes and upper airways but prolonged contact of these solvents with the skin can result in extreme dryness and fissuring with associated infection. This syndrome is secondary to the "degreasing" effects of these materials on the skin. The incidence of sensitization is very low. Immersion of the fingers in methylene chloride leads to severe pain with transient numbness; pain with trichloroethylene and carbon tetrachloride is less severe; with methyl chloroform and perchloroethylene it is minimal.

References

Aviado DM, Belej MA: Toxicity of aerosol propellants on the respiratory and circulatory systems. I. Cardiac arrhythmia in the mouse. *Toxicology* 1974;2:31–42.

Gehring PJ: Hepatotoxic potency of various chlorinated hydrocarbon vapours relative to their narcotic and lethal potencies in mice. *Toxicol Appl Pharmacol* 1968;13:287–298.

Plaa GL, Evans EA, Hine CH: Relative hepatotoxicity of seven halogenated hydrocarbons. *J Pharmacol Exp Ther* 1958;123:224–229.

Reinhardt CF, Azar A, Maxfield ME, et al: Cardiac arrhythmias and aerosol "sniffing." *Arch Environ Health* 1971;22:265–279.

Stewart RD, Gay HH, Erley DS, et al: Human exposure to 1,1,1-trichloroethane vapor. Relationship of expired air and blood concentrations to exposure and toxicity. *Am Ind Hyg Assoc J* 1961a;22:252–262.

Stewart RD, Gay HH, Erley DS, et al: Human exposure to tetrachloroethylene vapor. Relationship of expired air and blood concentrations to exposure and toxicity. *Arch Environ Health* 1961b;2:516–522.

Zimmerman HJ: *Hepatotoxicity.* New York, Appleton-Century-Crofts, 1978, p. 310.

Methyl chloride Methyl chloride (CH_3Cl; monochloroethane), a colorless gas at room temperatures, is handled in industry under pressure in the liquid state. It is used almost exclusively in the chemical industry as a methylating agent in the production of silicones, butyl rubber, and tetramethyl lead. Its use as a domestic and industrial refrigerant, the most common source of intoxication in the past, has almost entirely ceased although accidental poisonings continue to be reported (Spevak et al., 1976).

Methyl chloride is a potent narcotic that causes headache, drowsiness, giddiness, ataxia, and ultimately convulsions, coma, and respiratory failure. One follow-up study of persons exposed in a fishing trawler refrigeration leak revealed persistent neurological abnormalities 13 years after the accident (Gudmundsson, 1977). Chronic intoxication, primarily with neurological symptoms, has been seen in recent years in methyl chloride and foam plastic workers (Scharnweber et al., 1974). Cases of long-standing neuropsychiatric alterations have also been described, with depression, irritability, change of personality, insomnia, and disturbances of vision.

The current permissible exposure limit is 100 ppm.

References

Gundmundsson G: Methyl chloride poisoning 13 years later. *Arch Environ Health* 1977; 32:236–237.

Sacharnweber HC, Spears GN, Cowles SR: Chronic methyl chloride intoxication in six industrial workers. *J Occup Med* 1974;16:112–113.

Spevak L, Nadj V, Fellé D: Methyl chloride poisoning in four members of a family. *Br J Ind Med* 1976;33:272–278.

Methylene chloride Methylene chloride (CH_2Cl_2; dichloromethane) is used as a solvent and extracting agent where a high degree of volatility is desired. It is a common ingredient in paint strippers. It is the least toxic of the four chlorinated methanes but, because of its high volatility, it is easy to achieve air levels that result in "drunkenness" and associated unreliable behavior. Two cases of intoxication led a manufacturer to discontinue the use of methylene chloride in lacquer production because its use led to headache, stumbling, irritability, and stupidity in the workers (Collier, 1936).

It is of additional importance that exposures to this compound are followed by increases in the carboxyhemoglobin level, presumably as a result of the metabolism of this solvent to carbon monoxide. Experimental exposure of human subjects to methylene chloride at 1000 ppm for two hours resulted in carboxyhemoglobin saturation levels in excess of those permitted in the workplace from exposure to carbon monoxide alone (Stewart et al., 1972). Consequently, the dangers of carbon monoxide poisoning from the home use of paint removers that contain methylene chloride have been stressed by Stewart and Hake (1976).

Acute exposures of volunteers to concentrations of methylene chloride as low as 500 ppm produced decreased manual performance and, more importantly, attention lapses ascribed to short microsleeps (Winneke and Fodor, 1976). Physical exercise increases the absorption of methylene chloride, its conversion to carbon monoxide, the level of carboxyhemoglobin, and the pulmonary excretion of CO (DiVincenzo and Kaplan, 1981). Engström and Bjurström (1977) showed that obese male volunteers exposed to 750 ppm for one hour had greater amounts of methylene chloride in the total adipose tissue than did slim subjects. That serious cerebral deterioration can occur from chronic exposure to methylene chloride was shown by the case described by Barrowcliff and Knell (1979). A 60-year-old man, who presumably had stored methylene chloride in the body as a result of exposure for over 20 years to concentrations calculated to have been between 500 and 1000 ppm, developed serious dementia. Endogenous production of carbon monoxide from stored methylene chloride was thought to account for the cerebral damage.

Another hazard is the danger of phosgene poisoning from the combustion of methylene chloride, although reports of such accidents have been infrequent (Gerritsen and Buschmann, 1960; English, 1964).

While the permissible exposure limit for methylene chloride is 500 ppm averaged over an eight-hour workshift, with ceiling levels of 1000 ppm for five minutes in any two-hour period, NIOSH (1976) has recommended that the limit be lowered to 75 ppm with further lowering of the ceiling when concomitant CO levels are more than 9 ppm.

References

Barrowcliff DF, Knell AJ: Cerebral damage due to endogenous chronic carbon monoxide poisoning caused by exposure to methylene chloride. *J Soc Occup Med* 1979;29:12–14.

Collier HE: Methylene dichloride intoxication in industry—A report of two cases. *Lancet* 1936; 1:594–595.

DiVincenzo GD, Kaplan CL: Effect of exercise or smoking on the uptake, metabolism, and excretion of methylene chloride vapor. *Toxicol Appl Pharmacol* 1981;59:141–148.

English JM: A case of probable phosgene poisoning. *Br Med J* 1964;1:38.

Engström J, Bjurström R: Exposure to methylene chloride. Content in subcutaneous adipose tissue. *Scand J Work Environ Health* 1977;3:215–224.

Gerritsen WB, Buschmann CH: Phosgene poisoning caused by the use of chemical paint removers containing methylene chloride in ill-ventilated rooms heated by kerosine stoves. *Br Ind Med* 1960;17:187–189.

NIOSH: *Criteria for a Recommended Standard . . . . Occupational Exposure to Methylene Chloride.* Washington, DC, National Institute for Occupational Safety and Health (NIOSH 76-138), 1976.

Stewart RD, Fisher TN, Hosko MJ, et al: Experimental human exposure to methylene chloride. *Arch Environ Health* 1972;25:324–348.

Stewart RD, Hake CL: Paint-remover hazard. *J Am Med Assoc* 1976;235:398–401.

Winneke G, Fodor GG: Dichloromethane produces narcotic effect. *Occup Health Safety* 1976; 34–49, Mar/Apr.

Chloroform Chloroform (CHCl₃; trichloromethane) is no longer used as an anesthetic but it still has industrial applications as a solvent and extractant, as an intermediate in the production of dyes and drugs, and in the manufacture of fluorocarbons for refrigerants, propellants, and plastics. Its effects are similar to those of carbon tetrachloride, but its hepatotoxic action is less potent than CCl₄ (Zimmerman, 1978). Unlike CCl₄, chloroform depletes hepatic glutathione (Docks and Krishna, 1976), and a low protein diet does not inhibit its toxicity.

Adverse effects from occupational exposure are uncommon. General lassitude, dry mouth and thirst, gastrointestinal discomfort, urinary frequency, and a feeling of being dazed were prominent symptoms among a group of workers exposed to chloroform vapors in a confectionery factory producing medicinal lozenges (Challen et al., 1958).

The permissible exposure limit is 50 ppm (244 mg/m³), although NIOSH (1974) proposed a value of 10 ppm determined as a time-weighted average for a 10-hour workday, 40-hour workweek, and a 50 ppm limit for any 10-minute period.

References

Challen PJR, Hickish DE, Bedford J: Chronic chloroform intoxication. *Br J Ind Med* 1958;15: 243–249.

Docks EL, Krishna G: The role of glutathione in chloroform-induced hepatotoxicity. *Exp Molec Pathol* 1976;24:13–22.

NIOSH: *Criteria for a Recommended Standard . . . . Occupational Exposure to Chloroform.* Washington, DC, National Institute for Occupational Safety and Health (NIOSH 75-114), 1974.

Zimmerman HJ: *Hepatotoxicity.* New York, Appleton-Century-Crofts, 1978, p 210.

Carbon tetrachloride Carbon tetrachloride (CCl₄; tetrachloromethane) has lost its early predominance as an inexpensive nonflammable solvent for use in degreasing, dry cleaning, and extracting. Less toxic compounds such as tri- and tetrachloroethylene now serve as acceptable substitutes. For many years carbon tetrachloride was also used in the "Pyrene" fire extinguisher, but this application has been almost universally discontinued because of the toxic properties of the compound and its degradation products. Nor is it used any longer as a vermifuge or as a waterless shampoo. Most of the current industrial output goes into the synthesis of chlorofluoromethane refrigerants, solvents, and aerosol propellants. Relatively smaller amounts continue to be used as laboratory solvents (such as in chromatography), in the recovery of tin from scrap metal, as a grain fumigant, and as an addition to solvent mixes to lower their flammability.

Accumulating evidence over the years has shown carbon tetrachloride to be one of the most toxic of the common solvents. The earlier literature has been collected and summarized by Hardin (1954), Browning (1965), and NIOSH (1975). It is readily absorbed from the lungs on inhalation as well as from the gastrointestinal tract after ingestion, and it is stored in the body principally in adipose tissue, liver, bone marrow, brain, and kidneys (McCollister et al., 1951). It is eliminated slowly and may be detectable unchanged in the exhaled breath by infrared spectrophotometry or by vapor phase chromatography as long as three weeks after ingestion (Stewart et al., 1963). A portion of the absorbed CCl₄ is metabolized to CO_2, partly perhaps by way of chloroform, with both the trichloromethyl free radical, ·CCl₃, and carbonyl chloride (phosgene) as intermediates that may account for the toxic effects (Recknagel and Glende, 1973; Shah et al., 1979).

Carbon tetrachloride is a potent narcotic and, as such, has properties that resemble the other compounds in the chlorohydrocarbon series. Central nervous system depression that occurs after ingestion or inhalation is manifested by dizziness, blurring of vision, headache, giddiness, fatigue, and, in more severe cases, coma (Stevens and Forster, 1953). Farrell and Senseman (1944) considered their case of polyneuritis to have resulted from absorption of CCl₄ through the skin. Bilateral constriction of visual color fields, toxic amblyopia, and optic atrophy have also been reported (Wirtshafter, 1933; Gray, 1947; Smith, 1950). Parkinsonism as a consequence of chronic CCl₄ exposure has also been observed (Melamed and Lavy, 1977).

The specific toxic effects of carbon tetrachloride, however, involve the liver and kidneys. When exposure has been of sufficient magnitude, the liver and kidneys are commonly both affected, although not always to the same degree. Renal injury was once considered to be the principal manifestation of poisoning after inhalation, with hepatic damage predominant after ingestion. The evidence does not support this view. Nausea, vomiting, and abdominal cramps have been considered to be the presenting symptoms, primarily suggesting liver injury. That such symptoms have appeared in the absence of altered liver function tests, however, suggests that in some situations these complaints may represent a nonspecific effect. Nausea and vomiting usually appear within hours after exposure, although a delay up to six days has been noted, probably depending on the amount and rate of absorption. The abdominal pain has been misinterpreted as indicative of acute appendicitis.

Liver damage from carbon tetrachloride consists primarily of centrizonal necrosis and steatosis (Zimmerman, 1978), which may occur promptly after exposure, but clinical evidence of hepatic disease may not appear for from two to four days. Hepatocellular jaundice develops in half of the cases and there is a rapid increase in serum bilirubin levels. Serum glutamic oxaloacetic transaminase (SGOT) and serum glutamic pyruvic transaminase (SGPT) can be enormously elevated. In severe injury the liver is enlarged and tender, and hepatic failure with ammonia intoxication may ensue.

The mechanism of carbon tetrachloride hepatotoxicity has been examined in detail by Recknagel (1967). It appears that the two principal pathologic alterations, fatty degeneration and necrosis, are independent toxic events and have distinct pathogeneses. The hepatic accumulation of lipid is related to the injury of the endoplasmic reticulum and the disruption of the mechanism for moving lipid out of the liver cells by impairment of the coupling of triglycerides to the lipoprotein carrier. The precise mechanism for the necrosis has not been clearly established but it may be the result of injury to cell membranes with intracellular release of destructive lysosomal enzymes, loss of energy sources because of injury to the mitochondria, and general metabolic chaos subsequent to the loss of cytoplasmic enzymes and coenzymes. The fact that a wide variety of compounds (such as cerium chloride, cobaltous chloride, propylthiouracil, dithiocarb, chlorpromazine, and others) protect against carbon tetrachloride exposure serves to indicate the complexity of the biochemical pathogenetic processes that are involved.

While the intact carbon tetrachloride molecules may injure the hepatic cell wall, prime damage is caused by the metabolites of the solvent, perhaps, as already noted, by ·CCl_3 radicals and phosgene. Cells that do not actively metabolize carbon tetrachloride have been shown to be relatively resistant to this solvent. Conversely, measures that enhance metabolic activity by stimulating endoreticular expansion and enzyme induction also enhance carbon tetrachloride toxicity (Garner and McLean, 1969). The increased vulnerability of alcoholics to the hepatotoxicity of carbon tetrachloride may be due to the fact that ethanol leads to the induction of metabolizing enzymes of the endoreticular system.

Renal impairment is common and may exist in the absence of demonstrable hepatotoxicity (Guild et al., 1958). It reaches its peak in the second and third week after exposure. Costovertebral pain is common, proteinuria is characteristic, and oliguria may occur one to seven days after an acute exposure and may progress to anuria that may persist for one or two weeks. Examination of the urine sediment may reveal evidence of acute tubular necrosis: red and white blood cells; hyaline, granular, and red cell casts; and renal tubular epthelial cells. Early elevation of blood urea nitrogen (BUN) and nonprotein nitrogen (NPN) may represent extrarenal azotemia as a result of nausea, vomiting and dehydration. Frank azotemia from tubular necrosis develops soon thereafter and may be aggravated by concomitant liver damage. The observed nephrotoxicity appears to be due to the direct effects of carbon tetrachloride upon the proximal tubule and loop of Henle, although the distal tubule may be affected to a lesser degree.

The development of the uremic syndrome or of potassium intoxication are indications for hemodialysis. The prognosis in severe cases of carbon tetrachloride intoxication has improved markedly since dialysis has become commonly available. The simultaneous presence of hepatic failure with impaired urea synthesis and ammonia intoxication is obviously unfavorable. Recovery may require months but may eventually be complete.

There is no general agreement as to whether or not acute hepatorenal injury or prolonged exposure without acute effects may result in chronic impairment. There have been enough cases of cirrhosis after long exposures, however, to suggest that there may be a causal relationship in specific instances (McDermott and Hardy, 1963). Small chronic doses of CCl_4 have resulted in micronodular cirrhosis in many species of laboratory animals that resembles Laennec's cirrhosis in man, with portal hypertension, collateral venous circulation, ascites, and abnormal liver function tests (Zimmerman, 1978).

Hepatocellular carcinoma developing seven years after acute carbon tetrachloride intoxication has also been reported (Tracey and Sherlock, 1968), and this compound is a potent carcinogen in animals, although the rarity of metastases from CCl_4-induced liver tumors suggests that they may not be very malignant. It is, of course, possible that regeneration in itself in these cases is the precancerous lesion and that carbon tetrachloride is not a specific carcinogenic material.

A bleeding tendency with impaired coagulation as a result of hypoprothrombinemia and decreased levels of plasma clotting factors has been observed in many cases of acute carbon tetrachloride poisoning. The evidence that CCl_4 is a direct bone marrow poison is not indisputable, but cases have been reported in which the nature of the exposure and the sequence of events are reasonably convincing (Straus, 1954).

Since 1962, the permissible occupational exposure limit in the United States has been 10 ppm (63 mg/m³) for the usual workweek. NIOSH (1975) has recommended a limit of 2 ppm determined as a time-weighted average for up to a 10-hour workday, 40-hour workweek.

References

Browning E: *Toxicity and Metabolism of Industrial Solvents.* New York, Elsevier, 1965, pp 173–188.

Farrell CL, Senseman LA: Carbon tetrachloride polyneuritis — A case report. *Rhode Island Med J* 1944;27:334, 346.

Garner RC, McLean AE: Increased susceptibility to carbon tetrachloride poisoning in the rat after pretreatment with oral phenobarbitone. *Biochem Pharmacol* 1969;18:645–650.

Gray I: Carbon tetrachloride poisoning — Report of seven cases with two deaths. *NY State J Med* 1947; 47:2311–2315.

Guild WR, Young JV, Merrill JP: Anuria due to carbon tetrachloride intoxication. *Ann Intern Med* 1958;48:1221–1227.

Hardin BL Jr: Carbon tetrachloride poisoning — A review. *Ind Med Surg* 1954;23:93–105.

McCollister DD, Beamer WH, Atchison GJ, et al: Absorption, distribution and elimination of radioactive carbon tetrachloride by monkeys upon exposure to low vapor concentrations. *J Pharmacol Exp Ther* 1951;102:111–124.

McDermott WV, Hardy HL: Cirrhosis of the liver following chronic exposure to carbon tetrachloride. *J Occup Med* 1963;5:249–251.

Melamed E, Lavy S: Parkinsonism associated with chronic inhalation of carbon tetrachloride. *Lancet* 1977;1:1015.

NIOSH: *Criteria for a Recommended Standard . . . . Occupational Exposure to Carbon Tetrachloride.* Washington, DC, National Institute for Occupational Safety and Health (NIOSH 76-133), 1975.

Recknagel RO: Carbon tetrachloride hepatotoxicity. *Pharmacol Rev* 1967;19:145–208.

Recknagel RO, Glende EA Jr: Carbon tetrachloride hepatotoxicity: An example of lethal cleavage. *CRC Crit Rev Toxicol* 1973;2:263–297.

Shah H, Hartman SP, Weinhouse S: Formation of carbonyl chloride in carbon tetrachloride metabolism by rat liver *in vitro. Cancer Res* 1979; 39:3942–3947.

Smith AR: Optic atrophy following inhalation of carbon tetrachloride. *Arch Ind Hyg Occup Med* 1950;1:348–351.

Stevens H, Forster FM: Effect of carbon tetrachloride on the nervous system. *Arch Neurol Psychiatry* 1953;70:635–649.

Stewart RD, Boettner EA, Southworth RR, et al: Acute carbon tetrachloride intoxication. *J Am Med Assoc* 1963;183:994–997.

Straus B: Aplastic anemia following exposure to carbon tetrachloride. *J Am Med Assoc* 1954; 155:737–739.

Tracey JP, Sherlock P: Hepatoma following carbon tetrachloride poisoning. *NY State J Med* 1968;68:2202–2204.

Wirtshafter ZT: Toxic amblyopia and accompanying physiological disturbances in carbon tetrachloride intoxication. *Am J Publ Health* 1933;23:1035–1038.

Zimmerman HJ: *Hepatotoxicity.* New York, Appleton-Century-Crofts, 1978.

Ethyl chloride Ethyl chloride (CH_3CH_2Cl; monochloroethane) is a gas at room temperature; however, it is easily liquefied and is familiar to physicians as a local anesthetic agent that freezes the skin when it is applied as a spray. Ethyl chloride is used in industry almost entirely as a chemical intermediate in the synthesis of tetraethyl lead and other ethyl compounds, but it is also used as a solvent in making perfumes. The physiological properties of ethyl chloride are

232

related to its anesthetic effect and perhaps to its cardiotoxic action as a sensitizer of the myocardium to endogenous epinephrine. Generally, it is less toxic than methyl chloride (monochloromethane). As far as is known, ethyl chloride is excreted via the lungs without significant metabolic alteration in the body. The permissible exposure limit is 1000 ppm (2600 mg/m³).

Ethylene dichloride   The ethylene dichloride ($C_2H_4Cl_2$), or ethylene chloride, of industry is 1,2-dichloroethane. Its isomer, 1,1-dichloroethane, is commonly known as ethylidene dichloride or ethylidene chloride. These are saturated compounds, chlorinated ethanes, and should not be confused with the dichloroethenes, commonly known as dichloroethylenes.

While both dichlorinated ethanes are used as solvents, degreasers, and as chemical intermediates, the bulk of occupational medical experience seems to have been with the 1,2-dichloroethane isomer. This compound is principally used in the production of vinyl chloride and other halogenated hydrocarbons as well as a lead scavenger, as a consequence of which it becomes a component of leaded fuels. In those cases of intoxication that have been reported, the anticipated anesthetic effects have been observed along with headache, dizziness, nausea and vomiting, weakness, trembling, and epigastric cramps. These symptoms have been followed in severe cases by collapse, coma, and death from respiratory and circulatory failure. In severe and fatal cases, hepatic and renal injury have been noted. Cases of acute inhalation exposure, with and without fatalities, have been collected by NIOSH (1976).

More recently, concern has developed over the potential carcinogenicity of 1,2-dichloroethane because of malignant tumors that have been found in force-fed rats and mice (NCI, 1978). Because of these findings, NIOSH (1978) has proposed that its previous recommendations (1976) be revised downward from 5 ppm (20 mg/m³) to 1 ppm determined as a TWA for up to a 10-hour workshift, and that the ceiling concentration not exceed 2 ppm determined over a 15-minute sampling period. These proposals represent a drastic lowering of the current permissible exposure limit of 50 ppm. The existing limit for ethylidene chloride (1,1-dichloroethane) is 100 ppm. Caution should prevail in setting exposure standards on the basis of extrapolation from experience with small laboratory animals.

References

NCI: Report on carcinogenesis bioassay of 1,2-dichloroethane (EDC). National Cancer Institute. *Am Ind Hyg Assoc J* 1978;39:A26–A30.

NIOSH: *Criteria for a Recommended Standard . . . . Occupational Exposure to Ethylene Dichloride (1,2-Dichloroethane)*. Washington, DC, National Institute for Occupational Safety and Health (NIOSH 76-139), 1976.

NIOSH: *Revised Recommended Standard . . . . Occupational Exposure to Ethylene Dichloride (1,2-Dichloroethane)*. Washington, DC, National Institute for Occupational Safety and Health (NIOSH 78-211), 1978.

Methyl chloroform   Methyl chloroform (CH_3CCl_3; 1,1,1-trichloroethane) is a chlorohydrocarbon solvent that, because of its very low toxicity (Stewart, 1971), is being used at an accelerated rate. It is widely utilized as a solvent, vapor degreaser, and dry cleaning agent. Like many chlorohydrocarbons, methyl chloroform is somewhat unstable, and small amounts of stabilizing substances are added to the solvent sold in commerce. Such stabilizers or inhibitors may be various ketones, alcohols, esters, or nitrogen compounds that do not change the toxicity of the commercial product.

Methyl chloroform is a narcotic and skin defatting solvent as are the chlorohydrocarbons in general. Exposures to high air concentrations of methyl chloroform may lead to narcosis with central nervous system depression and even fatal respiratory depression under conditions of grossly negligent overexposure (Stewart, 1971). Necropsies of workers fatally overcome by methyl chloroform exposures showed pulmonary congestion and edema (Stahl et al., 1969; Hatfield et al., 1970). There is no evidence that this solvent causes the severe hepatic and renal injury that is characteristic of carbon tetrachloride, but elevated urinary urobilinogen has been reported in occasional experimental subjects (Stewart et al., 1961). Experimental work (Reinhardt et al., 1971; Aviado and Belej, 1974) and clinical experience with antitussive preparations containing trichloroethane have identified serious cardiotoxic properties of this compound, and deaths have been attributed to cardiac arrhythmias, probably as the result of epinephrine sensitization.

1,1,2-Trichloroethane ($CHCl_2CH_2Cl$; vinyl trichloride), an isomer of methyl chloroform, is a more potent anesthetic agent, an irritant to mucous membranes, a significant hepato- and nephrotoxin, and possibly a carcinogen, since it produces hepatocellular carcinomas and pheochromocytomas in mice (but not in rats) (NIOSH, 1978).

The permissible exposure limit for 1,1,1-trichloroethane is 350 ppm (1910 mg/m³), but NIOSH (1976) recommended that this level be a ceiling value as determined by a 15-minute sample. The permissible exposure limit for the beta isomer, 1,1,2-trichloroethane, by contrast, is only 10 ppm (55 mg/m³), because of its carcinogenicity in experimental mice.

References

Aviado DM, Belej MA: Toxicity of aerosol propellants on the respiratory and circulatory systems. I. Cardiac arrhythmia in the mouse. *Toxicology* 1974;2:31–42.

Hatfield TR, Maykoski RT: A fatal methyl chloroform (trichloroethane) poisoning. *Arch Environ Health* 1970;20:279–281.

NIOSH: *Criteria for a Recommended Standard . . . . Occupational Exposure to 1,1,1-Trichloroethane (Methyl Chloroform)*. Washington, DC, National Institute for Occupational Safety and Health (NIOSH 76-184), 1976.

NIOSH: Chloroethanes: Review of toxicity. *Current Intelligence Bulletin 27*, Washington, DC, National Institute for Occupational Safety and Health (NIOSH 78-181), 1978.

Reinhardt CF, Azar A, Maxfield ME, et al: Cardiac arrhythmias and aerosol "sniffing." *Arch Environ Health* 1971;22:265–279.

Stahl CJ, Fatteh AV, Dominguez AM: Trichloroethane poisoning—Observations on the pathology and toxicology in six fatal cases. *J Forensic Sci* 1969;14:393–397.

Stewart RD: Methyl chloroform intoxication: Diagnosis and treatment. *J Am Med Assoc* 1971; 215:1789–1792.

Stewart RD, Gay HH, Erley DS: Human exposure to 1,1,1-trichloroethane. Relationship of expired air and blood concentrations to exposure and toxicity. *Am Ind Hyg Assoc J* 1961;22:252–262.

Tetrachloroethane Industrial references to tetrachloroethane, also known as acetylene tetra-

chloride, are invariably to the symmetrical isomer, 1,1,2,2-tetrachloroethane (HCl₂CCHCl₂). Clinical evidence indicates that this compound is by far the most poisonous of the chlorohydrocarbons used as industrial solvents. Its toxic manifestations resemble those of carbon tetrachloride; however, the hepatotoxicity of tetrachloroethane is much more severe. Unfortunately from the health point of view, it is an excellent solvent, often the best available for many applications. Early utilization of tetrachloroethane as a solvent for cellulose acetate in the so-called "dope" to cover airplane fabrics led to numerous severe and fatal cases of toxic hepatitis and atrophy of the liver (Gurney, 1943, 1947). Hepatic injury from tetrachloroethane consisted of acute or subacute zonal necrosis and steatosis, with hepatomegaly, jaundice, and ascites. Outcome was frequently fatal in those workers who had continued exposure after the onset of gastrointestinal and neurologic complaints, such as anorexia, nausea, constipation, drowsiness, numbness of toes and fingers, paresthesias, hand tremors, and plantar pain (NIOSH, 1976).

The recognized toxicity of tetrachloroethane has caused it to be eliminated from most industrial uses unless its specific solvent properties are necessary. The use of this compound is now rarely justified. NIOSH (1976) estimated that no more than 5000 workers in the United States are now exposed to 1,1,2,2-tetrachloroethane, for which the permissible exposure limit is 5 ppm (35 mg/m³). NIOSH has recommended further lowering of this limit to 1 ppm determined as a time-weighted average for up to a 10-hour workday, 40-hour workweek.

References

Gurney R: Tetrachloroethane intoxication. Early recognition of liver damage and means of prevention. *Gastroenterology* 1943;1:1112–1126.

Gurney R: Useful procedures in the early diagnosis of liver damage following exposure to the chlorinated hydrocarbons. *NY State J Med* 1947;47:2566–2568.

NIOSH: *Criteria for a Recommended Standard . . . . Occupational Exposure to 1,1,2,2-Tetrachloroethane*. Washington, DC, National Institute for Occupational Safety and Health (NIOSH 77-121), 1976.

Dichloroethylene 1,2-Dichloroethylene (HClC = CHCl; acetylene dichloride) is handled in industry as a mixture of the trans and cis isomers. It is used as a low temperature extracting agent for heat-sensitive substances such as perfumes and caffeine in coffee. Aside from the narcotic properties of this solvent, toxic effects have not been noted in the rather small scale industrial usage that exists. It is hepatotoxic when inhaled by small laboratory animals at levels of 200 ppm (790 mg/m³), the permissible exposure limit (Freundt et al., 1977), although these experimental animals may be more susceptible than man at this exposure level.

The 1,1-isomer ($H_2C = CCl_2$; vinylidene chloride) is used almost entirely as a monomer in the manufacture of copolymeric plastics. Experience from the synthetic plastics industry and studies with experimental animals indicate that 1,1-dichloroethylene has toxic properties that are similar to those of carbon tetrachloride, i.e., there is significant hepato- and nephro-toxicity (Jenkins et al., 1972; Lee et al., 1977; Reynolds et al., 1975, 1980). Exposures of mice and rats to 55 ppm of vinylidene chloride have resulted in hepatic hemangiosarcoma and bronchoalveolar adenomas in the mice and mesenteric lymph node and subcutaneous hemangiosarcomas in the rats (Lee et al., 1977, 1978). This experience with laboratory animals appears to be related to the more strongly established carcinogenic potential of vinyl chloride in man and animals.

References

Freundt KJ, Liebaldt GP, Lieberwirth E: Toxicity studies on trans-1,2-dichloroethylene. *Toxicology* 1977;7:141–153.

Jenkins LJ Jr, Trabulus MJ, Murphy SD: Biochemical effects of 1,1-dichloroethylene in rats: Comparison with carbon tetrachloride and 1,2-dichloroethylene. *Toxicol Appl Pharmacol* 1972;23:501–510.

Lee CC, Bhandari JC, Winston JM, et al: Inhalation toxicity of vinyl chloride and vinylidene chloride. *Environ Health Persp* 1977;21:25–32.

Lee CC, Bhandari JC, Winston JM, et al: Carcinogenicity of vinyl chloride and vinylidene chloride. *J Toxicol Environ Health* 1978;4:15–30.

Reynolds ES, Moslen MT, Szabo S, et al: Hepatotoxicity of vinyl chloride and 1,1-dichloroethylene: Role of mixed function oxidase system. *Am J Pathol* 1975;81:219–236.

Reynolds ES, Moslen MT, Boor PJ, et al: 1,1-Dichloroethylene hepatotoxicity. Time course of GSH changes and biochemical aberrations. *Am J Pathol* 1980;101:331–344.

Trichloroethylene Trichloroethylene (HClC = CCl₂; trichloroethene) is utilized in very large quantities as a metal degreaser and dry cleaning agent, applications requiring over 90% of the amount produced. Minor quantities of the solvent have been used in the extraction of fats from fish meal and caffeine from coffee, in the manufacture of adhesives and industrial paints, and in the dewaxing of lubricating oils. Trichloroethylene is often used as a substitute for carbon tetrachloride, which has significantly greater toxic properties. Because of its relatively low toxicity and nonflammability, trichloroethylene has been used in clinical medicine as a surgical anesthetic agent. This use has been largely abandoned because of the availability of better anesthetic agents and because of several anesthesia accidents related to the generation of dichloroacetylene, a neurotoxic substance, when trichloroethylene was passed through a closed-circuit apparatus in which a soda-lime carbon dioxide absorber was used. In some situations where brief analgesia is helpful, such as in minor surgery and in obstetric analgesia where it has often been self-administered by the woman in labor, trichloroethylene has been useful. It is contraindicated as an anesthetic agent for children or together with epinephrine because of the high risk of ventricular fibrillation (Osol and Pratt, 1973).

Trichloroethylene is readily absorbed from the lungs and gastrointestinal tract (Waters et al., 1977); some absorption may also occur through intact skin (Stewart and Dodd, 1964). After it is absorbed, trichloroethylene disappears rapidly from the blood, a large percentage being exhaled unchanged (Daniel, 1963) and the remainder either metabolized or stored in fatty tissues. Biotransformation in the liver involves its oxidation to chloral hydrate, which in turn is rapidly reduced to trichloroethanol or is oxidized to trichloroacetic acid. The former is either oxidized to the latter by the mixed function oxidases or more often is conjugated with glucuronic acid (Müller et al., 1974). The urinary metabolites, then, consist of trichloroacetic acid, trichloroethanol, and trichloroethanol glucuronide. Details of the studies that established these reaction pathways have been summarized by Smith (1966) and by Waters et al. (1977).

Since trichloroacetic acid may be detectable in

the urine for several weeks after exposure has terminated, urine assays for it and for trichloroethanol have been widely used in Europe and Japan in the medical surveillance of workers exposed to trichloroethylene (Ikeda et al., 1972; Gubéran, 1977). It has been the more common practice in the United States to estimate the atmospheric concentrations of this compound in the workers' breathing zones by use of properly calibrated halide meters or detector tubes. In situations where the ambient air levels or exposures vary widely, it is possible to monitor the trichloroethylene concentrations in the exhaled breath of exposed persons (Stewart et al., 1970). Trichloroethylene is excreted exponentially via the lungs, most of the absorbed amount being exhaled during the first 24 hours after exposure. Samples of expired breath are easily collected in plastic bags and analyzed by infrared spectroscopy or gas chromatography. By making serial evaluations during the postexposure period, it is possible to obtain sufficient information to establish the excretion rate and an estimate of the previous vapor exposure. Stewart et al. (1970) have presented evidence that the data thus obtained are more accurate, more useful, and more easily acquired than those derived from determination of urinary metabolites.

The narcosis produced by acute exposure to trichloroethylene cannot be distinguished from that produced by the absorption of other chlorohydrocarbons. There may be an excitatory or euphoric stage that in some cases has led to "addiction" and the repeated intentional inhalation of the vapor (Harenko, 1967). There may be lack of coordination, dizziness, confusion, drowsiness, and eventual loss of consciousness. While most of these symptoms clear promptly with the breathing of uncontaminated air and the excretion of the compound by the lungs, residual neurological disturbances may appear in the form of persistent headache or hallucinations, although these have been ascribed to contaminants (Smith, 1966). Peripheral nerves may be involved as well as the central nervous system. Feldman and Mayer (1968) have demonstrated a slowing of conduction time in peripheral nerves that is reversible over the course of months. Chronic exposure, such as may be found among degreasers, may lead to fatigue, headache, loss of memory, intolerance to alcohol and tobacco, and depression (Grandjean et al., 1955). Various psychosomatic complaints and uncommon toxic psychoses have also been described.

There is some dispute in the clinical literature as to the extent to which trichloroethylene can produce toxic effects apart from nonspecific chlorohydrocarbon narcosis. Enzyme and urine urobilinogen studies after exposures to 200 ppm have not indicated any hepatotoxicity. On the other hand, the report of acute, fatal toxic hepatitis in a man operating a trichloroethylene degreaser (Priest and Horn, 1965) as well as the hepatorenal disease reported among "sniffers" (Baerg and Kimberg, 1970; Clearfield, 1970) suggest that there is a potential hepato- and nephrotoxicity of this solvent. The concurrent ingestion of alcohol has been described as contributory and may be accounted for by the well-known intolerance of ethanol during trichloroethylene exposure. The presence of ethanol in the blood also elevates blood trichloroethylene, perhaps because of competitive inhibition between these compounds for mixed function oxidases (Müller et al., 1975). In the usual occupational exposure, however, it would be inaccurate to depict trichloroethylene as a potent hepatotoxin.

Evidence that trichloroethylene is a nephrotoxin was presented by Gutch et al. (1965), who described acute renal failure and toxic myocarditis in a man who had used this solvent in cleaning floors with the rag and bucket technique. Other reports of similar cases are not known. Convincing evidence of hematopoietic damage is also absent.

Sudden death in young workers exposed to trichloroethylene has been described by a number of observers (Kleinfeld and Tabershaw, 1954). In spite of the lack of supporting anatomic information, the inference that these deaths were due to ventricular fibrillation is reasonable. Increased cardiac output in workers exposed to trichloroethylene has been attributed to elevated epinephrine levels. Bradycardia and cardiac muscle conduction abnormalities have been reported in long-term employees of a dry cleaning facility.

Trichloroethylene vapors are mildly irritating to the eyes and upper airways of some individuals. In many cases these subjective complaints disappear with repeated or continuing exposure. Trichloroethylene can act on the skin as a primary irritant or as a sensitizer and, because of its defatting properties, it may aggravate existing eczematous lesions. Open flames and heated surfaces may cause the pyrolysis of this compound to the highly toxic gas, phosgene.

The current permissible exposure limit is 100 ppm for an eight-hour time-weighted average, 200

236

ppm for a ceiling concentration, and 300 ppm for a maximum peak provided that it occurs not oftener than five minutes in any two hours. NIOSH (1973) agreed that the 100 ppm time-weighted average value would protect most workers, but since, in its view, the margin of safety would be small, it further recommended that no worker be exposed to a peak concentration over 150 ppm as measured by a 10-minute sample.

References

Baerg RD, Kimberg DV: Centrilobular hepatic necrosis and acute renal failure in "solvent sniffers." *Ann Intern Med* 1970;73:713–720.

Clearfield HR: Hepatorenal toxicity from sniffing spot remover (trichloroethylene). *Am J Dig Dis* 1970;15:851–856.

Daniel JW: The metabolism of ^{36}Cl-labelled trichloroethylene and tetrachloroethylene in the rat. *Biochem Pharmacol* 1963;12:795–802.

Feldman RG, Mayer RF: Studies of trichloroethylene intoxication in man. *Neurology* 1968;18:309.

Grandjean E, Münchinger R, Turrian V, et al: Investigations into the effects of exposure to trichloroethylene in mechanical engineering. *Br J Ind Med* 1955;12:131–142.

Gubéran E: Proposed biological threshold limit values for industrial exposure to trichloroethylene vapor. *Scand J Work Environ Health* 1977; 3:80–90.

Gutch CF, Tomhave WG, Stevens SC: Acute renal failure due to inhalation of trichlorethylene. *Ann Intern Med* 1965;63:128–134.

Harenko A: Two peculiar instances of psychiatric disturbance in trichloroethylene poisoning. *Acta Neurol Scand* 1967;43(suppl 31): 139–144.

Ikeda M, Ohtsuji H, Imamura T, et al: Urinary excretion of total trichloro-compounds, trichloroethanol, and trichloroacetic acid as a measure of exposure to trichloroethylene and tetrachloroethylene. *Br J Ind Med* 1972;29:328–333.

Kleinfeld M, Tabershaw IR: Trichloroethylene toxicity: Report of five fatal cases. *Arch Ind Hyg Occup Med* 1954;10:134–141.

Müller G, Spassowski M, Henschler D: Metabolism of trichloroethylene in man: II. Pharmacokinetics of metabolites. *Arch Toxicol* 1974; 32:283–295.

Müller G, Spassowski M, Henschler D: Metab-olism of trichloroethylene in man: III. Interaction of trichloroethylene and alcohol. *Arch Toxicol* 1975;33:173–189.

NIOSH: *Criteria for a Recommended Standard . . . . Occupational Exposure to Trichloroethylene.* Washington, DC, National Institute for Occupational Safety and Health (NIOSH 73-11025),1973.

Osol A, Pratt R (eds): *United States Dispensatory,* ed 27. Philadelphia, JB Lippincott, 1973, pp 1209–1210.

Priest RJ, Horn RC: Trichloroethylene intoxication: A case of acute hepatic cirrhosis possibly due to this agent. *Arch Environ Health* 1965; 11:361–365.

Smith GF: Trichlorethylene: A review. *Br J Ind Med* 1966;23:249–262.

Stewart RD, Dodd HC: Absorption of carbon tetrachloride, trichloroethylene, tetrachloroethylene, methylene chloride, and 1,1,1-trichloroethane through the human skin. *Am Ind Hyg Assoc J* 1964;25:439–446.

Stewart RD, Dodd HC, Gay HH, et al: Experimental human exposure to trichloroethylene. *Arch Environ Health* 1970;20:64–71.

Waters EM, Gertsner HB, Huff JE: Trichloroethylene: I. An overview. *J Toxicol Environ Health* 1977;2:671–707.

Tetrachloroethylene   Tetrachloroethylene ($Cl_2C = CCl_2$; tetrachloroethene; perchloroethylene) is the principal commercial dry cleaning solvent for clothing and is commonly used as well in metal degreasing operations. It is also used as a grain fumigant and is a constituent of some veterinary anthelminthics.

The toxicological properties of tetrachloroethylene are similar to those of trichloroethylene. Toxic effects have been most frequently demonstrated in dry cleaning shops with ineffective ventilation or solvent recovery equipment (see for example Saland, 1967; Lukaszewski, 1979). An unfortunate number of cases of fatal central nervous system and respiratory depression has resulted from the use of sleeping bags that had not been thoroughly cleared of the solvent prior to use.

Vapors of tetrachloroethylene are rapidly absorbed through the pulmonary alveolar epithelium and are largely excreted by the same route, with a rapid component succeeded after the first day by a slow exponential component that probably represents a washout of the poorly metabolized stores in fatty tissues (Stewart et al., 1970). Even persons residing near dry cleaning shops have been shown to have appreciable tetrachloroethylene in alveolar air in concentrations that dwindled with distance from the facilities (Verberk and Scheffers, 1980). Absorption may occur through skin but to a minimal extent (Stewart and Dodd, 1964). Some of the absorbed tetrachloroethylene is metabolized to trichloroacetic acid, which can be detected in the urine (Leibman and Ortiz, 1977).

Absorption may cause lightheadedness, confusion, and the entire spectrum of narcotic effects. Careful studies have failed to demonstrate any neurologic or behavioral abnormalities that could be specifically attributed to chronic exposure to perchloroethylene (Stewart et al., 1977). In one study, earlier exposure to Stoddard's solvent seems to have been a factor in some of the abnormal neurologic scores (Tuttle et al., 1977). The vapor may have a direct, mildly irritating effect upon the eyes and upper airway. Direct skin contact with liquid tetrachloroethylene has produced erythema, burns, and vesiculation. The evidence for hepatorenal toxicity is similar to that for trichloroethylene. Stewart (1969) noted abnormal liver function tests after exposure, with SGOT and SGPT levels reaching peaks in about three days. Asymptomatic individuals, who had totally recovered, showed elevated urinary urobilinogen and total serum bilirubin levels seven to 10 days after exposure. Stewart raised the question as to whether acute renal failure, rarely observed in cases of overexposure, may be due to shock after peripheral vascular collapse during deep central nervous system depression.

Exposure is evaluated either by environmental monitoring or by determining the level of solvent in exhaled breath (Stewart et al., 1961). Alveolar breath analysis permits the identification as long as two weeks after exposure, and serial determinations can provide an estimate of the magnitude of the exposure. The current permissible limit for tetrachloroethylene is 100 ppm (678 mg/m³), but NIOSH (1976) has recommended lowering this value to 50 ppm in order to provide a greater margin of safety against eye and airway irritation and to prevent possible neurologic effects.

References

Leibman KC, Ortiz E: Metabolism of halogenated ethylenes. *Environ Health Persp* 1977;21:91–97.

Lukaszewski T: Acute tetrachloroethylene fatality. *Clin Toxicol* 1979;15:411–415.

NIOSH: *Criteria for a Recommended Standard . . . . Occupational Exposure to Tetrachloroethylene (Perchloroethylene)*. Washington, DC, National Institute for Occupational Safety and Health (NIOSH 76-185), 1976.

Saland G: Accidental exposure to perchloroethylene. *NY State J Med* 1969;67:2359–2361.

Stewart RD: Acute tetrachloroethylene intoxication. *J Am Med Assoc* 1969;208:1490–1492.

Stewart RD, Baretta ED, Dodd HC, et al: Experimental human exposure to tetrachloroethylene. *Arch Environ Health* 1970;20:224–229.

Stewart RD, Dodd HC: Absorption of carbon tetrachloride, trichloroethylene, tetrachloroethylene, methyl chloride, and 1,1,1-trichloroethane through the human skin. *Am Ind Hyg Assoc J* 1964;25:439–446.

Stewart RD, Gay HH, Erley DS, et al: Human exposure to tetrachloroethylene vapor. *Arch Environ Health* 1961;2:516–522.

Stewart RD, Hake CL, Wu A, et al: *Effects of Perchloroethylene/Drug Interaction on Behavior and Neurological Function*. Cincinnati, National Institute for Occupational Safety and Health (NIOSH 77-191), 1977.

Tuttle TC, Wood GD, Grether CB: *A Behavioral and Neurological Evaluation of Dry Cleaners Exposed to Perchloroethylene*. Cincinnati, National Institute for Occupational Safety and Health (NIOSH 77-214), 1977.

Verberk MM, Scheffers TML: Tetrachloroethylene in exhaled air of residents near dry cleaning shops. *Environ Res* 1980;21:432–437.

Other Aliphatic Chlorohydrocarbons

Allyl chloride   Allyl chloride ($H_2C = CCH_2Cl$; 3-chloropropene) is a liquid with a pungent odor that is used in glycerol production and as an intermediate in the chemical industry. Its principal derivative is epichlorhydrin, which in turn is used in the manufacture of epoxy resins. Results of inhalation studies with animals suggest that it may be hepato- and nephro-toxic at levels of exposure as low as 8 ppm (Torkelson et al., 1959). Exposure at higher concentrations resulted in extensive lung and kidney damage (Adams et al., 1940). Occupational experience with allyl chloride has been limited but NIOSH (1976) has collected evidence of eye irritation at 50 to 100 ppm and nasal irritation and airway discomfort at less than 25 ppm.

238

Skin contact produces persistent deepseated pain.

The permissible exposure limit is 1 ppm (= 3 mg/m³) for a 10-hour workday, 40-hour work-week. NIOSH (1976) also suggested a ceiling concentration of 3 ppm for any 15-minute sampling period. Periodic examinations of employees should include pulmonary and liver function tests.

References

Adams EM, Spencer HC, Irish DD: The acute vapor toxicity of allyl chloride. *J Ind Hyg Toxicol* 1940;22:79–86.

NIOSH: *Criteria for a Recommended Standard . . . . Occupational Exposure to Allyl Chloride.* Washington, DC, National Institute for Occupational Safety and Health (NIOSH 76-204), 1976.

Torkelson TR, Wolf MA, Oyen F, et al: Vapor toxicity of allyl chloride as determined on laboratory animals. *Am Ind Hyg Assoc J* 1959;20: 217–223.

Epichlorohydrin   Epichlorohydrin (C_3H_5OCl; 1-chloro-2,3-epoxypropane; 2-chloropropylene oxide), a colorless liquid with a distinctive odor at room temperatures, is a reactive molecule that has uses as an alkylating agent and that forms stable cross-linkage bonds such as those in epoxy resins. It is used in the manufacture of synthetic glycerin, epoxy resins, surface active agents, agricultural chemicals, pharmaceuticals, coatings, adhesives, solvents, plasticizers, and many other products (NIOSH, 1976).

Epichlorohydrin is highly irritating and can produce severe burns, especially since it penetrates leather and rubber, and vapors at 20 ppm lead to burning sensations of the eyes and nose. There have been no reports of serious pulmonary or systemic injury in man. However, because this compound can cause renal damage in experimental animals, persons handling epichlorohydrin should be under surveillance (Gage, 1959). Additional caution is indicated by the findings that epichlorohydrin is mutagenic for bacteria and *Drosophila*, and may be carcinogenic for mice when it is injected subcutaneously (Van Duuren et al., 1974).

The permissible exposure limit for workplace air is 5 ppm (19 mg/m³), but NIOSH (1976) has recommended a more stringent standard of 0.5 ppm (2 mg/m³) for up to a 10-hour workday, 40-hour workweek, with a ceiling concentration of 5 ppm determined by a 15-minute sample.

References

Gage JC: The toxicity of epichlorhydrin vapour. *Br J Ind Med* 1959;16:11–14.

NIOSH: *Criteria for a Recommended Standard . . . . Occupational Exposure to Epichlorohydrin.* Washington, DC, National Institute for Occupational Safety and Health (NIOSH 76-206), 1976.

Van Duuren BL, Goldschmidt BM, Katz C, et al: Carcinogenic activity of alkylating agents. *J Nat Cancer Inst* 1974;53:695–700.

Chlorinated paraffins   This group of compounds is derived from *n*-paraffins that contain between 10 and 30 carbon atoms and that are variously chlorinated to between 40% and 70% by weight. They are used as plasticizers, additives for cutting oils and fire retardants, and in paints and electrical insulators. There are no reports of adverse effects of exposure in industry or in studies with animals, and they appear to be relatively safe compounds to work with (Birtley et al., 1980).

Reference

Birtley RDN, Conning DM, Daniel JW, et al: The toxicological effect of chlorinated paraffins in mammals. *Toxicol Appl Pharmacol* 1980;54: 514–525.

Aromatic Chlorohydrocarbons

Chlorinated biphenyls and chlorinated naphthalenes   Chlorinated biphenyls (polychlorinated biphenyls; PCBs) and chlorinated naphthalenes are prepared from biphenyl and naphthalene that are reacted to varying degrees with chlorine to produce a number of compounds designated by a variety of trade names. These compounds vary from oily liquids to waxy or hard solids. Because of their chemical stability, nonflammability, and high dielectric constants, they are widely used as insulating coolants in electrical transformers, capacitors, and electromagnets. They are also used for coatings such as paints, plastics, and varnishes, and in high pressure lubricants that are subject to oxidizing conditions, high temperatures, or submersion. Heat transfer media may also contain compounds of this type as may certain cutting fluid additives and carbonless copy paper systems.

The compounds found in industry are usually mixtures of specific molecules, and the commercial product is often described in terms of the relative proportion of chlorine. High degrees of chlorination are generally associated with higher toxicities. Since the toxicologic properties of the chlorinated biphenyls and chlorinated naphthalenes are not notably dissimilar, mixtures are considered to have biological properties that are common to the components.

Polychlorinated biphenyls are readily absorbed, but they are poorly metabolized, and they consequently accumulate in tissues. Chlorinated biphenyls and chlorinated naphthalenes, along with chlorobenzodioxins, chlorodibenzofurans, and chloroazobenzenes, are potent inducers of chloracne, which may develop after weeks or months of cutaneous exposure. Lesions appear first lateral to the eyebrows and then on the chin, cheeks, forehead, arms, chest, abdomen, thighs, or buttocks. A prior history of acne vulgaris is not necessary but direct local contact with the compounds over a period of time will be evident in the lesions that are primarily papules and yellowish cysts surrounded by mild erythema. Comedones, a common feature of acne vulgaris and oil folliculitis, are usually absent, as is melanosis. Pruritis is common. Chloracne, known among workers as "cable rash," is the clinical manifestation of a specific effect of these compounds on the pilosebaceous unit. The differentiation of sebaceous gland cells is altered so that keratinocytes form to plug the unit and create keratin-containing cysts.

The therapy of chloracne is based upon cessation of exposure to the offending materials and application of the dermatologic measures commonly used to control acne. Prevention by the use of protective clothing, showers, and appropriate clean clothing and lockers is necessary. Barrier creams have been of little, if any, utility in the control of chloracne.

When compounds of this group are used in poorly ventilated areas and especially when heat is applied, such as in welding and cable splicing, there may be significant systemic absorption of toxic vapors. The target organ is primarily the liver and cases of fatal acute yellow atrophy have occurred (Drinker et al., 1937). The biochemical mechanism of this toxic effect is not understood.

Workers who are exposed to these compounds, especially to the more highly chlorinated ones and particularly when volatilizing temperatures are encountered, should be monitored with periodic liver function tests. Elevation of serum triglycerides in sewage plant workers exposed to PCB-contaminated sludge suggests that these compounds may alter lipid metabolism at subclinical levels (Baker et al., 1980).

Their stability has led to environmental dissemination of the chlorinated biphenyls, and the presence of these materials in plant and animal tissues has become a matter of great international concern, particularly since these compounds have entered the food chain of higher animals (Kolbye, 1972). More than half of the people in the United States are now thought to contain levels of PCBs in their bodies in excess of 1 ppm (Price and Welch, 1972; Yobs, 1972). While the full significance of this contamination is yet to be established, clinical experience with toxic exposures of nonoccupational origin emphasizes the basis for concern. In 1968 an epidemic of "Yusho" ("rice oil disease") occurred in Japan and resulted from the contamination of rice bran oil with polychlorinated biphenyls. The disease was marked by swelling of the upper eyelids, meibomian gland discharges, chloracne, hyperpigmentation of the skin, nails, and mucous membranes, and nonspecific digestive and neurologic symptoms (Kuratsune et al., 1972). Recovery from "Yusho" has been slow, and the disorder, which has affected over 1000 persons, has been a major medical and social problem in several prefectures in western Japan.

Compounds of this group have also been associated with systemic disease in cattle and poultry. The extent to which these disease phenomena in man and animals may be due to substances other than polychlorinated biphenyls and naphthalenes that may be present as contaminants remains to be established (Kimbrough, 1972). Such contaminants that have come under suspicion include tetrachlorodibenzofurans and tetrachlorodibenzodioxins. Adverse reproductive effects have been noted in birds, mink, and monkeys, and fatty degeneration of the liver and hepatocellular carcinomas have been found in laboratory rats and mice (Lloyd et al., 1976).

The current permissible exposure limits for PCB vapors are 1 mg/m^3 for mixtures containing 42% chlorine and 0.5 mg/m^3 for mixtures containing 54% chlorine, determined as time-weighted averages for 8-hour workdays. NIOSH

(1977) has recommended that the TWA concentrations in the breathing zones of workers be maintained at or below the minimally detectable concentration of 1 $\mu g/m^3$ because of potential liver damage, adverse reproductive effects, and carcinogenicity.

References

Baker EL Jr, Landrigan PJ, Glueck CJ, et al: Metabolic consequences of exposure to polychlorinated biphenyls (PCB) in sewage sludge. *Am J Epidemiol* 1980;112:553-563.

Drinker CK, Warren MF, Bennett GA: The problem of possible systemic effects from certain chlorinated hydrocarbons. *J Ind Hyg Toxicol* 1937;19:283-311.

Kimbrough RD: Toxicity of chlorinated hydrocarbons and related compounds. *Arch Environ Health* 1972;25:125-131.

Kolbye AC: Food exposures to polychlorinated biphenyls. *Environ Health Persp* 1972;1:85-88.

Kuratsune M, Yoshimura T, Matsuzaka J, et al: Epidemiologic study on Yusho, a poisoning caused by ingestion of rice oil contaminated with a commercial brand of polychlorinated biphenyls. *Environ Health Persp* 1972;1:119-128.

Lloyd JW, Moore RM JR, Woolf BS, et al: Polychlorinated biphenyls. *J Occup Med* 1976;18:109-113.

NIOSH: *Criteria for a Recommended Standard . . . . Occupational Exposure to Polychlorinated Biphenyls* (PCBs). Washington, DC, National Institute for Occupational Safety and Health (NIOSH 77-225), 1977.

Price HA, Welch RL: Occurrence of polychlorinated biphenyls in humans. *Environ Health Persp* 1972;1:73-78.

Yobs AR: Levels of polychlorinated biphenyls in adipose tissue of the general population of the nation. *Environ Health Persp* 1972;1:79-81.

Paradichlorobenzene   Paradichlorobenzene in the form of white or colorless crystals or compressed cakes is commonly available as a "moth-proofing" material to protect woolen garments. Naphthalene, a less effective but strongly aromatic compound, has also been used for this purpose but has been largely superseded. At high concentrations, the vapors of paradichlorobenzene are strongly irritating to the eyes and upper airway, a property that serves to limit exposure to high concentrations of this volatile compound. There is evidence of hepatic and renal injury in experimental animals, but similar effects in humans have not been documented. Cataracts, attributed in rare instances to "moth-proofing" materials, are probably better related to naphthalene than to paradichlorobenzene. One case of aplastic anemia has been reported in a resale clothing shop worker who had an acute, severe exposure to both paradichlorobenzene and naphthalene (Harden and Baetjer, 1978). The permissible exposure limit for paradichlorobenzene is 75 ppm (450 mg/m³).

Reference

Harden RA, Baetjer AM: Aplastic anemia following exposure to paradichlorobenzene and naphthalene. *J Occup Med* 1978;20:820-822.

7 • Other Halogenated Hydrocarbons

The vast majority of industrial halogenated hydrocarbons are those that contain chlorine, usually without, but occasionally with, other halogen constituents. Fluorinated compounds are found in a relatively small number of specific materials, although the growth of the fluoro-organic chemical industry has been impressive. Industrial bromine-containing organic compounds are even less common, and the iodine derivatives are rare.

Fluorohydrocarbons

Those fluorine-containing hydrocarbons that have industrial and commercial applications include the simple compounds that often contain chlorine and bromine as well as those that are formed into a variety of polymers. The former are used as refrigerants, fire extinguishants, solvents for special or critical applications, and, until recently, as propellants in aerosol "bombs" or can dispensers. Recent concern over the possible action of chlorofluorocarbons in depleting the stratospheric ozone layer that filters the ultraviolet radiation reaching the earth has led to moves to prohibit the use of these chlorofluoroalkanes as propellants in self-pressurized containers.

As a group these compounds have been thought to lack biological properties or to have mild, reversible corticodepressive effects on the central nervous system. Halothane ($CF_3CHClBr$) has been used as an inhalation anesthetic agent since 1954. The fluoroalkanes are not pulmonary irritants, and they diffuse readily through cell membranes, including pulmonary alveoli, because of their lipid solubility (Back and Van Stee, 1977). A number of investigators have drawn attention to the cardiotoxic effects, manifested as arrhythmias, that are associated with pulmonary exposure to fluoro-carbons, especially trichlorofluoromethane (fluorocarbon 11), dichloromonofluoromethane (fluorocarbon 21), and trichlorotrifluoroethane (fluorocarbon 113). Sensitization of the heart to epinephrine is implicated in most of the arrhythmias (Reinhardt et al., 1971) but the process is incompletely understood. Sudden death from aerosol propellant "sniffing" may be explained by this mechanism (Bass, 1970). In experimental animals, variable degrees of cardiodynamic effects that include tachycardia, myocardial depression, and hypotension have been described.

Polymerized fluoroethylene and fluorochloro-compounds that are used in plastics are described in that section. Low molecular weight organofluorine compounds that decompose or may be metabolized to monofluoroacetic acid have a specific inhibitory effect on the tricarboxylic acid cycle and may be extremely toxic.

Workers exposed to fluorochemicals may have higher than normal levels of blood organic fluorine, but no ill effects of this exposure have been detected (Ubel et al., 1980). Another study of 50 workers exposed to trichlorotrifluoroethane at levels from 46 to 4700 ppm at the Kennedy Space Center similarly failed to reveal complaints or adverse clinical findings, except for one case of dry skin (Imbus and Adkins, 1972). However, repeated episodes of severe cardiac palpitation were reported in surgical pathology residents exposed to monochlorodifluoromethane (fluorocarbon 22) in the preparation of frozen sections. Electrocardiograms of these physicians showed premature beats of atrial and ventricular origin, and atrial fibrillation (Speizer et al., 1975).

References

Back KC, Van Stee EW: Toxicology of haloalkane propellants and fire extinguishants. *Ann Rev Pharmacol Toxicol* 1977;17:83–95.

Bass M: Sudden sniffing death. *J Am Med Assoc* 1970;212:2075–2079.

Imbus HR, Adkins C: Physical examinations of workers exposed to trichlorotrifluoroethane. *Arch Environ Health* 1972;24:257–261.

Speizer FE, Wegman DH, Ramirez A: Palpitation rates associated with fluorocarbon exposure in a hospital setting. *N Engl J Med* 1975;292: 624–626.

Ubel FA, Sorenson FD, Roach DE: Health status of plant workers exposed to fluorochemicals—A preliminary report. *Am Ind Hyg Assoc J* 1980;41:584–589.

Brominated Hydrocarbons

Methyl bromide Methyl bromide (CH_3Br; bromomethane) is a heavy colorless gas that has a chloroform-like odor at high concentrations. It is used in fumigating warehouses, homes, grain stores, the soil, and enclosed areas or spaces that can be sealed off with impervious plastic sheeting. Since the gas has a density over three times that of air, it tends to collect in low places. It penetrates easily into bales or sacks of material and is, therefore, a highly effective nonresidual pesticidal material. It also penetrates rubber and adhesive tape readily. The gas is highly toxic to man and has most commonly caused injury among fumigators and others who enter structures while the gas is still present prior to adequate posttreatment ventilation. The compound has also been involved in occupational accidents in the course of its use as a methylating agent in chemical synthesis operations and as a fire extinguisher in special or now obsolete appliances. Methyl bromide was formerly used as a refrigerant gas but it has now been superseded for this purpose by ammonia or the fluorohydrocarbons.

At lower concentrations, the gas gives no warning, and those that use it are well-advised to have suitable monitoring instruments and thoroughly tested personal protective equipment (Rathus and Landy, 1961). Methyl bromide is readily absorbed through the lungs. Transcutaneous absorption may also occur (Longley and Jones, 1965), but it is not ordinarily of significance in occupational poisoning.

Acute exposure to excessive concentrations of methyl bromide produces headache, nausea, and vomiting. The gas is a delayed lung irritant and it can produce bronchitis, pneumonitis, and pulmonary edema that may proceed to death. At lower concentrations, neurologic effects are more common, are often severe, and are frequently characterized by a prolonged clinical course. Such effects may be delayed in onset by a latent period that follows the termination of exposure by hours or even days, the delay possibly determined by the amount inhaled. In cases of mild exposure, neurologic phenomena may consist of giddiness, ataxia, vertigo, diplopia, paresthesias, weakness, and behavioral and emotional disturbances. Twitchings, tremors, and epileptic seizures may occur, the latter frequently of the Jacksonian type. More severe episodes are associated with status epilepticus, prolonged loss of consciousness, and pyramidal and extrapyramidal signs (Rathus and Landy, 1961). The presenting symptoms of confusion, irritability, drowsiness, and uncooperativeness may be misinterpreted as a psychosis (Zatuchni and Hong, 1981). In children, the combination of encephalopathy and hepatomegaly may lead physicians to suspect Reye syndrome (Shield et al., 1977). The neurologic manifestations may be very slow to resolve, and ataxia and seizures may persist for months or years. In some cases, a fatal outcome or permanent neurologic or psychiatric impairment may result.

Neurologic reactions occur at levels of exposure that are insufficient to produce acute or delayed pulmonary manifestations. The biochemical and physiological bases for methyl bromide poisoning are not understood, although there has been speculation that the clinical manifestations represent an unusual form of bromidism in which the action of inorganic bromide is related to hydrolysis of the organic compound after it has been distributed. Irish et al. (1941) suggested, however, that the effects were due to the alkyl halide molecule and not to hydrolysis products, while Lewis (1948) and Rathus and Landy (1961) concluded that methyl bromide attaches itself to sulfhydryl groups in proteins to produce irreversible changes in the brain and elsewhere.

Apart from indicated supportive treatment for pulmonary edema and epileptic seizures, specific antidotal attempts that have had some success include dimercaprol (BAL) (Rathus and Landy, 1961) and acetylcysteine (Zatuchni and Hong, 1981).

Splashes of liquid methyl bromide on the skin may produce a freezing sensation. Repeated splashes or prolonged exposure may lead to superficial burns with vesicle formation, and erythema and swelling of the surrounding skin (Butler et al., 1945). Vapors that become absorbed to clothing and shoes represent a relatively potent source of skin contact. Direct contamination of shoes may cause severe burns (Clarke et al., 1945).

The permissible exposure limit for methyl bromide is 20 ppm (80 mg/m³).

References

Butler ECB, Perry KMA, Williams JRF: Methyl bromide burns. *Br J Ind Med* 1945;2: 30–31.

Clarke CA, Roworth CG, Holling HE: Methyl bromide poisoning. *Br J Ind Med* 1945;2:17–23.

Irish DD, Adams EM, Spencer HC, et al: Chemical changes of methyl bromide in the animal body in relation to its physiological effects. *J Ind Hyg Toxicol* 1941;23:408–411.

Lewis SE: Inhibition of SH enzymes of methyl bromide. *Nature* 1948;161:692–693.

Longley EO, Jones AT: Methyl bromide poisoning in man. *Ind Med Surg* 1965;34: 499–502.

Rathus EM, Landy PJ: Methyl bromide poisoning. *Br J Ind Med* 1961;18:53–57.

Shield LK, Coleman TL, Markesbery WR: Methyl bromide intoxication: Neurologic features, including simulation of Reye syndrome. *Neurology* 1977;27:959–962.

Zatuchni J, Hong K: Methyl bromide poisoning seen initially as psychosis. *Arch Neurol* 1981;38:529–530.

Ethylene dibromide Ethylene dibromide ($BrCH_2CH_2Br$; 1,2-dibromoethane) is a scavenger for lead in antiknock additives for gasolines. It is also used as a grain and citrus fumigant, fire extinguishant, solvent, gauge fluid, and as an ingredient in many pesticides. Occupational medical experience with this compound is limited, but it is a severe skin irritant and vesicant and is a central nervous system depressant. Ethylene dibromide has a low vapor pressure, a property that tends to limit air levels. However, it is known to penetrate a variety of materials used in protective clothing, including natural rubber and neoprene, and these items should be discarded immediately after they become contaminated (Sansone and Tewari, 1978). Inhalation by workers has led to severe eye and throat irritation, headache, depression, and loss of appetite.

Rats and mice given ethylene dibromide by gavage have developed squamous cell carcinomas of the forestomach (Olson et al., 1973; Powers et al., 1975). For this reason, as well as the finding of the mutagenicity of this compound for bacteria, plants, fruit flies, and mammalian cell cultures, NIOSH (1977) has recommended that occupational exposure not exceed 1.0 ppm (0.13 mg/m³) as a ceiling determined by a 15-minute sample. The current exposure limit is 20 ppm (154 mg/m³).

References

NIOSH: *Criteria for a Recommended Standard . . . . Occupational Exposure to Ethylene Dibromide.* Washington, DC, National Institute for Occupational Safety and Health (NIOSH 77-221), 1977.

Olson WA, Habermann RT, Weisburger EK, et al: Induction of stomach cancer in rats and mice by halogenated aliphatic fumigants. *J Nat Cancer Inst* 1973;31:1993–1995.

Powers MB, Voelker RW, Page NP, et al: Carcinogenicity of ethylene dibromide (EDB) and 1,2-dibromo-3-chloropropane (DBCP) after oral administration in rats and mice. *Toxicol Appl Pharmacol* 1975;33:171–172.

Sansone EB, Tewari YB: Penetration of protective clothing by 1,2-dibromo-3-chloropropane, ethylene dibromide, and acrylonitrile. *Am Ind Hyg Assoc J* 1978;39:921–922.

Acetylene tetrabromide Acetylene tetrabromide ($CHBr_2CHBr_2$; 1,1,2,2-tetrabromoethane) is a very dense organic compound used as an ore flotation agent and as a gauge fluid. It is a central nervous system depressant but since it has a very low vapor pressure at ambient temperatures, clinical problems are not generally anticipated. The permissible exposure limit is 1 ppm (14 mg/m³).

Polybrominated biphenyls Polybrominated biphenyls (PBBs) and their oxides (PBBOs) have had industrial applications as fire retardants. They may contain from four to seven or more bromine atoms per molecule, but the hexabromobiphenyl compound appears to be the most commonly used. Since these compounds are highly lipotropic and are not readily metabolized, they accumulate in adipose tissues when absorbed.

Polybrominated biphenyls attracted public attention in 1973 when they were accidentally substituted for magnesium oxide in the preparation of a special feed supplement for lactating

244

cows in Michigan. Toxic effects that included swelling of the joints, persistent mastitis, subcutaneous abscess formation, wasting, and death involved many dairy herds (Jackson and Halbert, 1974), and swine and poultry stocks were also adversely affected. Although thousands of cattle and 1.5 million chickens were destroyed, meat and daily products containing PBB were widely consumed in Michigan (Bekesi et al., 1978). These compounds were subsequently found in the serum and adipose tissues of quarantined dairy farm families, and to a lesser extent in other persons in Michigan (Budd et al., 1978). The situation with respect to humans has engendered considerable controversy, for some investigators have maintained that there has been no clinical confirmation of PBB as an etiological agent in human disease (Kay, 1977) despite anecdotal reports of symptoms. On the other hand, there have been more recent reports of abnormal lymphocytes in Michigan dairy farmers not correlated with plasma PBB levels, (Bekesi et al., 1978) and an increased prevalence of hypothyroidism in a group of workers at a PBB chemical manufacturing plant (Bahn et al., 1980). Ongoing studies of exposed persons in Michigan is planned by state and federal agencies for at least another 10 to 15 years.

References

Bahn AK, Mills JL, Snyder PJ, et al: Hypothyroidism in workers exposed to polybrominated biphenyls. *N Engl J Med* 1980;302: 31–33.

Bekesi JG, Holland JF, Anderson HA, et al: Lymphocyte function of Michigan dairy farmers exposed to polybrominated biphenyls. *Science* 1978;199:1207–1209.

Budd ML, Hayner NS, Humphrey HEB, et al: Polybrominated biphenyl exposure—Michigan. *Morbidity Mortality Weekly Rep* 1978;27:115–121.

Jackson TF, Halbert FL: A toxic syndrome associated with the feeding of polybrominated biphenyl-contaminated protein concentrate to dairy cattle. *J Am Vet Med Assoc* 1974;165: 437–439.

Kay K: Polybrominated biphenyls (PBB) environmental contamination in Michigan, 1973–1976. *Environ Res* 1977;13:74–93.

8 • *Aromatic Hydrocarbons*

The aromatic series of compounds is based upon benzene and molecules that incorporate one or more benzene rings. Many of the most common members of the series were obtained initially from the distillation of coal in the coking process. The industrial demand for benzene regularly exceeded the supply available from coal carbonization by the early 1950s, and an increasing proportion of the aromatic compounds is now derived from petroleum materials. At the present time the petrochemical industry is the major source of aromatic compounds. Both coal- and petroleum-derived aromatics are produced in ways that lead to complicated mixtures of many compounds in the series. Accordingly, crude distillates and unpurified commercial products may contain substances not indicated on the label, which often reflects only the principal constituents. Minor ingredients in industrial or technical grade solvents distributed without adequate warning have been, however, important causes of toxic reactions.

Benzene

Benzene, the parent member of the series, has been the most significant from the toxicological point of view. In many instances of intoxication the compound responsible for the disease has not been identified as benzene, although hazardous amounts of this compound have been present in technical grade "toluene" or other solvent mixes. The European practice of using crude benzene to improve the antiknock properties of gasolines was utilized in the United States until about 1950 and led to cases of benzene intoxication in persons using this blended motor fuel for solvent purposes. Motor fuels in this country still have small amounts (less than 2%) of benzene (Runion, 1977), while the amounts in Europe range from 4% to 8% (Brief et al., 1980).

Although benzene continues to be an important solvent, over 90% of benzene production goes into the synthesis of other organic compounds, such as polymers, detergents, pesticides, and intermediates in chemical and pharmaceutical manufacture. It is also used in the preparation of chlorinated solvents, in the making of printing inks, and as a degreaser and cleaning agent. Benzene is the primary raw material for styrene used in synthetic rubber, for nylon intermediates, for phenol, and for synthetic detergents. Solvent benzene used in rubber cements and paint strippers have been a frequent cause of injury inasmuch as these materials have been used often under hazardous circumstances by people unaware of the presence or properties of this compound. Benzene used in laboratory extractions and in chromatographic separations is often done so under hazardous conditions.

A lack of precision in terminology is a serious problem in recognizing benzene hazards. There has been confusion with the term "benzine," which is a low-boiling petroleum fraction of predominantly aliphatic compounds and is similar to ordinary gasoline. Benzine, if uncontaminated with benzene, does not have the hematopoietic effects characteristic of chronic benzene poisoning. The term "benzol," which has been gradually losing in popularity, has usually been associated with crude aromatic mixtures, predominantly benzene. In cases of suspected benzene poisoning or when effective health conservation measures are to be applied, it is urgent to learn, by chemical analysis if necessary, whether or not benzene is present and, if so, in what concentration. Since usage in industry varies at different periods as a result of costs and technical needs, it may be necessary to repeat benzene assays at intervals.

Metabolism Benzene enters the body primarily by inhalation and only rarely by percutaneous absorption unless liquid benzene is in direct contact with the skin. Diffusion from lungs to blood occurs rapidly and, because of its solvent properties, benzene accumulates in fatty tissue such as bone marrow, central nervous system, and fat deposits. Cessation of exposure results in elimination by pulmonary exhalation and by enzymatic action in the liver. Benzene metabolites in the urine consist primarily of phenol along with hydroquinone, pyrocatechol, and phenyl mercapturic acid. Although total phenol excretion in the urine has been used for many years to monitor exposure to benzene, Fishbeck et al. (1975) have shown that two common over-the-counter medications that contain phenyl salicylate can elevate urine phenol values to levels in excess of 75 mg/L (=ppm) without any exposure to benzene.

Toxic effects Like most organic solvents, benzene is a central nervous system depressant at high concentrations and may cause acute narcotic reactions. These are nonspecific and may extend, depending on the extent of exposure, from mild manifestations such as lightheadedness, headache, and excitement to more severe problems such as respiratory paralysis and death with or without convulsions. A pattern of apparent drunken behavior due to benzene has been called "benzol jag" by industrial workers and consists of euphoria, unsteady gait, and confusion. Other effects resulting from inhalation of low concentrations of benzene include drowsiness, vertigo, headache, and nausea. Recovery from acute benzene narcosis is complete unless the levels and duration of exposure produce pathologic changes.

Chronic benzene poisoning is of far greater toxicologic significance. In most cases, chronic benzene poisoning has followed repeated exposures to unsafe air levels of benzene vapor over the course of months or years. Its incidence has been gradually decreasing over recent years with improvement of industrial hygiene measures and a thoughtful and effective search for technically satisfactory and less toxic benzene substitutes. Chronic intoxication is characterized primarily by a disturbance of the hematopoietic system that can affect every cell line. The clinical picture may vary from person to person. It is often not possible to establish a firm relationship between the character of the benzene exposure and the disease.

The view that women are more susceptible than men and that the young are more vulnerable than older persons is traditional but not well supported by sound epidemiological data, although this sex difference has been observed in laboratory animals (Ikeda, 1964). While the anemia characteristic of women due to demands on the bone marrow by menstruation and pregnancy may make them more vulnerable to benzene, Sato and his colleagues (1975) have shown that benzene elimination is in fact slower in human females than in males. These investigators attributed this phenomenon to the greater amounts of body fat in women, as well as in female rats, and the high affinity of fatty tissues for benzene, toluene, and other organic solvents.

Clinical manifestations of chronic benzene poisoning tend to be insidious in onset, and most recorded cases have been well advanced at the time of diagnosis (Hunter, 1939; Mallory et al., 1939). Classical signs of major hematopoietic injury, such as purpura and overwhelming agranulocytosis, are rarely noted in the more recent literature, however. The more common initial findings tend to be nonspecific and include fatigue, loss of appetite, headache, and nausea. Hematologic evaluation may show anemia, leukopenia, thrombocytopenia, or a pancytopenia, although all three cell lines are not always affected or involved to the same degree. Immature cells may be found in the peripheral blood, and there may be an eosinophilia or leukocytosis. The bone marrow may be hypoplastic, hyperplastic, or relatively unchanged. These findings do not correlate well with the clinical picture, the character of the exposure, or the prognosis. In some workers with chronic benzene poisoning there may be evidence for shortened red cell survival or for extramedullary hematopoiesis. From the clinical point of view, idiopathic aplastic anemia and bone marrow failure due to benzene cannot be distinguished from each other.

In addition to frequently producing fatal aplastic anemia, chronic benzene exposures of sufficient severity may eventuate in acute and chronic leukemias that can appear with or without an antecedent history of aplastic anemia (Vigliani and Saita, 1964; Vigliani and Forni, 1976). The conversion of aplastic anemia to leukemia is not uncommon in cases in which the cause of the anemia is not known. Chronic myelogenous leukemia appears to be the most common type associated with benzene exposures, but acute myelogenous and acute and chronic lymphocytic varieties have been reported as well (Aksoy et al., 1976; Infante et al., 1977). Erythroleukemia with prominent proliferation of the erythroblastic elements of the marrow has also been associated with benzene exposure (Rozman et al., 1968). On the other hand, Rushton and Alderson (1981) concluded from their study of refinery workers that there was no overall excess of leukemia deaths in comparison with national rates in the United Kingdom, and that if there were an increased risk of leukemia from benzene exposure, it could only have affected a very small proportion of men in the refinery work force. This conclusion is consistent with the summary by Brief et al. (1980) that no increase in leukemia incidence has been noted in workers in largely outdoor situations such as the petrochemical industries, while increased incidence of this group of diseases has been reported among workers in industries such as shoemaking and rubber manufacture where exposure to benzene and other solvents occurred indoors and in unventilated situations.

Interest in lymphocyte cultures and chromosome aberrations over the last two decades has led to their use in studies of benzene-exposed individuals (Tough and Court Brown, 1965; Forni et al., 1971a, 1971b, Picciano, 1979). Abnormal chromosome patterns have been demonstrated among former benzene workers with no exposure for over two years. This approach may ultimately shed light on the nature of the long latent periods that have been described in persons without exposure for many years but who eventually develop aplastic anemia or leukemia.

Aksoy (1980) has recently suggested that other serious diseases of the hematopoietic system, such as malignant lymphoma, multiple myeloma, paroxysmal nocturnal hemoglobinuria, and myeloid metaplasia, may also result from chronic occupational exposure to benzene, and that perhaps even bronchiogenic carcinoma may have been a consequence of such exposures. Teratological and other fetotoxic effects that have been noted in laboratory animals, reported for example by Green et al. (1978) and by Kuna and Kapp (1981), raise the question of possible effects, hitherto undetected in humans, of benzene exposure in relation to reproductive risks.

Therapy and control   Therapy for chronic benzene poisoning manifested either as aplastic anemia or as leukemia is the same as that used when these diseases occur without known cause.

The prevention of acute and chronic benzene poisoning is based upon control of levels of benzene in air. Convenient survey detector tubes and other instruments are available for measuring benzene in ambient atmospheres. The permissible exposure limit for benzene has dropped repeatedly in the last several decades (Zenz, 1978), and is now set at a concentration of 10 ppm (32 mg/m³) TWA for an eight-hour workday and a 40-hour workweek. For a 15-minute exposure the ceiling value is 25 ppm (80 mg/m³), and the peak permissible exposure is set at 50 ppm.

It is also possible to measure metabolites of benzene in the urine of workers and thereby establish an estimate of exposure. The urinary sulfate ratio has been used for years to express the portion of urinary sulfate that is present in ionic form, normally at least 80% (Elkins, 1959). In excessive benzene exposure, the excretion of phenol sulfate increases so that the proportion of inorganic sulfate drops to less than 80%. Other organic sulfates of nonoccupational origin, such as from the ingestion of bananas, smoked fish or meats, or phenolic drugs, may distort the estimate of benzene exposure derived by this method.

Phenol concentrations in the urine can also be determined, the normal range being 20 to 30 mg/L (Docter and Zielhuis, 1967), less than 20 mg/L (Lauwerys, 1976), or about 10 mg/L (Piotrowski, 1977). Again, these values will be affected by the ingestion of salicylates or ethanol, and by skin applications of phenol-containing topical preparations.

Direct measurement of benzene in exhaled air may be a more reliable test for benzene exposure: an eight-hour exposure to 10 ppm should give a level of 0.12 ppm in expired air 16 hours after exposure has ceased (Brief et al., 1980). Berlin and his co-workers (1980) have taken a more stringent view and have suggested that control measures be instituted when a morning breath sample has a benzene concentration that exceeds 10 ppb (0.01 ppm).

References

Aksoy M: Different types of malignancies due to occupational exposure to benzene: A review of recent observations in Turkey. *Environ Res* 1980; 23:181–190.

Aksoy M, Erdem S, Dinçol G: Types of leukemia in chronic benzene poisoning. A study in thirty-four patients. *Acta Haemat* 1976;55:65–72.

Berlin M, Gage JC, Gullberg B, et al: Breath concentration as an index of the health risk from benzene. Studies on the accumulation and

248

clearance of inhaled benzene. *Scand J Work Environ Health* 1980;6:104–111.

Brief RS, Lynch J, Bernath T, et al: Benzene in the workplace. *Am Ind Hyg Assoc J* 1980;41:616–623.

Docter HJ, Zielhuis RL: Phenol excretion as a measure of benzene exposure. *Ann Occup Hyg* 1967;10:317–326.

Elkins HB: *The Chemistry of Industrial Toxicology,* ed 2. New York, John Wiley and Sons, 1959.

Fishbeck WA, Langner RR, Kociba RJ: Elevated urinary phenol levels not related to benzene exposure. *Am Ind Hyg Assoc J* 1975;36:820–824.

Forni AM, Cappellini A, Pacifico E, et al: Chromosome changes and their evolution in subjects with past exposure to benzene. *Arch Environ Health* 1971a;23:385–391.

Forni A, Pacifico E, Limonta A: Chromosome studies in workers exposed to benzene or toluene or both. *Arch Environ Health* 1971b;22:373–378.

Green JD, Leong BKJ, Laskin S: Inhaled benzene fetotoxicity in rats. *Toxicol Appl Pharmacol* 1978;46:9–18.

Hunter FT: Chronic exposure to benzene (benzol). II. The clinical effects. *J Ind Hyg Toxicol* 1939;21:331–354.

Ikeda M: Enzymatic studies on benzene intoxication. *J Biochem (Tokyo)* 1964;55:231–243.

Infante PF, Wagoner JK, Rinsky RA, et al: Leukaemia in benzene workers. *Lancet* 1977;2:76–78.

Kuna RA, Kapp RW Jr: The embryotoxic/teratogenic potential of benzene vapor in rats. *Toxicol Appl Pharmacol* 1981;57:1–7.

Lauwerys R: Review of the biological monitoring methods for evaluating exposure to benzene. *International Workshop on Toxicology of Benzene.* Paris 1976.

Mallory TB, Gall EA, Brickley WJ: Chronic exposure to benzene (benzol). III. The pathologic results. *J Ind Hyg Toxicol* 1939;21:355–393.

Picciano D: Cytogenetic studies of workers exposed to benzene. *Environ Res* 1979;19:33–38.

Piotrowski JK: Exposure tests for organic compounds in industrial toxicology. Cincinnati, Ohio, National Institute for Occupational Safety and Health (NIOSH 77-144), 1977.

Rozman C, Woessner S, Saez-Serrania J. Acute erythromyelosis after benzene poisoning. *Acta Haemat* 1968;40:234–237.

Runion H: Benzene in gasoline II. *Am Ind Hyg Assoc J* 1977;38:391–393.

Rushton L, Alderson MR: A case-control study to investigate the association between exposure to benzene and deaths from leukaemia in oil refinery workers. *Br J Cancer* 1981;43:77–84.

Sato A, Nakajima T, Fujiwara Y, et al: Kinetic studies on sex difference in susceptibility to chronic benzene intoxication—with special reference to body fat content. *Br J Ind Med* 1975;32:321–328.

Tough IM, Court Brown WM: Chromosome aberrations and exposure to ambient benzene. *Lancet* 1965;1:685.

Vigliani EC, Forni A: Benzene and leukemia. *Environ Res* 1976;11:122–127.

Vigliani EC, Saita G: Benzene and leukemia. *N Engl J Med* 1964;271:872–876.

Zenz C: Benzene—Attempts to establish a lower exposure standard in the United States. *Scand J Work Environ Health* 1978;4:103–113.

Phenol

Phenol (monohydroxybenzene; carbolic acid) is the simplest member of the class of organic acids characterized by an OH group attached directly to a benzene ring. Other compounds in this class are derived from phenol by replacement of one or more of the hydrogen atoms with other atoms or groups. Phenols that contain more than one hydroxyl group bound to the benzene ring are called polyhydric phenols. Dihydric phenols, also known as benzenediols, include catechol, resorcinol, and hydroquinone. Pyrogallol, used as a photographic developer, is a trihydric phenol.

Phenol is used chiefly in the manufacture of phenol-formaldehyde resins and plastics and as a raw material in the preparation of a variety of more complex phenols that are used as drugs, antiseptics, fungicides and insecticides, wood and other preservatives, and in the manufacture of dyes, detergents, plasticizers, and epoxy resins. Phenol is produced either by the fractional distillation of coal tar or by a variety of synthetic processes.

Lister reported on his use of phenol as a surgical disinfectant in 1867 and he found that it produced painless tissue destruction. In the early 1900s a number of reports appeared that described ochronosis, a discoloration of collagenous tissue, acquired as a result of applications of 5% to 10%

phenol dressings to skin ulcerations. Sporadic reports appeared in the first half of this century documenting severe and sometimes fatal poisoning from the accidental absorption of phenol through intact skin (Hamilton, 1917; Smith, 1922; McCord and Minster, 1924; Winkler, 1939; Evans, 1952). In addition to skin burns, the victims variously experienced euphoria, headache, tinnitus, vertigo, tachycardia, depression, collapse, and coma. Winkler's patient, a chemical worker, also showed transient albuminuria and phenoluria. That severe reactions to occupational exposure still occur is evidenced by a recent report of marasmus in a laboratory technician who had a chronic exposure to phenol over a 13-year period (Merliss, 1972). The world literature on phenol poisoning has been summarized by Deichmann (1949) and by NIOSH (1976).

While phenol is readily absorbed through the lungs, volunteer individuals retaining 60% to 88% of the phenol to which they were exposed (Piotrowski, 1971), skin is the primary route of entry for phenol in vapor, liquid, or solid form. Some detoxification occurs in the liver, and both free and conjugated phenol are excreted in the urine to the extent of almost 100% within 24 hours after acute exposure (Ruedemann and Deichmann, 1953; Piotrowski, 1971). Urine analysis for phenol is complicated by the ingestion of certain foods and by salicylates, and is further confused by the British practice of normalizing urine specific gravity to 1.016 while American investigators use 1.024.

Laboratory animals differ in their responses to phenol, cats being more susceptible than dogs, pigs, and goats. Urinary metabolites consist of free phenol, phenylsulfate, and phenylglucuronide (Oehme and Davis, 1970).

Treatment of persons exposed to skin contact with phenol needs to be rapid in view of its quick absorption. Such absorption may increase with some dilution of the phenol, and the copious flooding of the skin with water may actually increase the toxicity of the phenol (Freeman et al., 1951). Conning and Hayes (1970) recommended removal of all clothing as quickly as possible (with care on the part of first aid personnel to avoid contaminating themselves), swabbing all the contaminated skin with absorbent cotten soaked in either glycerol or polyethylene glycol, and removal of the patient to a place equipped with resuscitation equipment for observation for 24 hours. Their studies with rats showed per-

cutaneous toxicity of phenol to be increased by applications of water, denatured alcohol, or olive oil.

The maximum permissible exposure limit has been set at 5 ppm (19 mg/m³). NIOSH has essentially concurred with its recommendation of 20 mg/m³ in air determined as a time-weighted average (TWA) for up to a 10-hour workday, 40-hour workweek, and a 15-minute ceiling exposure of 60 mg/m³.

References

Conning DM, Hayes MJ: The dermal toxicity of phenol: An investigation of the most effective first-aid measures. Br J Ind Med 1970;27:155–159.

Deichmann WB: Local and systemic effects following skin contact with phenol—A review of the literature. J Ind Hyg Toxicol 1949;31:146–154.

Evans SJ: Acute phenol poisoning. Br J Ind Med 1952;9:227–229.

Freeman MV, Draize JH, Alvarez E: Cutaneous absorption of phenol. J Lab Clin Med 1917;38:262–266.

Hamilton A: Industrial poisons encountered in the manufacture of explosives. J Am Med Assoc 1917;68:1445–1451.

Lister J: On a new method of treating compound fracture, abscess, etc., with observations on the condition of suppuration. Lancet 1867;2:326,357,387,507.

McCord CP, Minster DK: Phenol poisoning from ink. J Am Med Assoc 1924;83:843.

Merliss RR: Phenol marasmus. J Occup Med 1972;14:55–56.

NIOSH: Criteria for a Recommended Standard . . . . Occupational Exposure to Phenol. Washington, DC, National Institute for Occupational Safety and Health (NIOSH 76-196), 1976.

Oehme FW, Davis LE: The comparative toxicity and biotransformation of phenol. Toxicol Appl Pharmacol 1970;17:283.

Piotrowski JK: Evaluation of exposure to phenol: Absorption of phenol vapour in the lungs and through the skin and excretion of phenol in urine. Br J Ind Med 1971;28:172–178.

Ruedemann R, Deichmann WB: Blood phenol level after topical application of phenol-containing preparations. J Am Med Assoc 1953;152:506–509.

Smith RE: Absorption of carbolic acid through the skin. *Lancet* 1922;2:1359.

Winkler A: Phenolverätzung beider Augen und Allgemeinfolgen nebst einigen Bemerkungen über die Therapie von Augenverätzungen. *Klin Monatsbl Augenheilkunde* 1939;102:810–815.

___

Hydroquinone

Of the three dihydroxybenzenes, only hydroquinone has a history of adverse effects from occupational exposure. Catechol and resorcinol generally resemble phenol in their toxic effects (Flickinger, 1976). Hydroquinone is a reducing agent and constitutes a reversible oxidation-reduction system with quinone. Its reducing properties make it useful as a photographic developer and as an oxidation inhibitor.

The toxic effects of exposure to hydroquinone consist of injury to the skin and to the eyes. Depigmentation of the skin from wearing a brand of rubber gloves containing free hydroquinone as an antioxidant was reported by Oliver et al. in 1939. This leukoderma was found to be slowly reversible upon cessation of exposure. These observations led to a number of studies on the use of hydroquinone-containing creams to reduce pathologic hypermelanosis (Spencer, 1965; Arndt and Fitzpatrick, 1965; Findley et al., 1975; Bentley-Phillips and Bayles, 1975).

Eye injuries have resulted from occupational exposure to quinone vapor and hydroquinone dust. In their study of 50 cases of injury among workers exposed to these hazards, Sterner and his associates (1947) found both corneal and conjunctival damage. The former consisted of either a superficial greenish-brown stain confined to the interpalpebral fissure or grayish-white opacities of various sizes that involved all layers of the cornea. Conjunctival lesions also involved abnormal pigmentation varying from a diffuse brownish tinge to larger areas of brownish-black particles. In some cases there was an appreciable loss of vision. This pigmentation developed gradually over a span of several years, and removal from exposure led to some fading of the staining but not of the corneal opacities (Anderson and Oglesby, 1958). Naumann (1966), in his histopathologic review of the corneal damage seen in hydroquinone workers, found degenerative changes in the anterior half of the corneal stroma in addition to two distinctly different forms of pigmentation.

No systemic effects have been noted in occupationally exposed persons, but acute exposures from accidental or suicidal ingestion have resulted in hemolytic anemia, convulsions, coma, and death (NIOSH, 1978). The permissible exposure limit for hydroquinone dust is 2 mg/m^3, while that for quinone vapor is 0.1 ppm (0.4 mg/m^3). Flickinger (1976) suggested a threshold limit value (TLV) of 10 ppm, or even 20 ppm, for resorcinol, 5 ppm for catechol, and he agreed with the current limit of 2 mg/m^3 for hydroquinone.

References

Anderson B, Olgesby F: Corneal changes from quinone-hydroquinone exposure. *Arch Ophthalmol* 1958;59:495–501.

Arndt KA, Fitzpatrick TB: Topical use of hydroquinone as a depigmenting agent. *J Am Med Assoc* 1965;194:965–967.

Bentley-Phillips B, Bayles, MAH: Cutaneous reactions to topical application of hydroquinone—Results of a 6-year investigation. *So Afr Med J* 1975;49:1391–1395.

Findley GH, Morrison JGL, Simson IW: Exogenous ochronosis and pigmented colloid milium from hydroquinone bleaching creams. *Br J Dermatol* 1975;93:613–622.

Flickinger CW: The benzenediols: Catechol, resorcinol and hydroquinone—A review of the industrial toxicology and current industrial exposure limits. *Am Ind Hyg Assoc J* 1976;37:596–606.

Naumann G: Corneal damage in hydroquinone workers. A clinicopathologic study. *Arch Ophthalmol* 1966;76:189–194.

NIOSH: *Criteria for a Recommended Standard . . . . Occupational Exposure to Hydroquinone.* Washington, DC, National Institute for Occupational Safety and Health (NIOSH 78-155), 1978.

Oliver EA, Schwartz L, Warren LH: Occupational leukoderma. *J Am Med Assoc* 1939;113: 927–928.

Spencer MC: Topical use of hydroquinone for depigmentation. *J Am Med Assoc* 1965;194:962–964.

Sterner JH, Oglesby FL, Anderson B: Quinone vapors and their harmful effects. I. Corneal and conjunctival injury. *J Ind Hyg Toxicol* 1947;29: 60–73.

___

Alkylbenzenes

The alkylbenzenes that are important for occupational medicine are toluene, the xylenes, mesitylene, and pseudocumene. Styrene, the simplest of the alkenylbenzenes, is discussed in the chapter on plastics. In general, the alkylbenzenes are obtained by extraction from coal tar derived from coking or are synthesized from petroleum alkanes by catalytic processes.

Toluene Toluene (methylbenzene; toluol; methylbenzol; phenylmethane) is a liquid that boils at 110.4°C. Commerical toluene contains variable amounts of benzene, up to 25% according to NIOSH (1973). About 70% is used for conversion to benzene, and the remainder is used in the production of other organic compounds, as a solvent for gums, fats, and adhesives, as a paint thinner and remover, as a solvent for neoprene, and as a component of gasolines.

Toluene vapor is absorbed rapidly from the lungs, and liquid toluene is taken up readily from the gastrointestinal tract but poorly through the skin. In the body toluene is deposited in adipose tissue and in the central nervous system. Carlsson and Lindqvist (1977) found that toluene uptake was directly proportional to the amount of body fat. Part of the absorbed toluene is exhaled unchanged and most of the remainder is metabolized to benzoic acid, which in turn is conjugated with glycine in the liver and is excreted in the urine as hippuric acid (Browning, 1965; Kira, 1977; Wilczok and Bieniek, 1978), excretion being practically complete within 14 hours after cessation of exposure (von Oettingen et al., 1942). Urine hippuric acid levels may also be elevated by the ingestion of sodium benzoate used as a food preservative and of fruits and vegetables that contain benzoic acid as a natural constituent. A small fraction of inhaled toluene is metabolized to arene oxides that rearrange to form *o*- and *p*-cresol. Pfäffli et al. (1979) have devised a sensitive gas chromatographic method to test for *o*-cresol in urine as a guide to the amount of toluene inhaled. In contrast to benzene, toluene does not produce a reduction in the ratio of inorganic sulfates excreted in the urine.

Although it was once thought that the methylbenzenes had a toxic effect on the hematopoietic system, the current view is that this adverse influence is entirely attributable to contamination with benzene, especially in those preparations derived from coal tar distillation. However, isolated cases of bone marrow injury as a concomitant of toluene exposure do exist. Gattner and May (1963) reported the case of a 16-year-old boy who was exposed over the course of nine months to benzene-free toluene used in cleaning printing presses. He developed fatigue, weakness, and dizziness and was found to have leukopenia as low as 1500 cells/mm³ and a platelet count of 63,000 cells/mm³. Although a clear causal connection was not established, the evidence associating toluene with myelotoxic changes, although unusual, cannot be ignored.

Toluene exposure principally affects the central nervous system. Von Oettingen and his colleagues (1942) tested the effect of toluene vapor on three normal persons by subjecting them to concentrations from 50 ppm up to 800 ppm for daily periods up to eight hours. No definite changes were found in the white blood cell counts, in the circulation, or in the respiration even by exposures to the highest concentrations of toluene. At 200 ppm there was a slight, but definite, impairment of coordination and reaction time, changes that could bring about a greater liability toward accident. With concentrations over 200 ppm these effects became increasingly severe, and at 600 to 800 ppm three hours' exposure resulted in severe fatigue, extreme nausea, confusion, lack of self control, incoordination, and a staggering gait. Since evidence of neurological impairment occurred at a toluene concentration of 200 ppm, the continuing use of this threshold limit value has been questioned, and a reduction to 100 ppm has been recommended (NIOSH, 1973).

The effects of toluene on the central nervous system, such as dizziness, weakness, confusion, and incoordination, are not specific for toluene and are typical of the action of many organic solvents. The euphoria that is typical of toluene toxicity is attractive to certain individuals who have made a practice of sniffing glue, paint thinner (Weisenberger, 1977), or toluene itself, the latter instance resulting in a schizophreniform psychosis in one case (Tarsh, 1979). Sniffing of toluene has also resulted in some cases in life-threatening metabolic acidosis characterized by a high anion gap (Fischman and Oster, 1979) or by hyperchloremia and other findings consistent with renal tubular acidosis (Taher et al., 1974).

Recent studies of industrial populations exposed to toluene have not revealed any adverse effects of chronic exposure but instead have largely been concerned with toluene uptake in relation to ambient air concentrations (Övrum et al., 1978). Other investigations have looked for possible genetic effects by examining lymphocytes for chromosome aberrations. While Funes-Cravioto et al. (1977) did find an excess of these abnormalities among workers in a rotoprinting factory, Forni et al. (1971) and Mäki-Paakkanen et al. (1980) failed to detect chromosome aberrations or sister chromatid exchanges in workers exposed to toluene in this trade.

Xylene Xylene (dimethylbenzene) exists in three isomeric forms: *ortho-, meta-,* and *para*-xylene. Commercial xylene, called xylol, consists of a mixture of all three isomers plus ethylbenzene. Xylene is used as a solvent for gums, resins, rubber, and paints, as a cleaning agent and degreaser, as a starting material for the preparation of phthalic and terephthalic acids used in the manufacture of plastics and synthetic fibers, and as a constituent of gasolines (Browning, 1965).

Like toluene, some xylene is exhaled after it has been absorbed from the lungs. Åstrand et al. (1978) have shown that about 60% of xylene supplied to the lungs is taken up by the body, 95% of which is metabolized. Uptake by the body is highly correlated with the amount of body fat (Engström and Bjurström, 1978) and xylene that is stored in adipose tissue is eliminated slowly (Riihimäki and Savolainen, 1980). Absorbed xylene is converted in the body largely to toluic acid, which is excreted in the urine either in free or in conjugated form, usually as methylhippuric acid. The absence of adverse effects on the hematopoietic system is attributed, as with toluene, to the alkylation of the benzene ring and the consequent absence of the phenol metabolites that are produced from benzene.

Xylene acts on the skin and mucous membranes as a defatting agent to produce drying, erythema, and even blistering. When it is inhaled at high concentrations it acts as an irritant and as a narcotic, with dizziness, excitement, incoordination, and gait disturbances as initial effects. Psychophysiological tests have shown impairment of performance abilities, especially when uptake was increased by physical work (Gamberale et al., 1978). More serious effects from occupational exposure have not been widely recorded because, as has been suggested, workers will not voluntarily tolerate the highly irritant vapor at toxic levels.

Scattered reports of toxic effects of occupa-tional exposure to xylene gathered by Browning (1965) and NIOSH (1975) include instances of corneal microvesiculation, of headache, gastric discomfort, vomiting, throat dryness, giddiness, and slight drunkenness, of possible provocation of latent epilepsy, and of loss of consciousness and death (with hepatic impairment, renal failure, and petecchial hemorrhages in the brain). Careful review of cases with hematopoietic involvement has shown that the presence of benzene in the exposure mixture could not be excluded so that the myelotoxic effects could have resulted from benzene exposure rather than xylene.

The maximum permissible exposure level for xylene has been set at 100 ppm (435 mg/m³) in air with NIOSH (1975) further recommending a ceiling concentration of 200 ppm determined in a 10-minute sampling period.

Other alkylbenzenes Mesitylene (1,3,5-tri-methylbenzene; TMB), pseudocumene (1,2,4-tri-methylbenzene), and ethylbenzene (phenylethane) have industrial uses as solvents, paint and lacquer thinners, and as constituents of motor fuel because of their antiknock properties. Ethylbenzene is a skin irritant and has central nervous system effects in high concentrations, but no toxic systemic effects have been reported from occupational exposure (Browning, 1965). Knowledge of the toxicity of the trimethylbenzenes is based largely on experience with the commercial solvent "Fleet-X-DV-99" reported by Bättig et al. (1956a,b). Exposure to this mixture resulted in bleeding from the gums and nose, thrombocytopenia in some cases, mild anemia, asthmatic bronchitis, and headache, fatigue, and drowsiness.

The maximum permissible exposure level for ethylbenzene, like that for xylene, is 100 ppm (435 mg/m³) in air.

References

Åstrand I, Engström J, Övrum P: Exposure to xylene and ethylbenzene. I. Uptake, distribution and elimination in man. *Scand J Work Environ Health* 1978;4:185–194.

Bättig K, Grandjean E, Turrian V: Gesundheitschäden nach langdauernder Trimethylbenzol Exposition in einer Malerwerkstatt. *Z Prävent Med* 1956a;1:389–403.

Bättig K, Turrian V, Grandjean E: Toxikologische und arbeitsmedizinische Untersuchungen über Trimethylbenzol. *Z Unfallmed Berufskrankh* 1956b;49:265–266.

Browning E: *Toxicity and Metabolism of Industrial Solvents*. New York, Elsevier, 1965, pp 66–129.

Carlsson A, Lindqvist T: Exposure of animals and man to toluene. *Scand J Work Environ Health* 1977;3:135–143.

Engström J, Bjurström R: Exposure to xylene and ethylbenzene. II. Concentration in subcutaneous adipose tissue. *Scand J Work Environ Health* 1978;4:195–203.

Fischman CM, Oster JR: Toxic effects of toluene. A new cause of high anion gap metabolic acidosis. *J Am Med Assoc* 1979;241:1713–1715.

Forni A, Pacifico E, Limonta A: Chromosome studies in workers exposed to benzene or toluene or both. *Arch Environ Health* 1971;22:373–378.

Funes-Cravioto F, Kolomodin-Hedman B, Lindsten J, et al: Chromosome aberrations and sister chromatid exchange in workers in chemical laboratories and a rotoprinting factory and in children of some laboratory workers. *Lancet* 1977;2:322–325.

Gamberale F, Annwall G, Hultengren M: Exposure to xylene and ethylbenzene. III. Effects on central nervous function. *Scand J Work Environ Health* 1978;4:204–211.

Gattner H, May G: Panmyelopathie durch toluoleinwirkung. *Zbl Arbeitsmed* 1963;13:156–157.

Kira S: Measurement by gas chromatography of urinary hippuric acid and methylhippuric acid as indices of toluene and xylene exposure. *Br J Ind Med* 1977;34:305–309.

Mäki-Paakkanen J, Husgafvel-Pursiainen K, Kalliomäki P-L, et al: Toluene-exposed workers and chromosome aberrations. *J Toxicol Environ Health* 1980;6:775–781.

NIOSH: *Criteria for a Recommended Standard . . . . Occupational Exposure to Toluene*. Washington, DC, National Institute for Occupational Safety and Health (NIOSH 73-11023), 1973.

NIOSH: *Criteria for a Recommended Standard . . . . Occupational Exposure to Xylene*. Washington, DC, National Institute for Occupational Safety and Health (NIOSH 75-168), 1975.

Övrum P, Hultengren M, Lindqvist T: Exposure to toluene in a photogravure printing plant. Concentration in ambient air and uptake in the body. *Scand J Work Environ Health* 1978;4:237–245.

Pfäffli P, Savolainen H, Kalliomäki P-L, et al: Urinary o-cresol in toluene exposure. *Scand J Work Environ Health* 1979;5:286–289.

Riihimäki V, Savolainen K: Human exposure to m-xylene. Kinetics and acute effects on the central nervous system. *Ann Occup Hyg* 1980;23:411–422.

Taher SM, Anderson RJ, McCartney R, et al: Renal tubular acidosis associated with toluene "sniffing." *N Engl J Med* 1974;290:765–768.

Tarsh MJ: Schizophreniform psychosis caused by sniffing toluene. *J Soc Occup Med* 1979;29:131–133.

von Oettingen WF, Neal PA, Donahue DD: The toxicity and potential dangers of toluene. *J Am Med Assoc* 1942;118:579–584.

Weisenberger BL: Toluene habituation. *J Occup Med* 1977;19:569–570.

Wilczok T, Bieniek G: Urinary hippuric acid concentration after occupational exposure to toluene. *Br J Ind Med* 1978;35:330–334.

Cresol

Cresols are monomethyl phenols (or hydroxy derivatives of toluene) and exist in three isomeric forms: *ortho-, meta-,* and *para*-cresol; these occur together in mixtures. Cresylic acids, in turn, are mixtures of cresols, xylenols, and phenol. Creosol is a methoxy compound of o-cresol. Creosote, a wood preservative, is a mixture of phenol and phenol derivatives, including cresols, obtained from the distillation of coal and wood tars. Cresols are used in the production of wire enamel solvents, phenolic resins, and tricresyl phosphate, and are also used as disinfectants and ore-flotation agents.

Occupational exposure to cresol may be hazardous to skin, eyes, and respiratory tract. Exposure of skin to aerosols or liquid cresol can result in severe chemical burns, as with phenol. Such effects are known more from household accidents (see, for example, Arthurs et al., 1977; Wiseman et al., 1980) and suicide attempts (Isaacs, 1922) than from industry. Nevertheless, NIOSH (1978) has collected manufacturers' reports of cases of chemical burns of the skin and eyes, with erythema, dermatitis, localized anesthesia, and brown discoloration of the skin. One death occurred in an industrial accident in which a worker fell into a vat containing a cresylic acid derivative. He had burns over 15% of his body, and he developed fatal anuria and congestive heart failure (Cason, 1959). Nonoccupational skin exposures have demonstrated that cresols are absorbed rapidly through the skin and

254

produce hemorrhages and necrosis in brain, liver, kidneys, and heart.

Inhalation of cresol vapors is unusual unless they are processed at high temperatures. One study cited by NIOSH (1978) found headaches, tremors, and hypertension in a small group of French workers in a plant that used cresol at high temperatures to produce synthetic resins. Cresol vapor has an unpleasant odor and can be irritating to the upper respiratory tract. The maximum permissible exposure is 5 ppm (22 mg/m³), but NIOSH (1978) has recommended a more stringent limit of 2.3 ppm (10 mg/m³) determined as a time-weighted average concentration for up to a 10-hour workday, 40-hour workweek.

Triorthocresyl phosphate (TOCP) is used as a plasticizer, a high temperature lubricant, and as an additive to gasoline. Its neurotoxic properties were dramatically illustrated in the epidemic of paralyses in 1930 when it was used as an adulterant in an illicit extract of Jamaica ginger ("jake"). Peripheral neuritis as well as upper motor neuron disease developed in thousands of persons who drank this preparation, and abnormal neurological findings have persisted for as long as 47 years in some survivors (Morgan and Penovich, 1978). Although it is generally accepted that the neurotoxicity of TOCP is due to esterase inhibition by the phosphorylated phenols in the molecule, this explanation does not account for the delayed effects (Bischoff, 1977). Although the polyneuropathy of shoe factory workers in Italy and Japan has been attributed to n-hexane, Cavalleri and Cosi (1978) have suggested that the reduction of red cell acetylcholinesterase that they found in 37 female workers in an artificial leather shoe factory could more properly be accounted for by exposure to tricresylphosphate.

References

Arthurs GJ, Wise CC, Coles GA: Poisoning by cresol. *Anaesthesia* 1977;22:642–643.

Bischoff A: Tri-ortho-cresyl phosphate neurotoxicity, in Roizin L, Shiraki H, Grčević N, (eds): *Neurotoxicology*. New York, Raven Press; 1977, pp 431–441.

Cason JS: Report on three extensive industrial chemical burns. *Br Med J* 1959;1:827–829.

Cavalleri A, Cosi V: Polyneuritis incidence in shoe factory workers: Cases report and etiological considerations. *Arch Environ Health* 1978;33:192–197.

Isaacs R: Phenol and cresol poisoning. *Ohio State Med J* 1922;18:558–561.

Morgan JP, Penovich P: Jamaica ginger paralysis. *Arch Neurol* 1978;35:530–532.

NIOSH: *Criteria for a Recommended Standard . . . . Occupational Exposure to Cresol.* Washington, DC, National Institute for Occupational Safety and Health (NIOSH 78-133), 1978.

Wiseman HM, Turner WML, Volans GN: Acute poisoning due to Wright's Vaporizing Fluid. *Postgrad Med J* 1980;56:166–168.

Diphenyl and Diphenyl Oxide

Diphenyl (biphenyl; phenyl benzene) and diphenyl oxide are used in industry primarily as heat transfer media. Such use is found in nylon manufacture and in organically cooled and moderated nuclear reactors. High temperatures and radiation fields modify diphenyl and diphenyl oxide to produce a variety of high-boiling residues that must be removed from the coolant streams. Diphenyl is also used as a fungistatic agent in the preservation of citrus fruits.

Leaks from heat transfer systems may obviously produce thermal burns. Vapors of these compounds are irritating to the eyes and upper airway. The experience of Häkkinen et al. (1973) implicates diphenyl exposure in the production of central and peripheral nervous system damage and liver injury. Workers producing diphenyl-impregnated fruit wrapping paper under poor hygienic conditions complained of headache, polyneuritis with pain and numbness, and nonspecific gastrointestinal symptoms. In addition to the changes observable in electroencephalograms and electroneuromyograms, there were biochemical abnormalities in hepatic function, hepatic cell abnormalities in liver biopsy samples, and evidence that the death of one of the exposed workers was due to acute yellow atrophy of the liver.

The maximum permissible exposure limit for diphenyl has been set at 0.2 ppm (1 mg/m³) in air.

Reference

Häkkinen I, Siltanen E, Hernberg S, et al: Diphenyl poisoning in fruit paper production. A new health hazard. *Arch Environ Health* 1973;26:70–74.

Naphthalene

Naphthalene, familiar as "moth balls" (and not to be confused with paradichlorbenzene also used for mothproofing), is used primarily as a chemical intermediate in the production of phthalic acid and derivatives for the dye and plastics industries. The vapors produce eye irritation, headache, and a warm feeling of the skin with profuse sweating. Lenticular opacities have been observed in a number of workers exposed to high concentrations (Ghetti and Mariani, 1956). High levels of exposure, such as may be associated with accidental ingestion in children, can cause an acute hemolytic anemia and hemoglobinuria especially in individuals with an erythrocyte deficiency of glucose-6-phosphate dehydrogenase (Zuelzer and Abt, 1949). A single case of aplastic anemia has been reported in a woman occupationally exposed to high levels of both naphthalene and paradichlorbenzene (Harden and Baetjer, 1978).

The maximum permissible exposure level for naphthalene is 10 ppm (50 mg/m^3).

References

Ghetti G, Mariani L: Alterazione oculare da naftalina. *Med lavoro* 1956;47:533–538.

Harden RA, Baetjer AM: Aplastic anemia following exposure to paradichlorbenzene and naphthalene. *J Occup Med* 1978;20:820–822.

Zuelzer WW, L Abt: Acute hemolytic anemia due to naphthalene poisoning. *J Am Med Assoc* 1949;141:185–190.

9 • *Aromatic Nitro and Amino Compounds*

Aromatic nitro and amino compounds comprise a varied group of substances that are fundamental to industries producing explosives, pharmaceuticals, rubber chemicals, and "aniline" or "coal tar" dyes. Other compounds in this group are intermediates in the synthesis of pesticides, plastics, and paints. While certain members of the nitro ($-NO_2$) and amino ($-NH_2$) aromatic group have relatively specific toxic effects, there are general properties that are characteristic of the group. Many of these compounds produce methemoglobin, some are bladder carcinogens, and others uncouple oxidation from phosphorylation. There are also unusually potent sensitizers in the group. Liquid nitro- and amino-aromatics are readily absorbed through the intact skin.

Methemoglobinemia

Methemoglobinemia is considered to be the outstanding acute reaction to most nitro and amino aromatic compounds (Bodansky, 1951). It is not clear whether all the manifestations of methemoglobinemia in man reflect hypoxemia exclusively or whether the chemical compound implicated (e.g., aniline) has a specific, direct pharmacologic effect on the body. While it is probable that the chemically active compounds of this group do have direct organ and tissue effects, it is difficult to provide convincing demonstrations because the presence of severe methemoglobinemia tends to obscure other manifestations of direct toxicity.

In biochemical terms, methemoglobin is the chemical analogue of hemoglobin in which the iron of the heme moiety has become oxidized from the normal Fe^{++} (ferrous) state to the abnormal Fe^{+++} (ferric) state. Oxygen bound to methemoglobin is so firmly attached that it is not available to tissues and, in fact, can be separated

from the carrier pigment only by rather drastic nonphysiologic means. Consequently, methemoglobin is not an oxygen-transporting pigment. Tissue hypoxia is thus the consequence of hemoglobin oxidation, *not* oxygenation, to methemoglobin. Methemoglobin also distorts the oxygen dissociation curve of normal hemoglobin so that it interferes with the release of oxygen from normal hemoglobin. Consequently, hypoxia is more severe than the methemoglobin levels might suggest (Darling and Roughton, 1942).

Organic and inorganic nitrites, organic nitrates, and quinones form methemoglobin directly; inorganic nitrates on ingestion may produce methemoglobin through the action of intestinal bacteria that yields nitrites. In most cases it is probable that metabolites of the aryl nitro and amino compounds are the proximate cause of blood pigment oxidation. Phenylhydroxylamines and nitroso compounds are prime possibilities as methemoglobin-producing metabolites. Clinical observations indicate that nitro compounds are associated with a more insidious onset of methemoglobinemia and a more prolonged course than is the case with the corresponding amino compounds. These observations may reflect a somewhat slower conversion of the nitro compounds into the actual methemoglobin producer.

Methemoglobin is normally present in man in a low concentration, usually below 2%. An equilibrium exists between hemoglobin and methemoglobin, the latter being continually reduced by an intracellular methemoglobin reductase known as diaphorase (Smith, 1969). Glycolysis is adequate to drive this mechanism at a rate sufficient to handle normal pigment loads. But with massive chemical exposure, this mechanism is inadequate to handle the load of abnormal oxidized pigment, and clinical cyanosis becomes evident. An auxiliary reducing mechanism can participate in the reduction of methemoglobin when methylene blue is administered therapeutically. The precise biochemical nature of each step in this reduction is not yet clear, but the evidence is good that methylene blue can be of great value in the clinical treatment of methemoglobinemia (Wuertz et al., 1964). Industrial experience with methylene blue has been limited, a fact that is probably related to existing reports that methylene blue is itself a methemoglobin producer. More recent interpretations support the view that methylene blue does not produce methemoglobin in most laboratory animals and probably not in man.

Aniline, nitrobenzene, and indeed most of their homologues (e.g., dinitrobenzene, nitroaniline) generate methemoglobin. Many of these compounds penetrate the skin, and as vapors or dusts they are rapidly absorbed in the lungs. The onset of cyanosis is usually insidious, and the time required is a function of the absorption rate and the specific compound absorbed. Nitrobenzene and other nitro compounds generate methemoglobin more slowly, but cyanosis is more persistent.

The onset of cyanosis is often first noted in the lips ("blue lip") and ears. The color is more violet, lilac, or "huckleberry pie" than the cyanosis associated with unoxygenated normal hemoglobin. Symptoms may be absent although euphoria, flushed facies, and headache are common. Cyanosis is usually detectable when the proportion of converted hemoglobin approximates 15%. At methemoglobin levels above 40%, headache may become severe and weakness, ataxia, and lightheadedness occur. With increasing concentrations of methemoglobin, dyspnea, tachycardia, and alarming cyanosis are noted. Even at levels of 75%, however, recovery without specific therapy has been the rule.

Treatment In most cases of occupational methemoglobinemia the most useful therapeutic procedure is simply a prompt and thorough cleansing of the patient with soap and warm water with special attention to the hair and nails. Contaminated footwear must be discarded. There are numerous examples of "blue lip" after an apparently cured patient put on clean clothing and steps into his old shoes, a source of absorbable aniline or nitrobenzene. Bed rest may be indicated. Headache is often relieved by the administration of oxygen, although this procedure has no effect on methemoglobin reduction.

That these conservative procedures need to be supplemented with active therapeutic measures is not clear. Better industrial practice suggests,

however, that intravenous methylene blue is indicated when methemoglobin levels exceed 40%. The usual dose of the dye is 1 to 2 mg/kg body weight as a 1% solution in saline. Ascorbic acid, a reducing agent, has also been used, but it appears to be less effective than methylene blue, principally because it acts too slowly to be effective in a crisis. From time to time the possibility of exchange transfusions has been raised, especially when the offending agent also produces hemolysis, but this step is seldom, if ever, considered necessary.

Recovery is usually rapid, and spontaneous disappearance of cyanosis may occur in hours. With high levels of methemoglobin and when the agent involved is a nitro compound, 24 or more hours may be required. When recovery is slow, the physician must consider the possibility that toxic compounds are still being absorbed through the skin.

The management of methemoglobinemia is facilitated by prompt and accurate determinations of blood methemoglobin levels. Heinz bodies, small refractile granules in the erythrocytes, have been attributed to exposure to aromatic amines and nitro compounds and to nitrates and nitrate esters (Harley and Mauer, 1961).

Hepatic injury related to aryl amino compounds has been rare. There are reports of acute hepatic disorders in benzidine workers, but the effects in this population are presumably due to heavy exposures.

Trinitrotoluene and Dinitrobenzene

Nitro compounds of the trinitrotoluene (TNT) and dinitrobenzene type have a history of prominent hepatotoxic effects that are often associated with aplastic anemia. The data come to a large degree from the British munitions industry in both World Wars and to a lesser extent from similar American sources. Both compounds are readily absorbed through the skin, especially when it is exposed and wet with sweat. Hepatic injury is manifested by jaundice, which is often demonstrable only in the conjunctivae, since the skin of workers with this degree of exposure may already be dyed yellow by the compounds in question. Unfortunately, jaundice is a late sign of hepatic injury and is not satisfactory in the prevention of acute yellow atrophy. Earlier symptoms are not sufficiently specific to be very useful in prevention. Other medical problems have included gastritis, dermatitis, anemia, peripheral neuritis, myocardial irregularities, pancreatic dysfunction, and cataract formation (Hathaway, 1977). Workers with a glucose-6-phosphate dehydrogenase (G6 PD) deficiency are particularly susceptible to acute hemolytic episodes (Djerassi and Vitany, 1975).

McConnell and Flinn (1946) reported 22 cases of fatal TNT poisoning that occurred in American industry in World War II. Of these, 13 were due to aplastic anemia, eight were due to acute yellow atrophy of the liver, and one was due to hepatitis followed by aplastic anemia. The number of nonfatal cases during the same period was not reported, but recovery from either toxic hepatitis or toxic aplastic anemia is rare. It is very probable that TNT-related disease was much more common than these data suggest, especially during World War I. There is reason to believe that a somewhat better health record in the TNT industry in World War II may have been due to the fact that tetranitromethane, a toxic and irritating impurity of crude TNT, was removed during that period (Sievers et al., 1947). But even at exposures below the permissible exposure limit of 1.5 mg/m³, workers in an ammunition plant producing TNT had significant elevations of serum glutamic oxalacetic transaminase and lactic dehydrogenase (Morton et al., 1976). These and other results argue for a lowering of the current permissible exposure limits.

Dinitrobenzene is some 20 times as potent a methemoglobin producer as is TNT. Consequently, the appearance of cyanosis provides a warning of exposure to this potent hepatotoxin.

Picric Acid and Tetryl

Other aromatic nitro explosives, picric acid (trinitrophenol) and tetryl (methyltetranitroaniline) do not pose major industrial health hazards except during the very high exposures such as are encountered in wartime. Tetryl is highly irritating to the skin and mucous membranes and may cause severe upper respiratory tract irritation with coughing and epistaxis. The compound stains the skin and hair yellow. Picric acid produces a similar contact dermatitis and staining. There is evidence that heavy exposures to tetryl may cause liver damage (Hardy and Maloof, 1950).

Trimethylenetrinitramine

Trimethylenetrinitramine, called cyclonite or RDX, is a military high explosive. It has been found to cause convulsions in men working under poor conditions of hygiene (Barsotti and Crotti, 1949). Typical epileptiform seizures may be preceded by a few days of irritability, insomnia, or restlessness. No sequelae have been observed after cessation of exposure (Kaplan et al., 1965). Primary and sensitizing dermatitis may also be caused by RDX or, more likely, by impurities or chemical intermediates associated with its production. RDX does not induce methemoglobinemia or nitrate effects. Its relative safety when compared to TNT is evidenced by failure to detect any adverse health effects in workers exposed to RDX up to 1.57 mg/m³ (Hathaway and Buck, 1977).

Dinitrochlorobenzenes

The dinitrochlorobenzenes are almost universal skin sensitizers; a minute contact will sensitize approximately three fourths of all persons tested. The reaction may vary from a small area of pruritic vesiculopapular eruption to a generalized exfoliative dermatitis. The 2,4-isomer is used in experimental sensitizations; presumably it combines with lysine in cutaneous proteins to form a complete antigen.

Dinitrophenols and Dinitro-o-cresol

The dinitrophenols (DNPs) and dinitro-o-cresol (DNOC), which have uses as pesticides, are distinctive from the toxicological point of view in that they are compounds with marked effects upon energy-producing metabolic mechanisms. Upon absorption, these compounds uncouple oxidation from phosphorylation so that energy made available by oxidation is not converted into active phosphate but is expended in raising body temperature. Cataracts may occur in cases in which extreme elevations of body temperature are achieved, and fatal hyperpyrexia has been reported (Bidstrup and Payne, 1951). In the mid-1930s in the United States, the availability of 2,4-dinitrophenol as an over-the-counter anti-obesity agent resulted in several hundred cataracts (Horner, 1942).

Diphenylamines

The diphenylamines are compounds in which the substitute groups in the 3 and 3′ positions may be H (to give benzidine), CH$_3$ (*o*-tolidine), Cl (dichlorobenzene), OH (dihydroxybenzidine), OCH$_3$ (dianisidine), and others. *o*-Tolidine (3,3'-dimethyl, 4,4'-diamino diphenyl) should not be confused with *o*-toluidine (*o*-methylaniline; *o*-aminotoluene). The former is used as a dye and as a dye intermediate, as a component in trypan blue, and in chlorine test kits for water companies and swimming pools. It is an irritant of nasal mucosa but not of skin (NIOSH, 1978). Its toxicological importance lies in its possible bladder carcinogenicity, especially in combined exposures with benzidine. Both compounds are absorbed through human skin, both have similar metabolic biotransformations, and both are excreted in urine either unchanged or as chemically similar metabolites.

The so-called "aniline tumors" of the bladder are currently believed to be related to the absorption of any one of the following four aromatic compounds: 2-naphthylamine (β-naphthylamine), 4-aminodiphenyl (xenylamine), 4-nitrodiphenyl, and 4,4-diaminodiphenyl (benzidine). The disease was first reported in the German dye industry by Rehn in 1895 who described four cases of tumor of the bladder in dye workers. He concluded that vapors of aniline, used in the production of the dye fuchsin, were responsible. Aniline itself is no longer believed to be carcinogenic (Barsotti and Vigliani, 1952) and the term "aniline tumors" has largely been abandoned. Although Berenblum reviewed the problem in 1932, not until 1934 did the first American report appear and it described the discovery of 27 cases during the cystoscopic examination of 587 men (Ferguson et al., 1934). Sixteen other cases were found in which there were hemorrhagic areas in the bladder. The age of the men affected ranged from 30 to 60 years, and the duration of exposure from 4 to 18 years. Except for two α-naphthylamine workers, all of the men had been exposed to either β-naphthylamine or benzidine. No tumors were detected in workers exposed exclusively to aniline. The evidence is convincing that the tumors in the α-naphthylamine workers were actually due to contamination by the β-isomer.

The fact that many aromatic amines and related compounds are present in those segments of the chemical industry in which occupational bladder tumors have arisen has produced speculation as to relative toxicities of compounds, the proximate carcinogen(s), and the mechanism of malignant transformation. The compounds listed in the previous paragraph are known to produce bladder tumors in man. Dianisidine and dichlorbenzidine have also been implicated (Scott and Williams, 1957). Studies with dogs have indicated the carcinogenetic potential of other aromatic amines: 2-acetylaminofluorine, N:N-dimethyl-4-aminoazobenzene, and 4-amino-3:2'-azotoluene. It must be presumed that these compounds are carcinogenic in man as well, although there has been limited industrial exposure. It should be noted that these compounds may not be carcinogenic for they fail to produce tumors when implanted directly into the bladders of experimental animals. However, man and dogs both appear to have the necessary biochemical mechanisms for transforming these compounds into the proximate carcinogen (Troll and Belman, 1967). Carcinogenic metabolites have been isolated from the urine of dogs, and they can induce tumors in the rat bladder, whereas the parent amine cannot, either by direct implantation or by parenteral administration.

Occupational tumors of the bladder usually follow a long latent period averaging about 18 years, with reported extremes of one and 48 years. Durations of exposure have also varied widely from less than one year to many years. Age is not clearly a factor in the development of malignant disease. Once initiated, the course of occupational bladder tumors is similar to those arising in the general population. The tumors may first be noted as benign papillomas, simple noninvasive, nonmetastasizing growths of the bladder wall. In other cases, they may first be found as invasive carcinomas. There are all patterns of intermediate categories. In all instances there is a tendency to recurrence with complications from hemorrhage and infection. Primary tumors in the renal pelvis and ureters have also been observed, but there is no evidence that these carcinogenic aromatic compounds produce tumors outside of the urinary system.

Treatment is surgical. In a number of cases the bladder has been excised and the ureters have been connected to an intestinal bladder. Medical surveillance is based upon exfoliative cytological examination of urinary sediment and on periodic cystoscopy. For men who have been exposed to known bladder carcinogens there does not appear to be an alternative to these procedures. The obvious solution in the case of unexposed workers is the enclosure and control of the relevant industrial processes. In some jurisdictions the production of β-naphthylamine has been made illegal.

Toluidines and Chlortoluidines

Occasionally, hematuria may be observed in workers handling toluidines and chlortoluidines. There may be a hemorrhagic cystitis with painful and frequent micturition. This acute problem does not have long-term significance and clears promptly upon cessation of toxic exposure. If hematuria persists, the question of other urinary tract pathology must be considered. The cystitis related to these compounds is not involved in aromatic amine carcinogenesis.

Para-phenyldiamine and Para-aminophenol

Para-phenyldiamine and para-aminophenol are dye intermediates that give a brown or black color when applied to furs. These compounds are potent skin and respiratory allergens and can produce severe bronchial asthma among workers in the fur-dyeing industry. Dermatitis from properly finished fur is rare, however, since these dyes are well fixed to the hairs and do not cause reactions even in highly sensitized persons. In addition, p-aminophenol can generate methemoglobin when absorbed.

Dimethylnitrosamine

Two cases of poisoning from dimethylnitrosamine (DMN) were found by Alice Hamilton in the course of a survey of a large automobile factory. The toxic effect was on the liver and resulted in jaundice and ascites. The first patient was violently ill but survived; the second was less affected and was recovering when he developed an infection from paracentesis and died. The liver was cirrhotic with areas of regeneration. The hepatotoxic action of DMN has been confirmed in animal studies by Barnes and Magee (1954). Zimmerman (1978) described DMN and its congeners as important models of hepatotoxicity and liver carcinogenicity. Since DMN has these potent properties, exposure should be reduced to a minimum.

References

Barnes JM, Magee PN: Some toxic properties of dimethylnitrosamine. *Br J Ind Med* 1954; 11:167–174.

Barsotti M, Crotti G: Attacchi epilettici come manifestazione di intossicazione professionale da trimetilentrinitroamina. *Med lavoro* 1949;40: 107–111, Abstracted in *Br J Ind Med* 1950;7:47.

Barsotti M, Vigliani EC: Bladder lesions from aromatic amines. Statistical considerations and prevention. *Arch Ind Hyg Occup Med* 1952;5: 234–241.

Berenblum I: Aniline cancer. *Cancer Rev* 1932; 7:337–355.

Bidstrup PL, Payne DJH: Poisoning by dinitro-ortho-cresol. Report of eight fatal cases occurring in Great Britain. *Br Med J* 1951;2:16–19.

Bodansky O: Methemoglobin and methemoglobin-producing compounds. *Pharmacol Rev* 1951; 3:144–196.

Darling RC, Roughton FJW: The effect of methemoglobin on the equilibrium between oxygen and hemoglobin. *Am J Physiol* 1942;137:56–68.

Djerassi LS, Vitany L: Haemolytic episode in G6 PD deficient workers exposed to TNT. *Br J Ind Med* 1975;32:54–58.

Ferguson RS, Gehrmann GH, Gay DM: Symposium on aniline tumors of the bladder. *J Urology* 1934;31:121–148 (three papers).

Hardy HL, Maloof CC: Evidence of systemic effect of tetryl. *Arch Ind Hyg* 1950;1:545–555.

Harley JD, Mauer AM: Studies on the formation of Heinz bodies. II. The nature and significance of Heinz bodies. *Blood* 1961;17:418–433.

Hathaway JA; Trinitrotoluene: A review of reported dose-related effects providing documentation for a workplace standard. *J Occup Med* 1977;19:341–345.

Hathaway JA, Buck CR: Absence of health hazards associated with RDX manufacture and use. *J Occup Med* 1977;19:269–272.

Horner WD: Dinitrophenol and its relation to formation of cataract. *Arch Ophthalmol* 1942; 27:1097–1121.

Kaplan AS, Berghout CF, and Peczenik A: Human intoxication from RDX. *Arch Environ Health* 1965;10:877–883.

McConnell WJ, Flinn RH: Summary of 22 trinitrotoluene fatalities in World War II. *J Ind Hyg Toxicol* 1946;28:76–86.

Morton AR, Ranadive MV, Hathaway JA: Biological effects of trinitrotoluene from exposure below the threshold limit value. *Am Ind Hyg Assoc J* 1976;37:56–60.

NIOSH: *Criteria for a Recommended Standard . . . . Occupational Exposure to o-Tolidine.* Washington, DC, National Institute for Occupational Safety and Health (NIOSH 78-179), 1978.

Scott TS, Williams MHC: The control of industrial bladder tumors. A code of working practice recommended by the British dyestuffs industry for the manufacture and use of products causing tumours of the bladder. *Br J Ind Med* 1957;14: 150–163.

Sievers RF, Rushing E, Gay H, et al: Toxic effects of tetranitromethane; Contaminant in crude TNT. *Publ Health Rep* 1947;62:1048–1061.

Smith RP: The significance of methemoglobinemia in toxicology. *Essays in Toxicology* 1969; 1:83–113.

Troll W, Belman S: Studies on the nature of the proximal bladder carcinogens, in Deichmann WB, Lampe KF (eds): *Fifth Inter-American Conference on Toxicology and Occupational Disease, 1966.* Birmingham, Alabama, Aesculapius, 1967, pp 35–44.

Wuertz RL, Frazee WH Jr, Hume WG, et al: Chemical cyanosis-anemia syndrome. *Arch Environ Health* 1964;9:478–491.

Zimmerman HJ: *Hepatotoxicity.* New York, Appleton-Century-Crofts, 1978.

10 • *Carbon Disulfide*

Carbon disulfide, CS_2, is said to have been first discovered by Lampadius of Freiburg in 1796. It was recommended as a remedy for a great variety of diseases and was actually used in medicine during the following half century. It has been used industrially as an insecticide, and in the production of regenerated cellulose (viscose rayon and cellophane). It is a solvent for waxes, resins, gums, and rubber, and a substantial amount is used in the manufacture of carbon tetrachloride. For many years it played a very important part in the rubber industries in European countries, somewhat less in England, and much less in the United States. In rubber manufacture the crude latex must be made into an elastic, heat-resistant solid, and this is done by incorporating sulfur, a process known as vulcanizing. This change may be accomplished by adding flowers of sulfur to the mass that is then subjected to heat and pressure, a method that is known as the "heat cure." Or it may be done by exposing rubber to the action of sulfur chloride either in vapor form or by dipping it into the liquid, or by painting. The solvent or carrier for sulfur chloride usually has been carbon disulfide. American manufacturers have always preferred the heat cure for rubber, while Europeans have used the so-called cold or acid cure with carbon disulfide. It is this last compound that gave to European rubber manufacture a very bad reputation, and the older literature is full of reports of carbon disulfide poisoning in rubber workers.

When the process of making an artificial silk called viscose rayon was worked out in Switzerland, France, and England, reports began to appear describing cases of carbon disulfide poisoning in this new industry. In the production of viscose rayon, the starting point is cellulose from wood pulp or cotton linters, which is treated with an alkali to form flake-like "white crumbs" of alkali cellulose. This substance is changed to an orange-yellow, rubbery mass, known as cellulose xanthate, by treatment with carbon disulfide in revolving churns or "barattes" or "tumbling barrels." From the churns the xanthate goes to viscose mixing machines. The most severe exposure to CS_2 fumes takes place in the churn room, from leaking pipes and churns, from discharging the churns and scraping out the xanthate that sticks to the walls, and from conveying the xanthate to the viscose mixers and dumping it.

A lesser exposure occurs in the spinning process. The thick viscose syrup, which is sodium cellulose xanthate, comes from the mixers and is forced through spinnerets of different degrees of fineness according to the weight of the thread desired, into the spinning bath of sulfuric acid, sulfates, and other chemicals. Here, regenerated pure cellulose filaments are drawn out as threads and wound on bobbins. There is some production of CS_2 vapors caused by the "ripening" of the cellulose xanthate in the spinning bath, with the formation and escape of H_2S and CS_2. Poisoning from the latter is not as frequent or as severe as in the churn room. Since the recognition of carbon disulfide poisoning as a compensable occupational disease, these industrial processes have been elaborately safeguarded by ventilation systems, and air analyses are routinely made to check on the efficiency of these systems.

Worker Illness

Carbon disulfide was recognized as an industrial poison by the French almost 100 years before psychiatrists in the United States were willing to do so. Payen, who first described its action in 1851, was followed by Delpech in 1856 who described 24 cases in rubber workers as well as experimental poisoning in animals. Constensoux and Heim, in 1910, gave a detailed picture of CS_2

poisoning in French rubber workers, with loss of appetite, dyspepsia, disturbance of vision, sensory disturbances, and sexual impotence. Two very important studies came from Germany: In 1899 Laudenheimer published the medical histories of no less than 50 patients with carbon disulfide insanity. The early symptoms consisted of headache, dizziness, increasing sense of weariness, loss of strength, transient excitement, and slight delirium, very much like alcohol intoxication. Later came deep depression and loss of memory, increasing indifference, and apathy. The latter might change suddenly to acute mania or to delusions of persecution with hallucinations. Such cases usually developed early, during the victim's first months of work. Some ended in recovery, others in incurable dementia.

Koester in 1904 described a slower form, usually a toxic polyneuritis, with paralysis and atrophy. He believed carbon disulfide poisoning to be as varied in its manifestations as poisoning from lead. Probably because of this variability and because so many of its victims were young girls, the French, led by Pierre Marie, maintained for some time that CS_2 was not primarily a cause of nervous derangement but an "agent provocateur" of hysteria in those predisposed to it. However, the work of Koester disposed of that theory, for he found, in experimental animals, degenerative changes in the cerebral cells and in those of the spinal ganglia after CS_2 exposure. A necropsy performed on a worker who had acute CS_2 delirium revealed severe diffuse changes in the cerebral cortex and in the ganglion cells.

The first two papers on CS_2 poisoning in United States rubber workers were published in 1892 but they attracted little attention. Peterson (1892) gave the histories of three male rubber vulcanizers who were sent to a State Hospital for the Insane suffering from acute mania that subsided after a few weeks. Bard (1892) reported two incidents that eventuated in severe personality transformations and mental derangement. In 1902, a third United States paper appeared that described a case of amblyopia in a woman who spliced inner tubes with CS_2 (Heath, 1902). By 1914, United States plants in the rubber industry were using CS_2. Foremen reported cases of intoxication with irritability, depression, apathy, sudden outbursts of rage or fear, with hallucinations and even maniacal seizures. Yet no physician in rubber centers knew of such occurrences or that CS_2 was a poison to which rubber workers were exposed. In spite of the wealth of foreign literature on CS_2 poisoning in rubber workers, almost no notice was taken of the striking, if rare, cases occurring in American plants.

Jump and Cruice (1904) were the first to call American attention to the viscose rayon industry as a source of CS_2 poisoning. They reported three cases in churn-room men that attracted little attention. Alice Hamilton (1925) saw two cases of CS_2 poisoning. The first man had just returned to work in a viscose plant after a week on sick leave. He was very nervous, excitable, irritated by questions, and unable to bear any opposition. He had no wish to exaggerate his disability; on the contrary, he wanted to get back to his job in the churn room, provided he could sit down, for he had a distinct loss of power in his legs and he had a certain degree of ataxia. The second man was in the hospital with symptoms of acute psychosis. He seemed to be on the verge of bursting into tears and suffered keen mortification over his loss of self control, saying, "I was all right, doctor, till you came and stirred me up again."

A few years later, reports of CS_2 poisoning in viscose workers came from Europe, especially from Italy, where exposure was apparently excessive and mechanization little developed. In 1933, Ranelletti reviewed the published histories of 80 cases of CS_2 poisoning and found that 52% of these had acute psychoses, and 17% anemia and exhaustion. The psychoses were mainly of a maniacal type, with psychomotor excitement, delirium, hallucinations, distraught condition, and so-called dementia. The early stage, appearing after some months or even years of exposure, was usually one of depression, but there were sudden attacks of excitement with hallucinations. Seventeen percent of the workers had various forms of neuritis, especially involving the motor nerves. The peroneal muscles were sometimes affected so that gait was labored and dragging. Amblyopia was noted, and in one case a retrobulbar neuritis. Recovery took place, according to Ranelletti, with surprising rapidity, as a rule, when the victim was removed from exposure, even if the intoxication had resulted in "insanity."

During the Second World War, the blackout interfered with ventilation, and workers suffered from malnutrition. Vigliani (1954) studied 100 cases of chronic intoxication under wartime stress and found that 88% had polyneuritis, 28% had gastric symptoms, and headaches and vertigo each occurred in 18%. He also found that 160 to 800 ppm of CS_2 in workroom air led to signs of poisoning in a few months. Paluch (1948) reported 148 cases in two epidemics of CS_2 poisoning in Poland under the conditions of enemy occupation. He too emphasized the prevalence of polyneuritis, affecting especially the legs, never the arms alone. Biopsy showed myopathy, with both hypertrophy and atrophy of fibers. Mild cases usually recovered in two to three months, severe cases in six to eight months. If recovery was not noted in that time, it probably did not take place. An earlier belief that carbon disulfide polyneuritis is a temporary affliction with a favorable prognosis was not true in all cases.

In spite of the great growth of viscose manufacture in the United States in the 1930s, this danger to employees was very tardily recognized. Indeed, as late as 1946 psychiatrists in state institutions for the mentally ill were entering in their records items such as "etiology occupational," or "unknown," or "exogenous poison," but making no mention of CS_2, which apparently was not accepted as a cause of mental disease. In the most thorough early study of CS_2 poisoning in the United States, Lewey (1941) examined 120 men who were employed at the time as churn-room men and spinners. Mild forms of poisoning were found in 60% of spinners, whose exposure was not high, while in churners, whose exposure was much greater, severe poisoning was found in 20% in one plant, in 44% in the other. Lewey found that chronic carbon disulfide intoxication may involve all parts of the central and peripheral nervous systems, beginning with psychic symptoms, followed later by peripheral neuropathy and damage to the cranial nerves, decrease in corneal and pupillary reflexes as well as pyramidal and extrapyramidal signs. A variety of clinical pictures very much like Parkinson's disease was also observed. Kujelová et al. (1979) have suggested that CS_2 induces a pyridoxine deficiency, evidenced by reduced urine levels of 4-pyridoxic acid in rayon mill workers, that contributes to the development of the polyneuropathy.

Summary of Clinical Syndromes

Although the chronic form of poisoning is far more serious, acute cases are seen in which the concentrated vapors cause irritation to the eyes, nose, and skin. In chronic carbon disulfide poisoning the nervous system bears the brunt of the damage. Neuritis affecting peripheral or cranial nerves (optic and auditory) is very common. Usually the trouble begins with a sensation of crawling over the skin, formication, a tendency for the arms and legs to "go to sleep," a sensation of coldness and heaviness, and a curious feeling that the hand and foot belong to someone else. Pain and tenderness along the nerve trunks are associated with these symptoms, and at the same time tests may show touch, pain, and temperature sense to be heightened, rarely diminished. There is usually constant or paroxysmal pain in the distribution of one or several nerves and, during the night, pain in the legs may reach an intolerable intensity. Any of the nerves may be affected, but those that are more usually involved are the radial and ulnar, the sciatic, and the external peroneal. These symptoms are soon followed by signs of motor nerve involvement. The worker complains of fatigue, increased loss of strength and weakness in the legs. The reflexes are most often diminished. Reduced peripheral nerve conduction velocities have been demonstrated in rats (Knobloch et al., 1979) and in patients with chronic CS_2 poisoning. The earlier susceptibility of sensory fibers has permitted the diagnosis of polyneuropathy to be made in the subclinical stage, according to Vasilescu (1976).

The course of carbon disulfide neuritis is slow —slower than that of alcoholic, rheumatic, or syphilitic origin. Recovery proceeds with extreme slowness, and the prognosis must be guarded because the atrophy, pain, paresthesias, and other manifestations may persist even if the victim quits his job.

The most striking and the most disastrous effects of carbon disulfide poisoning are upon the brain. The mental symptoms run the gamut from simple irritability and depression to manic-depressive insanity. Increased rates of suicide have been reported for some populations of viscose rayon workers (Mancuso and Locke, 1972). If the basal ganglia are involved, Parkinsonian palsy occurs. In typical cases the attack of active or violent mental disturbance comes on fairly suddenly, but careful questioning of the family and fellow workers will always bring to light an earlier stage of emotional upset, irritability, depression, and complaint of loss of memory. Even in milder poisoning, changes in personality are evident, especially in the worker's relations with his or her spouse and children, and the victims realize this but are powerless to help it. Sleeplessness, dreams, and loss of memory are frequent complaints. Disturbances of vision, though rarely of a pronounced character, are often present and give valuable aid in the diagnosis. Central scotoma for color, abnormal color vision, loss of visual acuity, and paralysis of accommodation have been described (Gordy and Trumper, 1943). Retinopathy in the form of microaneurysms and small dot hemorrhages have been reported by Sugimoto et al. (1978). Impaired color discrimination in viscose rayon workers has been attributed to a reduction of retinal ganglion cell receptiveness or to a toxic demyelination of optic nerve fibers (Raitta et al., 1981).

Gastric disturbances are common in some reports with symptoms that mimic those of peptic ulcer. Heart, liver, and kidney damage have been described as associated with high and continuous CS$_2$ exposure. Beginning in 1950, chronic poisonings were reported that presented symptoms very similar to those found in pre-senile cerebral arteriosclerosis. Workers in the age group from 42 to 55 are usually affected, and they often have associated kidney damage. While some cases present only one aspect of the atherosclerotic process, some present a complete picture of cerebral, renal, and myocardial sclerosis (Browning, 1965). Von Rechenberg in 1957 and Vigliani and Cazzullo (1950) reported that workers exposed to CS$_2$ first noted pain in the calf of the leg, with difficulty in walking. In some cases, electrocardiograms suggested previous myocardial infarctions (Brieger, 1961). At autopsy, atheromatous plaques were found along with general arteriosclerosis, with retinal vessel changes resembling those in hypertension and glomerulosclerosis. A 10-year cohort mortality study of viscose rayon workers in Finland suggested that CS$_2$ exposure along with elevated blood pressures were the prominent risk factors for coronary heart disease in these workers (Tolonen et al., 1979). In contrast, Lieben et al. (1974), in their study of three rayon plants in the United States, found hypertension to be the only significant finding and these blood pressure values were not correlated with increased CS$_2$ exposures, perhaps because concentrations above 20 ppm were rare, especially after 1958.

While some of these reports are old and describe European experience in rubber factories, exposures continue because CS$_2$ is used as a raw material in the manufacture of viscose rayon and has excellent solvent properties. According to Kleinfeld and Tabershaw (1955) poisoning has been rare in the United States. Brieger (1961) reviewed the knowledge of CS$_2$ toxicity derived from laboratory animal studies as well as occupational illness. The biological behavior of CS$_2$ has had the attention of a number of research laboratories, especially in Italy and Czechoslovakia, and their work was summarized in a conference held in Prague in 1966 (Brieger and Teisinger, 1967). The details of the effects of absorbed CS$_2$ are to be found in Brieger's review (1961), Browning (1965), Cooper (1976), and NIOSH (1977). Briefly stated, CS$_2$ has been shown to have a toxic action on protein metabolism. In addition, by hepatic damage, CS$_2$ produces nervous system disease and hypercholesterolemia that leads to early arteriosclerosis.

Direct measurement of blood and urine for carbon disulfide levels gives some evidence of intensity of exposure. A more specific chemical test is available to evaluate exposure by measuring CS$_2$ metabolites in urine by using the iodine-azide method (Djurić et al., 1965).

At the present time, the permissible exposure limit in the United States is 20 ppm. Limits in other countries vary from about 20 ppm (60 mg/m^3) in Hungary, Japan, and the Federal Republic of Germany down to 3 ppm (10 mg/m^3) in Poland and the USSR. NIOSH (1977), however, recommended a limit of 1 ppm (3 mg/m^3) as a time-weighted average for up to a 10-hour workshift, 40-hour workweek, and a 15-minute ceiling concentration of 10 ppm (30 mg/m^3).

References

Bard CL: Insanity due to bisulphide of carbon. *South Cal Pract* 1892;7:476–485.

Brieger H: Chronic carbon disulfide poisoning. *J Occup Med* 1961;3:302–308.

Brieger H, Teisinger J (eds): *Toxicology of Carbon Disulphide.* Amsterdam, Excerpta Medica, 1967.

Browning E: *Toxicity and Metabolism of Industrial Solvents.* New York, Elsevier, 1965, pp 702–721.

Constensoux MG, Heim MF: Fréquence relative des stigmates nerveux dans le sulfocarbonisme chronique. Question VI. *2me Congr Intern Mal Prof,* Brussels, 1910.

Cooper P: Carbon disulphide toxicology: The present picture. *Food Cosmet Toxicol* 1976;14:57–59.

Delpech A: *Memoir sur les Accidents que Développe Chez les Ouvriers en Caoutchoue l'Inhalation du Sulfure de Carbone en Vapeur.* Paris, Labe, 1856.

Djurić D, Surdučki N, Berkeš I: Iodine-azide test on urine of persons exposed to carbon disulphide. *Br J Ind Med* 1965;22:321–323.

266

Gordy ST, Trumper M: Carbon disulfide poisoning, with a report of six cases. *J Am Med Assoc* 1938;110:1543–1549.

Hamilton A: *Industrial Poisons in the United States.* New York, MacMillan, 1925, pp 360–370.

Heath FC: Amblyopia from carbon bisulphide poisoning. *Arch Ophthalmol* 1902;11:4–8.

Jump HD, Cruice JM: Chronic poisoning from bisulphide of carbon. *Univ Penn Med Bull* 1904; 17:193–196.

Kleinfeld M, Tabershaw IR: Carbon disulfide poisoning: Report of two cases. *J Am Med Assoc* 1955;159:677–679.

Knobloch K, Stetkiewicz J, Wrońska-Nofer T: Conduction velocity in the peripheral nerves of rats with chronic carbon disulphide neuropathy. *Br J Ind Med* 1979;36:148–152.

Koester G: Ein klinischer Beitrag zur Lehre von der Chronischen Schwefelkohlenstoffvergiftung. *Deutsch Zeitschr Nervenh* 1904;26:1–56.

Kujalová V, Sperlingová I, Hromádka M: Urinary level of 4-pyridoxic acid in chronic exposure to carbon disulphide. *Med lavoro* 1979;70: 388–390.

Laudenheimer R: *Die Schwefelkohlenstoffvergiftung der Gummiarbeiter.* Leipsig, Veit, 1899.

Lewey FH: Neurological, medical and biochemical signs and symptoms indicating chronic industrial carbon disulphide absorption. *Ann Intern Med* 1941;15:869–883.

Lieben J, Menduke H, Flegel EE, et al: Cardiovascular effects of CS_2 exposure. *J Occup Med* 1974;16:449–453.

Mancuso TF, Locke BZ: Carbon disulphide as a cause of suicide. Epidemiological study of viscose rayon workers. *J Occup Med* 1972;14:595–606.

NIOSH: *Criteria for a Recommended Standard . . . . Occupational Exposure to Carbon Disulfide.* Washington, DC, National Institute for Occupational Safety and Health (NIOSH 77-156), 1977.

Paluch EA: Two outbreaks of carbon disulfide poisoning in rayon staple fiber plants in Poland. *J Ind Hyg Toxicol* 1948;30:37–42.

Peterson F: Three cases of acute mania from inhaling carbon bisulphide. *Boston Med Surg J* 1892;127:325–326.

Raitta C, Teir H, Tolonen M, et al: Impaired color discrimination among viscose rayon workers exposed to carbon disulfide. *J Occup Med* 1981; 23:189–192.

Ranelletti A: *Il Solfocarbonismo professionale.* Turin, Italy, La Grafica Moderna, 1933.

Sugimoto K, Goto S, Kanda S, et al: Studies on angiopathy due to carbon disulfide. Retinopathy and index of exposure doses. *Scand J Work Environ Health* 1978;4:151–158.

Tolonen M, Nurminen M, Hernberg S: Ten-year coronary mortality of workers exposed to carbon disulfide. *Scand J Work Environ Health* 1979;5:109–114.

Vasilescu C: Sensory and motor conduction in chronic carbon disulphide poisoning. *Eur Neurol* 1976;14:447–457.

Vigliani EC: Carbon disulphide poisoning in viscose rayon factories. *Br J Ind Med* 1954;11: 235–244.

Vigliani EC, Cazzulo CL: Alterazioni del sistema nervoso centrale di origine vascolare nel solfocarbonismo. *Med lavoro* 1950;41:49–63.

von Rechenberg HK: Das vasculäre Spätsyndrom der chronischen Schwefelkohlenstoffvergiftung. *Helv Med Acta* 1957;24:510–513.

SECTION FIVE
ORGANIC HIGH POLYMERS

1 • *Introduction*

The organic high polymers, regardless of their ultimate applications, are similar to the extent that they are based upon the structural repetition of smaller units (monomers), and they often contain additional substances that are not actually part of the polymer itself. Toxic phenomena associated with the high polymers may be related to their unreacted or underreacted constituents, to various auxiliary substances, or to degradation products. It is uncommon for a fully reacted or "cured" polymer to cause illness since most of these materials have a high degree of biological inertness and insolubility.

Plastics are usually defined as high molecular weight materials that are soft enough during manufacture to be molded by heat or pressure but are solid and permanently deformed in the finished state. The term elastomers is applied to those polymers, such as natural and synthetic rubbers, that can be stretched easily and that return to their original dimensions when the stressing force is removed. Elasticity is thus a capacity to be reversibly deformed. Linear macromolecules with high longitudinal mechanical strength and lateral flexibility can be utilized to form synthetic fibers for textile applications.

The toxicology of plastics has been reviewed by Lefaux (1968), by Eckardt and Hindin (1973), and by Eckardt (1976).

References

Eckardt RE: Occupational and environmental health hazards in the plastics industry. *Environ Health Persp* 1976;17:103–106.

Eckardt RE, Hindin R: The health hazards of plastics. *J Occup Med* 1973;10:808–819.

Lefaux R: *Practical Toxicology of Plastics.* Cleveland, CRC Press, 1968.

2 • Plastics

The term *resin* has an imprecise meaning in the plastics industry and may be used interchangeably with the term *plastic*. In some applications, resins are short-chain uncured polymers that are subjected to further polymerization and hardening. In other applications, resins are granular, fully cured thermoplastics that can be heated for extrusion, molding, or calendering.

The principal plastics may be divided into two groups: 1) *thermosets*, which cannot be reformed or melted after the initial "cure" and are generally obtained by polycondensation, and 2) *thermoplastics*, which can be reheated and reshaped repeatedly and are usually obtained by polymerization. A simple list is given in Table 8.

Table 8
Principal Plastics

Thermosets	
Aminos (urea and melamine)	Polyesters and alkyds
	Polyurethanes
Epoxys (ethoxylin)	Silicones
Phenolics	
Thermoplastics	
Acetals	Polyvinyl chloride
Acrylics	Nylons
Acrylonitrile-butadiene-styrene	Polycarbonates
	Polyethylene
Cellulosics (cellulose acetate propionate, butyrate)	Phenylene oxide
	Polypropylene
	Polystyrene
Fluoroplastics	Polyvinylidene chloride
Polyvinyl alcohol	

Thermosetting Resins

Amino resins The amino resins are formed by the condensation of aldehydes with amines and are almost entirely based upon urea-formaldehyde and melamine-formaldehyde. They are typically used for electrical switch housings, knobs, molded dinnerware, adhesives, plywood glues, coatings, and industrial laminates. Crease-resistant garments are produced by pressing textiles impregnated with suitable amino resins into the desired shape. Hexamethylenetetramine, called "hexa," is used as a stabilizer in amino resin systems to prevent premature hardening. It decomposes to form formaldehyde and is a possible source of irritating and sensitizing skin reactions, but it has never been a major problem in the plastics or the explosives industries. Acetic acid accelerators similarly do not present unusual problems.

The component of principal toxicologic interest is formaldehyde (CH_2O), which is present in the production of the resin and in incompletely cured products. Pure monomeric formaldehyde is a pungent colorless gas that polymerizes readily in aqueous or alcoholic solutions. It also reacts with water to form methylene glycol. Its toxic properties are discussed in the chapter on aldehydes.

Epoxy resins Cured epoxy resins have outstanding resistance to heat and chemicals and find wide application in reinforced plastics, coatings, adhesives, and in casting, "potting," and encapsulation. The typical resin is prepared by condensation of epichlorhydrin with a diphenol in the presence of a curing agent. Epoxy resins are cured by cross-linking agents known as "hardeners," such as the polyamines (diethylenetriamine, triethylenetetramine, piperazine) or the acid anhydrides and polybasic acids (phthalic anhydride, adipic acid). Catalysts perform a similar curing action but do not themselves act as cross-linking agents. Common catalysts include various polyamides, monoethylamine, and tertiary amines, such as triethylamine and benzyl-dimethylamine. Diluents—phenyl, allyl, and butyl glycidyl ether, styrene oxide, styrene, and other epoxides—may be utilized to reduce the viscosity of uncured resin systems.

Epichlorhydrin, bisphenol A, and liquid epoxy resins are skin irritants and sensitizers, as are the reactive diluent ethers and the related epoxy compounds. Epichlorhydrin is discussed in the chapter on chlorinated hydrocarbons. It has been pointed out that the epoxy group may be associated with radiomimetic effects that presumably reflect biological alkylation (Kotin and Falk, 1963). There is no evidence, however, that these substances are comparable to the nitrogen mustards in this regard, or that there is an industrial hazard related to this action.

Industrial health problems most frequently arise from exposure to aliphatic polyamine hardeners, which can cause severe primary irritative as well as hypersensitivity dermatitis and asthmatic reactions. These amines are strongly alkaline (pH 13-14) and can produce chemical burns of the skin. Some contain dye bases that may yellow the skin. Cutaneous amine reactions include erythema, intolerable itching, and severe facial swelling. Blistering may occur with weeping of serous fluid, crusting, and scaling. An apparently permanent hypersensitive state may develop as an extreme reaction to amines. Cases are recorded of persons with previous amine dermatitis who experienced a dramatic return of symptoms upon minute re-exposure. Highly sensitive persons may also react to cured resins containing small amounts of unreacted amine hardeners.

Although pulmonary reactions in the modern plastics industry are most commonly associated with components of polyurethane systems, amine hardeners for epoxy resins do cause bronchospasm and coughing episodes that may persist for several days after cessation of exposure. Repeated attacks of acute amine-induced respiratory disease are often associated with increased responsiveness to these compounds, for faint traces of amine vapors in the air have been sufficient to trigger the return of intense symptoms in persons with a history of amine asthma.

Acid anhydrides and polyamide hardeners and catalysts are contact irritants, but industrial problems related to their use have been uncommon. Diluents such as xylene or the ketones do not sensitize but may defat the skin with repeated contact. Glass fibers used in many applications are mechanically irritating and cause pruritis, and they may be released when inert laminates or other forms are cut or tooled. Sawing, machining, and other manipulations of solid cured resins that produce heat may give rise to degradation products that contain free amines or unreacted epichlorhydrin.

Prevention of problems from epoxy exposure is based upon meticulous cleanliness of work areas. Mixing of resin and hardener and the application of the liquid formulations should be done with appropriate ventilation. Material that is spilled on the skin should be removed promptly with soap and water. Organic solvents used for this purpose tend to spread contamination and irritate the skin.

Reference

Kotin P, Falk H: Organic peroxides, hydrogen peroxide, epoxides, and neoplasia. *Radiation Res* 1963 (suppl 3);193–211.

Phenolics The modern plastics industry is based on Baekeland's discovery in 1909 of phenol-formaldehyde thermosetting materials. The term *phenolic resins* now encompasses a variety of similar products made by the polycondensation of phenols with aldehydes. The "phenols" used for this purpose include phenol, cresol, xylenol, p-t-butylphenol, and resorcinol. The aldehydes involved include formaldehyde, paraformaldehyde, and furfural. Alkaline catalysts include hexamethylenetetramine (called "hexa"), ammonia, and various other amines. The applications of phenolic resins are similar to those of the amino resins, which have similar structures and properties. Large quantities of phenol-formaldehyde resins are used in bonded brake linings and clutch facings and as bonding agents for foundry sand models.

Important industrial health effects are dermatitides. Phenol is a potent primary irritant, and resorcinol, furfural, and formaldehyde are both irritants and sensitizers. Furfural, in addition, is a photosensitizer. In some applications, cashew nut shell oil has been used as a phenolic component in the resin formulation. This oil is chemically related to poison ivy resins, but the oil used in industry is said to have been treated to render it safe for handling. Nevertheless, persons highly sensitive to *Rhus*-type oleoresins may be reactive. Workers handling finely divided molding powder may be exposed to dusts that are irritating to the skin and that sometimes cause allergic dermatitis.

270

Polyesters and alkyds Materials of the polyester and alkyds group are fundamental to reinforced plastic technology, which has become increasingly important in the boat and automotive body industry and in the manufacture of structural panels, electric appliances, and home furnishings. The reinforcement is generally provided by glass fiber textiles, and the typical structure consists of laminations of polyester and textile. The polyesters are derived by the reactions of polyfunctional alcohols (e.g., propylene glycol, ethylene glycol, pentaerythritol) with polyfunctional acids (e.g., phthalic or maleic anhydride). Polyesters are dissolved in styrene and stabilized with an inhibitor, such as hydroquinone, to form a viscous syrup-like liquid that does not solidify readily. When gelation is desired, a catalyst, usually a peroxide (e.g., benzoyl peroxide or methyl ethyl ketone peroxide), is added. To accelerate this cross-linking solidification, promoters or accelerators (dimethylaniline or cobalt salts) may also be added. While styrene is generally the reactive solvent and cross-linking group between the polyester macromolecules, other equivalent compounds may be used for special purposes. Methylmethacrylate increases resistance to weathering, diallyl phthalate resists polymerization of the uncatalyzed syrup, and triallyl cyanurate increases resistance to elevated temperatures.

The acid phthalates can cause burns when applied to damp skin. The dusts are irritating to the eyes and upper airway, but there is no important systemic toxicity. The organic peroxides are highly irritating to epithelial tissues and are flammable oxidizing agents. There is also evidence that benzoyl and methyl ethyl ketone peroxides are skin sensitizers, as are dimethylaniline and cobalt naphthenate. Dimethylaniline can produce most of the effects of aniline. Although the allyl group has well-known toxic properties, serious occupational hazards have not been associated with diallyl phthalate and triallyl cyanurate, both of which are irritants. Polyester dusts produced by grinding operations can result in cough, dyspnea, and eye and throat irritation in exposed workers, who may also have marked reduction in expiratory flow rates (Zuskin et al., 1979). Generally, however, industrial health problems from the polyester group are infrequent, except for the direct effects of styrene, and most of them may be attributed to the mechanical effects of glass fibers on the skin.

Styrene (vinylbenzene; phenylethylene) is an oily liquid that is soluble in most organic solvents. It can be taken up by the bloodstream by inhalation and by percutaneous absorption. It and its metabolite, styrene oxide, are converted eventually to mandelic, hippuric, and phenylglyoxylic acids, which are excreted in the urine and can be used for biological monitoring of exposure (Fields and Horstman, 1979; Wilson et al., 1979). The acute toxicity of styrene involves irritation of the skin, eyes, and airway, and depression of the nervous system (Leibman, 1975; Härkönen, 1978). "Styrene sickness" consists of nausea and vomiting, headache, fatigue, dizziness, and drowsiness (Wilson, 1944). Workers exposed to styrene showed an appreciable incidence of prenarcotic symptoms and signs of incipient peripheral neuropathy as evidenced by distal lower limb hypesthesia and reduced peroneal nerve conduction velocity (Lilis et al., 1978). Some studies have detected chromosome aberrations in peripheral lymphocytes in workers in the reinforced plastics industry, presumably as the result of exposure to styrene (Bardoděj, 1978; Meretoja et al., 1978; Högstedt et al., 1979). Laboratory studies have shown styrene oxide to be mutagenic, although the mutagenicity of styrene itself could be demonstrated only after metabolic or immunologic manipulation (Loprieno et al., 1976; Vainio et al., 1976). The irritant properties of styrene are usually sufficiently potent to protect workers against serious effects, but perception of the characteristic odor diminishes with continued exposure. The permissible exposure limit for styrene vapor is 100 ppm.

References

Bardoděj Z: Styrene, its metabolism and the evaluation of hazards in industry. *Scand J Work Environ Health* 1978 (suppl 2);95–103.

Fields RL, Horstman SW: Biomonitoring of industrial styrene exposures. *Am Ind Hyg Assoc J* 1979;40:451–459.

Härkönen H: Styrene, its experimental and clinical toxicology. *Scand J Work Environ Health* 1978 (suppl 2);104–113.

Högstedt B, Hedner K, Mark-Vendel E, et al: Increased frequency of chromosome aberrations in workers exposed to styrene. *Scand J Work Environ Health* 1979;5:333–335.

Leibman KC: Metabolism and toxicity of styrene. *Environ Health Persp* 1975;11:115–119.

Lilis R, Lorimer WV, Diamond S, et al: Neurotoxicity of styrene in production and polymerization workers. *Environ Res* 1978;15:133-138.

Loprieno N, Abbondandolo A, Barale R, et al: Mutagenicity of industrial compounds: Styrene and its possible metabolite styrene oxide. *Mutation Res* 1976;40:317-324.

Meretoja T, Järventaus H, Sorsa M, et al: Chromosome aberrations in lymphocytes of workers exposed to styrene. *Scand J Work Environ Health* 1978 (suppl 2);259-264.

Vainio H, Pääkkönen R, Rönnholm K, et al: A study on the mutagenic activity of styrene and styrene oxide. *Scand J Work Environ Health* 1976;3:147-151.

Wilson HK, Cocker J, Purnell CJ, et al: The time course of mandelic and phenylglyoxylic acid excretion in workers exposed to styrene under model conditions. *Br J Ind Med* 1979;36:235-237.

Wilson RH: Health hazards encountered in the manufacture of synthetic rubber. *J Am Med Assoc* 1944;124:701-703.

Zuskin E, Saric M, Bouhuys A: Airway responsiveness in workers processing polyester resins. *J Occup Med* 1979;21:825-827.

Polyurethanes Urethane polymers are formed by polyaddition reactions between a diisocyanate and either a polyhydroxy compound, a polyester, or a polyether. Polyurethanes are used in coatings, elastomers, and foam cushions and flotation devices. Catalysts used to promote the reaction include organotin compounds, cobalt naphthenate, or various amines. In the course of polymerization, carbon dioxide is evolved to give rise to bubbles or foam. To obtain additional gas, foaming or blowing agents may be included to supplement the gases evolved in the basic reaction. Polyurethane foams are typically poured or sprayed into position, where the so-called final cure occurs.

Although amines are irritating and sensitizing, the main health problem associated with polyurethane plastics arises from the diisocyanates, most commonly toluene diisocyanate (TDI) and to some extent methylene diphenyl diisocyanate (MDI). TDI is employed in making flexible foams while the less volatile MDI is used for rigid foams. Vapors of these compounds invariably become airborne in polymerization reactions, especially since heat and gases are evolved. Clinical experience with TDI shows that it is a potent irritant of the eyes and upper airway. With prolonged exposure there may be significant respiratory distress wth dry painful cough, chest pain, and occasional blood-streaking of scant sputum. In some cases, fever, cyanosis, and general feeling of distress have been noted. The chest x-ray in these situations has usually been normal, although diagnoses or descriptions of bronchitis, "increased markings," or "reticulation" have been made (Brugsch and Elkins, 1963).

Acute, severe exposures to TDI have led to gastrointestinal distress and to neurological complaints that have included euphoria, ataxia, and loss of consciousness, and to lingering problems of poor memory, personality changes, irritability, and depression (Le Quesne et al., 1976). Continued or repeated exposures to TDI have resulted in bronchospasm, sometimes very severe, chest tightness, wheezing, cyanosis, and collapse. Chronic exposure has also been shown to result in loss of pulmonary function, as measured by $FEV_{1.0}$, that was correlated with the degree of exposure (Wegman et al., 1977). Some workers become exceedingly sensitive to TDI vapors and react dramatically to minute amounts of this material in the air (Dodson, 1971). While the nature of the sensitivity to TDI has not been clearly established, there is clinical evidence for the involvement of antigen-antibody mechanisms as shown by the presence of TDI-specific IgE antibodies and the development of positive skin test reactions to TDI-conjugates with human serum albumin (Butcher et al., 1977; Karol et al., 1978, 1979; Karol, 1980). It is also not clear whether chronic injury occurs, either in response to repeated acute episodes or to low-level long-term exposures without prominent symptoms. Nonspecific mechanisms may also be involved, especially in persons with a high degree of specific sensitivity (O'Brien et al., 1979).

There is evidence that the already low level threshold level value (TLV) of 0.02 ppm is not sufficiently low to preclude the development of bronchospastic reactions in sensitized persons (Wegman et al., 1977). Peters and his associates (1965) showed that TDI concentrations of one tenth of the TLV may cause significant depressions in the forced vital capacity and forced expiratory volume in one second. NIOSH (1978) recommended that no employee be exposed to vapor concentrations of any of the diisocyanates greater than 0.005 ppm (5 ppb) for a 10-hour workshift, 40-hour workweek, and that 20 ppb be a ceiling concentration for a 10-minute sampling period.

Treatment of these pulmonary problems is based

almost entirely upon control of exposure. For highly sensitive persons, work with polyurethane foams must be eliminated. Engineering measures are essential to the adequate control of vapors. Bronchospasm responds to bronchodilators; oxygen may be indicated in severe cases.

References

Brugsch HG, Elkins HB: Toluene di-isocyanate (TDI) toxicity. *N Engl J Med* 1963;268:353–357.

Butcher BT, Jones RN, O'Neil CE, et al: Longitudinal study of workers employed in the manufacture of toluene-diisocyanate. *Am Rev Resp Dis* 1977;116:411–421.

Dodson VN: Isocyanate anhelation. *J Occup Med* 1971;13:238–241.

Karol MH: Study of guinea pig and human antibodies to toluene diisocyanate. *Am Rev Resp Dis* 1980;122:965–970.

Karol MH, Ioset HH, Alarie YC: Tolyl-specific IgE antibodies in workers with sensitivity to toluene diisocyanate. *Am Ind Hyg Assoc J* 1978; 39:454–458.

Karol MH, Sandberg T, Riley EJ, et al: Longitudinal study of tolyl-reactive IgE antibodies in workers hypersensitive to TDI. *J Occup Med* 1979;21:354–358.

Le Quesne PM, Axford AT, McKerrow CB, et al: Neurological complications after a single severe exposure to toluene di-isocyanate. *Br J Ind Med* 1976;33:72–78.

NIOSH: *Criteria for a Recommended Standard . . . . Occupational Exposure to Di-isocyanates.* Washington, DC, National Institute for Occupational Safety and Health (NIOSH 78-215), 1978.

O'Brien IM, Newman-Taylor AJ, Burge PS, et al: Toluene di-isocyanate-induced asthma. II. Inhalation challenge tests and bronchial reactivity studies. *Clin Allergy* 1979;9:7–15.

Peters JM, Murphy RLH, Pagnotto LD, et al: Respiratory impairment in workers exposed to "safe" levels of toluene diisocyanate (TDI). *Arch Environ Health* 1965;20:364–367.

Wegman DH, Peters JM, Pagnotto L, et al: Chronic pulmonary function loss from exposure to toluene diisocyanate. *Br J Ind Med* 1977;34: 196–200.

Silicones   Silicones are composed of chains of alternate atoms of oxygen and silicon. Various organic groups can be attached to the silicon atoms, and the amount of cross-linkage between chains by these groups determines whether the polymer will be hard, an elastomer, or a fluid. The fully reacted polymers are remarkably inert and thus find use in heart valves, prostheses, heart-lung machines, and artificial kidneys. Major industrial uses are in lubricants, encapsulations, dielectric laminates, and "non-stick" release compounds.

The biological properties of the silicone intermediates have not been studied. Of the silicones, the chlorosilanes are corrosive to mucous membranes while the ethoxysilanes are less so. Various metallic soaps, acetic acid, and toluene solvents may be used in final applications.

Thermoplastics

Acetal resins (polyformaldehyde)   Acetal resins, also known as polyformaldehyde, are polymers of very pure formaldehyde and are materials of unusually good mechanical properties. They are resistant to elongation and impact and replace light metals in many applications. They may be thermally degraded, e.g., in an overheated molding machine, to formaldehyde with its well-recognized irritant and sensitizing properties that have already been discussed.

Acrylics   Acrylic plastics, such as Lucite and Plexiglas, are based upon methyl and ethyl acrylate and methacrylate; methyl methacrylate is the major constituent. These substances are respiratory and cutaneous irritants, the acrylates more so than the methacrylates. Acrylic monomers can be sensitizers, and allergic dermatitis has been described in printers handling light-sensitive acrylics (Rycroft, 1977). Methyl methacrylate vapors can produce headache, irritability, and other nonspecific symptoms. In experimental animals, inhalation of these vapors leads to weight loss, reduced adipose tissue, and inhibition of gastrointestinal motor activity (Tansy et al., 1976, 1977). Embryotoxicity and fetotoxicity have also been reported in rats (Nicholas et al., 1979). Acrylic paints are comprised of a water emulsion of acrylic polymers that have no known biological importance.

References

Nicholas CA, Lawrence WH, Autian J: Embryotoxicity and fetotoxicity from maternal inhalation of methyl methacrylate monomer in rats. *Toxicol Appl Pharmacol* 1979;50:451–458.

Rycroft RJG: Contact dermatitis from acrylic compounds. *Br J Dermatol* 1977;96:685–687.

Tansy MF, Kendall FM, Benhayem S, et al: Chronic biological effects of methyl methacrylate vapor. I. Body and tissue weights, blood chemistries, and intestinal transit in the rat. *Environ Res* 1976;11:66–77.

Tansy MF, Martin JS, Benhaim S, et al: GI motor inhibition associated with acute exposure to methyl methacrylate vapor. *J Pharm Sci* 1977; 66:613–619.

Acrylonitrile-butadiene-styrene The materials of this mixture can be varied in relative quantity and treatment to produce a family of plastics suited to home appliances, automobile instrument panels, boats, recreational vehicle bodies, and a heterogeneous group of other applications.

The monomeric reactants all have biological properties that are absent in the finished product. Butadiene is a weak irritant and narcotic gas that is combustible and explosive. It is used primarily in the production of synthetic rubber. Acronitrile (vinyl cyanide) is a flammable volatile liquid that can be absorbed through the skin, lungs, and intestinal mucosa. Its biological properties are those of cyanide, and the intensity of intoxication appears to be correlated with the blood level of cyanide ion. Medical therapy for acute acrylonitrile poisoning is the same as that for cyanide poisoning. Some workers handling acrylonitrile for 20 to 45 minutes have developed headache, chest fullness, mucous membrane irritation, apprehension, and irritability. Several cases developed mild jaundice, low grade anemia, and leucocytosis (Wilson and McCormick, 1954). Since acrylonitrile can pass through the intact skin, special attention to decontamination and the clean-up of spills is especially important. The compound can also penetrate various types of rubber, and gloves may not provide suitable protection. Chronic acrylonitrile intoxication apparently does not occur among workers in acrylic fiber factories (Sakurai et al., 1978) but there is some epidemiologic indication that this compound may be carcinogenic for man (O'Berg, 1980).

References

O'Berg MT: Epidemiologic study of workers exposed to acrylonitrile. *J Occup Med* 1980;22: 245–252.

Sakurai H, Onodera M, Utsunomiya T, et al: Health effects of acrylonitrile in acrylic fibre. *Br J Ind Med* 1978;35:219–225.

Wilson RH, McCormick WE: Toxicology of plastics and rubber—Plastomers and monomers. *Ind Med Surg* 1954;23:479–486.

Cellulose derivatives (cellulosics) Cellulose acetate, propionate, and butyrate have almost entirely replaced cellulose nitrate, which is highly flammable and is a source, when burned, of nitrogen dioxide gas. Modern cellulosics are used in nontoxic films and coatings in small parts such as knobs, eyeglass frames, and pencil barrels. Toxicity is not associated with these polymers. The synthetic process may involve exposure to solvents and organic acid compounds that may result in skin reactions.

Fluoroplastics Fluoroplastics vary somewhat in composition and include polytetrafluoroethylene, polyfluorinated ethylenepropylene, and polyvinylidene fluoride. These materials have high thermal stability, are extremely inert biologically, and can be used for human organ prostheses as well as for highly resistant insulations, chemical piping, containers, gaskets, and coatings. The widely used Teflon is a fluoroplastic.

Harmful worker exposures are not commonly related to the production of the polymers themselves inasmuch as the reactions are conducted in closed systems. The chemical intermediates include fluorohydrocarbons of the so-called Freon type, which are relatively inert or have only narcotic properties at high concentrations. More active reactants may occur in the polymerization process and these may be highly corrosive and possibly nephrotoxic, but exposures to them are highly unlikely. Illness resulting from exposure to the pyrolysis of fluorohydrocarbons is similar to influenza and was first described by the term "polymer-fume fever" by Harris (1951). Subsequent reports, among others by Lewis and Kerby (1965) and Wegman and Peters (1974), describe the symptoms that appear some four to five hours after exposure to sublimates or thermal decomposition products of fluoroplastics. These consist of chest tightness and dyspnea, followed rapidly by general malaise, aching, weakness, headache, and cough. Chills and fever to 40°C follow the onset of symptoms by about 12 hours. The acute illness may be alarming and uncomfortable when it is severe, but it is of short duration and without known sequelae.

In most situations the toxic material is generated when polymer dust contaminates smoking tobacco. The temperature of burning tobacco, 875°C, or equivalent heat sources is sufficient to cause pyrolysis of the otherwise inert polymer, and most cases have been associated with smoking on the job. The composition of the thermal decomposition products is complex and includes carbonyl fluoride, which is converted to hydrogen fluoride in the presence of water vapor. Other products include tetrafluoroethylene, hexafluoropropylene, octofluorocyclobutane, and octofluoroisobutylene (Arito and Soda, 1977). Under some circumstances, transient pulmonary edema has been observed, a finding that is not surprising since hydrogen fluoride and other highly irritating materials are contained in the pyrolysis fume. There is no evidence, however, of chronic illness in man from this cause.

Control of whatever problem exists is accomplished through warnings to the workers, prohibition of smoking in the work place, hand washing, and attention to airborne dust and to heat sources. NIOSH (1977) recommended that its proposals for standards for inorganic fluorides and for hydrogen fluoride also be followed.

References

Arito H, Soda R: Pyrolysis products of polytetrafluoroethylene and polyfluoroethylenepropylene with reference to inhalation toxicity. *Ann Occup Hyg* 1977;20:247–255.

Harris DK: Polymer-fume fever. *Lancet* 1951; 2:1008–1011.

Lewis CE, Kerby GR: An epidemic of polymer-fume fever. *J Am Med Assoc* 1965;191:103–106.

NIOSH: *Criteria for a Recommended Standard . . . . Occupational Exposure to Decomposition Products of Fluorocarbon Polymers.* Washington, DC, National Institute for Occupational Safety and Health (NIOSH 77-193), 1977.

Wegman DH, Peters JM: Polymer fume fever and cigarette smoking. *Ann Intern Med* 1974;81: 55–57.

Polyamides Polyamides, such as the Nylons, are used in fibers, filaments, castings, and extrusions, and can be classified into two families: the diamine-dibasic acid type and the condensed amino acid type. The finished plastic in either group has no known toxic effects, although nylons are not entirely inert biologically. Diamine-dibasic acid nylons are prepared by reacting a diamine, such as hexamethylenediamine, with an acid, such as adipic or sebacic acid. The diamine has a primary irritant as well as a sensitizing effect on skin and is irritating to the eyes and upper airway. The dibasic acids are not a source of illness. Amino acid nylons are formed from the condensation of materials such as ε-caprolactam (cyclohexanone iso-oxime), which is a convulsant for experimental animals. It is not a skin irritant and it can be respired as a fine dust for long periods without adverse effects (Goldblatt et al., 1954). Furthermore, the low volatility of ε-caprolactam makes its inhalation as a vapor unlikely in workshops and factories. Rare skin reactions to virgin nylon products have been described and have been generally attributed to residual reactants or to low molecular weight polyamides (Morris, 1960). Dyes and finishes applied to nylon for wearing apparel have also been uncommon causes of contact dermatitis.

The most prominent air contaminant in many typical polycaprolactam nylon operations is derived from eutectic mixtures of diphenyl and diphenyl oxide, already discussed in the chapter on aromatic hydrocarbons. This material is heated and pumped under pressure as a heat transfer fluid. In such applications, the material may be heated to temperatures as high as 370°C (700°F) so that there is an obvious potential for severe burns. Small leaks may give rise to vapors and mists of which the workers complain because of the nausea induced, and extensive exposures under poor hygienic conditions have produced liver injury and nervous system changes.

References

Goldblatt MW, Farquharson ME, Bennett G, et al: ε-Caprolactam. *Br J Ind Med* 1954;11:1–10.

Morris GE: Nylon dermatitis. *N Engl J Med* 1960;263:30–32.

Polycarbonates Polycarbonates are polyesters formed by the polymerization of dihydric phenols through carbonate linkages. The plastic is used primarily for small mechanical parts such as gears and cams because of its strength. Biological properties have not been associated with the finished polymer. However, various synthetic manipulations to form the polycarbonates utilize potentially harmful compounds such as bisphenol A, phosgene, dioxane, and other solvents.

Polyolefins: polyethylene, polypropylene

Materials of this group of plastics are widely used in packaging, housewares, toys, and vapor barriers. The polymerizations take place in closed reaction vessels under the influence of catalysts such as benzoyl peroxide, metallic oxides, or active organometallic compounds such as triethyl aluminum. The latter compound, as well as other alkyl aluminums, are spontaneously flammable in air so that caution is required in handling them (Harris, 1959). The finished resin, which is used for thermoplastic molding, extrusion, and other applications, is essentially without biological properties. Under conditions of thermal stress above 250°C, polyolefins undergo degradation to compounds that are irritating and injurious.

Reference

Harris DK: Some hazards in the manufacture and use of plastics. *Br J Ind Med* 1959;16:221–229.

Polystyrene Polystyrene is prepared by the polymerization of styrene (vinyl benzene) under the influence of organic peroxides, such as benzoyl peroxide or lauroyl peroxide. Styrene can polymerize prematurely in storage. This tendency is controlled by the addition of inhibitors such as butylcatechol or hydroquinone, both sensitizers. Polystyrene is used in appliances, toys, furniture, and in a variety of packagings, especially for food products because of its chemical inertness.

Monomeric styrene is strongly irritating to the eyes, pharynx, and upper respiratory tract and it can produce headache, dizziness, nausea, vomiting, and primary skin irritation, as noted in the discussion of polyesters. No chronic toxicity has been associated with styrene exposure.

Vinyl polymers and copolymers The vinyl group of plastics include polyvinyl chloride (PVC) used in floor tiles, ducts, waterproof clothing and upholstery, insulations, and piping; polyvinyl acetate used in adhesives and coatings; polyvinyl alcohol; and polyvinylidene chloride. In all of these applications the finished plastic has been found to be without injurious properties, except for unusual incidents such as the development of squamous cell carcinoma of the buccal mucosa in a man who had a lifelong habit of chewing plastic materials (Casterline et al., 1977).

Until recently the monomeric precursors have not been thought to have toxicological importance, although it has been known that vinyl chloride (VC) and vinyl acetate may produce dizziness and confusion, and that vinyl chloride was investigated as a possible general anesthetic 50 years ago (Peoples and Leake, 1933). It has become apparent, however, that vinyl chloride has a number of toxic effects that include acro-osteolysis, angiosarcoma of the liver, hepatic fibrosis, pulmonary effects, portal hypertension, embryotoxicity and teratogenicity, mutagenicity, and chromosomal effects (Haley, 1975; Binns, 1979). There has been an explosive expansion of the toxicological literature dealing with vinyl chloride in the past 15 years, first dealing with acro-osteolysis and later with angiosarcomas in workers and in laboratory animals, along with results of investigations of vinyl chloride metabolism.

In the last 15 years a distinctive industrial disease, occupational acro-osteolysis, has been observed in men working as "polycleaners" in several PVC production facilities (Wilson et al., 1967; Dinman et al., 1971). The disease appears to affect only those persons who manually clean PVC reaction kettles in which polymerization occurs. The disease does not occur in those who handle the finished thermoplastic resin. The clinical syndrome includes Raynaud's phenomenon with discomfort and blanching of the fingers and sometimes the toes on exposure to cold, sometimes preceded by numbness and tingling. Scleroderma-like changes may affect the dorsal surfaces of the hands and the flexor distal thirds of the forearms. These changes may also be accompanied by microvascular abnormalities of the skin of the hands detectable by *in vivo* microscopy (Maricq et al., 1976, 1978). Unique roentgenographic changes occur in the distal phalanges of the hands and may be present in asymptomatic individuals. These changes consist of the loss of the cortex of one or more tufts or complete lysis of the tuft and a portion of the adjacent shaft. Removal from exposure results in gradual healing with a fragmentation of the affected area and union of the fragments, although Raynaud's phenomenon persists (Williams and McLachlan, 1976). The fingers themselves appear to be shortened and "clubbed." Since it is now possible to clean reaction vessels by techniques that do not require hand scraping, new cases of this disease should no longer occur unless longer experience demonstrates that the toxic agent is present in other operations. Nevertheless, new cases continue to be reported (Walker, 1975; Hahn et al., 1979).

Angiosarcoma of the liver, a rare malignant tumor, was first reported to occur among workers handling polyvinyl chloride by Creech and Johnson (1974). Other reports followed so that by 1977 NIOSH had collected 64 cases from 12 countries, including 23 from the United States, 10 from Canada, 9 from the Federal Republic of Germany, and 8 from France (Spirtas and Kaminski, 1978). The most frequent histological pattern of this tumor was characterized by multicentric focal dilatation of the liver sinusoids lined with sarcoma cells and accompanied by noncirrhotic periportal hepatic fibrosis (Thomas et al., 1975). Frequently these changes have been associated with splenomegaly and portal hypertension. Surveys of workers in VC/PVC polymerization plants have revealed elevations of carcinoembryonic antigen (CEA) in otherwise healthy individuals, but whether this test is useful in predicting increased risk is not known (Anderson et al., 1978). Standard liver function tests do not appear to be of value in screening exposed vinyl chloride workers (Lee et al., 1977), but grayscale ultrasonography may be useful in detecting enlarged portal veins, splenomegaly, and changes in hepatic texture (Williams et al., 1976). It has been suggested that vinyl chloride itself is not carcinogenic but is biotransformed in the body to chloroethylene epoxide, a highly reactive alkylating compound, that may be the carcinogenic and mutagenic metabolite responsible for the adverse effects attributed to exposure to the parent compound (Antweiler, 1976; Zajdela et al., 1980).

Vinyl chloride can be absorbed through the skin and most of it is then eliminated by the lungs (Hefner et al., 1975), but 42% of an inhaled dose of VC is retained in the lungs (Krajewski et al., 1980). Workers exposed to polyvinyl chloride dust may develop a PVC pneumoconiosis characterized by diffuse micronodular infiltrates (Arnaud et al., 1978; Mastrangelo, 1979). In some cases, slight pulmonary function impairment is associated with exposure to vinyl chloride vapors and polyvinyl chloride dusts (Miller, 1975; Soutar et al., 1980), although in some studies smoking rather than PVC dust is the major cause of reduced lung function (Chivers et al., 1980).

Thermal degradation products of vinyl polymers and copolymers include the monomers and hydrochloric acid gas. The latter is responsible for danger to firefighters because of the ubiquitous use of PVC products. In addition to HCl, pyrolysis of PVC results in something like 75 potentially toxic compounds (Dyer and Esch, 1976). A disease, "meat wrapper's asthma," has been reported repeatedly among persons exposed to thermal degradation of PVC film (see, for example, Polakoff et al., 1975; Falk and Portnoy, 1976; Vandervort and Brooks, 1977; Brooks and Vandervort, 1977). More recent work suggests that the principal causal agent in meat wrapper's asthma may be phthalic anhydride emitted from heated price labels (Pauli et al., 1980), although direct challenge studies incriminate dicyclohexylphthalate and 2,5-di-tert-amyl quinone, which are also breakdown products of heated labels (Levy et al., 1978).

Monomeric vinyl chloride is produced by several processes, one of which is based upon the addition of hydrogen chloride to acetylene in the presence of mercuric chloride. This process has been responsible for the introduction of mercury compounds into natural bodies of water, from which methylmercury is eventually absorbed by fish, including those species used by man as food.

Exposure to vinylidene chloride (1,1-dichloroethylene) without concomitant exposure to vinyl chloride has not resulted in occupational illness (Ott et al., 1976). Nevertheless, vinylidene chloride is a hepatotoxin in laboratory animals (McKenna et al., 1978) and induces angiosarcoma and renal adenocarcinoma in rodents (Bahlman et al., 1979).

References

Anderson HA, Snyder J, Lewinson T, et al: Levels of CEA among vinyl chloride and polyvinyl chloride exposed workers. *Cancer* 1978;42:1560–1567.

Antweiler H: Studies on the metabolism of vinyl chloride. *Environ Health Persp* 1976;17:217–219.

Arnaud A, Pommier de Santi P, Garbe L, et al: Polyvinyl chloride pneumoconiosis. *Thorax* 1978;33:19–25.

Bahlman LJ, Alexander V, Infante PF, et al: Vinyl halides: Carcinogenicity. Vinyl bromide, vinyl chloride, and vinylidene chloride. *Joint NIOSH/OSHA Current Intelligence Bull #28*, 1978. (Also published in *Am Ind Hyg Assoc J* 1979;40:A30–A40).

Binns CHB: Vinyl chloride: A review. *J Soc Occup Med* 1979;29:134–141.

Brooks SM, Vandervort R: Polyvinyl chloride

film thermal decomposition products as an occupational illness: 2. Clinical studies. *J Occup Med* 1977;19:192–196.

Casterline CL, Casterline PF, Jaques DA: Squamous cell carcinoma of the buccal mucosa associated with chronic oral polyvinyl chloride exposure. Report of a case. *Cancer* 1977;39:1686–1688.

Chivers CP, Lawrence-Jones C, Paddle GM: Lung function in workers exposed to polyvinyl chloride dust. *Br J Ind Med* 1980;37:147–151.

Creech JL Jr, Johnson MN: Angiosarcoma of liver in the manufacture of polyvinyl chloride. *J Occup Med* 1974;16:150–151.

Dinman BD, Cook WA, Whitehouse WM, et al: Occupational acroosteolysis. I. An epidemiological study. *Arch Environ Health* 1971;22:61–73.

Dyer RF, Esch VH: Polyvinyl chloride toxicity in fires. Hydrogen chloride toxicity in fire fighters. *J Am Med Assoc* 1976;235:393–397.

Falk H, Portnoy B: Respiratory tract illness in meat wrappers. *J Am Med Assoc* 1976;235:915–917.

Hahn E, Aderka D, Suprun H, et al: Occupational acroosteolysis in vinyl chloride workers in Israel. *Israel J Med Sci* 1979;15:218–222.

Haley TJ: Vinyl chloride: How many unknown problems? *J Toxicol Environ Health* 1975;1:47–73.

Hefner RE Jr, Watanabe PG, Gehring PJ: Percutaneous absorption of vinyl chloride. *Toxicol Appl Pharmacol* 1975;34:529–532.

Krajewski J, Dobecki M, Gromiec J: Retention of vinyl chloride in the human lung. *Br J Ind Med* 1980;37:373–374.

Lee FI, Harry DS, Adams WGF, et al: Screening for liver disease in vinyl chloride workers. *Br J Ind Med* 1977;34:142–147.

Levy SA, Storey J, Phashko BE: Meat worker's asthma. *J Occup Med* 1978;20:116–117.

Maricq HR, Johnson MN, Whetstone CL, et al: Capillary abnormalities in polyvinyl chloride production workers. Examination by in vivo microscopy. *J Am Med Assoc* 1976;236:1368–1371.

Maricq HR, Darke CS, Archibald R McL, et al: *In vivo* observations of skin capillaries in workers exposed to vinyl chloride. An English-American comparison. *Br J Ind Med* 1978;35:1–7.

Mastrangelo G, Manno M, Marcer G, et al: Polyvinyl chloride pneumoconiosis: Epidemiological study of exposed workers. *J Occup Med* 1979;21:540–542.

McKenna MJ, Zempel JA, Madrid EO, et al:

The pharmacokinetics of [¹⁴C] vinylidene chloride in rats following inhalation exposure. *Toxicol Appl Pharmacol* 1978;45:599–610.

Miller A: Pulmonary function defects in nonsmoking vinyl chloride workers. *Environ Health Persp* 1975;11:247–250.

Ott MG, Fishbeck WA, Townsend JC, et al: A health study of employees exposed to vinylidene chloride. *J Occup Med* 1976;18:735–738.

Pauli G, Bessot JC, Kopferschmitt MC, et al: Meat wrapper's asthma: Identification of the causal agent. *Clin Allergy* 1980;10:263–269.

Peoples AS, Leake CD: The anesthetic action of vinyl chloride. *J Pharmacol Exp Ther* 1933;48:284.

Polakoff PL, Lapp NL, Reger R: Polyvinyl chloride pyrolysis products. A potential cause for respiratory impairment. *Arch Environ Health* 1975;30:269–271.

Soutar CA, Copland LH, Thornley PE, et al: Epidemiological study of respiratory disease in workers exposed to polyvinylchloride dust. *Thorax* 1980;35:644–652.

Spirtas R, Kaminski R: Angiosarcoma of the liver in vinyl chloride/polyvinyl chloride workers. 1977 update of the NIOSH Register. *J Occup Med* 1978;20:427–429.

Thomas LB, Popper H, Berk PD, et al: Vinyl-chloride-induced liver disease. From idiopathic portal hypertension (Banti's syndrome) to angiosarcomas. *N Engl J Med* 1975;292:17–22.

Vandervort R, Brooks SM: Polyvinyl chloride film thermal decomposition products as an occupational illness. I. Environmental exposures and toxicology. *J Occup Med* 1977;19:188–191.

Walker A: Occupational acro-osteolysis (two cases). *Proc R Soc Med* 1975;68:343–344.

Williams DMJ, McLachlan MSF: Healing of phalangeal defects in acro-osteolysis. *J Soc Occup Med* 1976;26:98–99.

Williams DMJ, Smith PM, Taylor KJW, et al: Monitoring liver disorders in vinyl chloride monomer workers using greyscale ultrasonography. *Br J Ind Med* 1976;33:152–157.

Wilson RH, McCormick WE, Tatum CF, et al: Occupational acroosteolysis. Report of 31 cases. *J Am Med Assoc* 1967;201:577–581.

Zajdela F, Croisy A, Barbin A, et al: Carcinogenicity of chloroethylene oxide, an ultimate reactive metabolite of vinyl chloride, and bis(chloromethyl) ether after subcutaneous administration and in initiation-promotion experiments in mice. *Cancer Res* 1980;40:352–356.

Acrylamide Acrylamide is a vinyl monomer used in the production of special polymers. These have applications as flocculating aids for the precipitation of suspended solids in aqueous systems and as special chemical grouts. Although the polymer is nontoxic, the absorption of acrylamide through the skin or from dusts has been associated with serious neurologic consequences (Garland and Patterson, 1967). A variable neuropathy with motor and sensory impairment is marked by numbness, paresthesias, loss of certain reflexes, and muscle weakness and atrophy (Spencer and Schaumberg, 1975). Ataxia, tremor, dysarthria, and other central nervous system signs are consistent with mid-brain lesions. Although recovery over the course of months has been the rule in mild cases, permanent neurologic sequelae are observed in severe intoxications. Several acrylamide analogues also have neurotoxic effects on rats (Edwards, 1975).

References

Edwards PM: Neurotoxicity of acrylamide and its analogues and effects of these analogues and other agents on acrylamide neuropathy. *Br J Ind Med* 1975;32:31–38.

Garland TO, Patterson MWH: Six cases of acrylamide poisoning. *Br Med J* 1967;4:134–138.

Spencer PS, Schaumberg HH: Nervous system degeneration produced by acrylamide monomer. *Environ Health Persp* 1975;11:129–133.

Polyvinylpyrrolidone Bergmann et al. (1958) described pulmonary damage that followed exposure to polyvinylpyrrolidone hair sprays and named the disease thesaurosis. McLaughlin and his colleagues (1963) reviewed the literature and reported on 775 chest x-rays of British hairdressers while Cares (1965) presented the United States experience. The reported cases resembled sarcoid clinically, radiographically, and by histopathologic findings. Alternative diagnoses in the literature are interstitial fibrosis and foreign body granulomas. McLaughlin et al. concluded that it was possible to diagnose thesaurosis by chest x-ray, perhaps because of hair spray particles in the lung, but they could not correlate quantity of spray inhaled and clinical findings. Their single case in a hairdresser was thought to be an example of unusual hypersensitivity. Gowdy and Wagstaff (1972) described five cases with pulmonary in-

filtrates on chest x-ray and four with respiratory complaints, all exposed to a variety of aerosols and all cured by freedom from exposure. Four biopsies and lung function tests were nonspecific. Further, these investigators surveyed 227 beauty shop operators and found none ill but 11 with increased bronchovascular markings on chest x-ray. Thesaurosis, then, appears to be chiefly a problem in differential diagnosis. The cases seen by HLH, for example, proved to be Boeck's sarcoid with lesions in other organs in addition to lung, or chronic beryllium disease.

The material used in the United States is polyvinylpyrrolidone (PVP) rather than shellac, which is used in Britain. PVP has proved to be safe when used as a plasma expander. Oils and propellants used in hair sprays may have a detrimental effect but current evidence suggests that hair sprays are harmless, especially in view of the large amounts used by women.

References

Bergmann M, Flance IJ, Blumenthal HT: Thesaurosis following inhalation of air spray: A clinical and experimental study. *N Engl J Med* 1958;258:471–476.

Cares RM: Thesaurosis from inhaled air spray? *Arch Environ Health* 1965;11:80–85.

Gowdy JM, Wagstaff MJ: Pulmonary infiltration due to aerosol thesaurosis. A survey of hairdressers. *Arch Environ Health* 1972;25:101–108.

McLaughlin AIG, Bidstrup PL, Konstam L: The effects of hair lacquer sprays on the lungs. *Food Cosmet Toxicol* 1963;1:171–188.

Additives

The polymers discussed above are modified through the addition of materials that impart specific, desirable properties to the finished product. These additives, not being large and inert polymeric macromolecules, may have biological characteristics that far outweigh those of the basic plastic to which they are added. For the most part, the biological properties of these additives are not well established. The metallic and organometallic compounds do, however, present a known hazard. Exposure to additives tends to be small because they are introduced primarily in early steps of formulation, and relatively few workers are exposed.

279

Plasticizers Plasticizers are mixed into polymers to increase flexibility and workability. Phthalate esters account for approximately two thirds of total domestic plasticizer production and include di(2-ethylhexyl) phthalate, diisooctyl phthalate, and dibutyl phthalate. Adipate, sebacate, and azelate esters are also commonly used, especially when low temperature flexibility is desired. These esters have a very low order of toxicity. Polyester and epoxidized plasticizers are also of little industrial health importance, although the epoxy material can be sensitizers.

Phosphate esters, among the first plasticizers to be developed, impart flame resistance to polymers. Tricresyl phosphates have been the most important, and the ones used as plasticizers are generally free of the ortho isomer, which has prominent neurotoxic properties. Triphenyl phosphate, cresyl diphenyl phosphate, and octyl diphenyl phosphate are also used. The question of purity of materials in this group and freedom from neurotoxic components is often difficult to establish in an industrial setting. The low vapor pressure of the aromatic phosphate esters is a source of protection.

Other plasticizers include chlorinated paraffins and chlorinated biphenyls. The latter group is associated with chloracne and liver injury; the paraffins lack this toxicity.

Flame retardants Flame retardant properties can be inherent in certain plastics because of high chlorine content or, as in the case of the polycarbonates, because they evolve carbon dioxide on thermal decomposition. Flame retardant additives of hygienic interest include tricresyl phosphate, chlorinated di- and triphenyls, bromine compounds, halogenated phosphates, and antimony trioxide. Flame retardant intermediates that actually become incorporated in the polymer usually contain chlorine or bromine.

Stabilizers Stabilizers retard the natural degradation of plastics due to light and heat. Potentially hazardous stabilizers are lead salts or soaps, barium and cadmium compounds, and organotin compounds. Ultraviolet absorbers are added to protect polymers against those wave lengths that tend to disrupt bonds in organic material. Typical absorbers are found among the benzophenones, benzotriazoles, aryl esters of salicylic, benzoic, and terephthalic acids, and organonickel compounds. Antioxidants include alkylated phenols and bisphenols, amines, and organic phosphites.

Organic peroxides Organic peroxides are used to cure polyester resins, to initiate polymerization of vinyl and diene monomers, and to cross-link polymer chains such as polyolefins or silicones. More than 45 organic peroxide compounds are available for industrial use. Although not all peroxides are hazardous, they are, in general, strong oxidizing agents capable of causing skin irritation or burns and severe eye damage. Peroxides on the skin or in the eyes should be removed promptly with large amounts of water. The use of face shields and protective clothing is advisable for those who handle organic peroxides. These compounds tend to be unstable and to undergo spontaneous decomposition. Fires or explosions can result from the contamination or improper storage or organic peroxides.

Inert fillers and fibrous reinforcements Inert fillers and fibrous reinforcements are added to many formulations to improve their mechanical properties, to act as extenders to reduce costs, or to impart special properties to the plastic. The addition of silica, asbestos, talc, mica, glass flakes and fibers, and other materials is common. Some of these substances have inherent biological properties that may create an exposure hazard at the time of polymer formulation or when the finished plastic is cut or machined. Under these circumstances potentially injurious dusts may be generated. Rapid developments within the plastics industry have created high thermal conductivity polymers (beryllia-filled epoxy), antifriction elastomers (molybdenum-disulfide filled), radiation shields (lead-filled polyolefin), and plastics reinforced with exotic fibers (boron, sapphire). Adverse biological effects may be associated with the use of some of these materials.

Foaming agents Foaming agents may be added to increase the porosity of plastics that normally foam or to create foamed structures from plastics that have no inherent foaming properties. Foaming agents may generate gas by either physical or chemical means. Physical foaming agents are generally volatile liquids that become gaseous and create cells under the influence of exothermic reactions or externally applied heat. Aliphatic hydrocarbons of the petroleum ether, ligroin, or light spirits type are flammable but do not have prominent toxic properties. Halogenated aliphatic hydrocarbons, such as methyl chloride, methylene chloride, and trichloroethylene, are also used as foaming agents. The aliphatic fluorocarbons are essentially inert.

Chemical "blowing" agents that produce foam are compounds that decompose under the influence of heat to yield a gas, usually nitrogen. The most common chemical foaming agent in industry is azobisformamide. This compound has been considered to be nontoxic, but when it is inhaled as a dust it results in a nocturnal productive cough and transient decreases in pulmonary function (Ferris et al., 1977). Azobisisobutyronitrile, however, is definitely toxic since it releases nitrogen gas and a residue of tetramethyl succinic dinitrile that persists in the foam. The latter compound is a convulsant in animals and has been believed to be the cause of headache, nausea, and other ill-defined systemic complaints in workers. The substitution of other foaming agents has corrected the problem. Azobisisobutyronitrile may also be used in small amounts for the catalytic polymerization of vinyl plastics. Dinitrosotereph-thalamide, also used, has not been a source of industrial illness.

Reference

Ferris BG Jr, Peters JM, Burgess WA, et al: Apparent effect of an azodicarbonamide on the lungs. *J Occup Med* 1977;19:424–425.

3 • *Elastomers*

Elastomeric polymers are frequently constructed of the same monomers that are used in plastics. Proportions, minor constituents, catalysts, and reaction conditions are varied to yield a product with elastic properties. From the medical point of view, an important distinction between some synthetic elastomers and other macromolecular polymers is that "cured" rubbers can occasionally be a source of toxic ingredients in the formulation stage. Cured plastics are rarely associated with this type of problem. Elastomers of the silicone, polyurethane (spandex), and fluorinated groups do not present these problems typical of the more rubber-like elastomers.

Synthetic Elastomers

The synthetic elastomers include:

Acrylonitrile-butadiene copolymers
Chlorosulfonated polyethylenes
Ethylene-propylene copolymers
Fluorinated copolymers
Polychloroprene (neoprene)
Polyisobutylene
Polysulfide rubber
Polyurethane elastomers
Silicone rubbers
Styrene-butadiene copolymers.

Acrylonitrile-butadiene copolymers Elastomers of this group are highly resistant to common hydrocarbon solvents and oils, and are used for hoses, gaskets, and protective clothing. Nitrile rubber is frequently plasticized with organic phosphates, phthalic esters, or dibenzyl ether. Dibenzyl ether is not believed to have important toxic properties. The harmful properties of butadiene and acrylonitrile have been well established over many years of production of nitrile rubber, and are discussed in the preceding chapter.

Chlorosulfonated polyethylenes These synthetic rubbers are prepared by the reaction of sulfur dioxide and chlorine on polyethylene. They are used in white sidewall tires, hoses, tank linings, and elsewhere where resistance to heat, oxidation, and ozone is required. These polymers are cured with oxides of lead or magnesium. Accelerators include mercaptobenzothiazole, benzothiazolyl disulfide, and dipentamethylenethiuram tetrasulfide, which as a group are known skin sensitizers and may be present in the finished rubbers in toxic amounts.

Ethylene-propylene copolymers and terpolymers To produce an elastomeric polymer, alkenes (olefines) are reacted under the influence of a coordination catalyst such as vanadium oxychloride or diethylaluminum chloride. Peroxides may be used in the cure, although the incorporation of a third monomer, such as dicyclopentadiene, will permit the use of conventional sulfur vulcanization. The toxicity of this alicyclic hydrocarbon is not established but adverse effects are probably unlikely. Elastomers of this group are resistant to atmospheric and chemical attack and are used in hoses, belts, gaskets, and footwear.

Fluorinated elastomers Copolymers of vinylidene fluoride and chlortrifluoroethylene or perfluoropropylene are highly resistant elastomers used in gaskets, seals, and other applications where high-cost materials can be afforded. The elastomers are biologically inert, although extreme heating can produce harmful breakdown products such as HF, monofluoroacetic acid, and other fluorocarbons. Curing agents include diamines, peroxides, or ionizing radiation.

Neoprene Neoprene rubber is obtained by the emulsion condensation of chloroprene (2-chloro-1,3-butadiene), a colorless liquid that is a skin and respiratory tract irritant. Neoprene is highly resistant to weathering and to oil, as well as to solvents, oxygen, ozone, and heat. Its major uses are in mechanical and automotive applications such as cable sheaths, belts, hoses, seals, and gaskets.

Chloroprene produces a number of toxic effects that include central nervous system depression and injury to lungs, liver, kidneys, and skin (Lloyd et al., 1975; Haley, 1978). Temporary epilation occurs in chloroprene workers, but termination of exposure results in normal hair regrowth. Reports from the USSR, summarized by Haley (1978), implicate chloroprene as a skin and lung carcinogen in chloroprene-exposed workers. The frequency of chromosome aberrations in lymphocytes from this population is also increased over nonexposed control groups (Sanotskii, 1976). While the United States maximum permissible exposure concentration in air is 25 ppm (90 mg/m^3), the USSR has set its exposure limit at 4 mg/m^3. NIOSH (1977) has recommended 1 ppm (3.6 mg/m^3) as a ceiling concentration for a 15-minute sample during a 40-hour workweek.

Polyisobutylene   Butyl rubber is formed from the polymerization of isobutene (isobutylene) with small amounts of chloroprene or butadiene. The reaction is carried out in a closed system with an aluminum chloride catalyst. Butyl rubber is highly impervious to gases and finds its major uses in inner tubes, air chambers, and dielectrics. Isobutene is an anesthetic and asphyxiant gas, but it is a hazard only if concentrations are high enough to produce asphyxia. Under these circumstances a concurrent hazard of explosion exists.

Polysulfide rubber   Polysulfide elastomers are condensation products of sodium polysulfides and dichloro compounds, such as ethylene dichloride. More complex chlorinated hydrocarbons yield products with improved properties. This group of elastomers is plasticized with biologically active compounds such as tetramethylthiuram disulfide or benzothiazolyl disulfide. Organic peroxides and lead compounds may also be present. This group of elastomers is highly resistant to oils, solvents, and weathering and they are therefore found in coatings, caulking compounds, adhesives, and mechanical components. In most applications of the polysulfide rubbers, occupational health problems are related to sensitizing contact dermatitis.

Polyurethane   The so-called spandex fibers are polyurethane elastomers, which are biologically inert. They can be substituted for rubber by persons who have become sensitized to auxiliary compounds invariably present in natural and synthetic rubbers. All spandex formulations are not identical; many are based on polytetramethylene glycol, 2,4-toluene diisocyanate, other diisocyanates, and hydrazine. The solvent for extrusion is dimethylformamide. The toxicologic effects of the diisocyanates are well-known and have already been discussed; they constitute the principal health problem in the production of these fibers.

Silicone rubbers   Industrial medical problems have not been prominent in the preparation or use of silicone rubbers. Benzoyl peroxide may be used as a vulcanizer.

Styrene-butadiene copolymer rubbers   Rubbers of this group are prepared in large quantities for tire treads and other similar applications. The biological properties of styrene and butadiene are significant, but from the industrial health point of view various additives have been a far greater source of difficulty.

Additives in Elastomer Systems

Various substances added to rubber formulations in the course of production may cause skin reactions in persons who use the finished products as well as in industrially exposed workers. The additives are generally similar in the case of natural rubber, nitrile rubber, polybutadiene, neoprene, butyl rubber, and ethylene-propylene copolymers.

Vulcanizers are generally based on elemental sulfur, although zinc and magnesium oxides are important in the neoprene cure, and peroxides are used for ethylene-propylene systems. The rate of vulcanization is influenced by *accelerators,* which are potent sensitizers. Common accelerators include:

> benzothiazolyl disulfide
> mercaptobenzothiazole (MBT)
> tetraethyl thiuramdisulfide (disulfiram)
> tetramethyl thiuramdisulfide (thiram)
> thiocarbanilide
> dithiocarbamates (zinc dimethyl, zinc diethyl, zinc dibutyl, lead dimethyl compounds)

diphenylguanidine phthalate
hexamethylene tetramine
lead oxide (litharge).

Besides causing allergic contact dermatitis, the accelerators disulfiram and thiram can produce severe reactions when they are absorbed together with alcohol or paraldehyde. This reaction involves the inhibition of aldehyde dehydrogenase, presumably through the chelation of molybdenum, so that there is interference with the normal metabolic degradation of aldehydes. Aldehydes consequently accumulate and produce flushing, palpitations, dyspnea, nausea, and hypotension. These reactions do not involve sensitization. Disulfiram of pharmaceutical grade is used to produce distaste and intolerance in the treatment of alcoholism.

Antioxidants are used to protect rubbers against the destructive effects of atmospheric oxygen. Those most commonly used include:

monobenzylether of hydroquinone (agerite alba)
di-(β-naphthyl)-p-phenylenediamine
mono and dioctyl diphenylamines
phenyl α and β naphthylamines.

The monobenzylether of hydroquinone, in addition to being a sensitizer, is capable of producing loss of pigment in many individuals, often in the absence of any previous skin reaction. This reaction is most apparent in very dark-skinned persons in whom the response resembles vitiligo. Exposures to this compound have been sharply reduced through modifications in the rubber compounding process. Most of the amine antioxidants are potent sensitizers.

Pigments and *fillers* include carbon black, whiting (calcium carbonate), clay, silica, and asbestos. The properties of the fibrogenic dusts are well established and are discussed in a separate chapter. There has been some speculation that polycyclic aromatic carcinogens are absorbed to the carbon black particles handled in industry, but there is no evidence that the pigment itself has toxic properties.

References

Haley TJ: Chloroprene (2-chloro-1,3-butadiene)—What is the evidence for its carcinogenicity? *Clin Toxicol* 1978;13:153–170.

Lloyd JW, Decoufle P, Moore RM Jr: Background information on chloroprene. *J Occup Med* 1975;17:263–265.

NIOSH: *Criteria for a Recommended Standard .... Occupational Exposure to Chloroprene.* Washington, DC, National Institute for Occupational Safety and Health (NIOSH 77-210), 1977.

Sanotskii IV: Aspects of the toxicology of chloroprene: Immediate and long-term effects. *Environ Health Persp* 1976;17:85–93.

4 • *Synthetic Fibers*

Polymeric textiles resemble to a great extent many of the high polymers used in plastics and elastomers. Significant chemical and physical modifications in production provide those properties that are necessary for fibers and filaments. Virgin, unfinished synthetic textiles are remarkably free of biological properties.

The synthetic textiles include:

    Acetates
    Acrylics (polyacrylonitrile)
    Modacrylics
    Nylons (polyamides)
    Polyesters
    Rayons

Acetates

Cellulose acetate rayons are made from wood pulp or cotton linters treated with glacial acetic acid and acetic anhydride, along with sulfuric acid as a dehydrating agent. Both acetic acid and its anhydride have a pungent odor and are potent lacrimators. The anhydride is a severe skin and eye irritant, and it may occasionally be a sensitizer. This response is presumably due to its reaction with amino groups of cutaneous protein.

In the production of fibers, the cellulose acetate is dissolved in a solvent for extrusion. In the case of triacetate material the solvent can be methyl acetate, glacial acetic acid, dimethylformamide, dimethylacetamide, or dimethylsulfoxide. Dimethylformamide is a powerful solvent that is irritating to the eyes, mucous membranes, and skin. It can pass through intact skin or can be absorbed from the lungs and gastrointestinal tract. It can be hepatoxic, but it is rapidly metabolized by demethylation to monomethylformamide, the presence of which in the urine serves as a biological indicator of exposure (Maxfield et al., 1975).

The unpleasant fishy odor serves as a warning and tends to limit exposure. Dimethylsulfoxide has been suggested as a vehicle for transporting drugs through the skin, but the application of this compound to the skin may result in erythema, itching, and burning. For cellulose acetates other than the triacetate the conventional solvent is acetone, a compound of very low toxicity.

Acrylics (Polyacrylonitrile)

Acrylonitrile is the chief constituent of acrylic fibers. To improve the dye and working properties of the material, acrylonitrile is frequently copolymerized with small amounts of other monomers such as acrylates, amides, vinyl esters, and various hydrocarbons (e.g., styrene, isobutene). When the comonomer is vinyl chloride or vinylidene chloride and is present in quantities that are approximately equal to the acronitrile, the polymer is said to be modacrylic. Modacrylics are extruded in acetone. Acrylics are prepared for extrusion in solvents that may include dimethylformamide, dimethylsulfoxide, strong acids, and concentrated inorganic salt solutions. Although they are generally inert, penetration of the skin by acrylic fibers has been reported to lead to sarcoid-like granulomas (Pimentel, 1977).

Nylon

The polyamides known as nylon are used principally as fibers, and to a lesser extent as resins in the plastics industry. In fiber applications nylon may be modified by titanium dioxide, a delusterant, by manganese and phosphorus salts as light stabilizers, and by copper salts and acridine compounds as heat stabilizers. These substances are not released from the finished fiber. There are only scattered reports of ill effects among exposed workers, sarcoid-like granulomas of the lung having been reported in a woman who for 20 years was exposed to nylon dust in a fiber bag factory (Pimentel, 1977). That nylon fibers are not completely inert biologically has been shown by *in vitro* studies in which human granulocytes placed in contact with such fibers have a burst in glucose oxidation and become recognizable to other phagocytes (Klock and Stossel, 1977).

Polyesters

Fibers of this group are formed of polyethylene terephthalate. This polymer is produced from dimethyl terephthalate and ethylene glycol under the influence of catalysts that include oxides, carbonates, or acetates of zinc, antimony, manganese, cobalt, calcium, or magnesium. The terephthalates have few, if any, biological properties.

Rayon

Rayon in its finished form is essentially cellulose and is without intrinsic toxicological properties. The phases of production that have been hazardous are those in which there are opportunities for exposure to carbon disulfide. In the production of rayon, wood pulp is treated with sodium hydroxide to produce alkali cellulose. This material is then reacted with carbon disulfide to produce cellulose xanthate. So-called xanthate crumb, when dissolved in dilute sodium hydroxide to form viscose, is extrudable to form rayon fibers. In modern practice this process takes place in closed systems. Hazardous exposure is possible, however, when safe practice is ignored or if ventilation is defective. Carbon disulfide is not involved in the cuprammonium process, which is used on a limited scale.

References

Klock JC, Stossel TP: Detection, pathogenesis, and prevention of damage to human granulocytes caused by interaction with nylon wood fiber. *J Clin Invest* 1977;60:1183–1190.

Maxfield ME, Barnes JR, Azar A, et al: Urinary excretion of metabolite following experimental human exposures to DMF or to DMAC. *J Occup Med* 1975;17:506–511.

Pimentel JC: Sarcoid granulomas of the skin produced by acrylic and nylon fibres. *Br J Dermatol* 1977;96:673–677.

SECTION SIX
PESTICIDES

1 • *Introduction*

Pesticides are commonly equated with insecticides, although the latter are only one category of biocides that range from germicides to rodenticides. A pesticide is defined in the Federal Environmental Pesticide Control Act of 1972 as "... any substance or mixture of substances intended for preventing, destroying, repelling or mitigating any pest." A pest, in turn, can be thought of as "any organism that interferes with the convenience or well-being of man or another species he favors" (Hayes, 1975, p.485). Thus, there are fungicides, slimicides, herbicides, silvicides, nematocides, molluscicides, insecticides, acaricides, and rodenticides. In addition, for plants there are growth regulators, defoliants, and desiccants, and for animals there are repellants, sexual lures (pheromones), and specific parasites and predators that can be used for pest control.

It is the continuing objective of the chemical and agricultural industries to develop materials that control specific categories of pests and at the same time have minimal potentials for detrimental effects on man and desirable plant and animal species. Unfortunately, this goal has not yet been achieved and examples of clinical intoxication continue to appear, usually as the result of accidents, suicide attempts, or incorrect methods of distribution and application. The average annual death rate from accidental poisoning by pesticides in the United States has been estimated by Hayes (1945) to be less than one per million population. It is impossible, as Hayes pointed out, to be certain about the extent of nonfatal morbidity attributable to pesticides in the absence of systematic reporting.

Reference

Hayes WJ Jr: *Toxicology of Pesticides.* Baltimore, Williams & Wilkins, 1975.

287

2 • Insecticides

While there are literally hundreds of insecticides, their purposes, chemical structures, and toxicological properties permit these agents to be classified in groups by chemical nature and toxicity, as in Table 9 (after Milby, 1971; WHO, 1973). Specified materials are usually not pure compounds but may be complex, technical-grade mixtures that contain various isomers, by products, reactants, and contaminants. Trade name products may thus include in the formulation a combination of pesticides, synergists, diluents, and other substances, all of which may have biological properties. Moreover, the composition of such formulations may change without notice or a corresponding change in trade name.

Organophosphorus Compounds

Of the several pesticide categories, the group most commonly associated with toxic effects in man has been that containing the organophosphorus compounds. Materials of this type were originally developed as chemical warfare agents. Their mechanism of action, probably in both insects and vertebrates, is based upon their inactivation of acetylcholinesterase, a property also found in the carbamate insecticides.

Acetylcholine (AcCh), the natural substrate of this enzyme, is a primary neurohumoral transmitter substance of the nervous system. AcCh is necessary for impulse transmission between: 1) preganglionic and postganglionic fibers of the sympathetic and parasympathetic autonomic nervous systems; 2) postganglionic parasympathetic (cholinergic) nerves and effectors such as secretory cells, smooth muscle, and cardiac muscle; 3) motor nerves and motor endplates of striated muscle; and 4) certain components of the central nervous system. The normal transmission of an impulse by AcCh is followed by the rapid hydrolysis of the transmitter by the enzyme and thus by the limitation of the duration and intensity of the stimulus.

Organophosphorus compounds of suitable configuration, because of certain structural similarities to AcCh, become oriented to the surface of the AcCh-esterase molecules and undergo changes analogous to those undergone by AcCh, the natural substrate. In the case of the organophosphorus compounds, however, the bond to the enzyme is abnormally stable and is only slowly reversible so that the phosphorylated enzyme loses its normal function as an AcCh-esterase. AcCh consequently accumulates and causes sustained stimulation, increased function, and finally decreased function with greater accumulation.

There is a wide variation in the mammalian toxicity shown by members of this group of pesticides. Certain sulfur-substituted organophosphorus compounds require metabolic oxidation before toxicity develops. Since this *in vivo* reaction occurs more rapidly in insects than in man, this chemical property is useful in increasing mammalian safety while insecticidal potency is maintained. The oxidative conversion does occur in man but is offset to a variable degree by metabolic inactivation of biologically significant portions of the insecticide molecule. As long as the inactivation processes are capable of keeping up with the activation (i.e., oxidation) processes, intoxication does not occur. The human body deals effectively with small doses of parathion, an agent that requires metabolic oxidation to become toxic. But when the inactivation mechanism cannot handle the amount of toxic compound presented to it, symptoms occur. Since the balance between oxidation and inactivation varies among individuals, it is not surprising that variation in susceptibility to intoxication occurs.

For reasons that are not clearly understood, phenothiazine derivatives, especially when taken over a long period, may potentiate the toxicity of

Table 9
Insecticides

	Organophosphorus Compounds	Organochlorine Compounds
Most Dangerous	Tetraethyl pyrophosphate (TEPP) Phorate Disulfoton; thiodemeton; dithiosystox Paraoxon Thionazin Demeton Mevinphos Ethyl-*p*-nitrophenyl thionobenzene phosphonate (EPN) Schradan Methyl parathion Azinphosmethyl Monocrotophos Dicrotophos Chlorfenvinphos	Isobenzan Endrin Aldrin Dieldrin Toxaphene
Dangerous	Phosphamidon Carbophenothion Coumaphos Dichlorvos (DDVP) Diazinon Ethion Dioxathion; delnav	Endosulfan Dichlorodiphenyltrichloroethane (DDT) Heptachlor Benzene hexachloride (BHC) Strobane Chlordane Dimite Bandane Dicofol
Less Dangerous	Methyl demeton Dimethoate Naled Phostex Dicaphthon Trichlorfon	
Least Dangerous	Chlorthion Malathion Ronnel Abate	Chlorbenside Chlorobenzilate 1,1-dichloro-2,2-bis(*p*-chlorophenyl) ethane (TDE) Chloropropylate Methoxychlor

organophosphorus compounds (Arterberry et al., 1962). This phenomenon may be related to the inhibition of cholinesterase by pharmaceutical preparations of this type. Neurotropic amines, such as theophylline and aminophylline, may have a similar detrimental effect. The toxicity of organophosphorus compounds is also influenced by exposure to ultraviolet and visible light, which may result in more potent anticholinesterase agents than the parent compound. Thus, parathion exposed to light on plant surfaces is probably more toxic than the unirradiated insecticide (Milby et al., 1964).

Organophosphorus compounds that do not require a modification to become active are "direct" inhibitors of AcCh and generally are highly toxic with rapid onset of systemic symptoms. They may also cause local reactions (e.g., miosis) in the absence of systemic manifestations because absorption into the body and metabolism is not necessary for activity. Compounds in this group include tetraethyl pyrophosphate (TEPP) and phosdrin, both highly toxic, and dichlorvos (DDVP), which is readily detoxified in vertebrates and is consequently somewhat less hazardous.

Insecticides of the organophosphorus group can be absorbed into the body via the skin, lungs, or gastrointestinal tract. Oral exposure is rarely of occupational origin, but accidental poisoning of children is not uncommon, especially when pesticides are improperly stored, such as in soft drink bottles. Manifestations of absorption tend to occur most rapidly after respiratory exposure or after massive exposure directly to the eye. Organophosphorus insecticides are absorbed by the skin, but the rate tends to be slow except in the presence of dermatitis or high ambient temperatures. Moreover, the presence of extensive dermatitis may be the major sign of systemic organophosphorus poisoning (Bisby and Simpson, 1975). Poor hygiene, boots and gloves contaminated on the inside, and materials with severe dermal toxicity contribute to the intensity of the hazard.

The pattern of symptoms in man reflects the degree of cholinesterase inhibition and the rate at which the enzyme has become inactivated. The level of AcCh-esterase can be reduced to a level as low as Δ 0.2 pH/hr gradually over the course of months by repeated small doses without the development of obvious clinical symptoms. Field experience suggests that the gradual depression of AcCh-esterase by repeated low doses does not increase susceptibility to a challenge dose of insecticide. There is evidently a biochemical adaptation to low enzyme levels. On the other hand, repeated doses administered before physiological adjustment has occurred tend to produce cumulative effects. After clinical poisoning, physiological adaptation may be assumed to be complete only after the blood enzyme level has returned to normal.

Moderate systemic effects of acute absorption may occur within 30 minutes after exposure via the respiratory tract, within 45 minutes after ingestion, and within two or three hours after cutaneous exposure. Absorption from the gastrointestinal tract and skin may be prolonged. Symptoms normally reach their peak four to eight hours after onset and gradually diminish over a period as long as a week. Complete restoration of blood cholinesterase levels may require as long as three months, depending upon the degree of depression. With massive exposure or direct application of compounds to the conjunctivae, the onset of symptoms is almost instantaneous, and death may follow within minutes. If the onset of symptoms follows exposure by more than eight hours, the diagnosis of organophosphorus poisoning is open to serious question.

Clinical evidence of systemic inhibition of cholinesterase is not specific for individual compounds but is characteristic of the entire group. Systemic responses are usually heralded by the onset of effects as a result of parasympathetic stimulation in which the muscarinic effects are most evident. Since the muscarinic receptors for AcCh are in the heart, smooth muscle, and exocrine glands, early evidence of intoxication includes anorexia, nausea, sweating, substernal and epigastric tightness, heartburn, and belching. A greater degree of absorption produces vomiting, hyperperistalsis with cramps and diarrhea, increased salivation and lacrimation, profuse sweating, pallor, dyspnea, wheezing, and bradycardia. Miosis may be observed, but it is not a constant feature since mydriasis has been occasionally noted. Severe symptoms include involuntary defecation and urination, excessive bronchial secretions, and pulmonary edema. Nicotinic evidence of inhibited cholinesterase activity at the motor endplates of skeletal muscle usually occurs after the muscarinic effects have become relatively prominent. These nicotinic phenomena include easy fatigue, muscular twitching, fasciculations, cramps of skeletal muscle, and general weakness, especially on exertion. The muscles of respiration may be impaired so that dyspnea and cyanosis ensue. Nicotinic effects on autonomic ganglia include hypertension and hyperglycemia. If severe, the nicotinic effects may predominate over the muscarinic so that tachycardia occurs rather than bradycardia. Death in cases of heavy exposure is usually related to respiratory collapse that reflects depression of the respiratory center, weakness of the muscles of respiration, bronchoconstriction, and excessive pulmonary secretions. Ventricular fibrillation may ensue when atropine is given in the presence of hypoxia.

Central nervous system manifestations may include anxiety, emotional aberration, insomnia or somnolence, headache, tremor, and intellectual deterioration. Electroencephalographic evidence of CNS impairment may persist for long periods. The significance of these effects may be increased by the critical demands of certain jobs, such as piloting crop-dusting aircraft. Studies of workers with chronic exposures to organophosphates have revealed neurological deficits in the absence of obvious clinical signs of intoxication (Metcalf and Holmes, 1969). These have included slowness of thinking, memory defects, irritability, and delayed reaction times. Other investigators have noted impaired vigilance, reduced concentration, linguistic depression, and anxiety (Levin et al., 1976; Rodnitzky et al., 1978). The chronicity and the relationship of these clinical phenomena to cholinesterase levels has not been established, but electromyographic studies have demonstrated abnormal neuromuscular function in pesticide workers who did not have other detectable evidence of intoxication or lowered blood cholinesterase levels (Drenth et al., 1972; Roberts, 1976, 1977). An unusual neurologic consequence is illustrated by the case of Guillain-Barré syndrome in a man who accidentally splashed merphos, a cotton defoliant, on his skin; complete recovery occurred after 20 weeks (Fisher, 1977). Chronic organophosphate exposures have also been found to be correlated with frontal lobe impairment (Korsak and Sato, 1977).

Slight exposure to an aerosol of a direct inhibitor of cholinesterase may produce local physiological responses without systemic absorption. Local effects on the eye may include miosis, blurred vision, sensation of retrobulbar pressure, headache, and conjunctival hyperemia. These reactions may persist for as long as a day, but miosis has been noted to remain for five days or longer. Localized skin exposure may result in muscle fasciculation and circumscribed areas of sweating that develop within minutes and last for several hours. Contact sensitization may occur but is infrequent and primary irritant effects on the skin are usually negligible (Rycroft, 1977). Respiratory exposure to an aerosol or vapor may lead to increased bronchial secretions, a sensation of chest tightness, and occasional wheezing from bronchoconstriction, with or without subsequent systemic poisoning. Indirect inhibitors, on the other hand, cause poisoning only after they have been metabolized and consequently do not produce local effects.

Some cholinesterase-inhibiting organophosphorus compounds can produce permanent paralysis due to a demyelinating process in the spinal cord (Bidstrup et al., 1953). This process may not become apparent for as long as a month after exposure and is similar to the chronic neurologic phenomena associated with tri-*o*-cresylphosphate (TOCP). Phosphate triester neuropathy has been reported in a wide variety of vertebrates, but hens and man seem to be the most sensitive to this effect (Aldridge et al., 1969). However, most organophosphate insecticides do not have this property, and demyelination in man has been attributed only to mipafox, an insecticide used in Britain but not in the United States.

Late onset neuromuscular block may result from organophosphate poisoning despite the use of a cholinesterase reactivator (Gadoth and Fisher, 1978). In experimental rats, paraoxen induces a progressive myopathy of skeletal muscle, especially severe in the diaphragm, characterized by breakdown in fiber architecture, necrosis, and phagocytosis (Wecker and Dettbarn, 1976). This myopathy appears to be neurally mediated since denervation reduced the muscle fiber necrosis.

Treatment   Treatment in cases of cholinesterase inhibition is based upon the prompt administration of atropine in sufficient doses. Atropine does not influence the inactivation of cholinesterase, but instead limits the exaggerated muscarinic effects of accumulated acetylcholine. Atropine has no effect on the nicotinic manifestations of acetylcholine at the motor endplates and consequently does not influence weakness of the respiratory musculature. There is a clear danger of ventricular fibrillation in persons who receive atropine in the presence of hypoxia. Hence, while agreement is not unanimous, it is the general view that the cyanotic patient should receive oxygen and artificial ventilation to correct hypoxia before atropine is administered. It is desirable to achieve a mild degree of atropine toxicity such as tachycardia, dry flushed skin, or cessation of salivary secretion so that unusually large doses may be required. In severely poisoned persons, as much as 40 mg of atropine can be given in a single day without producing overatropinization. A single intravenous dose of 10 mg atropine sulfate has been inadvertently administered to normal adults with consequent signs of overdosage, but without causing a critical threat to life. The effects of intravenous atropine begin in one to four minutes and are maximal at eight minutes. The use of atropine as a prophylactic measure prior to anticipated exposure should be avoided.

Since atropine does not influence the integrity of the inactive phosphorylated enzyme complex, specific agents of the oxime type have been developed to accelerate cholinesterase reactivation. The oxime currently available in the United States is 2-pyridine aldoxime (2-PAM; pralidoxime chloride). Other agents, such as Pro-PAM and P2AM, have been developed, especially in Europe. The evidence is very good that treatment with both atropine and 2-PAM is more effective than treatment with atropine alone. 2-PAM is rapidly excreted so that repeated doses may be necessary, particularly in the case of parathion and other organophosphorus compounds that must undergo bioactivation before becoming toxic. Since 2-PAM is itself a weak anticholinesterase compound, facilities for assisted ventilation should be available. The efficacy of energetic therapy in cases of severe organophosphorus poisoning is attested to by the experience of Warriner et al. (1977) in which atropine and pralidoxime therapy was maintained for 23 days.

In severe cases of poisoning (coma, cyanosis) the recommended treatment is as follows:

1. Correction of hypoxia and cyanosis with oxygen and assisted ventilation; removal of secretions; maintenance of patent airway.
2. Intravenous administration of atropine sulfate, 2 to 4 mg. This dose should be repeated at five- to 10-minute intervals until signs of atropine toxicity appear (dry, flushed skin; tachycardia as high as 140/min, dry mouth). Some atropinization should be maintained for at least 48 hours.
3. Administration of 2-PAM, 1 g intravenously, slowly, preferably in an infusion of 100 to 250 ml saline over a 30-minute period. The dose can be repeated in an hour. In overwhelming exposures, the doses may be doubled.
4. Decontamination of skin and hair with alkaline soap and water; decontamination of the eyes with saline. Alcohol can be used to remove final traces of material from the skin. Evacuation of the stomach and gut is indicated if the poisoning has been by the oral route.
5. Symptomatic treatment.

In less severe cases, the following treatment is appropriate:

1. Atropine sulfate intravenously, 1 to 2 mg, if symptoms appear; repeated every 15 to 30 minutes until muscarinic symptoms are relieved or until evidence of mild atropine toxicity occurs.
2. Decontamination.
3. Administration of 2-PAM, 1 g intravenously, slowly, if response to atropine is not satisfactory.
4. Symptomatic treatment.

Further details may be found in Namba et al. (1971), Hayes (1975, pp. 391–417), Murphy (in Casarett and Doull, 1980, pp. 374–375), and, in addition, for 2-PAM, *AMA Drug Evaluations* (1980, pp. 357–358, 1455–1456). Opiates, theophylline, aminophylline, phenothiazine, and succinylcholine are contraindicated. Seizures are generally best prevented or controlled by adequate oxygenation and the outlined regimen. Intravenous thiopental can be used if necessary with extreme caution. Persons who are sufficiently ill to require atropine should remain under medical supervision for at least 24 hours since absorption and bioactivation may occur for a prolonged period after the initial exposure.

Prevention Prevention of occupational exposure can be accomplished by education, use of protective clothing, respirators, and air-conditioned cabs, along with control of worker reentry into sprayed areas. Careful maintenance of equipment is necessary, since boots, gloves, and overalls are readily contaminated and become sources of cutaneous exposure. Spray-soaked clothing should obviously be removed promptly. Contamination of foods and tobacco products must be avoided, and the hands and face should be washed with soap and water prior to eating or smoking. Actually, cigarettes may be contaminated to the extent of over 200 μg per cigarette, and for parathion, inhalation exposure may be as much as 28% of the contamination (Comer et al., 1977).

Worker re-entry into fields treated with pesticides is an important factor in farm- and orchard-worker safety with respect to potential exposure and its control. Guthrie et al. (1976) have shown that rainfall may reduce the water-soluble residues so that earlier reentry may be permitted without demonstrable changes in worker cholinesterase levels. In general, 48-hour minimum reentry intervals are observed for cotton fields (Burns and Parker, 1975), but safe practice depends on foliage residues since methyl parathion disappears rapidly but monocrotophos is more persistent (Ware et al., 1975). Safe reentry times for workers may vary from one day for malathion to 45 days for high levels of parathion. Nigg (1980) has maintained that a systematic approach to this problem can be developed by utilizing data derivable from current technology along with the use of suitable and tested mathematical models.

Blood analyses for cholinesterase activity are valuable in diagnosis and in medical surveillance of potentially exposed workers (Witter, 1963). Plasma cholinesterase levels drop to lower levels and recover more rapidly than do red cell cholinesterase values, which represent the true levels. Red cell cholinesterase recovers only as fast as new erythrocytes are formed, unless there has been treatment with oximes. The normal level for an individual is his preexposure level, and it is against this value that subsequent comparisons should be made. In the absence of preexposure information, group "normals" can be used but they are less satisfactory.

Colorimetric field procedures are available that permit the identification of those persons whose whole blood cholinesterase activity has fallen to below 50% of control levels, persons who should be removed from further exposure and whose previous exposure should be examined. This method is based upon the rate of pH shift in the sample as acetylcholine is hydrolyzed with the release of acetate. A testing paper yielding relatively crude approximations of plasma cholinesterase levels is available for diagnostic field and emergency room use. Instructions for use of all field methods must be followed exactly if errors are to be avoided. Various standard laboratory methods are available for more precise enzyme determinations, one of the newer ones of which measures cholinesterase in micromoles of -SH per minute per milliliter with acetylthiocholine as the substrate (Knaak et al., 1978). Micromodifications of the Michel glass electrode pH measurement technique are most common. Normal enzyme levels have been determined by Rider et al. (1957) and are given in Table 10.

Table 10
Normal Cholinesterase Levels in △ pH/hr

	Men	Women
Red cells		
Range	0.39 – 1.02	0.34 – 1.10
Mean ± SD	0.766 ± 0.081	0.750 ± 0.082
Plasma		
Range	0.44 – 1.63	0.24 – 1.54
Mean ± SD	0.953 ± 0.187	0.817 ± 0.187

For practical purposes, a cholinesterase level of 0.5 △ pH/hr for either cells or plasma represents depressed activity. Also, from the practical point of view, a significant reduction of cholinesterase activity can be caused only by exposure to organophosphorus or carbamate insecticides. When intoxication of at least moderate severity is suspected on clinical and epidemiologic grounds, enzyme assays should be regarded as confirmatory, and treatment should not be delayed until a laboratory report is received. Symptomatic persons should not be permitted to return to work with organophosphorus compounds until cholinesterase levels have returned to 75% of normal. Procedures for the collection, storage, and shipment of biological materials have been fully described (Morrison and Durham, 1971). An additional surveillance method is based upon the urinary excretion levels of p-nitrophenol and of alkyl phosphate metabolites of parathion and several related insecticides (Davies et al., 1966; Kuo and Fong, 1976; Morgan et al., 1977).

In addition to blood cholinesterase measurements, simple electromyographic methods have been developed to monitor worker exposure to organophosphorus pesticides (Roberts, 1979).

References

Aldridge WN, Barnes JM, Johnson MK: Studies on delayed neurotoxicity produced by some organophosphorus compounds. *Ann NY Acad Sci* 1969;160:314–322.

American Medical Association: *AMA Drug Evaluations,* ed 4. Chicago, AMA 1980.

Arterberry JD, Bonifaci RW, Nash EW, et al: Potentiation of phosphorus insecticides by phenothiazine derivatives. *J Am Med Assoc* 1962;182:848–850.

Bidstrup PL, Bonnell JA, Beckett AG: Paralysis following poisoning by a new organic phosphorus insecticide (mipafox). *Br Med J* 1953;1:1068–1072.

Bisby JA, Simpson GR: An unusual presentation of systemic organophosphate poisoning. *Med J Aust* 1975;2:394–395.

Burns JE, Parker RD: An investigation of the safety of cotton reentry after organophosphate application. *Arch Environ Contamin Toxicol* 1975;3:344–351.

Comer SW, Robbins AL, Staiff DC: Potential exposure from smoking parathion-contaminated cigarettes. *Arch Environ Contamin Toxicol* 1977;6:103–110.

Davies JE, Davis JH, Frazier JB, et al: Urinary p-nitrophenol concentrations in acute and chronic parathion exposures. Organic pesticides in the environment. *Adv Chem* 1966;60:67–78.

Drenth HJ, Ensberg IFG, Roberts DV, et al.: Neuromuscular function in agricultural workers using pesticides. *Arch Environ Health* 1972;25:395–398.

Fisher JR: Guillain-Barré syndrome following organophosphate poisoning. *J Am Med Assoc* 1977;238:1950–1951.

Gadoth N, Fisher A: Late onset of neuromuscular block in organophosphorus poisoning. *Ann Intern Med* 1978;88:654–655.

Guthrie FE, Domanski JJ, Chasson AL, et al:

Human subject experiments to estimate reentry periods for monocrotophos-treated tobacco. *Arch Environ Contamin Toxicol* 1976;4:217–225.

Hayes WJ Jr: *Toxicology of Pesticides.* Baltimore, Williams & Wilkins, 1975.

Knaak JB, Maddy KT, Jackson T, et al: Cholinesterase activity in blood samples collected from field workers and nonfield workers in California. *Toxicol Appl Pharmacol* 1978;45: 755–770.

Korsak RJ, Sato MM: Effects of chronic organophosphate pesticide exposure on the central nervous system. *Clin Toxicol* 1977;11:83–95.

Kuo T-L, Fong JM: Studies on parathion poisoning. I. Determination of urinary p-nitrophenol. *J Formosan Med Assoc* 1976;75: 674–680.

Levin HS, Rodnitzky RL, Mick DL: Anxiety associated with exposure to organophosphate compounds. *Arch Gen Psychiatry* 1976;33:225–228.

Metcalf DR, Holmes JH: EEG, psychological and neurological alterations in humans with organophosphate exposure. *Ann NY Acad Sci* 1969;160:357–365.

Milby TH: Prevention and management of organophosphate poisoning. *J Am Med Assoc* 1971;216:2131–2133.

Milby TH, Ottoboni F, Mitchell HW: Parathion residue poisoning among orchard workers. *J Am Med Assoc* 1964;189:351–356.

Morgan DP, Hetzler HL, Slach EF, et al: Urinary excretion of paranitrophenol and alkyl phosphates following ingestion of methyl or ethyl parathion by human subjects. *Arch Environ Contamin Toxicol* 1977;6:159–173.

Morrison G, Durham WF: Analytical diagnosis of pesticide poisoning. Collection, storage, and shipment of biological samples. *J Am Med Assoc* 1971;216:298–300.

Murphy SD: Pesticides, in Doull J, Klaassen CD, Amdur MO (eds): *Casarett and Doull's Toxicology,* ed 2. New York, MacMillan, 1980, pp 357–408.

Namba T, Nolte CT, Jackrel J, et al: Poisoning due to organophosphate insecticides. Acute and chronic manifestations. *Am J Med* 1971;50: 475–492.

Nigg HN: Prediction of agricultural worker safety reentry times for organophosphate insecticides. *Amer Ind Hyg Assoc J* 1980;41:340–345.

Rider JA, Hodges JL, Swader J, et al: Plasma and red cell cholinesterase in 800 "healthy" blood donors. *J Lab Clin Med* 1957;50:376–383.

Roberts DV: EMG voltage and motor nerve conduction velocity on organophosphorus pesticide factory workers. *Int Arch Occup Environ Health* 1976;36:267–274.

Roberts DV: A longitudinal electromyographic study of six men occupationally exposed to organophosphorus compounds. *Int Arch Occup Environ Health* 1977;38:221–229.

Roberts DV: Theoretical and practical consequences of the use of organophosphorus compounds in industry. *J Soc Occup Med* 1979;29:15–19.

Rodnitzky RL, Levin HS, Morgan DP: Effect of ingested parathion on neurobehavioral functions. *Clin Toxicol* 1978;13:347–359.

Rycroft RJG: Contact dermatitis from organophosphorus pesticides. *Br J Dermatol* 1977;97: 693–695.

Ware GW, Morgan DP, Estesen BJ, et al: Establishment of reentry intervals for organophosphate-treated cotton fields based on human data: III. 12 to 72 hours post-treatment exposure to monocrotophos, ethyl and methyl parathion. *Arch Environ Contamin Toxicol* 1975;3:289–306.

Warriner RA III, Nies AS, Hayes WJ Jr: Severe organophosphate poisoning complicated by alcohol and turpentine ingestion. *Arch Environ Health* 1977;32:203–205.

Wecker L, Dettbarn W-D: Paraoxon-induced myopathy: Muscle specificity and acetylcholine involvement. *Exp Neurol* 1976;51:281–291.

World Health Organization: WHO Technical Report Series No. 525, 1973.

Witter RF: Measurement of blood cholinesterase. *Arch Environ Health* 1963;6:537–563.

Carbamate Insecticides

Insecticides of the carbamate group are becoming increasingly popular because of their efficacy and relatively low order of mammalian toxicity. Carbamates are also used as fungicides and herbicides.

To a large extent, carbamates function in a manner similar to that of the organophosphorus compounds: there is an interference with the normal hydrolysis of acetylcholine (AcCh) by the enzyme cholinesterase. Since carbamates do not require metabolic activation, they are direct inhibitors of cholinesterase. The enzyme appears to be inactivated by carbamylation, a process analagous to phosphorylation. It may also be that carbamates act by competition with the AcCh substrate for the enzyme surface rather than by forming a stable bond with the enzyme. In either case, the clinical phenomena resulting from esterase inhibition are the same, and the signs and symptoms resemble those of organophosphate poisoning. However, the inactivating reaction is readily reversible in the case of the carbamates, and the normal enzyme is easily regenerated. In fact, the half-time for decarbamylation has been calculated to be between 30 and 40 minutes, so that cessation of exposure is followed almost immediately by restoration of cholinesterase within several hours. Since reversal is so rapid, measurements of blood cholinesterase in cases of poisoning are likely to be inaccurate and will appear as false-negatives unless special precautions are taken.

Most carbamates are readily hydrolyzed in mammalian organisms. Carbamates also vary in toxicity: carbaryl and Baygon are relatively safe but Temik (aldicarb) is so highly toxic that it is used only for limited greenhouse applications.

Most carbamates are absorbed via the lungs, skin, and gastrointestinal tract, but penetration through the skin is more common than poisoning by way of other routes (Kuhr and Dorough, 1976). When symptoms result from heavy exposure, atropine sulfate is the treatment of choice, as in the case of organophosphorus poisoning. The oximes are of no value in carbamate poisoning since they have no effect on decarbamylation of cholinesterase, and they may be harmful to the recovery of the patient. The use of 2-PAM, then, should be avoided in carbaryl and other carbamate intoxication.

The methylcarbamates, which comprise the bulk of the carbamate insecticides, alter a number of other enzyme systems in the body in addition to cholinesterase. Carbaryl, for example, depresses alkaline phosphatase in the liver, kidneys, and adrenal glands, although serum levels may be elevated. Other enzymes affected adversely include arginase, aldolase, glucose-6-phosphate dehydrase, phosphofructokinase, and transaminase. Phospholipid synthesis and metabolism are inhibited in liver, brain, and heart. In mammals, carbamate exposures may produce necrotic changes in the liver, but these have not been reported for man.

It has been suggested that in carbamate manufacturing and field applications the intensity of exposure may be evaluated by determinations of urinary metabolites such as 1-naphthol (Best and Murray, 1962). However, analytic methods for detection of carbamates and their phenol derivatives are not sufficiently reliable for biological monitoring (Kuhr and Dorough, 1976).

References

Best EM Jr, Murray BL: Observations on workers exposed to Sevin insecticide: A preliminary report. *J Occup Med* 1962;4:507–517.

Kuhr RJ, Dorough HW: *Carbamate Insecticides: Chemistry, Biochemistry, and Toxicology.* Cleveland, CRC Press, 1976.

Organochlorine Insecticides

The organochlorine insecticides consist mainly of 1) chlorinated ethane compounds, such as DDT and methoxychlor; 2) cyclodienes, such as aldrin, chlordane, dieldrin, endrin, heptachlor, and toxaphene; and 3) hexachlorocyclohexanes, such as lindane. Organochlorine compounds, very widely used in agriculture and malaria control programs for 20 years beginning in the mid-1940s, have declined in use since the mid-1960s (Ridgeway et al., 1978). The shift has been attributed to their persistence in the environment and their biomagnification in food chains as well as to serious toxic properties, such as mutagenicity, that have been found for certain of them.

The mechanism of action of chlorinated hydrocarbon insecticides in mammals and insects has never been clearly elucidated, although it is apparent that these compounds are neurotoxins. They are soluble in body fat, and numerous studies have measured the levels of chlorinated hydrocarbon insecticides in human tissues. Indeed, their fat solubility and slow degradation are the basis for their prolonged retention and accumulation in adipose tissue (Deichmann, 1973). Measurable concentrations of DDT and other agents have been found in normal human fat and even in neonatal tissues and are evidence of absorption by man from foods, particularly those of animal origin. These materials or their metabolites may often be identified in urine or milk.

Compounds of this group may be absorbed through ingestion and via the respiratory tract. Cyclodienes, in particular, can be absorbed through intact skin, and at least one, dieldrin, can be absorbed in this manner from a dry state without being in solution. DDT, on the other hand, is poorly absorbed through skin, and dusts containing 5% DDT have been applied to the skin in louse control programs for extended periods without untoward effects.

Diagnosis Manifestations of central nervous system stimulation from slight exposures include headache, anorexia, nausea, and irritability. With increasing intensity of exposure, weakness, paresthesias, tremors, and muscle fibrillation may develop. Paresthesias of the tongue, face, and lips have been noted in the course of DDT poisoning, and in severe cases paresthesias may occur in the extremities as well. Relatively high levels of absorption accelerate the onset of these symptoms, and seizures or coma may occur. In most overexposure situations, symptoms appear within several hours, and a delay of over eight hours would be unusual. Long-continued low-level exposures are not known to produce clinical phenomena that differ from those of the acute response to intense single exposures.

Diagnosis is based almost entirely upon the history and clinical picture. Laboratory techniques, especially gas-liquid chromatography, can identify insecticides or their metabolites in blood, urine, gastric contents, or body fat (Morrison and Durham, 1971). The correlation of these assays with the character of the illness is not very good, and it is apparent that these relatively sophisticated procedures have limited applicability in emergency situations.

Treatment Treatment is symptomatic and supportive, and no specific antidotes are available. Contaminated clothing must be removed, and material on the skin, in the hair, and under the nails must be washed away with soap and water. Emesis or gastric lavage is indicated if the toxic material has been ingested. Petroleum-based solvent vehicles present the additional hazard of aspiration pneumonia, although this danger is of less significance than the fact that large amounts of highly toxic material may have been ingested. Oil-based cathartics should not be used since they may increase absorption. To control convulsions, pentobarbital sodium 0.2 to 0.5 g may be given intravenously; repeated doses may be necessary. Diazepam intravenously may be preferable for this purpose since it produces less respiratory depression. After seizures have been stopped, phenobarbital will provide more prolonged control. In cases of severe intoxication, artificial ventilation and supplemental oxygen may be required.

Mild intoxication may be treated with oral phenobarbital alone. Symptoms of chlorinated hydrocarbon poisoning may persist as long as a week, and control of symptoms may be necessary for the entire period.

Whether or not delayed effects or chronic sequelae are related to the absorption of chlorinated hydrocarbon insecticides is not always clear. Occupational medical experience with organochlorine pesticides has been varied. Heavy exposures to DDT in manufacturing plants has failed to produce harmful effects (Laws et al., 1967; Deichmann, 1973; Morgan and Roan, 1973). Experience with cyclodienes such as aldrin, dieldrin, and endrin has been similar: except for cases of acute intoxication that occurred early in manufacture, no abnormalities have been found after long-term exposure. Despite extensive use of toxaphene, worker intoxication has not been reported. On the other hand, occupational exposure to chlordecone (Kepone) in a pesticide manufacturing plant produced an illness characterized by nervousness, generalized tremors, ocular flutter (opsoclonus), muscle weakness, gait ataxia, incoordination, pleuritic and joint pains, and oligospermia (Cannon et al., 1978; Taylor et al., 1978). Neuropathologic investigation established chlordecone as a neurotoxic agent principally affecting the Schwann cells of myelinated and unmyelinated fibers of peripheral nerves (Martinez et al., 1977), and Sanborn et al. (1979) found that it produced increased intracranial pressure as a result of impaired absorption of cerebrospinal fluid. Mirex, which is structurally related to chlordecone, has not been reported to have adverse effects on man, although it has been detected in human adipose tissue (Waters et al., 1977). Serious alterations in testicular function, involving oligospermia and azoospermia, have been reported for workers manufacturing 1,2-dibromo-3-chloropropane (DBCP), an organochlorine nematocide (Whorton et al., 1979).

In 1972, the use of DDT in the United States was severely restricted because of evidence of its carcinogenicity in laboratory animals, and in the same year aldrin and dieldrin were removed from the market for similar reasons. Chlordane and heptachlor have been incriminated as etiologic agents in cases of childhood neuroblastoma, aplastic anemia, and acute leukemias (Infante et al., 1978), while toxaphene has been found to be highly carcinogenic in rats and mice (Reuber, 1979). Aplastic anemias have also been reported to follow exposure to lindane, the gamma isomer of benzene hexachloride (BHC), but the hematological diagnoses, while certain, were not convincingly attributable to lindane exposure (Milby et al., 1968).

References

Cannon SB, Veazey JM Jr, Jackson RS, et al: Epidemic Kepone poisoning in chemical workers. *Am J Epidemiol* 1978;107:529–537.

Deichmann WB: The chronic toxicity of organochlorine pesticides in man, in *Pesticides and the Environment: A Continuing Controversy.* New York, Intercontinental 1973, pp 347–420.

Infante PF, Epstein SS, Newton WA Jr: Blood dyscrasias and childhood tumors and exposure to chlordane and heptachlor. *Scand J Work Environ Health* 1978;4:137–150.

Laws ER Jr, Curley A, Biros FJ: Men with intensive occupational exposure to DDT. *Arch Environ Health* 1967;15:766–775.

Martinez AJ, Taylor JR, Houff SA, et al: Kepone poisoning: Cliniconeuropathological study. in Roizin L et al (eds): *Neurotoxicology,* New York, Raven Press, 1977, pp 443–456.

Milby TH, Samuels AJ: Human exposure to lindane. Comparison of an exposed and unexposed population. *J Occup Med* 1971;13:256–258.

Morgan DP, Roan CC: Adrenocortical function in persons occupationally exposed to pesticides. *J Occup Med* 1973;15:26–28.

Morrison G, Durham WF: Analytical diagnosis of pesticide poisoning. Collection, storage, and shipment of biological samples. *J Am Med Assoc* 1971;216:298–300.

Reuber MD: Carcinogenicity of toxaphene: A Review. *J Toxicol Environ Health* 1979;5:729–748.

Ridgeway RL, Tinney JC, MacGregor JT, et al: Pesticide use in agriculture. *Environ Health Persp* 1978;27:103–112.

Sanborn GE, Selhorst JB, Calabrese VP, et al: Pseudotumor cerebri and insecticide intoxication. *Neurology* 1979;29:1222–1227.

Taylor JR, Selhorst JB, Houff SA, et al: Chlordecone intoxication in man. I. Clinical observations. *Neurology* 1978;28:626–635.

Waters EM, Huff JE, Gerstner HB: Mirex. An overview. *Environ Res* 1977;14:212–222.

Whorton D, Milby TH, Krauss RM, et al.: Testicular function in DBCP exposed pesticide workers. *J Occup Med* 1979;21:161–166.

Other Insecticides

Pyrethrum is extracted from the flowers of certain species of *Chrysanthemum* and is used in many insect sprays and powders, especially when a rapid "knock-down" is required. It is consequently found in many aerosol pressurized cans for home use. The pyrethrins are moderately potent skin sensitizers and cross react with other chrysanthemums and with ragweed. Systemic intoxication is not usually a problem, although severe anaphylactic reactions have occurred, and death from convulsions and paralysis have resulted from ingestion of large oral doses. The synthetic pyrethroids are said to be less allergenic.

Rotenone, a derivative of derris root, has properties that are similar to pyrethrum. Rotenone has been safely used against body ectoparasites on man but the dust may be toxic when inhaled.

Nicotine sulfate is a potent neurological poison that can be absorbed from the skin, lungs, or gastrointestinal tract. Systemic poisoning results in stimulation of nicotinic receptors of the autonomic nervous system with symptoms that are discussed in the section dealing with organosphosphate insecticides.

Piperonyl butoxide is not an insecticide but is a synergist that permits the reduction of concentrations of pyrethrum to 10% of levels that would otherwise be required. This synergist is comparatively nontoxic when tested alone by conventional techniques. It, and other piperonyl derivatives, synergize the action of a number of pesticides by inhibiting microsomal enzyme systems that are concerned with the metabolism of the primary agent. However, in the case of certain sulfur-containing organophosphorus insecticides that require metabolic activation, the enzyme-inhibiting synergists are in fact antagonistic to the development of normal pesticide potency. The applicability of these relationships to human health is not entirely clear (Conney et al., 1972), but there is little reason to doubt that insecticidal synergists influence the metabolic detoxification of agricultural chemicals, hormones, and pharmaceuticals.

Hydrogen cyanide and methyl bromide are used in homes, warehouses, and ships as fumigants. The arsenicals (e.g., Paris green, lead arsenate, and other inorganic compounds of arsenic) are used as insecticides with decreasing frequency.

Mites, such as the red spider mite, are not insects and are not controlled by the usual insecticidal agents. Such agents, in fact, tend to kill the insect predators of mites. Nevertheless, miticides (acaricides) are included in this section because they are applied in the same manner as are the insecticides and because their probable effects on man resemble those of certain groups of insecticides. The chemical compounds that are used, chlorbenzilate and chlorbenside, resemble the chlorinated hydrocarbon insecticides and have similar effects on animals. The mammalian toxicity of these agents is not great. Dinitrophenol and its derivatives are miticides of distinctly greater mammalian toxicity and are discussed in the section on herbicides.

Nematodes are roundworms that are ubiquitous, and some forms inhabit the soil as do certain insects, all of which are controlled by nematocidal soil fumigants. The best known of these agents is referred to as DD, a mixture of 1,2-dichloropane and 1,3-dichloropropene, which is an intense irritant to the eyes, skin, and respiratory tract mucosa. Other nematocides include methyl bromide, ethyl dibromide, and carbamates.

Reference

Conney AH, Chang R, Levin WM, et al: Effects of piperonyl butoxide on drug metabolism in rodents and man. *Arch Environ Health* 1972; 24:97–106.

3 • *Fungicides*

The classical agricultural fungicides, sulfur and inorganic copper, have never been of great toxicological significance to man. These agents, however, are being supplemented or superseded to an increasing extent by organic compounds, some of which are clearly hazardous.

Organomercury Compounds

Among the most useful organomercurial fungicides are those based on alkyl, alkoxyalkyl, and aryl mercury: phenyl mercury acetate, ethyl mercury phosphate, methoxyethyl mercury silicate, and a series of more complex compounds. Alkyl mercurials, which have been used as fungicidal seed dressings, are highly poisonous neurotoxins that, when absorbed, are capable of causing ataxia, constricted visual fields, and other manifestations of central and peripheral nervous system involvement. Aryl mercury compounds are used to control fungus diseases of turf, fruits, vegetables, and grain crops, but not under conditions that will leave measurable residues in food or animal feeds. The aryl, usually phenyl, derivatives are less toxic than the alkyl compounds, but they can cause similar neurological disease and an active dermatitis. These materials are also used as fungicides in paints and some leathers. Compounds of nickel, chromium, and tin may also be found in metal-based fungicides.

Dithiocarbamates

Dithiocarbamates are widely used in agriculture as foliage sprays. The principal compounds are the dimethyldithiocarbamates and the ethylene bis(dithiocarbamates). The former include the iron and zinc derivatives, ferbam and ziram, while among the latter are manganese, zinc, and sodium formulations, maneb, zineb, and nabam. These materials are not considered to have important systemic toxicities, although they may irritate the skin, eyes, and upper airway. Ethylene thiourea (ETU) is the principal impurity and metabolic degradation product in the ethylene bis(dithiocarbamates) (Fishbein, 1976). ETU is also used as an accelerator for neoprene (polychloropropane) rubber and in curing polyacrylate rubber. While ETU has antithyroid properties and is carcinogenic for many animals, as are many dithiocarbamates, the hazards to those occupationally exposed appears to be small. Thiram is tetramethylthiuram disulfide; it is a seed protectant and is also used in the rubber industry as an accelerator.

Phthalimides

The principal phthalimides, captan and folpet, which are found in many agricultural and home garden fungicides, have not presented significant hazards to man. Both agents have the phthalimide moiety of thalidomide and are teratogenic for chick and hamster embryos. While extrapolation of these observations to man are not reliable, the thalidomide experience in Europe suggests that caution be observed in the case of female workers of childbearing age.

Hexachlorobenzene

Hexachlorobenzene (HCB) has been used as a fungicidal seed dressing particularly because of unfortunate accidents that have resulted from the consumption of seed grains that have been treated with organomercurials. Nevertheless, the ingestion of food prepared from seeds treated with

300

HCB and intended for agriculture has led to outbreaks of acquired porphyria cutanea tarda, with bullous skin lesions, ulcerations, permanent pigmented scarring, and hypertrichosis (Courtney, 1979; Schmid, 1960). Workers handling HCB have also developed signs of porphyria cutanea tarda.

Hexachlorobenzene (C_6Cl_6) should not be confused with benzene hexachloride ($C_6H_6Cl_6$; BHC). The latter is an insecticide that is properly designated as hexachlorocyclohexane, the gamma isomer of which is lindane. Nor should hexachlorobenzene be confused with hexachlorobiphenyl, an isomer of polychlorinated biphenyl (PCB).

Pentachlorophenol

Pentachlorophenol (PCP) is an insecticide, herbicide, and fungicide that is used to control weeds and the deterioration of timber. It is not applied to food crops. The action of PCP in man is similar to that of the dinitrophenols and is based upon the uncoupling of oxidation and phosphorylation with a resultant marked increase in metabolic rate and elevation of body temperature. Rapid absorption through the skin has been demonstrated by unfortunate hospital nursery fatalities where pentachlorophenol residues in diapers resulted from its use as a laundry fungicide (Armstrong et al., 1969). Technical grade preparations may contain certain hexachlorinated and octachlorinated dibenzodioxins and dibenzofurans. Some of these chlorophenols become enriched in sawmill work environments where they present a hazard to workers (Levin et al., 1976).

Pentachlorophenol is also a potent skin, eye, and upper respiratory irritant, and clinical manifestations related to this irritation have been found in workers exposed to PCP (Klemmer et al., 1980). PCP residues have been detected in serum and urine samples of PCP handlers (Wyllie et al., 1975), and such workers have been found to have reduced glomerular filtration and tubular function during periods of exposure (Begley et al., 1977).

Karathane

Karathane is a member of the dinitrophenol group discussed in the section on herbicides and it

has potent fungicidal and miticidal properties. It is irritating to the eyes and upper airway, but is much less toxic systemically than 4,6-dinitro-*o*-cresol (DNOC).

Other Fungicides

Other fungicidal agents used in industrial applications include creosote that has value as a wood preservative. Creosote, which is a distillate of either coal tar or wood tar, may be a mixture of numerous compounds. It can produce painful skin burns and is highly toxic on ingestion. Paranitrophenol, a methemoglobin producer, is used in the preparation of leather.

References

Armstrong RW, Eichner ER, Klein DE, et al: Pentachlorophenol poisoning in a nursery for newborn infants. II. Epidemiologic and toxicologic studies. *J Pediatrics* 1969;75:317–325.

Begley J, Reichert EL, Rashad MN, et al: Association between renal function tests and pentachlorophenol exposure. *Clin Toxicol* 1977;11:97–106.

Courtney KD: Hexachlorobenzene (HCB): A review. *Environ Res* 1979;20:225–266.

Fishbein L: Environmental health aspects of fungicides. I. Dithiocarbamates. *J Toxicol Environ Health* 1976;1:713–735.

Klemmer HW, Wong L, Sato MM, et al: Chemical findings in workers exposed to pentachlorophenol. *Arch Environ Contam Toxicol* 1980;9:715–725.

Levin J-O, Rappe C, Nilsson C-A: Use of chlorophenols as fungicides in sawmills. *Scand J Work Environ Health* 1976;2:71–81.

Schmid R: Cutaneous porphyria in Turkey. *N Engl J Med* 1960;263:397–398.

Wyllie JA, Gabica J, Benson WW, et al: Exposure and contamination of the air and employees of a pentachlorophenol plant, Idaho—1972. *Pesticides Monit J* 1975;9:150–153.

4 • Herbicides

Herbicides are compounds that are used for extermination or control of noxious or otherwise undesirable plants. The wide variety of materials used for this purpose include inorganic as well as organic compounds (Brian, 1964). The former include arsenicals, cyanates, copper salts, and sodium chlorate. Inorganic arsenicals and sodium chlorate have been used to kill weeds and to sterilize soils for areas such as parking lots in which no vegetation is desired. More recent usage emphasizes organic compounds, many of which are selective herbicides that affect only certain types of vegetation. However, the use of sodium chlorate has continued and its hazard is evidenced by the cases of leucomelanoderma that have been reported in handlers (Matsushita et al., 1975).

Chlorphenoxy Group

This group includes 2,4-dichlorophenoxyacetic acid (2,4-D), 2,4,5-trichlorophenoxyacetic acid (2,4,5-T), 2-(2,4,5-trichlorophenoxy) propionic acid (silvex), 4-chloro-2-methyl-phenoxyacetic acid (MCPA). In most applications amine salts or esters are used to permit control of volatility and drift. Compounds of this group act as growth-regulating hormones in plants; however, no hormonal effects have been noted in animals. Skin absorption is slight, and toxicity by oral or inhalation routes has not been an agricultural health problem. Experimental exposures and suicidal ingestion have resulted in weakness, muscle twitching, myotonia, convulsions, and coma, the mechanisms for which are not known.

Compounds of this group can produce a contact dermatitis and chloracne (Kimmig and Schulz, 1957), and the features of porphyria cutanea tarda have occurred in chemical operators manufacturing 2,4-D and 2,4,5-T (Bleiberg et al., 1964; Poland et al., 1971). The presence of 2,3,7,8-tetrachlorodibenzodioxin (TCDD) as a production contaminant was thought to account for the chloracne in these exposures, and concern has been widely expressed about the use of 2,4,5-T because of this presence of TCDD, which is also porphyrinogenic in man and is a potent teratogen in experimental animals (Poland and Kende, 1976). In July 1976, a runaway reaction at a trichlorophenol production facility in Seveso, Italy resulted in the discharge of chemical materials that contained TCDD and their dispersion over 2.8 sq km area. Evacuation of persons living in the area was ordered because of the potential hazards of TCDD. However, careful studies of the exposed population have failed to uncover any pathologic disturbances except for transient chloracne in 12 persons that healed completely (Homberger et al., 1979; Reggiani, 1980). Nevertheless, the continued use of 2,4,5-T and TCDD remains controversial (Greig, 1979) and their use has been restricted, along with silvex, in the United States and elsewhere.

Dinitrophenols

A series of substituted dinitrophenols has been developed for use as eradicant herbicides along roadways and rights of way, as selective weed killers in fields, and as blossom thinners for fruit trees. In different formulations these compounds can also be used as fungicides, miticides, and insecticides, especially in dormant sprays for the control of overwintering insect eggs in fruit trees. The principal compounds include 4,6-dinitro-*o*-cresol (DNOC), 4,6-dinitro-*o*-sec-butylphenol (dinoseb), and 2,4-dinitrocyclohexylphenol. Each of these compounds, as well as others in the group, is readily absorbed by inhalation or ingestion. Most of them can be absorbed through the skin, although the cyclohexyl derivative is less

301

penetrating in this manner. Compounds of this group share a common toxic mechanism whereby oxidation at the mitochondrial level is uncoupled from phosphorylation. Oxidation not only continues but increases in response to the deficit of adenosine triphosphate.

Symptoms of acute poisoning in man include restlessness, anxiety, nausea and vomiting, flushed skin, deep and rapid respiration, tachycardia, hyperthermia, cyanosis, weakness, collapse, and coma. The increase in metabolic rate is proportional to the absorbed dose, and very high basal metabolic rates may be attained. Under such circumstances the production of heat exceeds the capacity to dissipate heat by a very great margin, and fatal hyperthermia may result. High ambient temperatures aggravate the problem of heat loss, while cold weather permits toleration of higher blood levels without the development of symptoms.

Chronic intoxication may be marked by fatigue, restlessness, excessive sweating, unusual thirst, and weight loss as well as by other symptoms of acute poisoning. There may be yellow staining of the skin by the dinitrophenol compounds, although staining is not indicative of poisoning. Cataract formation may occur as it did in the cases of the 1930s when dinitrophenols were used in weight-reducing drugs.

Treatment is symptomatic and is based on controlling the hyperthermia with cold baths. Oxygen and careful attention to fluid and electrolyte balance are indicated. Material on the skin should be removed with soap and water, but there is no reason to attempt to remove the fixed yellow stains of skin and hair. Atropine is absolutely contraindicated, and it is essential not to confuse the evidence for dinitrophenol poisoning with manifestations of cholinesterase inhibition.

Acute poisoning by the dinitrophenols usually runs a rapid course with either essentially complete recovery or death within 24 to 48 hours. The excretion of these compounds is very slow, however, and persons who have shown symptoms of intoxication should be shielded against risks of further absorption for at least six weeks.

Laboratory findings are not usually helpful with the exception of the basal metabolic rate, which is elevated. Tests are available for determining blood and urine levels of dinitrophenols. Blood DNOC values that exceed 20 ppm (20 μg/ml) indicate serious intoxication. Those who regularly apply dinitrophenols should be checked periodically for blood levels of these compounds. The permissible exposure limit for air concentrations of DNOC is 0.2 mg/m³.

Bipyridinium Compounds

Diquat and paraquat of the bipyridinium (or bipyridilium or quaternary ammonium) group are nonselective contact herbicides that have desiccant and defoliant effects. Paraquat is especially remarkable from the toxicological point of view in that it is capable, when absorbed into the body, of causing lung pathology resulting from the proliferation of alveolar macrophages, alveolar cells, pulmonary fibroblasts, and terminal bronchial cells. These changes lead to the thickening and fibrosis of the alveolar walls, respiratory insufficiency, and death. In man this response has been observed even after the ingestion of small amounts of paraquat and the onset of symptoms may be delayed for several days after acute exposure. Kidney disorders with renal failure (Vaziri et al., 1979) and hepatic necrosis have also been observed to accompany the development of pulmonary fibrosis. Toxicological information has largely come from accidental or suicidal ingestion and very little from inhalation (Haley, 1979).

Treatment of paraquat poisoning needs to be vigorous and is directed to minimizing absorption: gastric lavage, cathartics, and ingestion of a suspension of bentonite or Fuller's earth are recommended. Forced diuresis and hemodialysis or hemoperfusion through charcoal should be considered. Corticosteroids have not been helpful. Although oxygenation should be maintained, the use of oxygen may aggravate the underlying pathological mechanism that involves the generation of superoxide ions (Fairshter and Wilson, 1975).

Diquat is less toxic than paraquat in that the lung effects seen with the latter compound do not occur. In one instance, inhalation of diquat aerosol has produced fever, cough, lung consolidation, and jaundice from which the patient recovered (Wood et al., 1976). Nasal bleeding has occurred in field use, especially when spray mists have been encountered (Gage, 1968). Ingestion leads to gastrointestinal disturbances, and long-term feeding has produced cataracts in experimental animals.

In normal field use of these compounds it is prudent to avoid the mists generated by spraying since changes in the eyes and fingernails may be produced by contact, in addition to the lung changes that may result from inhalation, or even from skin contact (Newhouse et al., 1978).

Other Herbicides

Carbamate herbicides include compounds known by a variety of designations, such as propham. The phenylurea group includes monuron, diuron, and linuron. Simazine and atrazine are of the triazine group. None of these materials has been shown to have a high degree of acute toxicity for mammals. However, there is evidence from animal studies that some of the carbamates and phenylureas produce tumors after prolonged oral administration.

Dalapon is the sodium salt of 2,2-dichloropropionic acid. While it is not a great hazard to applicators, it has been reported to cause contact dermatitis (Matsushita et al., 1975).

Aminotriazole (amitrol), used mainly for the destruction of poison oak and poison ivy, has potent antithyroid properties and is goitrogenic when ingested over long periods, although the acute toxicity is low.

References

Bleiberg J, Wallen M, Brodkin R, et al: Industrially acquired porphyria. *Arch Dermatol* 1964; 89:793–797.

Brian RC: The classification of herbicides and types of toxicity, in Audus LJ (ed): *The Physiology and Biochemistry of Herbicides.* New York, Academic Press, 1964, pp 1–37.

Fairshter RD, Wilson AF: Paraquat poisoning: Manifestations and therapy. *Am J Med* 1975;59: 751–753.

Gage JC: Toxicity of paraquat and diquat aerosols generated by a size-selective cyclone: Effect of particle size distribution. *Br J Ind Med* 1968;25:304–314.

Greig JB: The toxicology of 2,3,7,8-tetrachlorodibenzo-*p*-dioxin and its structural analogues. *Ann Occup Hyg* 1979;22:411–420.

Haley TJ: Review of the toxicology of paraquat (1,1′-dimethyl-4,4′-bipyridinium chloride). *Clin Toxicology* 1979;14:1–46.

Homberger E, Reggiani G, Sambeth J, et al: The Seveso accident: Its nature, extent and consequences. *Ann Occup Hyg* 1979;22:327–370.

Kimmig J, Schulz KH: Occupational chloracne caused by aromatic cyclic ethers. *Dermatologica* 1957;115:540–546.

Matsushita T, Arimatsu Y, Misumi J, et al: Skin disorders caused by herbicides sodium chlorate and sodium 2,2-dichloropropionate. *Kumamoto Med J* 1975;28:164–169.

Newhouse M, McEvoy D, Rosenthal D: Percutaneous paraquat absorption. An association with cutaneous lesions and respiratory failure. *Arch Dermatol* 1978;114;1515–1519.

Poland A, Kende A: 2,3,7,8-tetrachlorodibenzo-*p*-dioxin: Environmental contaminant and molecular probe. *Fed Proc* 1976;35:2404–2411.

Poland AP, Smith D, Metter G, et al: A health survey of workers in a 2,4-D and 2,4,5-T plant. *Arch Environ Health* 1971;22:316–327.

Reggiani G: Acute human exposure to TCDD in Seveso, Italy. *J Toxicol Environ Health* 1980; 6:27–43.

Vaziri ND, Ness RL, Fairshter RD, et al: Nephrotoxicity of paraquat in man. *Arch Intern Med* 1979;139:172–174.

Wood TE, Edgar H, Salcedo J: Recovery from inhalation of diquat aerosol. *Chest* 1976;70:774–775.

5 • *Rodenticides*

A variety of rodenticides are used in baits and inaccessible places, such as rodent runways, so that environmental contamination is minimal. Toxic effects in man are almost never occupational and usually result from accidental or suicidal ingestion.

Inorganic rodenticides include arsenic trioxide, elemental phosphorus, thallium sulfate, and zinc phosphide.

Warfarin is a coumarin derivative that has anticoagulant properties that are familiar to physicians who use similar preparations in clinical medicine. Single doses of warfarin do not seriously inhibit prothrombin synthesis but chronic ingestion, as in the case of a family eating baited cornmeal for two weeks, can lead to death from severe hemorrhagic complications.

Sodium fluoroacetate (Compound 1080) and fluoracetamide (Compound 1081) are extremely toxic metabolic poisons that block the metabolism of citrate in the tricarboxylic acid cycle so that citrate accumulates in the tissues and there is a general inhibition of oxidative energy metabolism. Sodium fluoroacetate is readily absorbed from the gastrointestinal tract. In man the clinical consequences include apprehension, nausea and vomiting, cyanosis, convulsions, ventricular fibrillation, and death. Therapy is mainly nonspecific, although there is evidence from animal experimentation that an extrinsic supply of acetate ions (as glycerol monoacetate) may be helpful. The main protection against poisoning is the limitation of use to specially qualified exterminators. These compounds, as well as thallium sulfate, should not be available to householders for the control of rodents.

SECTION SEVEN
RADIANT ENERGY

1 • *Infrared Radiation*

The infrared region of the electromagnetic spectrum is intermediate in wavelength and frequency between the visible and the microwave regions. The range of infrared wavelengths is from 0.75 μm to 3000 μm. All objects emit infrared radiation to other objects of a lower surface temperature. The higher the temperature of an object, the shorter the emitted infrared wavelength. With extremely high temperatures (e.g., the sun), visible and even ultraviolet radiation is emitted.

Baking, drying, and heating are the three most common industrial applications of infrared radiation. Baking is used for curing paints, enamels, varnishes, and lacquered finishes in the automobile industry. In various other industries, drying of water and other liquids from paper, cloth, leather, wood, rubber, and porcelain is a common practice. Infrared spectroscopy has applications in chemical analyses and studies of molecular structure. In medicine, infrared physiotherapy treatments are a routine practice. The military services use infrared radiation for signalling, photography, and anti-intruder weapons, while infrared photography is widely used by meteorology services for earth surface photography from satellites.

The initial biological effect of infrared radiation is the heating of exposed tissues. Three biologically significant infrared spectral bands have been defined by the International Commission on Illumination (CIE): (1) IR-A: 780 to 1400 nm, sometimes referred to as the "near infrared;" this radiation penetrates skin and to some extent the media of the eye to reach the retina. (2) IR-B: 1.4 μm to 3μm; this radiation is almost completely absorbed by the upper layers of the skin and eye. (3) IR-C: 3μm to 1μm; together with IR-B, this band is referred to as the "far infrared." IR-C is absorbed by the very superficial layers of tissue and does not penetrate beyond them.

The sensation of heat produced by infrared radiation on the sensory endings of the skin and eye usually provides adequate warning of potentially harmful exposure. However, the lens of the eye is of particular concern with respect to occupational overexposure to infrared radiation. Many European workers, exposed to hot metals or glass, developed cataracts after an average latent period of 25 years. Various names, such as "furnaceman's cataract," "glass-blower's cataract," "bottle-worker's cataract," and "chain-maker's cataract," were used to designate the opacities that resulted (Hunter, 1978). Infrared radiation in the IR-A band is especially effective in inducing cataracts, since the other bands are absorbed by the cornea. Corneal burns can be produced by intense infrared radiation above 2000 nm, but they rarely occur in industry because the accompanying pain results in an aversion response (Sliney and Wolbarsht, 1980).

Prolonged exposure to infrared radiation, along with elevated ambient temperatures, may lead to heat stress. Such stress may progress from local edema and prickly heat to heat syncope, heat exhaustion, and eventually to hyperthermia and heat stroke (Collins, 1977; Dukes-Dobos, 1981; Shibolet et al., 1976).

Control of infrared overexposure to the skin is readily achieved by the use of reflective and/or thermal insulation shielding. Protective lenses or goggles containing mineral oxides will absorb approximately 90% of the incident infrared radiation, but the selection of such eye shields should be governed by the nature of the incident radiation. Use of protective goggles by United States workers exposed to high infrared intensities has virtually eliminated infrared-induced cataracts in the occupationally exposed population.

References

Collins KJ: Heat illness: Diagnosis, treatment

and prevention. *The Practitioner* 1977;219:193–198.

Dukes-Dobos FN: Hazards of heat exposure. A review. *Scand J Work Environ Health* 1981;7:73–83.

Hunter D: *Diseases of Occupations,* ed 6. London, Hodder & Stoughton, 1978.

Shibolet S, Lancaster MC, Danon Y: Heat stroke: A review. *Aviat Space Environ Med* 1976;47:280–301.

Sliney D, Wolbarsht M: *Safety with Lasers and Other Optical Sources.* New York, Plenum Press, 1980.

2 • *Microwave and Radiofrequency Radiation*

The microwave region of the electromagnetic spectrum is intermediate in wavelength and frequency between the conventional radio region and the infrared region. The microwave band lies between 30 and 300,000 MHz (10 m and 1 mm wavelengths) while the radiofrequency (RF) boundaries are put at 0.01 and 30 MHz (10 km and 10 m wavelengths). The energy content per photon for microwaves is very low. One photon of ultraviolet radiation at 253.7 nm has 400,000 times as much energy as one photon of 10-cm microwave radiation. Like ultraviolet radiation, microwave and radiofrequency radiation energy levels are below those needed to cause ionization. The only biological effects produced at the molecular level by microwave radiation are those associated with heating and electric field effects.

Before 1950, the use of microwave devices was essentially limited to radar and diathermy applications. Now, microwave devices are used in communications, telemetry, navigation, and in a variety of industrial processes that require heating and drying, such as drying of photographic film, newsprint, and glue binders in plywood. Some commercially prepared foods are also dried and otherwise processed by the use of microwave heating: potato chips, precooked bacon, chicken. Microwave ovens are widely used in restaurants, hospitals, self-service food vending machines, and increasingly in homes. Occupational exposures can occur in a variety of activities in the manufacture and use of microwave equipment. RF heaters and sealers generally operate at frequencies between 10 and 70 MHz, although some wood gluing devices operate at 3 to 6 MHz, and some RF heaters used for plastics have frequencies as high as 300 to 400 MHz. NIOSH and OSHA (1979) have issued a joint bulletin listing the occupations that may involve the use of these applications with the warning that the adverse effects seen in laboratory animals may occur in humans at comparable or even lower exposure levels.

Most of the biological effects of microwave and radiofrequency radiation can be attributed to local or general hyperthermia. The effect of microwaves on the human body varies with the wavelength or frequency. At the lower microwave frequencies that approach radio waves, the body is transparent to the radiation so that no appreciable absorption occurs. At 3000 MHz approximately 40% of the incident energy is absorbed and the depth of penetration is about 1 cm (Ricketts, 1978). This portion of the energy range is potentially the most hazardous with respect to whole body heating since there is very little heating of the skin. Ordinarily, except for the eyes, a sensation of warmth provides a warning that may be absent with microwaves.

Those body organs that are least able to dissipate heat are the ones that are most susceptible to microwave radiation. The ability of an organ to dissipate heat depends chiefly on the magnitude of its blood flow. Since the eyes and the testes are the organs with the least blood flow, they are the most vulnerable to microwave radiation. The lens of the eye with no cooling system and inability to repair itself is in turn the part of the eye most susceptible to microwave radiation. Overexposure of the lens results in the formation of opacities in animals and man (McRee, 1972). Hirsch and Parker (1952) were the first to report cataract formation in a technician operating a microwave generator at frequencies of from 1500 to 3000 MHz.

Overexposure of the testes to microwave radiation results in a reduction of spermatocytes and damage to the cells lining the seminiferous tubules. Although temporary sterility can occur, the condition does not appear to be permanent and recovery will occur.

At the present time, the radiation protection

guide for the United States and Great Britain is 10 mW/cm² averaged over any 0.1 hour period. For shorter periods, the permissible exposure is somewhat greater. The Soviet Union and its satellite countries have more stringent standards: from 2.5 mW/cm² to 1 mW/cm², depending upon the length of exposure. The United States standard is based solely on heating effects, while that of the USSR is based upon low-energy effects that are essentially free from heating. These effects are usually referred to as "athermal" and are reported to include central nervous system disturbances such as headache, fatigue, hyperactivity, and even disturbances of heartbeat, at levels below 10 mW/cm². Until recently, United States scientists had not taken the Russian data seriously, but some investigators in the United States are now reporting behavioral effects in animals at levels below 10 mW/cm² (Eakin and Thompson, 1965), although full agreement has been lacking on effects at these energy levels (Tyler, 1975).

Devices emitting microwaves should be checked periodically by experienced personnel with microwave detection instruments. Physical barriers with appropriate signs, microwave shielding enclosures, protective clothing, and interlocks should be utilized where applicable. In addition to the direct hazard from microwave and RF exposure, one must consider the possibilities of associated hazards of the equipment, such as x-rays and electric shock.

References

Eakin SK, Thompson WD: Behavior effects of stimulation by UHF radio fields. *Psych Rep* 1965;17:595–602.

Hirsch FG, Parker JT: Bilateral lenticular opacities occurring in a technician operating a microwave generator. *Arch Ind Hyg Occup Med* 1952;6:512–517.

McRee DI: Environmental aspects of microwave radiation. *Environ Health Persp* 1972;2:41–53.

NIOSH/OSHA: Radiofrequency (RF) sealers and heaters: Potential health hazards and their prevention. *Joint NIOSH/OSHA Current Intelligence Bulletin 33,* Washington, DC, National Institute for Occupational Safety and Health; Occupational Safety and Health Administration, 1979.

Ricketts CR: Nonionizing radiations. *J Soc Occup Med* 1978;28:125–133.

Tyler PE, ed: Biological effects of nonionizing radiation. *Ann NY Acad Sci* 1975;247:1–545.

3 • *Ultraviolet Radiation*

The ultraviolet region of the electromagnetic spectrum is intermediate in wavelength and frequency between the x-ray and visible regions. The limits of the ultraviolet portion are not clear-cut but are generally considered to occupy that portion of the spectrum between 4 nm (millimicron, mμ) and 400 nm (or 40 angstroms [Å] to 4000 Å).

Ultraviolet radiation has been divided by the International Commission on Illumination (CIE) into three spectral bands that do not quite correspond to the biological action regions. The UV-A region extends from 315 to 400 nm and is also referred to as the "black light" region or the "near UV" or "long UV." It slightly overlaps the visible portion of the spectrum. Most of the solar ultraviolet radiation reaching the earth's surface falls within this range since atmospheric ozone filters out all wavelengths shorter than 290 nm. Wavelengths in the black light region are generally not considered to be biologically active except in the production of skin pigmentation and photoreactions (Pathak et al., 1962) and thermal skin burns. Radiation in this region does not cause injury to the eyes.

The next region, UV-B, between 280 and 315 nm is referred to as the "mid-UV" or erythemal region. Skin, when moist, is more susceptible to erythema induction than when dry. The lips, since they are frequently moist, are particularly susceptible (Urbach, 1969). The relationship between erythema and skin cancer, if any, is obscure. Photokeratitis is produced by ultraviolet radiation in this region and region UV-C.

The UV-C band, from 100 to 280 nm, is the "far UV" or "short UV" region, and is germicidal and viricidal. Low-pressure mercury discharge lamps designed to emit 90% or more of their ultraviolet radiation at 253.7 nm, which is the peak of maximum bactericidal activity, are used extensively in industry, medicine, and research to destroy surface bacteria, viruses, yeasts, and molds. The portion of UV-C between 170 and 220 nm is generally referred to as the ozone region. This is the most efficient wavelength range for the production of atomic oxygen, which, in turn, combines with diatomic oxygen to form ozone. The production of ozone is the only significant biological effect in this region.

Sources of ultraviolet radiation range from the sun to a number of artificial sources, including lasers. In industry, ultraviolet radiation is the byproduct of welding, plasma-torch operations, glass blowing, and hot metal manipulations. Any radiant black body at a temperature of 1000°C or greater will emit most of its electromagnetic radiation as ultraviolet radiation. Some of the common applications that utilize ultraviolet lamps are food, water, and air sterilization, and medical therapy. Fluorescence and phosphorescence result from the absorption of ultraviolet radiation and are used in fluorescent lamps, fluorescent pigments and dyes, phosphors, and ultraviolet photography. The use of ultraviolet-cured inks is a recent industrial development that has been reported to result in the development of photosensitivity in workers (Emmett et al., 1977).

The skin and the eyes are very susceptible to damage from ultraviolet radiation. The cornea and aqueous humor absorb essentially all of the ultraviolet radiation incident on the eye and very little penetrates as far as the lens. Solar retinitis can occur, however, and may not be entirely attributable to thermal effects (Clarke and Behrendt, 1972; Naidoff and Sliney, 1974). Exposure of the eyes can result in blepharitis, conjunctivitis, keratitis, and keratoconjunctivitis (Buessler, 1968). Welders, who number about 50,000 in the United States, comprise the largest group of potentially exposed workers, although flash burns experienced by other persons in the vicinity may be a greater hazard (Kinsey et al., 1943). Universal use of protective eye shields has made skin rather than eyes the major occupational target organ in welding.

Acute exposure of skin leads to erythema and sunburn, and eventually to tanning by pigment deposition. Chronic exposure of the skin to solar ultraviolet radiation results not only in tanning but in solar elastosis that consists of dry, leathery, deeply wrinkled skin. Such changes are commonly seen in outdoor workers, such as farmers and sailors, and result from degeneration of the dermis collagen. Nonmelanoma skin cancer incidence has been correlated with latitude and UV exposure in the United States, most recently by Scotto et al. (1974) and Fears et al. (1977). The carcinogenic aspects of ultraviolet radiation have been reviewed by Blum (1959), Green et al. (1976), Urbach et al. (1976, 1980), Summer (1980), and by WHO (1979), among others.

Control of ultraviolet radiation is easily accomplished since shielding is easy. Ordinary window glass will filter out all wavelengths below about 320 nm. A light layer of clothing will eliminate all wavelengths from reaching the skin. This weak penetration ability limits the usefulness of ultraviolet radiation as a bactericidal or viricidal agent, but it also allows the human body to protect itself from ultraviolet radiation except for superficial effects. When occupational exposure to ultraviolet radiation is required, appropriate protective clothing and eye shielding must be used.

References

Blum HF: *Carcinogenesis by Ultraviolet Light*, Princeton, NJ, Princeton University Press, 1959.

Buessler JA: Ultraviolet irradiation in medicine: Ophthalmological aspects. *Missouri Med* 1968;65:293–296.

Clarke AM, Behrendt T: Solar retinitis and pupillary reaction. *Am J Ophthalmol* 1972;73:700–703.

Emmett EA, Taphorn BR, Kominsky JR: Phototoxicity occurring during the manufacture of ultraviolet-cured ink. *Arch Dermatol* 1977;113:770–775.

Fears TR: Scotto J, Schneiderman MA: Mathematical models of age and ultraviolet effects on the incidence of skin cancer among whites in the United States. *Am J Epidemiol* 1977;105:420–427.

Green AES, Findley GB Jr, Klenk KF, et al: The ultraviolet dose dependence of non-melanoma skin cancer incidence. *Photochem Photobiol* 1976; 24:353–362.

Kinsey VE, Cogan DG, Drinker P: Measuring eye flash from arc welding. *J Am Med Assoc* 1943;123:403–404.

Naidoff MA, Sliney DH: Retinal injury from a welding arc. *Am J Ophthalmol* 1974;77:663–668.

Pathak MA, Riley FJ, Fitzpatrick TB, et al: Melanin formation in human skin induced by long-wave ultraviolet and visible light. *Nature* 1962;193:148–150.

Scotto J, Kopf AW, Urbach F: Non-melanoma skin cancer among Caucasians in four areas of the United States. *Cancer* 1974;34:1333–1338.

Summer W: Photo-carcinogenicity: The physical basis of its exogenous causes. *Br J Dermatol* 1980;102:611–619.

Urbach F (ed): *The Biologic Effects of Ultraviolet Radiation.* New York, Pergamon Press; 1969.

Urbach F, Forbes PD, Davies RE, et al: Cutaneous photobiology: Past, present and future. *J Invest Dermatol* 1976;67:209–224.

Urbach F, Bailar JC III, Gori GB, et al: Ultraviolet radiation and skin cancer in man. *Prevent Med* 1980;9:227–230.

WHO: *Environmental Health Criteria 14: Ultraviolet Radiation.* Geneva, World Health Organization, 1979.

4 • *Lasers*

Lasers or optical masers are devices that can produce visible, ultraviolet, or infrared radiation of a practically uniform wavelength. The term "laser" is an acronym that represents "light amplification by stimulated emission of radiation." Lasers can be operated in a continuous mode or in pulses, which may be as short as 10^{-11} seconds. Output power levels range from milliwatts to kilowatts for continuous operation and up to 10^{12} watts in pulsed operations.

Laser technology has had a rapid growth since its beginnings in 1960. Numerous devices utilizing various laser radiation properties of high power, short pulse lengths, monochromaticity, and collimation have been developed for application in a wide range of scientific activities. In industry, lasers are used for such applications as drilling, cutting, and welding. High power pulsed lasers can drill tiny holes in diamonds in a fraction of the time required by mechanical means. In medicine, lasers have been used for repair of retinal detachments and for treatment of tumors.

Most biological effects of laser radiation are attributable to the heating of tissue, and skin and eye are the principal organs of hazard. Overexposure of the skin will produce a burn, with severity depending upon the radiation wavelength, intensity, and duration of exposure. Of critical importance is potential damage to the eye (Marshall, 1978). The ability of the lens of the eye to focus near-ultraviolet, near-infrared, and visible laser radiation onto the retina results in energy densities at the retina that are several orders of magnitude greater than the radiation intensity at the cornea. Consequently, for these wavelengths, a relatively low radiation exposure incident on the cornea can produce a retinal lesion and subsequent impairment of vision, especially if the macula is damaged. With laser radiation in the far-infrared and far-ultraviolet regions of the spectrum, the iris and the lens may be injured by local heating. Depending upon the amount of the heating and its duration, inflammation of the iris and lenticular cataract formation are possible. The literature contains case reports of severe ocular damage resulting from accidental exposure to laser radiation (Rathkey, 1965; Zweng, 1967; Friedmann and Graham, 1969).

Concern over the hazards of exposure to laser radiation has resulted in the establishment of guidelines for human exposure by several agencies, such as the American Conference of Governmental Industrial Hygienists (1976), the American National Standards Institute (1976), and the International Electrotechnical Commission (IEC) (1978). Current guides are based upon the minimum dose required to produce a visible lesion. These threshold values may vary with the criteria by which they are measured. For the eye, threshold damage has been determined by such varying means as ophthalmoscopy, light microscopy, histopathology, histochemical studies, and electroretinography (Goldman, 1966).

Lasers have been classified into four categories that represent the degree of potential hazard: Class I or "Exempt" lasers will not produce radiation damage and require no control measures. Class II lasers are low powered and may be viewed directly under controlled exposure conditions, but they must bear a cautionary label since continual staring at the source may be harmful. Class III lasers are medium powered and require controls that prevent viewing of the direct beam since eye damage can occur before the protective blink reflex can take place. Class IV lasers are high powered and must have controls to prevent damage to personnel. Hazard analysis is based upon output and maximum permissible exposure levels.

The control of occupational hazards that may occur with the use of lasers has been widely

312

described. Older papers are listed in the *Laser Hazards Bibliography* (1967). More recent discussions are to be found in Chisum (1979), Harlen (1978), and in the encyclopedic handbook by Sliney and Wolbarsht (1980). In addition to direct beam and scattered radiation exposure, other potential hazards of laser operations include contact with cryogenic agents such as liquid nitrogen, fire, airborne contaminants, noise, electric shock, exposure to gases such as ozone, and explosions at capacitor banks, optical pump systems, and target areas. Safe laser use depends upon design characteristics, exposure control, and eye and skin protection.

References

ACGIH: *A Guide for Control of Laser Hazards.* Cincinnati, American Conference of Governmental Industrial Hygienists; 1976.

ANSI: *Safe Use of Lasers.* New York, American National Standards Institute, Standard Z-136.1, 1976.

Chisum GT: Laser eye protection for flight personnel, *Aviat Space Environ Med* 1979;50: 239–242.

Friedmann AI, Graham FE: A screening programme for personnel exposed to laser radiation. *Ann Occup Hyg* 1969;12:219–221.

Goldman L: *Laser Cancer Research.* New York, Springer-Verlag, 1966.

Harlen F: The development of laser codes of practice and maximum permissible exposure levels, *Ann Occup Hyg* 1978;21:199–211.

IEC: *Laser Equipment, Radiation Safety of Laser Products and Equipment Classification, Requirements and User's Guide.* Geneva, International Electrotechnical Commission, Technical Committee #76, Fifth Draft, 1978.

Laser Hazards Bibliography, U.S. Army Environmental Hygiene Agency, 1967.

Marshall J: Eye hazards associated with lasers. *Ann Occup Hyg* 1978;21:69–77.

Rathkey AS: Accidental laser burn of the macula. *Arch Ophthalmol* 1965;73:346–348.

Sliney D, Wolbarsht M: *Safety with Lasers and Other Optical Sources.* New York, Plenum Press, 1980.

Zweng HC: Accidental Q-switched laser lesion of human macula. *Arch Ophthalmol* 1967;78: 596–599.

5 • Ionizing Radiation

The potential for occupational illness arising from the use of radiant energy has become a more important problem with the increasing use of radiation and radioactive materials in laboratory investigation and in industry. The literature has become so enormous as to be unwieldy, but there exists sufficient information to establish safe industrial and medical utilization of ionizing radiation modalities that are capable of profound biological effects. The field of radiation protection has become a well-defined discipline and is also known as "radiation safety" or "health physics." National and international bodies have been organized to set standards of permissible radiation exposure that have undergone periodic revision as more information has been acquired.

The scientific development most relevant to this discussion began with the discovery of the x-ray in 1895 by Roentgen. Becquerel's discovery of radioactivity in the double sulfate of uranium and potassium shortly thereafter was followed two years later by the description of the radioactive properties of thorium by Schmidt and of thorium and uranium by M. Curie. M. and P. Curie isolated polonium from pitchblende (uranium oxide), and in 1902 they separated radium from this source material. Other phenomena of radioactivity were then discovered by Rutherford, Soddy, and the Curies. Mme Curie's initial radiochemical work in separating and identifying polonium and radium led to the development of modern nuclear physics and the use of radioactive isotopes.

Rutherford and others then elucidated the nature of radioactive decay, introduced the concept of "half-life," and established the notion of radioactive disintegration series. In 1913, Hevesy and Paneth used minute amounts of radium D (^{210}Pb) as tracers for the study of chemical problems, and in 1918 Paneth extended the use of naturally occurring lead and bismuth in chemical studies. Hevesy, in 1923, made the first use of radioactive tracers in a biological problem when he used thorium B (^{212}Pb) to study the uptake of lead by plants. Hevesy also initiated the use of artificial radioisotopes as tracers when he studied the absorption of phosphorus by plants in 1935.

The discovery of artificial radioactivity in 1934 by Joliot and Joliot-Curie gave rise to the applied nuclear physics of the late 1930s and subsequent years. At the present time, isotopes of all the chemical elements have been discovered and amount to approximately 1800 radionuclides. By developing the cyclotron, Lawrence made possible the production of a number of radioactive isotopes in quantity, and some of these were soon applied to biological and medical research and were used in therapy. The development of nuclear reactors in the United States and abroad has led to an enormous expansion of these activities, and a wide variety of reactor- and cyclotron-produced radioactive isotopes are now available commercially. The extensive use of radioactive materials for diagnosis and therapy has led to the development of a new discipline called nuclear medicine.

Meanwhile, the use of x-rays for diagnosis and therapy in medicine has flourished since the early 1900s, and x-rays and gamma rays have had applications in manufacturing by their use in industrial radiography. Ionizing radiation from x-ray beams as well as from radioactive sources has led to the development of methods of measurement and protection from overexposure in a special application of industrial hygiene and preventive medicine to these problems.

Brief Review of Radiation Physics

Radioactivity, natural or artificial, is the emission of radiation that results from the spontaneous or induced disintegration of atomic nuclei. The radiations that result from these nuclear transformations are of three principal types that have been designated as alpha rays, beta rays, and gamma rays. Other forms of emitted radioactivity are x-rays, neutrons, and heavy fragments produced by spontaneous or induced nuclear fission.

Roentgen rays or x-rays are electromagnetic radiations generated as a result of energy transitions of atomic electrons that are produced by the bombardment of high atomic weight materials by high-energy electrons. X-rays ionize gases and other materials through which they pass, penetrate solids of various thicknesses with differential absorption depending upon their density or atomic weights, and have application in the fact that they act on fluorescent screens and photographic plates. X-rays are widely used in industrial and medical radiography, radiotherapy, and in analytical techniques such as x-ray crystallography, x-ray diffraction, and x-ray fluorescence analysis.

Alpha particles are doubly charged helium ions and are produced when an atom emits a helium nucleus. This emission results in a change in the parent atom to one having an atomic number two units lower and an atomic mass four units lower (e.g., $^{226}_{88}Ra \rightarrow {}^{222}_{86}Rn$). In the example just given, the noble gas radon is produced when radium emits an alpha ray. Radon itself decays by the emission of another alpha particle to become transformed into radium A ($^{218}_{84}Po$). Radon is the heaviest member of the group of noble gases that contains helium, neon, argon, krypton, and xenon. This group of elements, long considered to be chemically inert, is now known to be capable of forming compounds under special conditions (Hyman, 1963). The path that an alpha particle may travel ranges from about 3 to 9 cm in air. The range in denser materials is very much less so that alpha particles are stopped by a few sheets of paper or a thin aluminum foil. In biological tissue, which is largely water, alpha rays penetrate up to 50 μm and are of serious concern because of the intense ionization produced along this short path (high linear energy transfer). The ingestion of radium or the inhalation of radium dust or of radon gas daughters will consequently expose the tissues of the organism to the highly localized effects of ionizing radiation wherever these substances are deposited or translocated.

Beta rays are electrons emitted from an atom that thereby changes in atomic number by one unit but does not change in atomic mass. All beta rays produced by natural radioactivity are nega-

tively charged (beta negatrons), and the parent atom increased in atomic number (e.g., $^{90}_{38}Sr \rightarrow {}^{90}_{39}Y$). However, in the laboratory a number of radionuclides have been found to emit positively charged beta rays (beta positrons), and in these cases the parent atom loses one unit of atomic number (e.g., $^{22}_{11}Na \rightarrow {}^{22}_{10}Ne$). Beta rays may travel several meters in air but they are stopped by a few millimeters of most solid material. They scatter readily and the small mass of the particle leads to much less energy transfer along the ionization path than is the case with alpha particles. Nevertheless, external exposure to beta ray sources can lead to radiation burns of the skin that can be quite severe.

Gamma rays are electromagnetic radiations that are similar to x-rays but have shorter wavelengths. Gamma rays are the result of transitions in the energy levels within the atomic nucleus while x-rays result from changes in the energy levels of the orbiting electrons. Gamma rays may accompany the emission of alpha and beta particles and are characterized by great powers of penetration, the range of which depends upon the energy and the atomic weights of the absorbing material. Solid materials and biological tissues reduce the intensities of the rays, but some "hard" gamma rays may penetrate up to several centimeters of lead. Each radionuclide that emits gamma rays has a distinctive gamma ray energy spectrum, a feature that enables the identification and quantitative measurement of such radionuclides by techniques of scintillation spectrometry.

Neutrons are elementary particles in the atomic nucleus that have no electric charge and are emitted only by the expenditure of energy equivalent to the binding energy of the nucleus. Such energy is afforded by bombardment with alpha particles, and a common neutron source consists of a radium-beryllium mixture, which leads to the production of a neutron beam when the alpha particles from the radium strike the beryllium nuclei. Neutrons can also be released from beryllium nuclei by the very energetic gamma rays of radioantimony, and such neutrons are called photoneutrons. Since they have no electric charge, neutrons interact only slightly with atomic electrons and have much greater penetrating power than charged particles with the same energy. They interact with matter by collision with nuclei, which in turn lose energy by ionizing surrounding atoms and by the production of heat. Neutrons are hence capable of producing profound biological damage and, because of their great penetrability, they lead to serious shielding problems for the protection of persons working in the vicinity of nuclear reactors and other neutron sources. Concrete walls several feet thick are required for biological shielding in these installations.

A chain of radioactive changes is called a "disintegration series" and continues until a stable product is formed. A short series is illustrated by the decay of strontium 90: $^{90}_{38}Sr \rightarrow ^{90}_{39}Y \rightarrow ^{90}_{40}Zr$. At the upper end of the periodic table, the naturally occurring radioelements of high atomic weight form three separate disintegration series: the *thorium* series, the *uranium* series, and the *actinium* series. A fourth series, the *neptunium* series, has been found in radionuclides produced artificially in the laboratory. The uranium series begins with $^{238}_{92}U$ and proceeds by a series of alpha and beta emissions through intermediaries to radium ($^{226}_{88}Ra$) to radon ($^{222}_{86}Rn$) through a series of isotopes of polonium, lead, astatine, bismuth, and thallium eventually to stable lead ($^{206}_{82}Pb$) as the end product. Radium is found in deposits of pitchblende where it is formed as a natural decay product from uranium. Thorium ($^{232}_{90}Th$) is found in monazite sands and thorite, and is the parent nuclide for the thorium series that passes through mesothorium 1 ($^{228}_{88}Ra$), radiothorium ($^{228}_{90}Th$), thorium X ($^{224}_{88}Ra$) and a series of isotopes of radon, polonium, lead, bismuth, and thallium to end in another stable isotope of lead ($^{208}_{82}Pb$).

Reference

Hyman HH (ed): *Noble-Gas Compounds.* Chicago, University of Chicago Press, 1963.

Biological Effects of Radiation

The impact of ionizing radiation on living systems forms the subject matter of radiobiology. The effects of radiation on water and on inorganic and organic molecules have been examined along with investigations at the genetic, cytologic, pathophysiologic, and organismic levels of biological organization. At the genetic level, radiation may produce gene mutations and may damage or otherwise alter chromosomes. At the cellular level, radiation may delay or critically impair cell division, and at higher doses it may interfere with cellular metabolic processes. Certain mammalian tissues, especially those that normally divide rapidly, are unusually radiosensitive; these include the blood-forming tissues, the mucosa of the gastrointestinal tract, the skin, and the gonads, along with the lens of the eye. However, radiation of sufficient intensity and duration may also affect less sensitive tissues such as the lungs, bone, endocrine glands, and the nervous system. Whole body or partial body irradiation may lead to the acute radiation syndrome and to delayed radiation injuries and the poorly understood phenomenon of life-span shortening. Radiation-induced injuries include lens opacities, radiation nephrosclerosis, myelogenous leukemia, and a number of specific cancers (Rubin and Casarett, 1968; Upton, 1969; Fry et al., 1970).

Acute radiation syndrome Of particular interest in the pathogenesis of the signs and symptoms of the acute radiation syndrome is the interaction between the hematopoietic and gastrointestinal systems (Patt and Brues, 1954). Radiation acts on the cellular elements of the blood to produce leukopenia (with lymphopenia preceding granulocytopenia), thrombocytopenia, and perhaps anemia. Increased capillary fragility and the reduced number of platelets lead to increased bleeding that partly accounts for the anemia. The leukopenia results in reduced resistance to infection and contributes to the development of bacteremia and septicemia. Radiation affects the gastrointestinal tract by injury of the lining cells, and this damage leads to altered secretions and disturbances in intestinal motility. These changes result in a series of interacting effects that include altered digestion and absorption, ulcerations, nausea and vomiting, diarrhea, dehydration, and bacterial invasion from the gut (which, in the presence of reduced immunity as a result of the leukopenia, also leads to bacteremia and septicemia). If the level of radiation is high, the central nervous system is also involved in the acute radiation syndrome.

In addition to this interacting set of events, radiation at sufficiently high doses may affect the skin by producing erythema, radiodermatitis, and temporary or permanent epilation. Irradiation of the gonads may produce transient or lasting sterility, while irradiation of the lens of the eye, especially by neutrons, may result in a characteristic form of radiation cataract.

The severity and time sequence of events of the acute radiation syndrome just described depend upon the amount and localization of the radiation received. For man, the LD_{50}, or median lethal dose, is thought to be between 400 and 500 rad, although this estimate can be raised to 600 rad in the presence of supportive measures and therapy, such as isolation of the patient, fluid, electrolyte, and blood replacement, antibiotics and chemotherapy, and nutritional support. Below an exposure of 100 rad there are no definite clinical signs or symptoms of the syndrome. Above whole body exposure of 100 rad, symptoms increase in severity and appear sooner with greater exposure to radiation. Hematopoietic signs (destruction of bone marrow and depletion of circulating blood cells) and their sequelae (hemorrhage, anemia, and agranulocytic ulcerations) appear earliest and account for the fatalities at 30 to 35 days in the region of the median lethal dose (500 to 700 rad) (Bond et al., 1965).

At greater radiation dose levels (900 to 2000 rad) the signs and symptoms are predominantly those of the gastrointestinal system, and include anorexia, nausea, vomiting, diarrhea, infection, fluid and electrolyte imbalance, dehydration, prostration, and death that occurs in 8 to 10 days (Sullivan, 1968). At still higher dose levels, above 5000 rad, death occurs earlier (at two days) and is due to central nervous system involvement that produces incoordination, disorientation, tremors, convulsions, shock, and coma (Bond et al., 1965). Where death does not occur, either because the radiation dose is too low to be fatal or because of successful vigorous supportive therapy that may include bone marrow transplantation, recovery occurs gradually. The duration of the convalescence is directly proportional to the size of the radiation dose.

Hempelmann et al. (1952) reviewed nine early atomic energy cases of acute radiation syndrome in great detail, and brought the case histories up to date 30 years later (Hempelmann et al., 1980). In a later dramatic incident, a laboratory worker exposed to an estimated whole body dose of 3900 to 4900 rad, with 12,000 rad, neutron plus gamma, to the upper abdomen, died after 35 hours with a clinical course consistent with the pattern of a fatal central nervous system syndrome after acute radiation exposure (Shipman, 1961). The medical aspects of accidental radiation injury resulting from nuclear criticality incidents in the United States, Russia, and Yugoslavia were reviewed by Thoma and Wald (1959). A worldwide overview of serious radiation accidents was provided more recently by Lushbaugh et al. (1980). The clinical data from these radiation accidents, along with experimental work with animals, have contributed greatly to our understanding of the acute radiation syndrome.

Long-term and delayed effects Long-term or delayed effects of radiation may result from acute and chronic radiation exposure. Leukemia was noted in the Hiroshima and Nagasaki survivors with a peak incidence of the chronic granulocytic form at five to eight years after the acute exposure in 1945 (Bizzozero et al., 1966). Cuzick (1981) has examined a number of cohorts of persons exposed to radiation medically and occupationally and has found an excess of myelomatosis, a tumor of B lymphocytes, in most groups with a preponderance of cases occurring 15 to 25 years after exposure.

Chronic or protracted irradiation may result from continuous or intermittent repeated exposures of the body to low levels of radiation or from internally deposited radionuclides. The classic cases of the latter situation occurred in the radium dial painters in the early 1920s (Martland, 1929), and long-term effects have continued to appear up to the present time in persons exposed 50 to 60 years ago. Also, at the present time, uranium miners may be experiencing a similar hazard while working in mines that have elevated radon levels. Plutonium has become a potential hazard in the atomic energy industry, although here it is a well-recognized danger, and is usually handled with great care and proper protective techniques. The occupational experiences with radium, uranium, and plutonium will be examined in some detail later in this chapter.

References

Bizzozero OJ Jr, Johnson KG, Ciocco A: Radiation-related leukemia in Hiroshima and Nagasaki, 1946–1964. I. Distribution, incidence and appearance in time. *N Engl J Med* 1966;274:1095–1101.

Bond VP, Fliedner TM, Archambeau JO: *Mammalian Radiation Lethality.* New York, Academic Press, 1965.

Cuzick J: Radiation-induced myelomatosis. *N Engl J Med* 1981;304:204–210.

Fry RJM, Grahn D, Griem ML, et al: *Late Effects of Radiation.* London, Taylor and Francis, 1970.

Hempelmann LH, Lisco H, Hoffman JG: The acute radiation syndrome. A study of nine cases and a review of the problem. *Ann Intern Med* 1952;36:279–510.

Hempelmann LH, Lushbaugh CC, Voelz GL: What happened to the survivors of the early Los

Alamos nuclear accidents? In Hübner KF, Fry SA, (eds): *The Medical Basis for Radiation Accident Preparedness,* New York, Elsevier, 1980, pp 17–32.

Lushbaugh CC, Fry SA, Hübner KF, et al: Total-body irradiation: A historical review and follow-up, in Hübner KF, Fry SA, (eds): *The Medical Basis for Radiation Accident Preparedness.* New York, Elsevier, 1980, pp 3–15.

Martland HS: Occupational poisoning in manufacture of luminous watch dials. *J Am Med Assoc* 1929;92:466–473, 552–559.

Patt HM, Brues AM: The pathological physiology of radiation injury in the mammal, in Hollaender A, (ed): *Radiation Biology.* New York, McGraw-Hill, 1954, vol 1, part II, pp 919–1028.

Rubin P, Casarett GW: *Clinical Radiation Pathology.* Philadelphia, WB Saunders, 1968, 2 vols.

Shipman TL, ed: Acute radiation death resulting from an accidental nuclear critical excursion. *J Occup Med* 1961;3:146–192.

Sullivan MF, ed: *Gastrointestinal Radiation Injury.* Amsterdam, Excerpta Medica, 1968.

Thoma GE, Wald N: The diagnosis and management of accidental radiation injury. *J Occup Med* 1959;1:421–447.

Upton AC: *Radiation Injury.* Chicago, University of Chicago Press, 1969.

Occupational Exposure

The use of radiation and radioactive isotopes has increased enormously since World War II, principally as a result of the development of atomic energy and its applications since that time. Occupational exposure to radiation can occur in industry, medicine, agriculture, and in laboratory research.

Apart from traditional diagnostic radiology in medicine, dentistry, and veterinary medicine, x-rays and gamma rays (e.g., from ^{60}Co) are used for therapy, as are electron beams from linear accelerators and protons and other particles from cyclotrons. A wide variety of radionuclides is used in nuclear medicine and they are potential hazards for inadvertent external irradiation and for radioactive contamination of professional and technical personnel.

In industry there is a wide spectrum of applications of radiation. Nuclear power plants and research reactors are carefully operated, but they present potential hazards for neutron and gamma-ray exposure, especially during transfer and chemical processing of fuel elements. Penetrating radiation from x-rays and gamma rays is used in industrial radiography for flaw detection (welding cracks; defects in reinforced concrete), for thickness gauging (in production line control of paper, aluminum, copper, tinplate, plastics, glass, rubber, and other items), for density gauging (tobacco in cigarettes; H/C ratios in analysis of hydrocarbons such as fuel oils and conduit pipe contents), and for liquid level gauges (measurement of height of molten metals). Reflection of radiation is used for measurement of thickness of coatings over base metal and for soil moisture and soil density studies in the selection of suitable sites for airfields, roadbeds, and dams. Self-luminescent markers are widely used for instrument panels and faces; beta-ray isotopes such as ^{90}Sr and ^{147}Pm are now used instead of alpha- and gamma-ray emitting radium and polonium since they are less hazardous and the phosphor deteriorates less rapidly. Ionization of the air by alpha particles to eliminate static electricity is one of the more recent industrial uses of radioactivity. This application is of importance, for example, in preventing fires in cotton mills, in eliminating static charges where paper is cut and handled by high speed processes, and in eliminating dust from developed photographic film. Radium was once used for this purpose, but since 1947 polonium has replaced radium. Polonium is less hazardous than radium because it emits alpha particles almost exclusively.

Radiation is used in chemical processing for the promotion of polymerization, for the initiation of cross-linking of long-chain polymers, for nuclear vulcanization of rubber, and for triggering halogenation and oxidation reactions. Radiation is also used for pasteurization and sterilization of pharmaceuticals and foodstuffs by the use of gamma rays to destroy bacteria, parasites, and enzymes, without significant elevation of temperature. A number of radioisotope batteries have been developed for the production of electric current, and radioisotopes have been used as tracers in detecting metal wear (such as in piston rings), in catalytic beads circulating in petroleum cracking processes, as boundary markers between two types of petroleum flowing in cross-country pipelines, in detection of water leaks, and in tracing pirate colors in the textile industry. Radiosulfur, for example, has been used to study vulcanization and polymerization in the manufacture of rubber and has been used in the steel industry to study the sources of sulfur impurities in finished steel products.

Occupational ill effects from external radiation

After the discovery of x-rays by Roentgen in December, 1895, the news traveled quickly around the world, and by the end of 1896 a number of investigators in Europe and North America were applying this technique in orthopedic surgery. Three reports illustrated early medical use in that year: Edwin B. Frost made the first diagnostic radiograph in North America when he demonstrated a fractured ulna in a youngster in Hanover, New Hampshire; John Cox demonstrated a bullet in the leg of a shooting victim in Montreal; and James Burry of Chicago was the first physician in America to remove a foreign body as a result of radiographic location of buckshot in a hand (Brecher and Brecher, 1969). Grubbé experimented with Crookes tubes in 1895 and treated a case of mammary carcinoma in the following year. He sustained an x-ray burn of the skin that became manifest as a typical radiodermatitis in 1896. He was one of the early martyrs to x-ray research inasmuch as the extensive burns and later cancer of the hands and face cost him his left arm (Hodges, 1964). Throughout 1896 investigators of x-rays reported loss of hair and skin burns that led to ulcerations. The first fatality from overexposure was Friedrich Claussen (1864–1900) who exposed his hands to x-rays over 1000 times in public demonstrations in Berlin and who died of generalized carcinomatosis after amputation of the right arm.

In 1902, Codman reviewed all the papers in the world literature that dealt with x-ray injuries and found less than 200 cases. He described two types of x-ray injuries to the skin. The first type, which he termed "skiagrapher's dermatitis," resulted from repeated short exposures to the hands, arms, and face, usually in industrial fluoroscopy. In mild form this chronic exposure led to cracking and roughening of the skin with the folds over the knuckles becoming swollen and stiff and the skin between the folds had lesions that resembled capillary hemorrhages. Nail development was distorted by marked longitudinal striations and increased brittleness. With continued exposure there was progression to ulceration and gangrene of the skin with eventual involvement of the tendon sheaths and joints. In severe cases, there was bleb formation, exfoliation of the skin and nails, joint destruction, intense pain, scar formation, and deformity. The second type of x-ray injury followed single short exposures, or perhaps several such exposures. In mild cases there was transient erythema that lasted a few days and was followed by scaling. Often there was a burning sensation or hyperesthesia, but there was no real pain. Localized epilation sometimes occurred. With deeper burns serous or purulent blisters formed, and sometimes the burn, instead of disappearing after a few weeks, became a penetrating ulcer. Here the progress was exceedingly slow and obstinate, and the lesion tended to progress and resist treatment.

As time passed after Codman's description, it was learned that the skin lesions of the slowly penetrating variety might go on to loss of deeper tissues from ulceration that necessitated repeated amputations of fingers and hands so that only a stump of a hand or arm was left. It also became evident that x-rays were capable of altering the tissues so that ulcerations underwent malignant transformation. These x-ray cancers metastasized early, especially if not treated promptly. A striking feature was the long latent period between the original severe lesions and the development of malignancy in the persistent ulcer. Surgical treatment brought relief from the severe pain promptly, but the lesions were very slow in healing. According to Wolbach (1909), if the injury was severe, complete repair was not to be expected because of the local degenerative changes in the blood vessels and intercellular substances. Warren (1961) summarized the pathological sequence of this early type of radiation injury that occurred largely to the skin and underlying structures: slowly developing and persistent skin burn; blistering and ulceration if the dose has been several thousand roentgens (R); epilation that is transient below 700 R, permanent if higher; local hyperpigmentation with lower doses, depigmentation with higher doses. Late radiodermatitis is characterized by atrophy, destruction of skin appendages, patchy ulceration, poor vascularization, but at the same time telangiectasia, frequent progression to cancer, usually epidermoid carcinoma, sometimes basal cell carcinoma.

These descriptions of the effects of irradiation of the skin can be extended to the rest of the body. Rubin and Casarett (1968) have described the pathological changes that occur in all of the tissues and organs of the body as a result of irradiation and have summarized the histopathological sequence of events as occurring in four phases:

1. Acute damage to sensitive cells and tissues, with inhibition of mitosis, destruction of parenchymal cells, hypoplasia and atrophy of radiosensitive tissues, along with damage to small blood vessels and connective tissue.
2. Recovery from acute damage by regenerative repopulation of lost parenchymal cells or by replacement fibrosis where cell regeneration is impaired, the latter process enhanced by spotty degeneration of supporting vasculature.
3. An intermediate phase of little or no change in parenchymal cellularity that varies inversely in duration with the magnitude of the radiation dose.
4. Delayed or late parenchymal degeneration, with either gradual premature involution of tissues (with hypoplasia, atrophy, and replacement fibrosis, seen in premature aging), or more rapid breakdown or necrosis of tissues (such as ulceration), or late malignant transformation.

These phases can be correlated with successive periods of clinical events that follow organ or whole body irradiation, such as may occur with radiation therapy or accidental exposure.

References

Brecher R, Brecher E: *The Rays: A History of Radiology in the United States and Canada.* Baltimore, Williams and Wilkins, 1969.

Codman EA: A study of the cases of accidental x-ray burns hitherto recorded. *Philadelphia Med J* 1902;9:438–442,499–503.

Hodges PC: *The Life and Times of Emil H. Grubbé.* Chicago, University of Chicago Press, 1964.

Rubin P, Casarett GW: *Clinical Radiation Pathology.* Philadelphia, WB Saunders, 1968, 2 vols.

Warren S: *The Pathology of Ionizing Radiation.* Springfield, IL, Charles C. Thomas, 1961.

Wolbach SB: The pathological histology of chronic x-ray dermatitis and early x-ray carcinoma. *J Med Res* 1909;16:415–449.

Radiation Accidents

With the development of the atomic energy industry since 1945 and the subsequent use of radioisotopes, nuclear energy, and other radiation sources on a vast scale, the fact that these potential hazards can be handled safely has been demonstrated by the unusually good safety record in the atomic energy industry in the United States, Great Britain, and elsewhere (Biles, 1969). Accidents, however, have taken place and continue to occur principally because of carelessness of trained personnel. Robbins et al. (1946), for example, reported burns of skin and eyes sustained by six men when the target was removed from a 12,000 kV electrostatic generator and a cathode-ray window was inserted in its place. This procedure was done to make a quick determination of the size and location of an error resulting from a wandering focal spot. In order to observe the fluorescent effect, these men looked for an estimated five seconds at the cathode-ray window at a distance of three to five feet from the central beam. Although the men were roentgenologists and medical students and should have known the danger, they received an overdose of scattered cathode rays (electrons) with delivered doses calculated to be between 1000 and 2000 R. Conjunctivitis, loss of hair, and skin burns of varying intensity resulted.

In another example, Rossi et al. (1962) reported a case of acute radiation syndrome from accidental exposure to high energy gamma rays from a 200-Ci cobalt-60 source. This exposure to a 33-year-old male graduate student occurred in a university laboratory when the cobalt source became detached from its holder, a mishap that was not noted by the patient. The greatest exposure was to the mid-portion of the body, and the total body dose was estimated to be between 250 and 300 rad. The severity of the clinical course of the patient was typical of the acute radiation syndrome and was consistent with the dose. Nausea and vomiting began one to two hours after exposure, and there were subsequent changes in the peripheral blood that were followed by acute bone marrow depression. Epilation, largely confined to the preumbilical area, began on the 37th day, and there were subsequent skin changes that culminated in an area of necrotic slough above the umbilicus one year later. This case is particularly interesting because it involved gamma rays alone in contrast to the atomic energy laboratory accidents that involved exposure to both neutrons and gamma rays.

That serious accidents can occur with highly sophisticated equipment is illustrated by the report of Lanzl and his colleagues (1967). An industrial worker was accidentally exposed when he walked into a room to place a mold on a conveyor belt near the output port of a 10-million electron volt (meV) beam of a linear accelerator during its operation. Reconstruction of the accident led to an estimated dose of 240,000 rad to the thumb and 420,000 rad to the little finger. The anterior and right lateral surfaces of the trunk of the body received doses ranging from 245 to 325 rad. The toes of the foot received an estimated 11,000 rad, the instep 29,000 rad, and the arch of the foot 300 rad. When the patient was seen at a university research hospital less than four hours after the accident had occurred, there was erythema of the dorsum of the right hand with greatest intensity at the thumb. The most prominent clinical observations were the development of swelling, erythema, blister formation, severe pain, and eventually necrosis. Pain in the hand and forearm became so severe by the 12th day that a percutaneous cervical tractotomy was performed. Over the next few months there was progressive necrosis of the deep structures, the muscles, tendons, and bones, of the hand and forearm. Amputation above the elbow was required 138 days after exposure.

These cases illustrate some of the clinical problems that arise as a result of accidental irradiation that usually results from carelessness. Indeed, the frequency of preventable overexposures to ionizing radiation is experienced more often by industrial radiographers than by any other category of Nuclear Regulatory Commission licensees in the United States according to Ross et al. (1980), who described an accident in which 11 persons were exposed to an industrial iridium 90 source.

The proceedings of an international symposium in 1969 on the handling of radiation accidents contains instructive descriptions of a number of such events in several countries (IAEA, 1969). Catlin of the United States reported that 68% were due to operator error such as failure to survey, failure to follow procedures, failure to use protective devices, and human error; 15% were due to failure of operating mechanisms, containers and pipes, regulating devices, ventilation systems, monitoring instruments, and protection equipment; and 8% were attributable to absent or inadequate procedures. The United States government has initiated a Radiation Incidents Registry (Mills and Segal, 1970). Of the 47 cases of occupational exposure to ionizing radiation listed in its first report, 24 were noted to have biological effects. The status of several radiation accident registries was described recently by Fry (1980).

Detailed reports on more recent radiation accidents are included in the proceedings of an international symposium held in 1979 (Hübner and Fry, 1980). These unfortunate events included whole body as well as localized exposures. These occurrences are in contrast to the results of the greatly publicized nuclear accident at Three Mile Island in March 1979, where the workers received radiation doses of 3 to 4 rem, amounts that slightly exceeded the maximum permissible quarterly dose of 3 rem, and where persons living within a 50-mile radius received an increment of radiation dose that was somewhat less than 1% of the annual background radiation (Fabrikant, 1981). Indeed, the principal health effect of that incident appears to have been the fright, mental distress, and demoralization that prevailed among the residents in the vicinity of the reactor (Moss and Sills, 1981).

References

Biles MB: Characteristics of radiation exposure accidents, in *Symposium on Handling of Radiation Accidents.* Vienna, International Atomic Energy Agency, 1969, pp 3–18.

Fabrikant JI: Health effects of the nuclear accident at Three Mile Island, *Health Phys* 1981;40: 151–161.

Fry SA: The U.S. radiation accident and other registries of the REACT/TS registry system: Their function and current status, in Hübner KA, Fry SA, (eds): *The Medical Basis for Radiation Accident Preparedness.* New York, Elsevier, 1980, pp 451–468.

Hübner KA, Fry SA (eds): *The Medical Basis for Radiation Accident Preparedness.* New York, Elsevier, 1980.

IAEA: *Symposium on Handling of Radiation Accidents,* Vienna, International Atomic Energy Agency, 1969.

Lanzl LH, Rozenfeld ML, Tarlov AR: Injury due to accidental exposure to 10 MeV electrons. *Health Phys* 1967;13:241–251.

Mills LF, Segal P: *Radiation Incidents Registry Report 1970,* Washington, DC, U.S. Public Health Service BRH/DBE 70-6, 1970.

Moss TH, Sills DL, eds: The Three Mile Island nuclear accident: Lessons and implications. *Ann NY Acad Sci* 1981;365:1–341.

Robbins LL, Aub JC, Cope O, et al: Superficial "burns" of the skin and eyes from scattered cathode rays. *Radiology* 1946;46:1–23.

Ross JF, Holly FE, Zarem HA, et al: The 1979 Los Angeles accident: Exposure to iridium 192 industrial radiographic source, in Hübner KA, Fry SA, (eds): *The Medical Basis for Radiation Accident Preparedness.* New York, Elsevier 1980, pp 205–221.

Rossi EC, Thorngate AA, Larson FC: Acute radiation syndrome caused by accidental exposure to cobalt-60. *J Lab Clin Med* 1962;59:655–666.

Other Occupational Radiation Disease

Mobile x-ray units formerly used in the United States for industrial and community surveys for tuberculosis and other chest lesions may also have constituted a real, although less dramatic, hazard for the technicians operating them. The greater quantity of radiation per exposure in such units, the difficulty of adequate protection in mobile equipment, and the scattered radiation within the vehicle resulted in a very real danger that may have been difficult to control (Birnkrant and Henshaw, 1945). The use of mobile equipment for mass chest x-ray surveys was largely discontinued after 1972.

The mortality experience of radiologists comprises an interesting aspect of the occupational effects of ionizing radiation. In the 1940s and afterward an excess of leukemia was noted in United States physicians when this group was compared with the general population (March, 1950, 1961). Warren (1956) then reported a shortened life-span as well as an excess incidence of leukemia among radiologists. Lewis (1963) analyzed the death certificates of 425 United States radiologists who died between the ages of 35 and 74 during the period from 1948 to 1961 and found a statistically significant excess of leukemia, multiple myeloma, and aplastic anemia. In a further study, Warren (1966) reported an improvement in life-span of American radiologists after 1950 with no impairment after 1960. In contrast with these United States studies, Court Brown and Doll (1958) found no evidence that occupational exposure to ionizing radiations caused a detectable shortening of life expectancy among British radiologists from 1897 to 1957. A study of 52 Japanese x-ray technicians who died between 1933 and 1963 suggested slightly higher death rates than expected in this group, but the leukemia incidence was not increased (Kitabatake and Komiyana, 1967). Awareness of the hazards of radiation and the installation of proper protection devices has reduced radiation exposure to most radiologists, dentists, veterinarians, and radiology and nuclear medicine technicians. There does remain a significant risk in these occupations, however, through ignorance, pressure of work, and carelessness.

References

Birnkrant MI, Henshaw PS: Further problems in radiation protection: Radiation hazards in photofluorography. *Radiology* 1945;44:565–568.

Court Brown WM, Doll R: Expectation of life and mortality from cancer among British radiologists. *Br Med J* 1958;2:181–187.

Kitabatake T, Komiyana K: Mortality and causes of death in x-ray technicians. *Ind Med Surg* 1967;36:135–138.

Lewis EB: Leukemia, multiple myeloma, and aplastic anemia in American radiologists. *Science* 1963;142:1492–1494.

March HC: Leukemia in radiologists in a 20-year period. *Am J Med Sci* 1950;220:282–286.

March HC: Leukemia in radiologists, ten years later. *Am J Med Sci* 1961;242:137–149.

Warren S: Longevity and causes of death from irradiation in physicians. *J Am Med Assoc* 1956;162:464–468.

Warren S: The basis for the limit on whole-body exposure—Experience of radiologists. *Health Phys* 1966;12:737–741.

Internal Emitters

The effects of radioisotope deposition within the body as a result of accidental or occupational exposure and the resulting need for therapy depend on a number of factors that include the amount and site of deposition, the chemical form of the isotope, the physical half-life of the radionuclide, the duration of retention in the critical organs, the subsequent transposition of the radionuclide and its radioactive daughters to other parts of the body, the rate of elimination from the body, the type and energy of the emitted radiation, the sensitivity of the critical organs and tissues to radiation injury, and the essentiality of the affected organs (Norwood, 1963). Evaluation of these factors requires knowledge of the radiation properties of the radionuclide(s), its physical

322

and chemical state, its metabolic and toxicologic properties, as well as of the medical condition of the patient.

Reference

Norwood WD: Medical therapy for internally deposited radioisotopes. *Am Ind Hyg Assoc J* 1963;24:492–496.

Radium   The earliest human experience with internal emitters was with radium (^{226}Ra), mesothorium (^{228}Ra), and thorium (^{224}Ra), work that dated back to the Curies in 1902. When Mottram and Clarke (1920) examined the workers in the London Radium Institute who prepared and tested radium applicators as well as the hospital personnel who applied them, they found a low white blood cell count in over 50%. Castle et al. (1925) examined the blood of users of radioactive dial paint and did not find a normal specimen in 22 individuals, the chief change consisting of granulocytopenia. Martland (1926) described fatal cases of "chronic leukopenic anemia" in young women who worked as radium dial painters.

In 1924 another form of injury from internal radiation came to light—namely, a rarifying osteitis that in most cases affected the bony mandible and was followed by suppuration, a condition resembling the familiar phossy jaw of match workers (see chapter on Phosphorus). Blum (1924), a dentist and a physician, described this lesion in the jaw of a radium dial painter and correctly attributed it to the radioactive material in the paint rather than to the phosphorus that had hitherto been implicated. Later, radiation osteitis of the femur and of the humerus were described by Martland (1929), and the same process in the cranium was noted by Flinn and Seidlin (1929). Martland's series of studies were all in women exposed to the ingestion of radium and mesothorium in the course of their work in which they applied a luminous paint containing radium on the numerals and dials of clocks by means of delicate hair brushes that they habitually shaped and pointed with their lips and tongues. The fact that these women used their mouths to shape their brushes is of the greatest importance, for this practice was done principally in a factory in New Jersey, a plant in Connecticut, and another in Illinois. In other establishments in the United States, Britain, and Switzerland, pointing of the brushes between the lips was not practiced, and in these places no serious harmful effects have been reported.

Martland's classic studies of radium workers in the 1920s revealed not only radiation osteitis of the mandible and long bones, but also aplastic anemia, myelogenous leukemia, spontaneous pathological fractures, and malignant bone tumors (Martland, 1931). Although the lesions were early attributed to the phosphorus in the luminous paint, it was soon shown that the women who licked their brushes swallowed small amounts of insoluble sulfates of radium, mesothorium, and radiothorium in the paint day after day during the years of their employment. Small amounts of these compounds were absorbed from the gut and eventually deposited in bone where they continued to emit alpha particles and gamma rays with consequent intense irradiation of the osteoblasts and the bone marrow. Martland's studies in the late 1920s (Martland and Humphries, 1929) were followed by other studies by later investigators that began in the 1950s and have continued to date. The possible effects of inhaled radon from workroom air has never been properly assessed in the dial paint industry.

In 1963, the Bureau of Radiological Health of the U.S. Public Health Service began to collect reports of incidents associated with exposure to radium since 1905 in the United States. By the end of 1968, 415 incidents were collected and analyzed: 83% occurred in medical facilities, perhaps because of greater faithfulness in recording untoward events in this setting. Contamination from ruptures of leaks of sealed sources, from mishaps in the processing and refining of radium, the operation of radon generators, and the use of luminous compounds containing radium accounted for 18%. Despite increasing knowledge and awareness of radiation hazards, almost each decade beginning with 1911 saw an increase in radium exposure over the preceding decade. Most of the occurrences could have been prevented by caution, common sense, and good accountability procedures. Over half of the recoveries of radium lost from hospitals occurred in their trash systems, and the lost radium was carried to municipal dumps or sanitary landfills. Such radiation incidents were not serious occupational hazards because radiation exposure was largely external.

According to Evans (1943), records show that several hundred people were killed through various types of internal exposure to radium prior to 1930. Since then, the number of persons engaged in the industrial handling and application of radium and other radioactive substances has increased enormously. Reports from a number of investigators in Britain demonstrated that radium and its compounds may be handled safely when engineering controls are adequate in the dial painting industry (Browning, 1944; Jones and Day, 1945). In the United States radium dial factories, the practice of pointing the brushes between the lips seems to have stopped after 1926. Since 1930, the manufacturing processes appear to have been consistent with fairly good industrial housekeeping practices and radiological protection, and the hazard of inhalation and ingestion has largely been eliminated (Finkel et al., 1969a).

A brief review of the metabolism of radium is necessary for an understanding of the more recent studies of the harmful effects of radium deposition in the human body. In 1915, Seil et al. studied the elimination of radium by living persons and found that it largely occurred in the feces. Similar results were reported by Schlundt and Failla in 1931, who found that radium in the feces averaged 82% of the total eliminated. Evans (1937), with more accurate measurements, reported that 91% of radium is eliminated in the feces while the remaining 9% is excreted in the urine, and he stated that this ratio was remarkably constant. All of these investigators noted that radium was eliminated very rapidly from the body when it is acquired orally or intravenously. Evans, for example, had reported earlier that only 10% remained after one week, and that after one year the amount of radium remaining in the body was largely fixed in the skeletal tissues with smaller concentrations in the lung, liver, spleen, and heart (Evans, 1933). When it is administered orally, radium behaves like lead and calcium (Aub et al., 1938).

A more sophisticated approach to the characterization of radium retention in man was provided by the studies of Norris et al. (1955). These investigators studied a group of mental hospital patients near Chicago who had been treated with intravenous radium in a series of studies by Schlundt et al. (1933). When the original measurements by Schlundt were combined with those on the same patients in 1951 and 1953, the radium retention data were found to be best described by a power function. The use of the power function to describe the retention of radioactive alkaline earths that are bone seekers was

generalized by Norris et al. (1958) to include strontium and calcium in addition to radium. The importance of the power function lies in its replacement of biological half-time as a mathematical description of retention of these substances by the body. In 1968, Miller and Finkel re-examined eight of the same patients that were studied by Norris. By this time, very accurate whole body measurement techniques were available that used a shielded iron room and scintillation-crystal gamma-ray spectrometry with multichannel analyzers. A new power function was derived that implied that, on the average, 30% of injected or absorbed radium is eliminated by the end of the first 24 hours.

Studies published in 1952 by Aub et al., summarizing earlier experiences, revealed that, despite wide variations in response to deposited radium, seven cases had carried more than $0.02\,\mu g$ and less than $0.5\,\mu g$ of radium for 7 to 25 years without the appearance of any clinical symptoms of chronic radium poisoning. A number of cases were known to these investigators where fatal results had occurred when the radium burden was between 1.2 and $2\,\mu g$ of radium. On the basis of those earlier observations, a committee convened in 1941 by the National Bureau of Standards tentatively established $0.1\,\mu g$ of radium fixed in the body as the tolerance value for man. This figure replaced tolerance values of such widely differing quantities as $10\,\mu g$ and $1\,\mu g$ that had been recommended earlier by individual observers before adequate physical methods were available for detecting smaller quantities of radium in living humans. Actually, this 1941 value has been maintained as a standard not only for radium itself but as a basis for calculating the permissible levels for body burdens of other radioactive isotopes deposited in the body. This standard was set forth by the National Council on Radiation Protection in the United States as well as in the recommendations of the International Commission on Radiological Protection in 1965.

The immediate and long-term effects of radium deposition in man have continued to be of interest and importance, not only because radium is the standard for computing many of the maximum permissible levels of deposition of radionuclides, but also because it has afforded the only bridge between studies of the clinical effects in man and the vast number of experimental studies with laboratory animals. As a consequence, studies have been pursued in New England, New Jersey, and Illinois on the surviving populations of former radium dial painters, and similar studies have been done in Britain, Switzerland, and Czechoslovakia. Detailed studies on a selected number of cases from the United States were reported by Aub et al. (1952) and Looney et al. (1955). Summary reviews dealing with larger numbers of cases were published in the 1960s (Evans, 1966; Evans et al., 1969; Finkel et al., 1969a,b; Hasterlik et al., 1970), and the investigations are still in progress (Sharpe, 1974; Rowland et al., 1978; Brues, 1980).

Such studies reflect not only an improvement in the analytical instruments for detecting and measuring radium but also a sharpened approach to the evaluation of the deleterious effects. For example, a spectrum of radiographic changes in the skeletal tissues was found to be roughly correlated with concurrently measured body levels of radium. These radiographic changes ranged from slight coarsening of trabeculation, through a series of abnormalities such as local areas of rarefaction of cortical bone and of isolated foci of parametaphyseal sclerosis, to more severe changes such as aseptic necrosis and pathological fractures, on to the most severe change, malignant bone tumors (Hasterlik and Finkel, 1965; Evans, 1967). The latter, for the most part, consisted of fibrosarcomas and osteogenic sarcomas.

Although cases of osteogenic sarcoma have appeared in persons exposed in the early 1920s after time intervals as long as 45 years (in 1967), a more recent set of serious long-term effects has been the development of epithelial carcinomas of the linings of the mastoid air cells and the paranasal sinuses. These malignancies are partly attributable to the close juxtaposition of epithelial cells and bone in these areas and partly to the accumulation of radon within these cavities. For example, in the Illinois study of approximately 300 persons, most of whom acquired radium burdens in the period from 1918 to 1933, 46 cases of malignant disease were noted by 1967. These included 23 bone sarcomas, 16 neoplasms of the skull that were principally mastoid and paranasal air-cell carcinomas, and 7 leukemias and aplastic anemias (Finkel et al., 1969b). When retrospective estimates of maximum radium burdens were made, it was found that the lowest estimated peak initial burden for the bone sarcoma cases was 6.7 μg ($-\mu$Ci in the case of Ra), while the comparable value for cases of carcinoma and leukemia attributable to radium in dial painters was estimated to be 5.7 μg, well above the maximum permissible level of 0.1 μg (Finkel et al., 1969a,b).

Loutit (1970), in his review of reports of radium toxicity, especially those of Martland (1931), has concluded that malignancy induced in the bone marrow is fully as important as that seen in bone. He emphasized that the classic reports of Martland support the presence of a syndrome that, in modern terms, has the features of atypical (aleukemic) leukemia. Loutit stressed the view that the terminal marrow dyscrasias in the early, as well as the more recent, cases of radium poisoning were refractory to treatment.

An interesting complication of occupational exposure to radium was provided by the report of Müller and his colleagues in Prague (1961). In 1958, they had found several cases of dermatitis involving the fingers of radium dial painters working in a factory in Prague. Since they had never seen these skin problems before, they investigated the factory conditions and discovered that a new type of paint had been introduced that contained 1.2 mCi of strontium 90 per gram of paint as well as a small amount of radium 226. A detailed survey of the workers revealed that there was considerable contamination of the homes of the workers as well as of the workshops. While the radium body burdens were determined in 10 patients to be less than 0.01 μg, the body burdens of strontium 90 were estimated to be of the order of tens of microcuries as a result of the contamination. Although no serious clinical illness was encountered in this group of radiation workers, hematological studies revealed signs of disturbed erythropoiesis, such as reticulocytosis and hyperplasia of the erythroblast series in the bone marrow. These findings are consistent with the point made by Loutit (1970) in support of the conclusions of the report of the International Commission on Radiological Protection (ICRP, 1968) that the beta rays of the radioactive alkaline earth fission products, strontium 89, strontium 90, and barium 140, should be considered to be at least as leukemogenic to the bone marrow as they are accepted to be sarcomatogenic to bone tissue.

References

Aub JC, Evans RD, Gallagher DM, et al: Effects of treatment on radium and calcium metabolism in the human body. *Ann Intern Med* 1938; 11:1443–1463.

Aub JC, Evans RD, Hempelmann LH, et al: The late effects of internally deposited radioactive materials in man. *Medicine* 1952;31:221–329.

Blum T: Osteomyelitis of the mandible and maxilla. *J Am Dent Assoc* 1924;11:802-805.

Browning E: Medical aspects of radiations used in industry. *Br J Ind Med* 1944;1:170-175.

Brues AM: Long-term follow-up of radium dial painters and thorium workers, in Hubner KF, Fry SA (eds): *The Medical Basis for Radiation Accident Preparedness.* New York, Elsevier, 1980, pp 441-450.

Castle WB, Drinker KR, Drinker CK: Necrosis of the jaw in workers employed in applying a luminous paint containing radium. *J Ind Hyg* 1925;7:371-382.

Evans RD: Radium poisoning, a review of present knowledge. *Am J Publ Health* 1933;23:1017-1023.

Evans RD: Radium poisoning. Quantitative determination of the radium content and radium elimination rate of living persons. *Am J Roentgenol* 1937;37:368-378.

Evans RD: Protection of radium dial workers and radiologists from injury by radium. *J Ind Hyg Toxicol* 1943;25:253-269.

Evans RD: The effect of skeletally deposited alpha-ray emitters in man. *Br J Radiol* 1966;39:881-895.

Evans RD: The radium standard for bone-seekers: Evaluation of the data on radium patients and dial painters. *Health Phys* 1967;13:267-278.

Evans RD, Keane AT, Kolenkow RJ, et al: Radiogenic tumors in the radium and meso-thorium cases studied at M.I.T. in Mays CW, et al (eds): *Delayed Effects of Bone-Seeking Radionuclides.* Salt Lake City, University of Utah, 1969, pp 157-194.

Finkel AJ, Miller CE, Hasterlik RJ: Radium-induced malignant tumors in man, in Mays CW, et al (eds): *Delayed Effects of Bone-Seeking Radionuclides.* Salt Lake City, University of Utah, 1969a, pp 195-225.

Finkel AJ, Miller CE, Hasterlik RJ: Radiobiological parameters in human cancers attributable to long-term radium deposition, in *Radiation-Induced Cancer.* Vienna, International Atomic Energy Agency, 1969b, pp 183-202.

Flinn FB, Seidlin SM: Parathormone in treatment of "radium poisoning." *Bull Johns Hopkins Hosp* 1929;45:269-275.

Hasterlik RJ, Finkel AJ: Diseases of bones and joints associated with intoxication by radioactive substances, principally radium. *Med Clin North Am* 1965;49:285-296.

Hasterlik RJ, Finkel AJ, Miller CE: Late effects of radium deposition in man, in Fry RJM, et al (eds): *Late Effects of Radiation.* London, Taylor and Francis, 1970, pp 173-190.

ICRP: *Radiosensitivity of the Tissues in Bone,* ICRP Publication 11, International Commission on Radiological Protection, Oxford, Pergamon Press, 1968.

Jones JC, Day MJ: Control of hazards in the luminous dial painting industry. *Br J Ind Med* 1945;2:202-208.

Looney WB, Hasterlik RJ, Brues AM, et al: A clinical investigation of the chronic effects of radium salts administered therapeutically (1915-1931). *Am J Roentgenol* 1955;73:1001-1037.

Loutit JR: Malignancy from radium. *Br J Cancer* 1970;24:195-207.

Martland HS: Microscopic changes of certain anemias due to radioactivity. *Arch Pathol* 1926;2:465-472.

Martland HS: Occupational poisoning in manufacture of luminous watch dials. *J Am Med Assoc* 1929;92:466-473, 552-559.

Martland HS: The observance of malignancy in radioactive persons. *Am J Cancer* 1931;15:2435-2516.

Martland HS, Humphries RE: Osteogenic sarcoma in dial painters using luminous paint. *Arch Pathol* 1929;7:406-417.

Miller CE, Finkel AJ: Radium retention in man after multiple injections: The power function re-evaluated. *Am J Roentgenol* 1968;103:871-880.

Mottram JC, Clarke JR: Leucocytic blood-content of those handling radium for therapeutic purposes. *Arch Radiol Electrother* 1920;24:345, also in *Proc R Soc Med* 1920;13:25.

Müller J, David A, Rejskova M, et al: Chronic occupational exposure to strontium-90 and radium-226. *Lancet* 1961;2:129-131.

Norris WP, Speckman TW, Gustafson PF: Studies of the metabolism of radium in man. *Am J Roentgenol* 1955;73:785-802.

Norris WP, Tyler SA, Brues AM: Retention of radioactive bone seekers. *Science* 1958;128:456-462.

Rowland RE, Stehney AF, Brues AM, et al: Current status of the study of [226]Ra and [228]Ra in humans at the Center for Human Radiobiology. *Health Phys* 1978;35:159-166.

Schlundt H, Failla G: The detection and estimation of radium in living persons. III. The normal elimination of radium. *Am J Roentgenol* 1931;26:265-271.

Schlundt H, Nerancy JT, Morris JP: The detection and estimation of radium in living persons. IV. The retention of soluble radium salts administered intravenously. *Am J Roentgenol* 1933;30: 515–522.

Seil HA, Viol CH, Gordon MA: The elimination of soluble radium salts taken intravenously and per os. *Radium.* 1915;5:40–44, also in *NY Med J* 1915;101:896–898.

Sharpe WD: Chronic radium intoxication — Clinical and autopsy findings in long-term New Jersey survivors. *Environ Res* 1974;8:243–383.

Uranium   Mining of metal ores in Central Europe in two regions of the Erz mountains, Schneeberg on the German side and Jáchymov (Joachimstal) 30 kilometers southeast on the Czechoslovakian side, had been known for some four centuries to have a strange and harmful effect on the lungs of miners. Mining has been continuous in this region since the 15th century for copper, iron, silver, and later for cobalt, arsenic, and nickel, and, at the end of the 19th century, for pitchblende. The Schneeberg miners were prone to die off in the prime of life from damaged lungs and a rapidly progressing cachexia. A thorough medical investigation of the nature of the illness was not reported until 1879 by Härtig and Hesse, who discovered lung cancer in 75% of the deaths. In 1913, Arnstein confirmed the presence of lung cancer in at least 40% of those miners who died between 1875 and 1912, and he found that the tumor was predominantly squamous cell carcinoma. The next study of the Schneeberg miners was made by Rostoski et al. (1926): 13 of 21 miners were shown to have lung carcinoma when necropsied.

It had long been a matter of wonder that no similar reports came from the Czechoslovakian side of the mountains, where similar ores were mined and where, according to the miners, "Bergkrankheit" (mountain illness) was as common as on the German side. After the discovery of radium, the Czechoslovakian mines became a famous source of pitchblende, but it was not until 1932 that the first cases of lung cancer were reported in the Jáchymov miners, and a 50% incidence of this condition was found (Pirchan and Šikl, 1932; Šikl, 1950).

Although it was long believed that arsenic, and possibly cobalt, in the ore was the cause of the tumors, after the discovery of radium it was suspected that the radioactivity of the ore and the presence of radon in the mine air were the responsible agents. Evans and Goodman (1940) and later Evans (1943) summarized the available data on the concentrations of radon in the air of the Schneeberg and Jáchymov mines. From these data they derived a value of 10 pCi/L of air as a safe working condition (1 pCi = 10^{12} Curie). Lorenz (1944) concluded from the same data plus small animal studies that radon was not the sole cause of lung cancer in these miners. He listed a number of contributing factors that included dust-induced pneumoconiosis, chronic irritation from respiratory diseases, arsenic, and a possible hereditary susceptibility as a result of inbreeding in the local populations. More recent work, however, has shown that the radon in the mines is the predominant factor and that the inhalation of the decay products of radon has more significance than the inhalation of radon itself, which is inhaled and exhaled during its brief physical half-life of 3.8 days. The radioactive daughters of radon (polonium 218, lead 214, bismuth 214, and polonium 214), which collectively have a half-life of about 30 minutes, become quickly attached to dust particles and other solid surfaces when they are formed in the air of a mine. When these dust particles along with the attached radionuclides are inhaled, the alpha particles and other radiation from them locally irradiate the mucosa of the nose, pharynx, and tracheobronchial tree. The radiation dose delivered in this manner has been estimated by Holaday et al. (1968) to be 20 times greater than that from the inhaled radon itself.

Corroborating evidence has been provided by the experience of a small fluorspar mining community in Newfoundland, Canada, where primary cancer of the lung accounted for 23 of 51 deaths that occurred there from 1952 to 1961 among males with at least one year of underground mining experience. Investigation revealed that radon and radon daughter products were in the mine air at concentrations well in excess of maximum permissible levels (de Villiers and Windish, 1964). Although only traces of uranium were present in the rock, the radon was apparently carried into the mines by the considerable seepage of ground water.

The concentration of radon in uranium mine air depends upon many factors, including the uranium concentrations in the exposed rock, the area and porosity of the exposed surface, the concentration and sizes of the particulates in the air, humidity, and the ventilation rates in the mines (Holaday et al., 1968). Problems of persistently changing working conditions and of inadequate instrumentation to measure mine radon concentrations have made it difficult to relate tumor incidence to exposure and to establish workable controls in the industry. The present standard used as a guide for the control of exposure in uranium mines is the potential alpha energy produced by a "Working Level" (WL), which is equivalent to 100 pCi of each of the four immediate daughters of radon per liter of air, or any airborne concentration of them that releases the same amount (1.3 × 10^5 meV) of alpha energy in their decay to RaD (^{210}Pb). The various mines listed here are thought to have had these ranges of radon daughter concentrations, expressed in terms of WL, according to Holaday (1969):

European uranium mines	10–180
United States uranium mines	2–200
Newfoundland fluorspar mines	2.5–10
United States metal mines	0.5–1.5

The measurements made in the mines in the Colorado Plateau during the decade from 1955 to 1966 have shown that, while prior to 1960 over 50% of the mines had WL values over 3.0, the majority of them had levels below that after 1961 (Holaday et al., 1968). By 1967, 70% of the mines were below 1 WL (Holaday, 1969). Problems have attended the setting of upper WL limits for uranium mines, and the standards continue to be in contention.

Among uranium miners in the United States, increased exposure in the mines has been associated with increased numbers of atypical cells in the sputum, increased respiratory symptoms and prevalence of emphysema and pneumoconiosis, and with decreased pulmonary ventilatory function as measured by expiration spirometry (Parsons et al., 1964). Most of the tumor deaths occurred 10 or more years after the onset of underground mining. Since those uranium miners who had smoked had an excess of lung cancer that was 10 times greater than that among nonsmoking miners, cigarette smoking appears to increase the cancer risk (Lundin et al., 1969; Archer et al., 1973). Saccomanno et al. (1965) have shown that among the Colorado Plateau miners dying of lung cancer the predominant cell was of the small undifferentiated type (57%). The remainder were of the epidermoid type. The tendency of the undifferentiated small cell tumors to metastasize early and extensively is thought to account for the rapid clinical course and early death after onset of symptoms in the United States uranium miners. The association of these small cell lung tumors with increasing exposure supports the relationship with exposure to airborne radiation. Further, the predominantly hilar origin of the tumors implies that the large bronchi received a higher carcinogenic dose than did other parts of the lung.

Uranium milling also provides a health risk to workers, although less than that encountered in uranium mining (Archer, 1981). In contrast with the experience of uranium miners, workers exposed to high average air levels of uranium dust in a conversion and enrichment plant at Oak Ridge, Tennessee, have not had increased mortality rates from lung cancer, leukemia, bone cancer, or diseases of the respiratory and genitourinary systems (Polednak et al., 1981).

Uranium has had other industrial uses in both the ceramics and steel industries. It has been used, for example, as an additive in dental porcelain to improve the appearance of ceramic teeth (FDA, 1976) and it has long been used in ceramic glazes. The use of uranyl acetate as a contrasting agent in electron microscopy constitutes a potential hazard to users of this technique (Darley and Ezoe, 1976).

Leconte in 1854 described chronic nephritis caused by uranium compounds and his observations have been confirmed since that time. Wilson and Smales (1946) reported finding from 2 to 10 µg/L of uranium in urine samples of six chemists who had contact with magnesium uranyl acetate for two months prior to the tests. The medical examinations of these chemists revealed no abnormalities. Apparently, it is necessary to have a soluble uranium compound to produce renal damage in man. According to Hodge (1956), who performed extensive studies with experimental animals in the 1940s, uranium is one of the most toxic elements chemically, but it is absorbed into the body with difficulty. A diffusible uranium-bicarbonate complex is formed in the blood and is filtered through the glomerulus, but the bicarbonate is resorbed in the proximal convoluted tubule and the liberated uranyl ions react with the protein membranes to produce injury. Rupture of the cells and discharge of their contents into the urine leads to albuminuria, aminoaciduria, and release of catalase and phosphatase. The major histological site of uranium injury is the distal third of the proximal convoluted tubule. Taking advantage of the release of catalase just described, Dounce (1947) developed a test using catalase in the urine as an index of uranium poisoning.

Natural uranium (uranium 238) is an alpha emitter that is only weakly radioactive because of its extremely long physical half-life, 4.5×10^9 years. Its toxic hazard resides not in its radiation effects but in its chemical action on the renal tubules. It is usually measured in bioassay samples by photofluorimetric rather than radiochemical techniques, and workers handling ordinary uranium are usually monitored by chemical determinations of urinary uranium and the associated presence or absence of albuminuria. Enriched uranium, containing ^{234}U and ^{235}U, is a radiation hazard if it is internally deposited, in which case it is measured by whole body *in vivo* counting methods based upon detection of the 186 keV gamma ray from uranium 235. Lung deposition was the so-called critical factor in 239 of 246 cases of internal deposition of enriched uranium reported in the United States from 1957 to 1966. These workers were engaged in production operations, and no harmful effects were reported (Ross, 1968).

References

Archer VE: Health concerns in uranium mining and milling. *J Occup Med* 1981;23:502–505.

Archer VE, Wagoner JK, Lundin FE Jr: Uranium mining and cigarette smoking effects on man. *J Occup Med* 1973;15:204–211.

Arnstein A: Ueber den sogennanten "Schneeberger Lungenkrebs." *Verh Deutsch Pathol Gesellsch* 1913;16:332–342, also in *Wien Klin Wchnschr* 1913;26:748–752.

Darley JJ, Ezoe H: Potential hazards of uranium and its compounds in electron microscopy: A brief review. *J Microscopy* 1976;106:85–86.

Dounce A: Catalasuria as a sensitive test for uranium poisoning. *Fed Proc* 1947;6:323.

Evans RD: Protection of radium dial workers and radiologists from injury by radium. *J Ind Hyg Toxicol* 1943;25:253–269.

Evans RD, Goodman C: Determination of the thoron content of air and its bearing on lung cancer hazards in industry. *J Ind Hyg Toxicol* 1940;22:89–99.

FDA: *Uranium in Dental Porcelain*. Washington, DC, Food and Drug Administration. FDA-76-8061, 1976.

Hodge H: Mechanism of uranium poisoning, in *Peaceful Uses of Atomic Energy* Geneva, United Nations, 1956;13:229–232.

Holaday DA: History of the exposure of miners to radon. *Health Phys* 1969;16:547–552.

Holaday DA, Archer VE, Lundin F: A summary of the United States exposure experiences in the uranium mining industry, in Kornberg HA, Norwood WD, (eds): *Diagnosis and Treatment of Deposited Radionuclides*. Amsterdam, Excerpta Medica, 1968, pp 451–456.

Lorenz E: Radioactivity and lung cancer: A critical review of lung cancer in the miners of Schneeberg and Joachimstal. *J Nat Cancer Inst* 1944;5:1–15.

Lundin FE Jr, Lloyd JW, Smith EM, et al: Mortality of uranium miners in relation to radiation exposure, hard rock mining and cigarette smoking—1950 through September 1967. *Health Phys* 1969;16:571–578.

Parsons WD, de Villiers AJ, Bartlett LS, et al: Lung cancer in a fluorspar mining community: II. Prevalence of respiratory symptoms and disability. *Br J Ind Med* 1964;21:110–116.

Pirchan A, Šikl H: Cancer of the lung in the miners of Jáchymov (Joachimstal): Report of cases observed in 1929–1930. *Am J Cancer* 1932; 16:681–722.

Polednak AP, Frome EL: Mortality among men employed between 1943 and 1947 at a uranium-processing plant. *J Occup Med* 1981; 23:169–178.

Ross DM: A statistical summary of United States Atomic Energy Commission contractors' internal exposure experience, 1957–1966, in Kornberg HA, Norwood WD (eds): *Diagnosis and Treatment of Deposited Radionuclides*. Amsterdam, Excerpta Medica, 1968, pp 427–434.

Rostoski, Saupe, Schmorl: Der Bergkrankheit der Erzbergleute in Schneeberg in Sachsen (Schneeberger Lungenkrebs). *Zeitschr Krebsforsch* 1926;23:360–384.

Saccomanno G, Archer VE, Saunders RP, et al: Lung cancer of uranium miners on Colorado Plateau. *Health Phys* 1965;10:1195–1201.

Šikl H: The present status of knowledge about the Jáchymov disease (cancer of the lungs in miners of the radium mines). *Acta Unio Internat Contra Cancrum* 1950;6:1366–1375.

de Villiers AJ, Windish JP: Lung cancer in a fluorspar mining community. I. Radiation, dust, and mortality experience. *Br J Ind Med* 1964;21:94–109.

Wilson HM, Smales AA: Uranium in urine. *Nature* 1946;158:590.

Plutonium   Plutonium was discovered in 1940 by Seaborg and his colleagues (Seaborg et al., 1946) and has subsequently been produced in increasing quantities for military and peaceful purposes. Although the problem of occupational exposure to plutonium has largely been confined to the atomic energy industry, the increasing use of plutonium in power reactors, especially those of the breeder type, will eventually expose a substantial number of persons to this relatively new toxic substance as a hazard of work. Those persons working with plutonium will be involved largely with fabrication and chemical processing of fuel elements. Similar exposures, although on a smaller scale, may be anticipated in the fabrication of plutonium-powered cardiac pacemakers.

The chief isotope of this new element is plutonium-239, which is mainly an emitter of alpha particles that have a range of about 40 μm in water and soft tissue and of some very soft gamma rays. Plutonium-239 has a physical half-life of 24,400 years. The oldest exposures on record occurred at the Los Alamos Scientific Laboratory in 1944 and 1945 when 27 workers accumulated plutonium body burdens of 0.1 μg or greater (Langham, 1959). Subsequent occupational exposures to plutonium-239 also occurred at other atomic energy laboratories in the United States, Canada, France, and Great Britain. In 1968 a plutonium registry was formed by the United States Atomic Energy Commission and is now called the United States Transuranium Registry. Its purpose is to collect and study cases of exposure to plutonium and other transuranic elements. No clinical illness has been attributed to long-term internally deposited plutonium as a result of occupational exposure (Hempelmann et al., 1973), and a mortality study of 224 plutonium workers at the Los Alamos Scientific Laboratory has shown no excess deaths from any cause (Voelz et al., 1980).

Langham (1959) summarized the biological properties of plutonium-239. When taken into the systemic circulation, plutonium deposits predominantly in the skeleton and liver. It is absorbed from the gastrointestinal tract only to the extent of 0.003%, and intact skin is a nearly complete barrier. Inhalation of contaminated air is the most important mode of exposure, although accidental subcutaneous injection may also occur. The amount absorbed and the metabolism of plutonium both depend upon its particle size, solubility, and chemical form. Radiochemical bioassay of urine has long been used to detect plutonium in the body and to estimate the extent of the burden; *in vivo* whole body counting techniques have been developed to supplement these estimates (Ramsden and Speight, 1968; Dolphin, 1971; Roesch

and Palmer, 1972). Similar devices have been designed to detect plutonium and americium-241 in wounds (Epstein and Johanson, 1966).

Once deposited in the body, plutonium is excreted extremely slowly with a biological half-time of about 200 years unless excretion is hastened by the use of chelating agents. The first such compound to be used successfully was ethylenediaminetetraacetic acid (EDTA) reported by Foreman et al. in 1954, although some increase in excretion was obtained earlier by the use of zirconium citrate. Since 1960, diethylenetriaminepentaacetic acid (DTPA) has replaced EDTA in the treatment of plutonium deposition because of its greater effectiveness in binding and mobilizing plutonium for urinary excretion. The trisodium calcium salt of DTPA administered intravenously soon after an accident is considered to be quite effective in removing soluble plutonium that has been inhaled or deposited in wounds (Norwood, 1962; Norwood et al., 1956; Kornberg and Norwood, 1968).

The possible nephrotoxicity of EDTA was pointed out early and proved to be reversible tubular nephrosis. The same reaction was noted after DTPA therapy (Norwood, 1960). The nephrotoxic effects from these two compounds occur with prolonged use or high dosages and may be due to a transient depletion of manganese in renal tubular tissue (Foreman and Nigrovic, 1968). From animal studies it is known that sufficiently concentrated amounts of plutonium in the body can produce symptoms of the acute radiation syndrome (Langham, 1959). On a weight basis, plutonium is one of the most toxic substances known to man. It is from four to 30 times as potent as radium in terms of tumorigenicity for small animals depending on the dose level (Finkel, 1953). Long-term studies with dogs that have been in progress since 1950 led to the production of osteosarcomas from 3.6 to 10 years after plutonium-239 was injected. Bile duct tumors and a frontal sinus epidermoid carcinoma have also been seen in these plutonium-treated dogs (Taylor et al., 1969). Precise interpretation of these laboratory findings and their direct application to human exposure is not yet possible.

References

Dolphin GW: The biological problems in the radiological protection of workers exposed to [239]Pu. *Health Phys* 1971;20:549–557.

Epstein RJ, Johanson EW: Apparatus for monitoring ^{239}Pu in wounds. *Health Phys* 1966; 12:29–35.

Finkel MP: Relative biological effectiveness of radium and other alpha-emitters in CF No. 1 female mice. *Proc Soc Exp Biol Med* 1953;83: 494–498.

Foreman H, Fuqua PA, Norwood WD: Experimental administration of ethylenediamine-tetra-acetic acid in plutonium poisoning. *Arch Ind Hyg* 1954;10:226–231.

Foreman H, Nigrovic V: Nephrotoxicity of chelating agents, in Kornberg HA, Norwood WD (eds): *Diagnosis and Treatment of Deposited Radionuclides.* Amsterdam, Excerpta Medica, 1968, pp 419–423.

Hempelmann LH, Langham WH, Richmond CR, et al: Manhattan Project plutonium workers: A twenty-seven year follow-up study of selected cases. *Health Phys* 1973;23:461–479.

Kornberg HA, Norwood WD (eds): *Diagnosis and Treatment of Deposited Radionuclides.* Amsterdam, Excerpta Medica, 1968.

Langham WH: Physiology and toxicology of plutonium-239 and its industrial medical control. *Health Phys* 1959;2:172–185.

Norwood WD: DTPA—Effectiveness in removing internally deposited plutonium from humans. *J Occup Med* 1960;2:371–376.

Norwood WD: Therapeutic removal of plutonium in humans. *Health Phys* 1962;8:747–750.

Norwood WD, Fuqua PA, Scudder BC: Treatment of acute plutonium poisoning. *Ind Med Surg* 1956;25:135–139.

Ramsden D, Speight RG: The measurement of ^{239}Pu *in vivo*: A progress report, in Kornberg HA, Norwood WD, (eds): *Diagnosis and Treatment of Deposited Radionuclides,* Amsterdam, Excerpta Medica, 1968, pp 171–188.

Roesch WC, Palmer HE: Detection of plutonium *in vivo* by whole-body counting. *Health Phys* 1962;8:773–776.

Seaborg GT, McMillan EM, Kennedy JW, et al: Radioactive element 94 from deuterons on uranium. *Physical Rev* 1946;69:366–367.

Taylor GN, Dougherty TF, Shabestari L, et al: Soft-tissue tumors in internally irradiated beagles, in Mays CW et al. (eds): *Delayed Effects of Bone-seeking Radionuclides,* Salt Lake City, University of Utah, 1969, pp 323–336.

Voelz GL, Stebbings JH Jr, Healy JW, et al: Studies on health risks to persons exposed to plutonium, in Hübner KF, Fry SA, (eds): *The Medical Basis for Radiation Accident Preparedness,* New York, Elsevier, 1980, pp 419–430.

Thorium   Thorium is found in ore such as thorianite in Madagascar and thorite and monazite in Brazil and India. Occupational exposure to thorium and its decay products occur in mining, ore concentration, extraction processing, reduction to metal, metallurgical procedures, and alloy preparation. The toxicology of thorium is complicated by the fact that some of the radionuclides in the thorium natural decay series have been involved in the harmful effects of radium after occupational, research, or iatrogenic exposure. This situation is particularly true of mesothorium 1 (MsTh₁), which is a weak beta-ray emitting isotope of radium (^{228}Ra) with a half-life of 6.7 years, and of radiothorium (RdTh), which is an alpha- and gamma-ray emitting isotope of thorium (^{228}Th). The earlier use of thorium in making gas mantles has been largely superseded by its applications in ceramics where it is used in the fabrication of highly refractory thorium oxide crucibles and other ceramic oxide components, and in nuclear power reactors where it is used in fuel elements for neutron capture. The principal hazards from thorium in industry are inhalation of thorium dust and of thoron gas and its decay products, and exposure to external beta and gamma radiation. The inhalation hazard is greatest in dusty operations such as grinding of metals, ceramics, handling of thorium powder, and contamination from thorium fires. Beta-gamma radiation hazards result from the condensation of volatilized radium-228 and radium-224 on cooler surfaces (Albert, 1966).

Thoron (Tn) is a noble gas produced in the thorium decay chain and is an alpha-particle emitting isotope of radon (^{220}Rn) with a physical half-life of 55.3 seconds. Evans and Goodman (1940) published a study of the thoron content of the air in the working environment in Welsbach thorium mantle factories. They discussed the lung cancer hazard on the basis of existing knowledge of radon exposures in industries handling radium. Definite standards were suggested that were calculated to eliminate any hazardous exposures to thoron. There have been no reports to date of pulmonary carcinoma in workers in thorium mantle factories. In 1954, Albert and his colleagues conducted a very thorough industrial hygiene and medical survey in a refinery where thorium and rare earths had been extracted from monazite ores for 30 years. The workers had been exposed to monazite ore dust, thorium dust, thorium salts, thoron gas and its daughters, and to external beta and gamma radiation. Medical examinations of 21 employees who had worked in the most contaminated areas of the plant for an average of eight years were negative except for four persons whose chest radiographs were interpreted as showing a mild amount of pulmonary fibrosis (Albert et al., 1955). Recent studies on former thorium refinery workers have shown that it is possible to detect thoron in the exhaled breath, presumably emanating from retained ^{232}Bi in the chest (Rundo et al., 1979).

Thorium dioxide has been used in the form of a colloidal suspension ("Thorotrast") as a contrast medium in x-ray diagnosis for purposes of arteriography of the liver and spleen, and of the viscera, and for visualizing sinus tracts. Thousands of patients received injections of this preparation between 1930 and 1945 (Abbatt, 1979). Reports of endothelial cell sarcoma of the liver and the development of fibrotic thorotrastomas as a result of leakage at the injection sites led to discontinuation of the clinical use of Thorotrast (MacMahon et al., 1947). In recent years there has been an extensive and growing literature describing the delayed serious effects from these clinical uses, and, while such cases do not represent industrial exposure, they are of significance in terms of delayed effects of internally deposited radionuclides. They are of particular interest because of the translocation of thorium decay products, radium-228 and radium-224, to the skeleton (Looney, 1960; Boyd et al., 1968; Janower et al., 1972; Curry et al., 1975; Falk et al., 1979; Mole, 1979; among many others).

References

Abbatt JD: History of the use and toxicity of Thorotrast. *Environ Res* 1979;18:6–12.

Albert RE: *Thorium, Its Industrial Hygiene Aspects.* New York, Academic Press, 1966.

Albert RE, Klevin P, Fresco J, et al: Industrial hygiene and medical survey of a thorium refinery. *Arch Ind Hyg* 1955;11:234–242.

Boyd JT, Langlands AO, MacCabe JJ: Long-term hazards of thorotrast. *Br Med J* 1968;2:517–521.

Curry JL, Johnson WG, Feinberg DH, et al:

Thorium-induced hepatic hemangioendothelioma. *Am J Roentgenol* 1975;125:671–677.

Evans RD, Goodman C: Determination of the thoron content of the air and its bearing on lung cancer hazards in industry. *J Ind Hyg Toxicol* 1940;22:89–99.

Falk H, Telles NC, Ishak KG, et al: Epidemiology of Thorotrast-induced hepatic angiosarcoma in the United States. *Environ Res* 1979;18:65–73.

Janower ML, Miettinen OS, Flynn MJ: Effects of long-term Thorotrast exposure. *Radiology* 1972;103:13–20.

Looney WB: An investigation of the late clinical findings following Thorotrast (Thorium dioxide) administration. *Am J Roentgenol* 1960;83:163–185.

MacMahon HE, Murphy AS, Bates MI: Endothelial cell sarcoma of liver following Thorotrast injections. *Am J Pathol* 1947;23:585–611.

Mole RH: Carcinogenesis by Thorotrast and other sources of irradiation, especially other α-emitters. *Environ Res* 1979;18:192–215.

Rundo J, Polednak AP, Brues AM, et al: A study of radioactivity and health status of former thorium workers. *Environ Res* 1979;18:94–100.

Tritium Tritium is an isotope of hydrogen with an atomic weight of 3 (^{3}H) that emits a weak beta ray and has a physical half-life of 12.26 years. It is manufactured in quantities that are sufficient to be a radiation hazard to persons working in plants where it is produced by the irradiation of lithium. It is also produced in heavy water (deuterium oxide) moderated nuclear reactors where it is a byproduct of neutron irradiation of D_2O. Tritiated water (HTO) enters the body by inhalation of the vapor and by percutaneous absorption (Pinson and Langham, 1957). Since it mixes with extracellular body water, tritium is distributed uniformly throughout the organism, and a urine specimen constitutes a readily obtainable aliquot for analysis. Early work had shown that tritium leaves the body rapidly and that the biological half-time is ordinarily 10 days, when water intake is roughly 2.7 L/day. Water loading by forced fluid intake up to 12.8 L/day can reduce the biological half-time to 2.4 days. Later work showed that the biological half-time is influenced by ambient temperature inasmuch as an 8.3 day half-time was found in spring and summer, while a 10.4 day half-time was encountered in fall and winter. Average biological half-times also decrease comparably with increasing age: 10.5 days for persons 20 to 29 years old, and 8.5 days for persons between 50 and 59 (Butler and Leroy, 1965).

Tritium is exchanged with organically bound hydrogen and is consequently retained selectively in certain tissues or "pools" of organic compounds. Sophisticated mathematical analysis of the data in terms of flow between idealized body compartments suggests that the dose contributed by organically bound tritium is less than that from body water tritium (Sanders and Reinig, 1968).

A study of exposures among U.S. Atomic Energy Commission contractors and licensees where tritium deposition exceeded 25% of the standard maximum permissible level revealed 116 cases, in all of which tritium entered the body by inhalation or through intact skin (Roeder, 1968). In 11 cases, the body tritium levels were high enough to require treatment by increased intake of fluids. No harmful effects were expected or reported in these cases, but Seelentag (1973) reported two fatal cases of panmyelophthisis that followed overexposure to tritium used in luminous compounds applied to watch dials.

Samuels et al. (1964), and more recently Feinendegen (1975), have called attention to the potential hazard from tritium when this isotope is used to label thymidine in cytological studies, a technique that is commonly used to investigate rates of mitosis in cell-renewal systems. These matters are more fully discussed in a recent NCRP publication (1979).

References

Butler HL, Leroy JH: Observations on the biological half-life of tritium. *Health Phys* 1965;11:283–285.

Feinendegen LE: Effects of tritium on the human organism. *J Belge Radiol (Belg Tijdschr Radiol)* 1975;58:147–155.

NCRP: *Tritium and Other Radionuclide-Labelled Organic Compounds Incorporated in Genetic Material.* Washington, DC, National Council on Radiation Protection and Measurements, NCRP Report No. 63 1979.

Pinson EA, Langham WH: Physiology and toxicology of tritium in man. *J Appl Physiol* 1957;10:108–126.

Roeder JR: A statistical summary of the United States Atomic Energy Commission licensees' internal exposure experience, 1957–1966, in Korn-

berg HA, Norwood WD (eds): *Diagnosis and Treatment of Deposited Radionuclides,* Amsterdam, Excerpta Medica, 1968, pp 435–450.

Samuels LD, Kisieleski WE, Baserga R: Tritiated thymidine toxicity in mammalian systems. *Atompraxis* 1964;10:144–148.

Seelentag W: Two cases of tritium fatality, in Moghissi AA, Carter MW (eds): *Tritium.* Phoenix, Messenger Graphics, 1973, pp 267–280.

Sanders SM Jr, Reinig WC: Assessment of tritium in man, in Kornberg HA, Norwood WD, (eds): *Diagnosis and Treatment of Deposited Radionuclides.* Amsterdam, Excerpta Medica, 1968, pp 534–542.

Radiation Protection Standards

In order to utilize the benefits of ionizing radiation and at the same time minimize its harmful effects, a number of successful control techniques have been developed. In addition, certain important committees have been at work, beginning with the International Commission on Radiological Protection (ICRP) formed in 1928. In 1934, the ICRP recommended a tolerance dose of 0.2 R per day. After 1950, the ICRP broadened the scope of its concerns so that it considered problems of radiation protection associated with high voltage accelerators, industrial radiography, and the operation of nuclear reactors and their related chemical and metallurgical facilities, in addition to the medical use of radiant energy. Most standards recommended by the ICRP have been applicable to occupational exposure, although in 1958 recommendations were made that related to the exposure of various population groups and of the population at large (ICRP, 1958).

The National Council on Radiation Protection and Measurements (NCRP) was organized by federal charter in the United States in 1964. The same acronym had applied to an organization named the National Committee on Radiation Protection that was organized in 1946, and that in turn grew out of an earlier group formed in 1929, called the Advisory Committee on X-ray and Radium Protection. The NCRP in 1934 adopted the value of 0.1 R per day as the maximum permissible dose level. In 1941, it established the first internal dose standard of 0.1 μg of radium-226 as the maximum permissible body burden. Apart from setting these basic standards of radiation exposure, the NCRP has also made recommendations for waste disposal of radioactive isotopes, the safe handling of cadavers containing radionuclides, the safe design of industrial beta-ray sources, radiation dose limits for pregnant employees, the management of accidentally contaminated persons, and many other topics of interest to occupational medicine and industrial toxicology (see Appendix for list).

The ICRP (1965) and the NCRP (1971) recommended maximum permissible dose equivalents for occupational exposure. For total body exposure, the annual permissible dose equivalent was set at 5 rem per year, with 3 rem permitted within a period of 13 weeks. The *rem* is a unit used to express human biological doses as a result of exposure to one or many types of ionizing radiation, so that the dose in rems is equal to the absorbed dose in rads times the relative biological effectiveness (RBE) factor of the type of radiation absorbed. The rem is consequently a unit of RBE dose. For a working lifetime, the maximum accumulated whole body dose equivalent (in rem) is given by the formula 5 (N-18), where N is the age of the worker. This formula is designed to allow 5 rem per year during the lifetime work span starting at age 18. For occupational exposure of the hands, the maximum permissible dose equivalent was set at 75 rem in any one year, of which not more than 25 rem is permitted in any one quarter. Similarly, the maximum permissible dose equivalent for occupational exposure to the forearms was set at 30 rem in any one year, with not more than 10 rem in any one quarter. For areas of the skin other than hands and forearms, the maximum permissible dose equivalent was set at 15 rem in any one year. For combined external and internal irradiation of any tissue, organ, or organ system not otherwise singled out, the recommendation was for 15 rem maximum in any one year. Occupational exposure of an expectant mother during the entire gestation period is not to exceed 0.5 rem.

For individual members of the public not occupationally exposed or for occasionally exposed individuals, the NCRP recommended that the dose limit for the critical organs (gonads, red bone marrow, lens of the eye) or whole body not exceed 0.5 rem in any one year in addition to the radiation received from natural background sources and from medical and dental exposures. For the entire population of the United States, the average dose limit for the whole body (possible somatic effects) as well as for the gonads (possible genetic effects) should not exceed a yearly average of 0.17 rem (170 mrem) per person.

The NCRP also made recommendations for exposures that lead to doses considerably in excess of the routine standards when recovery operations from an accident are necessary or major operational difficulty is encountered. Women in the reproductive age should not take part in these actions and volunteers generally should be above the age of 45. Planned doses to the whole body should not exceed 100 rem, although the hands and forearms may receive an additional 200 rem for a total of 300 rem. Participation in such life-saving overexposures should be limited to once in a lifetime.

The NCRP, in addition, considered the problems that related to accidental occupational exposures. Planned whole body doses up to 25 rem are acceptable for emergency operations, and accidental doses up to the same level should not cause major concern. Medical attention is recommended at higher levels. Contributions to the whole body dose from natural radiation background is not ordinarily included in maximum permissible dose equivalents for occupational exposure. Similarly, contributions from man-made devices outside the occupational environment, such as might be received from television sets, from radioactive fallout, and from environmental radiation in the vicinity of nuclear power plants, are also excluded. Exposures from the procedures of the healing arts, such as medicine and dentistry, are also excluded in occupational exposure calculations.

Of importance in this discussion is the background dose attributable to natural radiation. Such exposure comes from external sources of ionizing radiation and from internally deposited, naturally occurring radionuclides. The two principal sources of external radiation from natural sources are cosmic radiation and gamma radiation from the ground and from building materials. On the average, the annual cosmic ray dose equivalent in the United States is about 40 mrem. This value rises with increase in altitude above sea level to about 70 mrem per year at an elevation of one mile (1.6 km), as in Denver, Colorado. The average terrestrial radiation dose in the United States is estimated to be about 60 mrem per year outdoors and 55 mrem inside buildings. The whole body dose, then, is about 100 mrem per year from cosmic and terrestrial radiation combined. The contribution of radionuclides in food, drinking water, and air leads to internal deposition that provides about 25 mrem per year from uranium and thorium and their decay products, from radiopotassium (^{40}K) in red cells and other tissues, and from radiocarbon (^{14}C). Altogether, the natural radiation in the United States results in an average annual dose equivalent of about 125 mrem (NCRP, 1975).

References

ICRP: *Recommendations of the International Commission on Radiological Protection,* ICRP Publication 1. London, Pergamon Press, 1958.

ICRP: *Report of Committee II on Permissible Dose for Internal Radiation,* ICRP Publication 9. Oxford, Pergamon Press, 1965.

NCRP: *Basic Radiation Protection Criteria,* NCRP Report No. 39. Washington, DC, National Council on Radiation Protection and Measurements, 1971.

NCRP: Natural Background Radiation in the United States, NCRP Report No. 45, Washington, DC, National Council on Radiation Protection and Measurements, 1975.

Radiation safety procedures Protection against unnecessary exposure to occupational radiation involves the use of protective devices such as shielding appropriate to the intensity and type of radiation, protective clothing, enclosed dry boxes (also known as glove boxes), appropriate ventilation with high-efficiency filters interposed in the duct work, and the presence of safety showers in case of external contamination. Measurement of the amount of radiation that a person may have received is accomplished by the use of a variety of detectors, such as film badges, pocket dosimeters, and other devices. These may include permanently installed radiation monitors with signaling alarms when the radiation level exceeds a critical point. A variety of portable alpha and beta-gamma meters are also available. In cases of suspected internal contamination, whole body counting systems are exceedingly useful. Ordinarily, these pieces of equipment are quite cumbersome, but portable and less formidable modifications have been designed. Older techniques that involved the use of ionization chambers and Geiger-Müller tubes have been superseded by liquid, plastic, and crystal scintillation detectors and, more recently, by semiconductor detectors that possess remarkable properties in resolving the peaks and valleys of gamma-ray and x-ray energy spectra.

Bioassay monitoring When radionuclides are deposited internally in the body, it is necessary to have some measure of the amounts involved in order to estimate the internally delivered radiation dose. When the radionuclide emits a sufficiently penetrating gamma ray, *in vivo* whole body counting methods described above can be used for this purpose. When, however, the emitted radiation cannot be measured from outside the body, an estimate can be based upon measurements of the amount of radionuclide or of radioactive daughters in the exhaled breath, the excreta, or blood. Exhaled breath analysis is largely restricted to the noble gases, radon and thoron, although analyses of ^{14}C-labeled CO_2 are possible. Analyses of blood samples will give information on the circulating radionuclides that have not been excreted or deposited in specific tissues or organs. Examination of the feces presents a number of problems. A portion of inhaled insoluble materials is cleared from the tracheobronchial tree by the ciliary ladder and is then transferred to the gastrointestinal tract by swallowing. Radionuclides that are soluble or insoluble may enter the gastrointestinal tract directly by ingestion or secondarily by secretion with the digestive juices or more likely with the bile. Moreover, not all of the inhaled material is transferred to the GI tract, so that fecal analyses will not give a true estimate of the amount inhaled. For these reasons, fecal assay for amounts of radioactive material is not dependable as a biological control measure. In contrast, bioassay of urine samples is widely used both for routine monitoring and for estimates of body burden in cases of overexposure to internally deposited radionuclides.

Interpretation of the results of bioassay analyses requires a consideration of the physical and chemical state of the incorporated radionuclide, the route of entry into the body, and the patterns of absorption, translocation, deposition, and elimination from the body. Compartment models of varying degree of complexity have been devised to assist in the interpretation of bioassay data. Some of these that permit estimates of body burden on the basis of urine assay data are given by Dolphin and Jackson (1964) and by ICRP Publication 10 (1968). The latter report has a very succinct discussion of the problems of radionuclide metabolism as they relate to bioassay procedures.

References

Dolphin GW, Jackson S: Interpretation of bioassay data, in *Assessment of Radioactivity in*

Man. Vienna, International Atomic Energy Agency, 1964, vol 1 pp 329–354.

ICRP: *Report of Committee IV on Evaluation of Radiation Doses to Body Tissues from Internal Contamination due to Occupational Exposure*, ICRP Publication 10. Oxford, Pergamon Press, 1968.

Examination of the blood   Because of the known toxic effects of radiation on the hematopoietic system, especially in the acute radiation syndrome, white blood cell counts were used at one time to monitor working population exposure. With the realization that exposures of the order of 100 R were required to produce definitive hematologic effects, it was concluded in the early 1950s that the use of routine blood counts for monitoring personnel was probably without value, and the procedure was generally abandoned by 1955. Ingram (1952) discovered that the bilobed lymphocyte, a distinctly abnormal cell, was associated with radiation overexposure in cyclotron workers. However, the appearance of such cells is so infrequent that it is not feasible to use this observation as a means of monitoring personnel.

Chromosome aberrations   Analysis of lymphocyte chromosomes has become a means of evaluating the extent of radiation changes produced by external and by internal irradiation. Ionizing radiation has been found to produce chromosome aberrations in peripheral leukocytes, and these abnormalities have been found to be persistent. Such changes have been demonstrated in the lymphocytes of persons exposed to radiation from diagnostic x-rays (Bloom and Tijo, 1964), therapeutic x-rays (Court Brown et al., 1965; Warren and Meisner, 1965), radiation accidents (Bender, 1964), survivors of the bombing of Hiroshima and Nagasaki (Doida et al., 1965), and chronic occupational exposure (Court Brown et al., 1965; Norman et al., 1964). After Tough et al. (1960) had shown that therapeutic irradiation readily produced chromosome damage that was detectable in human white blood cells, Bender (1964) examined the chromosomes of peripheral blood leukocytes from a number of men who had been exposed to whole body, mixed gamma-ray and fission neutron irradiation, where the doses were estimated to range from 22.8 to 365 rad. In those persons whose dose exceeded 230 rad there was an increased frequency of aneuploid cells and grossly altered chromosomes with rings, dicen-

trics, and minutes. The gross chromosomal aberrations persisted and were seen 3½ years after the accident. Similar findings were noted by Norman et al. (1964) in chromosome studies made on a group of 33 radiation workers with a lifetime dose in excess of 10 R, accumulated at a median dose of 1.4 R per year. Here, the frequency of morphological changes was significantly higher than in the control population. Abnormalities were also seen with a higher frequency than normal in peripheral blood cells in Japanese atom bomb survivors where they persisted for as long as 18 years (Doida et al., 1965).

Boyd et al. (1966) studied the chromosomes in cell cultures of peripheral blood from women who were formerly dial painters in Britain. He found the incidence of structurally abnormal chromosomes to be higher in this group than in a nonexposed, randomly selected control population. A very careful study of a patient who had acquired a radium-226 body burden by inhalation and ingestion while working in a radium reprocessing plant for one year was reported by Brown et al. in 1968. Cytogenetic analysis revealed acentric and translocated chromosomes, but dicentric and ring forms were not present, a finding that confirmed the minimal body burden since the latter abnormalities are usually associated with relatively larger radiation doses.

While karyotype analysis of peripheral blood leukocytes is a laborious procedure, experience suggests that it has a role in the evaluation of previous exposure to radiation. It may be especially important after exposure to undetected external radiation that can no longer be measured or retrospectively estimated. The full biological and genetic significance of these changes in peripheral blood cells remains to be elucidated, especially since there is evidence of an efficient repair mechanism (Wolff, 1961). Whether chromosome abnormalities can be employed as a quantitative indicator of exposure to low doses of ionizing radiation will depend upon standardization of techniques of cell culture (Court Brown et al., 1965).

References

Bender MA: Chromosome aberrations in irradiated human subjects. *Ann NY Acad Sci* 1964; 114:249–251.

Bloom AD, Tijo JH: *In vivo* effects of diagnostic radiation on human chromosomes. *N Engl J Med* 1964;270:1341–1344.

Boyd JT, Court Brown WM, Vennart J, et al: Chromosome studies on women formerly employed as luminous-dial painters. *Br Med J* 1966; 1:377–382.

Brown CD, Porter IH, Gabay JJ: Chronic effects from radium-226 body burden on human chromosomes cultured in vitro. *NY State J Med* 1968;68:2641–2647.

Court Brown WM, Buckton KE, McLean AS: Quantitative studies of chromosome aberrations in man following acute and chronic exposure to x-rays and gamma rays. *Lancet* 1965;1:1239–1241.

Doida Y, Sugahara T, Horikawa M: Studies on some radiation-induced chromosome aberrations in man. *Radiat Res* 1965;26:69–83.

Ingram M, Adams M, Coonan L, et al: The occurrence of lymphocytes with bilobed nuclei in cyclotron personnel. *Science* 1952;116:706–708.

Norman A, Sasaki M, Ottoman RE, et al: Chromosome aberrations in radiation workers. *Radiat Res* 1964;23:282–289.

Tough IM, Buckton KE, Baikie AG, et al: X-ray-induced chromosome damage in man. *Lancet* 1960;2:849–851.

Warren S, Meisner L: Chromosomal changes in leukocytes of patients receiving irradiation therapy. *J Am Med Assoc* 1965;193:351–358.

Wolff S: Some postirradiation phenomena that affect the induction of chromosome aberrations. *J Cell Comp Physiol* 1961;58(suppl 1):151–162.

tion Against Radiation: A Practical Handbook. Springfield, IL, Charles C. Thomas, 1961.

Finkel AJ: Medical supervision of radiation workers. *Triangle* 1967;8:138–142.

IAEA: *Diagnosis and Treatment of Radioactive Poisoning,* IAEA Publication No. STI/PUB/65. Vienna, International Atomic Energy Agency, 1963.

IAEA: *Handling of Radiation Accidents,* IAEA Publication No. STI/PUB/229, Vienna, International Atomic Energy Agency, 1969.

IAEA: *Diagnosis and Treatment of Incorporated Radionuclides,* IAEA Publication No. STI/PUB/411. Vienna, International Atomic Energy Agency, 1976.

Kornberg HA, Norwood WD (eds): *Diagnosis and Treatment of Deposited Radionuclides.* Amsterdam, Excerpta Medica, 1968.

Lanzl LH, Pingel JH, Rust JH: *Radiation Accidents and Emergencies in Medicine, Research, and Industry.* Springfield, IL, Charles C. Thomas, 1965.

NCRP: *Management of Persons Accidentally Contaminated with Radionuclides,* NCRP Report No. 65. Washington, DC, National Council on Radiation Protection and Measurements, 1980.

Saenger EL: *Medical Aspects of Radiation Accidents.* Washington, DC, US Atomic Energy Commission, 1963.

WHO: *Medical Supervision in Radiation Work,* WHO Technical Report Series No. 196. Geneva, World Health Organization, 1960.

Medical Aspects of Occupational Exposure to Radiation

Detailed suggestions for the medical supervision of radiation workers have been published by WHO (1960), Abbatt et al. (1961), Finkel (1967), and Lanzl et al. (1965). The medical management of radiation accident victims and of persons accidentally contaminated with radioactive materials was discussed in publications by Saenger (1963), Lanzl et al. (1965), Kornberg and Norwood (1968), IAEA (1963,1969,1976), and NCRP (1980). Of great value to those having responsibility for the protection of radiation workers are many of the reports of the National Council on Radiation Protection and Measurements (NCRP), some of which are listed in the Appendix.

References

Abbatt JD, Lakey JRA, Mathias DJ: *Protec-*

SECTION EIGHT
DUSTS

1 • *Introduction*

The character of the inhaled dust is the critical factor in the production of identifiable industrial dust disease. Fundamental is the fact that only a very few particles of dust greater in diameter than 5 μm will be deposited in the respiratory tract while those inhaled particles with diameters less than 0.5 μm are immediately exhaled and so leave the lung without exerting local harmful effects. These rather simple limits hold for roughly spherical particles but they are inadequate for evaluating the respirability of fibers, where aerodynamic equivalents have to be considered (Gross, 1981). These equivalent diameters are calculated from fiber lengths and actual cylinder diameters (Timbrell, 1965), and have been reported by Gross for amosite and glass fibers. Nonrectilinear fibers, such as chrysotile, have aerodynamic equivalent diameters that increase in proportion to their deviations from rectilinearity. In addition, inhaled particles become deposited in the mouth and especially in the nasal passages and on nasal hair. This collection has been subjected to considerable experimental study in man, and statistical analyses have enabled calculations to be made of various deposition probabilities (Yu et al., 1981).

The amount of dust inhaled, the integrity of the normal anatomic defenses, and the rate at which the dust is introduced are important factors contributing to pathologic changes. The literature dealing with the pneumonoconioses requires that the reader keep in mind the variations of these etiologic factors, especially the differing kinds of dusts inhaled in different parts of the world. Certain underground mining operations, for example, require the use of sand for traction in transporting ore out of the mines, a practice causing silicosis. Other jobs in the same mine may involve little or no silica exposure but may involve the hazardous inhalation of finely divided coal dust and blasting fumes that cause a different but potentially disabling form of chronic chest disease. Knowledge of how much of what dust is capable of causing disease is scanty and imprecise. Methods of measurement of dust actually deposited in the lung and assay of tissue are not well worked out, and only in the past 60 years have serious efforts been made to develop such knowledge. Increasingly sophisticated instrumentation and international use of recommended safe levels of exposure are rapidly contributing much needed information in this field.

The terminology used in describing dust-induced diseases needs to be understood. The generic term for these diseases is "pneumonoconioses," derived from the words *pneumono* (lung) and *cono* (dust), with a terminal ending that denotes reaction to dust in the lung. A group of cases associated with the inhalation of a single or predominant etiologic dust is spoken of as a "pneumonoconiosis," usually shortened for convenience to "pneumoconiosis." Silicosis, asbestosis, baritosis, and siderosis are identified kinds of pneumoconioses. If the dust elicits no inflammatory reaction in the lung, it is referred to as a "benign pneumoconiosis," such as is the case with stannosis arising in tin mining. There are many dusty operations leading to chronic lung illness that involve exposure to more than one dust, each of which could cause pathologic changes that depend upon its character and the amount of respirable dust inhaled. The term "mixed dust pneumoconioses" is best used for this category. Some authors prefer to use a diagnostic term identifying the dust in terms of the offending agents, for example, anthracosilicosis for the disease of underground coal miners inhaling both silica and coal. The dust diseases are local respiratory tract diseases and the term "pneumoconioses" is best reserved for this group. It is not properly applied to systemic disease such as beryllium disease, which has been shown to affect a number of organs and biochemical systems.

337

References

Gross P: Consideration of the aerodynamic equivalent diameter of respirable mineral fibers. *Am Ind Hyg Assoc J* 1981;42:449–452.

Timbrell V: The inhalation of fibrous dusts. *Ann NY Acad Sci* 1965;132:255–273.

Yu CP, Diu CK, Soong TT: Statistical analysis of aerosol deposition in nose and mouth. *Am Ind Hyg Assoc J* 1981;42:726–733.

2 • Benign Dusts

Certain industrial operations, unless carefully controlled by ventilation, produce large quantities of dust of particle sizes known to reach the peripheral lung airways and alveoli. When they are composed of minerals, such dusts are opaque to x-rays and, if present in sufficient amounts, produce a chest roentgenogram of startling appearance. The term benign is used to describe such dusts because, especially if they are not mixed with free silica, they are not fibrogenic and lie within the reticulum framework of the lung without provoking inflammatory responses. However, if the amount of dust is excessive, as a result of either long exposure or intense exposure over a short period, such inert dust can produce damage by overwhelming the lymphatic drainage, by obstructing blood vessels, and by distorting the anatomy of the terminal bronchioles to cause infarction, necrosis, bronchiectasis, and atalectasis. Since the precise quality and quantity of inhaled dust is often unknown, the literature on the subject of benign dust disease is confusing. Few such pneumoconioses have been described in which groups of workers have been exposed to a single clearly identified dust. Yet, because of its relatively harmless character, it is essential that benign pneumoconiosis be correctly diagnosed. Workers can be made invalids or denied jobs because of striking chest roentgenograms that suggest, among other diagnoses, tuberculosis, silicosis, or metastatic disease.

Iron

Siderosis is caused by exposure to iron oxide dust. Chest x-ray changes of this pneumoconiosis are easily confused with those of silicosis, hemosiderosis, and a host of diseases producing bilateral densities. Workers using electric arc or oxyacetylene equipment in welding, cutting, grinding, or polishing are at risk, especially when working in closed spaces such as boilers, tanks, and below decks of ships. The high temperatures of welding operations produce a fume of iron oxide that is readily inhaled in the absence of complete protection. Because of the heat and physical effort required in this work, it is often impossible for the welder to wear a useful mask except for very short periods. Jeweller's rouge, which contains ferric oxide, is used for fine polishing and in high exposures can also cause siderosis. Other sources of siderosis include the manufacture of iron oxide, iron shot, sieving and bagging of powder from emery rock, and grinding with an emery wheel. Emery is an abrasive that is a mixture of corundum with either magnetite or hematite.

Well-studied series of workers with siderosis show no increase in morbidity or mortality from respiratory disease. If exposure ceases, the dramatic chest x-ray abnormalities disappear (Sander, 1944; Doig and McLaughlin, 1948; Morgan and Kerr, 1963). The few necropsy reports confirm the fact that the nodules of siderosis are collections of iron oxide particles with no fibrosis. Considerable dust may be caught in the respiratory tract defenses and expelled in sputum, well known to the worker because of its rust color. The remaining iron oxide accumulates in lymphoid tissue along bronchi, around blood vessels, or at the bifurcation of bronchi. If a worker exposed to iron oxide is short of breath or has abnormal lung function indices, it is important to discover whether or not he has also inhaled a fibrogenic dust such as silica in addition to the iron (Charr, 1956). HLH cared for a patient who developed a disabling respiratory disease as a result of sandblasting rust from locomotive engines. Necropsy confirmed the presence of both siderosis and severe silicosis. Meyer et al. (1967), reporting a case of pulmonary fibrosis in an arc

340

welder, pointed out that silica and metals in the coatings of electrodes and in the metals being welded may produce pathologic changes that overshadow the benign pneumoconiosis of siderosis.

The study of Faulds and Stewart (1956) revealed a significant increase in lung cancer among hematite (iron ore) workers in England. In contrast to other occupational lung tumors, these arose not in the larger bronchi but in the scar tissue of sidero-silicosis. In discussing this problem at length, Boyd et al. (1970) raised the possibility that the radioactive gas, radon, was responsible since it and its radioactive daughters are thought to be the carcinogenic agents in other groups of metal ore miners in Canada and the Colorado Plateau (see the discussion on uranium in an earlier chapter).

References

Boyd JT, Doll R, Faulds JS, et al: Cancer of the lung in iron ore (haematite) miners. *Br J Ind Med* 1970;27:97–105.

Charr R: Pulmonary changes in welders: A report of three cases. *Ann Intern Med* 1956;44:806–812.

Doig AT, McLaughlin AIG: Clearing of X-ray shadows in welders' siderosis. *Lancet* 1948;1:789–791.

Faulds JS, Stewart MJ: Carcinoma of the lung in haematite miners. *J Pathol Bact* 1956;72:353–366.

Meyer EC, Kratzinger SF, Miller WH: Pulmonary fibrosis in an arc welder. *Arch Environ Health* 1967;15:462–469.

Morgan WKC, Kerr HD: Pathologic and physiologic studies of welders' siderosis. *Ann Intern Med* 1963;58:298–304.

Sander OA: Further observations on lung changes in electric arc welders. *J Ind Hyg Toxicol* 1944;26:79–85.

Barium

Barium compounds have a wide variety of uses in industry in addition to the well-known use of insoluble barium sulfate as a contrast medium in diagnostic x-ray studies in medicine. Barium is obtained from two minerals: barite (barium sulfate and barium oxide) and, less commonly, witherite (barium carbonate and barium oxide). Barite is mined in the United States in Arkansas, Missouri, Colorado, and Nevada. Witherite is usually associated with galena and is found in England, Germany, and California. Barium compounds are used as weighting agents, in well drilling, as fillers in rubber, linoleum, and paints, and as a flux in glassmaking.

Barium miners and some workers handling barium sulfate develop, after long or intense exposure to the dust, a harmless pneumoconiosis termed baritosis, characterized by bilateral lung infiltrates seen on chest radiographs that resemble those of stannosis. Most of the early reports came from Italy (Doig, 1976). The chest x-ray abnormalities disappear after exposure ceases (Pendergrass and Greening, 1953; Doig, 1976). Some reports suggest that baritosis is accompanied by a significant increase in deaths from pneumonia and tuberculosis. Closer study makes it likely that there has been exposure to fibrogenic silica dust in such cases.

References

Doig AT: Baritosis: a benign pneumoconiosis. *Thorax* 1976;32:30–39.

Pendergrass EP: Greening RR: Baritosis: Report of a case. *Arch Ind Hyg Occup Med* 1953;7:44–48.

Tin

Stannosis due to inhalation of tin dust is recognized as a benign dust disease (Oyanguren et al., 1958; Robertson et al., 1961). Schuler et al. (1958) concluded from their studies that tin oxide fumes rather than the dust was the more likely cause of stannosis. The chest x-ray changes, like those of siderosis, are dramatic, with dense, bilateral nodular infiltrates. Because the atomic weight of tin is 119, its presence in the lung is demonstrated readily by x-ray in amounts less than in the case of iron, which has a lower atomic weight of 56. The few necropsies that have been done have shown no fibrosis around the tin deposits (Dundon and Hughes, 1950). Cases of stannosis were found in 121 of 215 tin smelter workers (Robertson and Whitaker, 1955).

There is no tin mining in the United States; case reports of stannosis in miners come from Britain, Bolivia, and certain areas in Asia. Exposures also occur in tinning and in scrap tin recovery operations. Stannosis has occurred in men working in tin processing and fettling. Organic tin compounds present an entirely different and serious hazard that does not occur in foundry operations (see earlier chapter on Tin).

References

Dundon CC, Hughes JP: Stannic oxide pneumoconiosis. *Am J Roentgenol* 1950;63:797–812.

Oyanguren H, Haddad R, Maass H: Stannosis: Benign pneumoconiosis owing to inhalation of tin dust and fume. I. Environmental and experimental studies. *Ind Med Surg* 1958;27:427–431.

Robertson AJ, Rivers D, Nagelschmidt G, et al: Stannosis: Benign pneumoconiosis due to tin oxide. *Lancet* 1961;1:1089–1093.

Robertson AJ, Whitaker PH: Radiological changes in pneumoconiosis due to tin oxide. *J Fac Radiol* 1955;6:224–233.

Schuler P, Cruz E, Guijon C, et al: Stannosis: Benign pneumoconiosis owing to inhalation of tin dust and fume. II. Clinical study. *Ind Med Surg* 1958;27:432–435.

Perlite

Perlite is a naturally occurring volcanic glass that contains abundant cracks that cause it to break into "pearls" or pebbles. When the finely divided crude ore is heated to 760° to 1100°C (1400° to 2000°F), the 2% to 5% contained moisture causes expansion or "popping" to produce a product 15 to 20 times the original volume. This product is used as a lightweight aggregate, as a soil conditioner, and in insulation, filters, and fillers. The ore and the expanded perlite are about 75% noncrystalline silicate, and the free silica concentrations are usually less than 5%.

Cooper (1975) examined the chest roentgenograms of 240 workers exposed to perlite dust for from one to 23 years, and he found no evidence of pneumoconiosis attributable to these exposures even though the nuisance dust levels of 30 mppcf had probably been exceeded. Nevertheless, he advised continued medical surveillance since some crude perlite ores contain as much as 6% crystalline silica (quartz).

Reference

Cooper WC: Radiographic survey of perlite workers. *J Occup Med* 1975;17:304–307.

Carbon Black

Carbon black consists of elemental carbon in the form of near-spherical colloidal particles and coalesced aggregates of such particles (ASTM, 1972). It is obtained by partial combustion or thermal decomposition of liquid or gaseous hydrocarbons. Different processes produce furnace black, thermal black, or channel black, and these forms of carbon black should not be confused with lampblack, acetylene black, charcoal, bone black, or graphite. Carbon black may contain traces of sulfur and of ash as well as from 0.1% to 1.5% adsorbed polycyclic aromatic hydrocarbons (PAHs) that include benzo(a)-pyrene (BaP) (Falk and Steiner, 1952).

Common soot is a form of carbon black that accumulates in the lungs to produce a blackened "anthracotic" appearance and measurable content (Lewis and Coughlin, 1973). These investigators found a significant association of cerebrovascular accidents and increased amounts of lung soot. However, soot deposition in the lungs does not date from the onset of the Industrial Revolution nor is it seen primarily in city dwellers. Paleopathology studies have demonstrated marked anthracosis of ancient lungs (in mummified materials) as a consequence of exposure to indoor fires for cooking and heating (Zimmerman et al., 1981).

Epidemiological studies in North America have revealed no unusual risk of malignancy or heart disease in carbon black workers (Robertson and Ingalls, 1980) despite the resport of Maisel et al. (1959) of a case of parotid duct cancer in a carbon black chemist. Russian studies, particularly those of Komarova (summarized in NIOSH, 1978) indicate that prolonged exposure to carbon black dust and carbon monoxide can lead to the development of a diffusely sclerotic pneumoconiosis.

The permissible exposure limit for all forms of carbon black has been set at 3.5 mg/m³ air for an eight-hour time weighted average measured as total dust. NIOSH (1978) has further recommended that this limit also include a maximum concentration of adsorbed polycyclic aromatic hydrocarbons of 0.1 mg/m³ air measured as the cyclohexane-extractable fraction.

References

ASTM: Standard definition of terms relating to carbon black, Designation D 3053-72. *Annual Book and ASTM Standards.* Philadelphia,

American Society for Testing and Materials, 1972, p 668.

Falk HL, Steiner PE: The identification of aromatic polycyclic hydrocarbons in carbon blacks. *Cancer Res* 1952;12:30–39.

Lewis GP, Coughlin L: Lung "soot" accumulation in man. *Atmos Environ* 1973;7:1249–1255.

Maisel B, Pearce C, Connolly J, et al: Carbon-black carcinoma of Stensen's duct. Report of a case. *Arch Surg* 1959;78:331–339.

NIOSH: *Criteria for a Recommended Standard . . . . Occupational Exposure to Carbon Black*. Washington, DC, National Institute for Occupational Safety and Health (NIOSH 78-204), 1978.

Robertson J McD, Ingalls TH: A mortality study of carbon black workers in the United States from 1935 to 1974. *Arch Environ Health* 1980;35:181–186.

Zimmerman MR, Trinkaus E, LeMay M, et al: The paleopathology of an Aleutian mummy. *Arch Pathol Lab Med* 1981;105:638–641.

3 • Fibrogenic Dusts

Silica (Silicon Dioxide)

Agricola observed in the mid-16th century that women living in the Carpathian mountains might each have as many as seven husbands since the men working in the local mines died of pulmonary disease at a young age. In the years since that time, reports of mineral dust diseases of the chest have come from all countries where mining is done. It is now known that such illness was in large part due to the fact that quartz, called silica (silicon dioxide, SiO_2), which is abundant in the earth, has fibrogenic properties and is unique in acting synergistically with acid-fast bacillary infections. The ubiquitous nature of lung disease resulting from exposure to silica is illustrated by the names for this condition collected by Corn (1980): dust consumption, ganister disease, grinders' asthma, grinders' rot, grinders' consumption, masons' disease, miners' asthma, miners' phthisis, potters' rot, sewer disease, stonemasons' disease, chalicosis, shistosis.

In 1932, the Committee on Silicosis of the American Public Health Association defined this illness as "a disease due to breathing air containing silica (SiO_2), characterized anatomically by generalized fibrotic changes and the development of miliary nodulations in both lungs, and clinically by shortness of breath, decreased chest expansion, lessened capacity for work, absence of fever, increased susceptibility to tuberculosis (some or all of which symptoms may be present) and by characteristic X-ray findings" (Lanza, 1963). There are few reliable data on the prevalence of silicosis in the United States, because of failure to recognize the disease and because, in addition, there is no requirement for central reporting. Trasko (1956) found records of 10,362 silicotics during the period from 1950 through 1954, about which she wrote "obviously an underestimate of the real condition."

Because there is such a great amount of silica in the earth's crust, all forms of tunnel construction and underground mining are associated with the risk of overexposure to this substance, a hazard that is very hard to control. Silica should be distinguished from silicates, which are based on SiO_4 units. Many silica-containing compounds are useful in industry, but it is those with free silica that are serious hazards because of the fibrogenic property of this mineral. Free forms of silica are used in industry because of their crystalline character. Actually, crystobalite and tridymite are more hazardous than quartz in the pathogenesis of silicosis. Industrially important silica-containing materials are quartzite, sandstone, flint, tripoli, and diatomaceous earth. Table 11, adapted in part from Ladoo (1925), provides a list of some of the industrial uses of crystalline silica (quartz). A number of operations listed here no longer carry a silica hazard since nonfibrogenic materials have been substituted; however, they are included because of the great delay in onset of symptoms after the last exposure in some cases.

Table 11
Industrial Uses of Silica

Abrasive manufacturing	Road construction
Abrasive blasting	Sandpaper
Boiler scaling	manufacturing
Ceramics manufacturing	Sandstone grinding
Foundry work	Shipyard sandblasting
Furnace and kiln lining	Silica flour manufacture
Glass grinding	Silicon alloy melting
Gold and other hardrock	Silver polishing
mining	Slate pencil cutting
Granite cutting and	Street sweeping
crushing	Tombstone grinding
Pottery and porcelain	Tunnel work
making	Vitreous enameling
Refractory manufacturing	

343

344

Clinical aspects The symptoms of silicosis are in no way unusual. Gradually increasing dyspnea and nonproductive cough, often thought by the patient to be due to smoking habits or to age, are the usual initial complaints. Well-studied groups of workers exposed to silica have established the fact that some of them who have no symptoms will show, on routine chest x-ray, densities in the lungs. Sander (1960) believed that such men will not develop progressive pulmonary disease if the amount of silica exposure is at or below the so-called safe level. HLH does not share this view because of the fibrogenic nature of silica. Slow development of silicosis at low doses and the great variation in individual awareness of symptoms help to explain such reports. Accidental deaths have made it possible to study such cases and silicotic nodules have been present in what appeared to be normal lungs on radiography. Exceptions to the usual course are cases of acute silicosis due to inhalation of heavy doses of finely divided silica generated, for example, in the manufacture of abrasive soap powders first reported by Chapman (1932). Such patients suffer an abrupt onset of violent coughing, severe dyspnea, and weight loss. Mechanization of certain mining and tunneling operations without complete protection, which is difficult to achieve, will produce amounts of fine silica particles that can also cause acute silicosis.

In the usual case of silicosis and in the absence of infection there is a slow deterioration of capacity for physical effort. If respiratory infection occurs, dyspnea and cough are often increased and become established at more severe levels after the infection has subsided. Vague chest tightness and clinically obvious pleurisy occur in some cases. Hemoptysis is unusual unless acid-fast infection complicates the silicosis. Asthmatic bronchitis characterized by wheezing and difficulty in expiring air often occurs. Chronic bronchitis, due to direct effect of finely divided silica dust, is a possibility that is hard to establish, but emphysema is a common complication of silicosis. Smoking habits, bacterial infection, and aging are all factors that can affect normal upper respiratory tract defenses or by themselves act as complicating etiologic factors. In addition, many jobs with silica exposure may involve the inhalation of irritant chemicals, such as oxides of nitrogen from blasting fumes or welding (Becklake et al., 1957; Stoeckle et al., 1962). Underground mining in hot, damp atmospheres and operations near furnaces create other modify-

ing or aggravating influences acting on respiratory function. Lanza (1963), a life-long student of silicosis, agreed with HLH that if enough is known about the quality and quantity of the dust inhaled by the worker-patient, the notion of differences in susceptibility becomes unnecessary, except in those cases where identifiable genetic factors have been shown to be present. Such factors have been described by Noweir et al. (1980) and have included the degree of consanguinity and blood groups O or AB. Bonnevie (1977) concluded from his studies of Danish foundry workers that individual variations in susceptibility are minor factors in the evolution of silicosis, at least in a country with a very low tuberculosis morbidity. Lanza also suggested that individual resistance may in fact be due to undetected intermittency of exposure.

Work exposure to silica does not carry a significant risk of pulmonary malignancy (James, 1955), but animal studies have confirmed human experience that a lung dusted with silica is extremely vulnerable to infection by tubercle bacilli (Gardner and Dworski, 1922; Gross et al., 1960). Where pulmonary tuberculosis is prevalent in a community, death rates among workers also exposed to silica climb dramatically. There has been a decline in cases of silicotuberculosis in countries where acid-fast infection has come under control as a result of public health measures and modern drugs. An additional factor is improvement in the engineering control of silica hazards. Rodnan et al. (1967) reviewed reports of an association between scleroderma (progressive systemic sclerosis) and occupational exposure to silica and they concluded from a study of 60 patients that silicosis may indeed be a predisposing cause of scleroderma. HLH studied two similar cases but the assay of skin lesions revealed no increase in silica content.

Physical signs are of little help in the diagnosis of silicosis. Diminution of breath sounds with dullness to percussion, prolonged expiration, inconstant râles, and rhonchi have been reported. Cyanosis, clubbing, orthopnea, or serious weight loss are not usually evident until the disease is advanced. Except in acute cases or those complicated by acid-fast infection, most cases of silicosis develop slowly clinically. Continued silica exposure may increase the rate of progression, but even with cessation of exposure the fibrogenic action of retained crystalline silica continues.

Laboratory studies are also of little help. Silica may be found in urine but its interpretation is difficult in diagnosis. Silica may be found in urine of non-exposed individuals since the present methods of measurement reflect all forms of the element silicon, some of which are harmless in contrast to the pathogenic compound, silicon dioxide. Furthermore, only fine particles below 1 μm in diameter will reach the urine. Such dust is not retained by the lung and is therefore probably harmless. Lung biopsy has no diagnostic value apart from histopathologic changes, on which there is not general agreement as to specificity. Further investigation is needed to establish the value of x-ray diffraction and spectrographic analyses of lung and lymph node samples. Large-sized samples of post-mortem tissue from proven silicotic patients have more silica in lung tissue than do control samples (Drinker and Hatch, 1954; Harrison et al., 1967). Sedimentation time, hematrocit, sputum culture, and tuberculin skin testing are obvious steps in the study of a case of suspected silicosis. Vectorcardiograms may be helpful in discovering early cor pulmonale.

Lung function studies can be helpful in assessing impairment but the literature is confusing and sometimes contradictory, and no functional test is specific for silicosis (Ziskind et al., 1976). It should be noted that silicosis may be seen on x-ray films without any measurable disturbance in lung function. Cugell et al. (1956) and Becklake et al. (1958) measured the diffusing capacity of silicotics and found a decrease during exercise in some cases. In cases of some years' duration, there may be a reduction in functional residual capacity with relatively normal air flow, results that reflect pulmonary fibrosis. When secondary emphysema develops to any degree, hyperinflation and decreased air flow are signs of declining lung function. In acute, rapidly developing silicosis associated with heavy doses of silica inhaled in a short period (such as in sandblasting in confined spaces and in mechanized coal mining operations) there may be at the onset the single defect of decreased diffusing capacity. Thus, to some degree the pattern of lung function change is some measure of the duration of the silicotic process and its character. The work of Theriault et al. (1974) showing the relationship of dose and disease as measured by lung function tests and chest x-ray films may prove to be useful in decisions to change a worker's job rather than have such decisions made by social and economic pressures. It is interesting that this study of granite shed workers showed that changes in measured ventilatory capacity occurred 13.5 years before opacities developed in the chest roentgenograms.

Roentgenographic features The chest x-ray changes associated with silicosis have interested many radiologists in the United States, especially Pancoast and Pendergrass (1934). The clinician can be overwhelmed by the diverse schemes and classifications that can be found in the literature, although the International Labor Office proposed a standard x-ray classification in 1960. This problem is especially difficult since in some jurisdictions compensation awards are made solely on the basis of chest x-ray changes, independently of patient complaints or lung function changes. A number of factors affect the diagnostic value of the x-ray findings. Examples are exposure to inert dusts like iron oxide, alone or simultaneously with silica; atypical host response to dust illustrated by the Caplan syndrome in workers with rheumatoid arthritis (Caplan, 1953); the rate at which silica enters the lung; and bacterial infection prior to dust exposure or infection superimposed on a dusted lung. Perhaps the most important factor in judging the chest x-ray film is knowledge of the stage of dust disease at which the film is taken, a matter best judged by the work history of the character and quantity of exposure to silica. It needs to be emphasized that there may be no delay or a period as long as 20 + years between exposure and radiographic changes.

The chest x-ray abnormalities are usually bilateral, the densities varying from fairly evenly distributed nodular opacities to asymmetrical shadows of all sizes. Calcification in lung and nodes are common, especially in cases of long duration, and pneumoliths have been reported (Morrow and Staskiel, 1959). It is thought from experimental evidence that silica can bind protein and calcium and this effect can explain the so-called egg-shell calcification (Scheel et al., 1954). Cavitation suggests complicating tuberculosis. Emphysema is commonly seen in the chest films except in cases of short duration after intense silica exposure. Visibly thickened pleurae are often seen. Because of mixed dust exposure, which may include a harmful silicate such as talc or an inert dustlike clay, the chest radiograph may be confusing indeed and the process may be indolent because the inert dust is thought to slow the fibrogenic action of the silica.

Most x-ray classifications of silicosis that have proved to be useful are those that have been kept simple without detailed description. Various stages of simple silicosis in published classifications refer to discrete opacities of varying sizes. As the fibrogenic process continues, opacities merge and are termed conglomerate. When infection is established the description becomes "complicated silicosis." The appearance of cavitation, emphysema, thickened pleurae, and enlarged right and left heart can best be described by a term such as "conglomerate silicosis with emphysema." The diagnosis of silicosis cannot be made by radiography alone. Miliary tuberculosis, sarcoidosis, chronic beryllium disease of the lung, hemosiderosis, and metastatic malignancies can present shadows that resemble silicosis at some stage. Careful medical and work histories are required to make a correct diagnosis of silicosis.

Pathogenesis It is an index of the importance of silicosis in causing impairment and death that many investigators in all parts of the world have been actively engaged in research on the mechanism of action of silica. Of the many theories that have been proposed, the most durable one is that the silicic acid liberated from quartz by the action of tissue fluids or phagocytes stimulates collagen formation. Studies with small animals have shown that silica provokes a rise in alkaline phosphatase and ribonucleic acid. Other studies have shown that quartz adsorbs certain globulins from the plasma (Scheel et al., 1954). Vigliani and Pernis (1958) speculated that silicosis is an immunologic disease, with acid-fast bacillus infection acting as an adjuvant. There is no agreement on the immunologic theory of silicosis although some antibodies have been found in the sera of both underground miners and dusted animals (Gross, 1960). Heppleston has suggested that the reaction of macrophages to silica involves nonlipid fibrogenic and lipid reticuloendothelial stimulating factors. The various views on pathogenesis and other aspects of silicosis have recently been summarized by Ziskind et al. (1976).

Descriptions of the pathologic changes in silicosis do not agree on the precise histopathologic picture probably because the inhaled dust is rarely silica alone. Furthermore, differences in prevalence of tuberculosis among a group of workers and the communities from which they came accounted for other descriptions of silicosis, because of the effect of silica and the tubercle bacillus acting synergistically to produce rapidly progressive damage. The unit lesion is the silicotic nodule, which, when present in sufficient numbers, is dense to x-rays and provides characteristic multiple opacities. These lesions are caused by the presence in the alveoli of finely divided silica particles that stimulate phagocytosis. The usual distribution of silicotic nodules in the upper lobes of the lung is thought to be due to the greater movement of the lower half of the lung that prevents dust deposition. Hilar lymphoid tissue retains a portion of the inhaled silica. The movement by macrophages of silica that has reached interstitial tissue accounts for the usual uneven distribution of the lesions of silicosis. Some particles of respirable size (0.5 to 5 μm in diameter) accumulate in parts of the lower respiratory tract. As a result of having penetrated the lung interstitium, silicotic nodules form outside the walls of fine respiratory bronchioles.

The silicotic nodule itself has the appearance of an onion because it is made up of concentrically arranged acellular collagen with a center of hyaline tissue made up of plasma proteins. The center of the silicotic nodule may become necrotic because of ischemia. The periphery of the nodule may be covered by a cellular layer, sometimes called the "reactive zone" (Gross, 1963). Silica particles may be stained or seen with polarized light. However, silica is constantly being removed from nodules and moved about in the lung. Such free silica may cause little reaction or may stimulate further nodule formation and confluent lesions that account for the progressive character of silicosis after dust exposure ceases.

The terms conglomerate, confluent, complicated silicosis are used to denote silicotic lesions of increasing size that displace the pattern of separate single nodules. Such lesions have been thought to be caused by mycobacterial infection only, but with increase over the years of improved control of pulmonary tuberculosis, it has become clear that this situation is not true. The confluence of nodules and the action of other bacterial infections (including those caused by photochromogenic mycobacteria) may account for the lesions of complicated silicosis in the absence of tuberculosis. It is important, however, to remember that a silicotic patient who develops active tuberculosis suffers from a severe and rapidly progressive disease. The confluent lesions consist of dense hyaline collagenous fibrosis, a few lymphocytes that usually contain silica, few blood vessels, and rarely a typical inflammatory reaction. Cavities commonly develop in the center of these massive lesions, and they may be due to infection with acid-fast bacilli or to ischemia, but because of avascularity, hemorrhage into cavities is rare. Morgan (1979) pointed out that the risk of tuberculosis persists for life in persons with silicosis and, on the basis of his experience, that chemotherapy for the infection needs to be continued for life.

The lesions of silicosis may be great enough in size to obstruct the larger bronchi (Vorwald, 1941). Secondary infection accompanying the pathologic changes of silicosis can lead to all degrees of bronchiectasis. In severe cases of silicosis, vascular changes may result from the invasion of small elastic muscular branches of the pulmonary arterial bed by silicotic nodules or from the pressure of massive lesions. Pulmonary hypertension and cor pulmonale are obvious complications. Clinically evident cor pulmonale may develop slowly partly because the patient is so dyspneic that little physical effort is possible.

Hilar lymph nodes invaded by silica-containing macrophages undergo fibrosis usually in a whorled pattern. Although it is rarely a clinical problem, the pleura may become thickened and adhesions develop. Varying degrees of emphysema, both at the bases or as bullae at the apices, are present, and may be due to the anatomic distortion produced by the pathologic changes of silicosis.

Treatment and control There is no satisfactory treatment for silicosis except that control of pulmonary infections is of critical importance. Appropriate chemotherapy should be used when tuberculosis is also involved. Decrease in tuberculosis in most parts of the world and improvements in drug therapy will continue to improve the prognosis. Steroids may be useful in cases of acute silicosis when the lung function abnormality is decreased diffusing capacity. It has been thought by some investigators that an inert dust inhaled before, during, and after silica exposure might alter or prevent silicosis. Aluminum dust has been proposed and tried both as prophylaxis and as therapy without demonstrable success in humans although studies with animals continue to be promising (Le Bouffant et al., 1977). Another suggestion has been to introduce aerosol sprays of water into the workers' breathing zone to agglomerate the silica particles to a size that would not reach the lower respiratory tract. There are unpublished accounts of the effectiveness of this procedure. Considerable interest has been aroused by the discovery that poly(2-vinylpyridine 1-oxide) can inhibit the fibrogenic action of quartz dust in animal lungs

and other tissues (Holt, 1971), but there have not been reports of the results of clinical trials with this compound.

Engineering controls such as wet drilling are first steps but rarely offer more than minimal protection. Complete individual protection by a well-fitted respirator is the ideal but in many silica-producing operations (for example, underground mining or sandblasting inside a boiler) compliance in respirator use is hard to achieve. If the job is physically exacting, a respirator that fits well and has adequate filtration is impossible for the worker to wear except for short periods. Completely enclosed protective clothing with an outside air supply may be the only safe control of some silica exposure hazards.

In the United States, the so-called tolerance limit for potentially hazardous silica exposure in a 40-hour workweek is now governed by a somewhat complicated formula: the limit for respirable crystalline silica is 10 mg/m³ of air divided by the percent SiO_2 + 2, averaged over an eight-hour workshift. This formula means that the percentage of crystalline silica in a dust sample that contains clays and organic binders, for example, has to be determined before the threshold limit value for that dust can be determined. At the present time there is no agreement on the amount of harmful silica that a worker may inhale safely. In the United States a series of formulas is in use for tolerance limit values and these involve methods of measurement, particle size distribution, and silica content (ACGIH, 1971). NIOSH (1975) proposed an exposure limit of 50 μg/m³ of respirable free silica in air averaged over a 10-hour workshift, 40-hour workweek. However, the approach of NIOSH in reaching this recommendation has provoked critical responses from Morgan (1975) and Levadie and Froines (1977).

There is divided opinion as to whether or not a worker should be removed from his job once the diagnosis of silicosis is made. Some authorities believe that periodic chest x-ray surveillance, if the respirable silica is kept at or below the so-called tolerance level, will allow men with simple silicosis to continue at the same job. However, because of the difficulty in controlling the amount of silica in the air in most jobs, the uncertainty of just how much silica can be tolerated without disabling pathologic changes, and the poor prognosis of complicated silicosis for which there is no treatment make this practice debatable. HLH has found it hard to defend further silica exposure once the diagnosis of silicosis has been made with

348

certainty. However, older skilled workers with little chance of alternative jobs should be allowed to remain at their work with as much dust control as possible.

References

ACGIH: *Documentation of the Threshold Limit Values,* ed 3. Cincinnati, American Conference of Governmental Industrial Hygienists, 1971.

Becklake MR, Goldman HI, Boxman AR, et al: The long-term effects of exposure to nitrous fumes. *Am Rev Tuberculosis* 1957;76:398–409.

Becklake MR, Du Preez I, Lutz W: Lung function in silicosis of the Witwatersrand gold miner. *Am Rev Tuberculosis* 1958;77:400–412.

Bonnevie A: Silicosis and individual susceptibility — Fact or myth? *Ann Occup Hyg* 1977; 20:101–108.

Caplan A: Certain unusual radiological appearances in the chest of coal miners suffering from rheumatoid arthritis. *Thorax* 1953;8:29–37.

Chapman EM: Acute silicosis. *J Am Med Assoc* 1932;98:1439–1441.

Corn JK: Historical aspects of industrial hygiene — II. Silicosis. *Am Ind Hyg Assoc J* 1980;41:125–133.

Cugell DW, Marks A, Ellicott MF, et al: Carbon monoxide diffusing capacity during steady exercise. *Am Rev Tuberculosis* 1956;74:317–342.

Drinker P. Hatch T: *Industrial Dust: Hygienic Significance, Measurement and Control,* ed 2. New York, McGraw-Hill 1954.

Gardner LU, Dworski M: Studies on the relation of mineral dusts to tuberculosis. *Am Rev Tuberculosis* 1922;6:782–797.

Gross P: An immunologic approach to the pneumoconioses. *Arch Ind Health* 1960;21:228–231.

Gross P: Pathology of silicosis, in Lanza AJ (ed): *The Pneumoconioses.* New York, Grune & Stratton, 1963, pp 40–47.

Gross P, Westrick ML, McNerney JM: Tuberculosilicosis, a study of its synergistic mechanisms. *J Occup Med* 1960;2:571–575.

Harrison EG Jr, Koves G, Andersen HA: X-ray diffraction and spectrographic analysis in pneumoconiosis. *Arch Environ Health* 1967;14: 412–423.

Holt PF: Poly(vinylpyridine oxides) in pneumoconiosis research. *Br J Ind Med* 1971;28: 72–77.

James WRL: Primary lung cancer in South Wales coal-workers with pneumoconiosis. *Br J Ind Med* 1955;12:87–91.

Ladoo RB: *Nonmetallic Minerals: Occurrence, Preparation, Utilization.* New York, McGraw-Hill, 1925.

Lanza AJ: Silicosis, in Lanza AJ (ed): *The Pneumoconioses.* New York, Grune & Stratton, 1963, pp 1–12.

Le Bouffant L, Daniel H, Martin JC: The therapeutic action of aluminium compounds on the development of experimental lesions produced by pure quartz or mixed dust. *Inhaled Particles IV* 1977 (part 1):389–401.

Levadie B, Froines JR: Comment on Criteria Document for quartz. *J Occup Med* 1977;19: 358–359.

Morgan EJ: Silicosis and tuberculosis. *Chest* 1979;75:202–203.

Morgan WKC: The walrus and the carpenter or the Silica Criteria standard. *J Occup Med* 1975;17:782–783.

Morrow CS, Staskiel LJ: Pneumoliths in profusion in silicosis. *Am Rev Tuberculosis* 1959; 79:512–517.

NIOSH: *Criteria for a Recommended Standard . . . . Occupational Exposure to Crystalline Silica.* Washington, DC, National Institute for Occupational Safety and Health (NIOSH 75-120), 1975.

Noweir MH, Moselhi M, Amine EK: Role of family susceptibility, occupational and family histories and individuals' blood groups in the development of silicosis. *Br J Ind Med* 1980; 37:399–404.

Pancoast HK, Pendergrass EP: Roentgenological aspects of simple silicosis and silicotuberculosis. *Am Rev Tuberculosis* 1934;29:43–60.

Rodnan GP, Benedek TG, Medsger TA, et al: The association of progressive systemic sclerosis (scleroderma) with coal miners' pneumoconiosis and other forms of silicosis. *Ann Intern Med* 1967;66:323–334.

Sander OA: Current concepts of pneumoconioses: Clinical aspects. *J Am Med Assoc* 1960; 172:1587–1590.

Scheel D, Smith B, van Riper J, et al: Toxicity of silica. II. Characteristics of protein films adsorbed by quartz. *Arch Ind Hyg Occup Med* 1954; 9:29–36.

Stoeckle JD, Hardy HL, King WB Jr, et al: Respiratory disease in United States soft-coal miners: Clinical and etiologic considerations. A study of 30 cases. *J Chron Dis* 1962;15:887–905.

Theriault GP, Peters JM, Johnson WM:

Pulmonary function and roentgenographic changes in granite dust exposure. *Arch Environ Health* 1974;28:23–27.

Trasko VM: Some facts on the prevalence of silicosis in the United States. *Arch Ind Health* 1956;14:379–386.

Vigliani EC, Pernis B: Immunological factors in the pathogenesis of the hyaline tissue of silicosis. *Br J Ind Med* 1958;15:8–14.

Vorwald AJ: Cavities in the silicotic lung: A pathological study with clinical correlation. *Am J Pathol* 1941;17:709–718.

Ziskind M, Jones RN, Weill H: Silicosis. *Am Rev Resp Dis* 1976;113:643–665.

Diatomaceous Earth

Diatomaceous earth, or diatomite, is a friable material composed of the fossil remains of diatoms, which are unicellular or colonial algae that have silicified cell walls of various shapes and microscopic sizes. Because of its physical characteristics that include low density, friability, and porosity and because of its chemical inertness, this mineral is used in many ways, especially as a filter and as an insulating material against cold, heat, and sound. Other uses are as fillers for paints, paper, insecticides, fertilizers, polishes, and concrete, and as an abrasive and to absorb water. There are three forms known to cause dust disease of the lungs in uncontrolled operations during crushing, screening, and preparing diatomaceous earth for industrial use. The dried crude material is called "natural powder." The second form is a calcined powder produced by passing the crude material through high temperatures (1000°C, 1800°F). When soda ash is added, the third form is known as fluxcalcined powder.

A study of the powders shows "natural powder" to be amorphous silica. High temperature and soda ash convert varying amounts of the amorphous noncrystalline powder to crystalline forms that are fibrogenic, an effect first noted by Vigliani and Mottura (1948). These fibrogenic forms of silica are cristobalite and tridymite. There are deposits of diatomite in various parts of the world, with large quantities in Germany, France, and California. Diatomaceous earth had been used for centuries but on a small scale until 1870 when Nobel discovered that a safe explosive, dynamite, could be made by combining this powder with nitroglycerin.

Medical studies of pneumoconiosis in diatomaceous earth workers appeared first in 1932 from the United States (Legge and Rosencrantz, 1932). Subsequent reports of pulmonary disease in diatomite workers from Germany, France, Italy, Sweden, and Denmark during the years from 1932 through 1956 were summarized by Ahlmark et al. (1960). The essence of these reports was that exposure to large amounts of the amorphous natural powder leads only to chest x-ray changes with little or no impairment. Similarly, amorphous silica dust produced from quartz vapors has been reported to produce granulomatous nodules and fibrosis in the lungs without impairment of pulmonary function (Vitums et al., 1977). These effects are obviously related to the lack of crystalline configuration of the particles.

In contrast to the "natural powder," the calcined or fluxcalcined forms, depending on the level and duration of exposure, cause dramatic chest x-ray changes and progressive pulmonary fibrosis, often with pleural involvement leading to pneumothorax, emphysema, and cor pulmonale (Cooper et al., 1958). The chief symptom is dyspnea, with no correlation between its severity and x-ray evidence of disease. Altered breath sounds, râles, and wheezes occur, with no single auscultatory change diagnostic. Cough, anorexia, and weight loss can be noted, but rarely clubbed fingers, which are characteristic of patients with chronic chest disease. Lung function abnormalities follow no consistent pattern, with diminished maximum breathing capacity most often recorded.

Chest x-ray patterns of diatomaceous earth pneumoconiosis have been described as being characteristically linear, nodular, or coalescent. There is a difference of opinion as to whether there is a progression through identifiable first, second, and third degree stages. Emphysematous blebs and bullae can often be seen except in the mild pneumoconiosis associated with exposures to natural powders only. When confluent x-ray densities appear and form coalescent masses, they are most often seen in the apices or upper third of the lung fields. Cases of delayed appearance of chest x-ray changes and of dyspnea as long as 11 years after last exposure are known. Before control of dust levels was achieved, morbidity and mortality were high.

Gross (1963) described the pathologic changes of diatomaceous earth pneumoconiosis as a combined effect of diffuse non-nodular, interstitial pneumonitis with alveolar wall thickening caused

350

by amorphous silica plus the fibrogenic effects of the crystalline forms, cristobalite and tridymite. As a consequence, the inhalation of fluxcalcined diatomite dust leads to dense collagenous, coalescent masses, especially in the upper lung fields. Smith (1963) and others believe that a low incidence of tuberculin reactivity in cases of coalescent diatomite pneumoconiosis supports the view that acid-fast infection is not important in the pathogenesis of the coalescent lesion. This position is difficult to reconcile with the well-known synergistic action of crystalline silica and the tubercle bacillus. Gross further described pulmonary vessel sclerosis due to dust infiltration of blood vessel walls and inflammatory changes in adjacent tissues. As is the case in other mineral dust diseases, some investigators believe that an antigen-antibody response provoked by dust plus infection explains the striking conglomerate masses seen on x-ray.

Cases of diatomaceous earth pneumoconiosis occur throughout the world wherever diatomite is mined and prepared for industrial use. Recognition of the disease depends on knowledge of its existence and interest in taking a careful occupational history. HLH once saw a case of chronic lung disease with a chest x-ray film that strongly resembled advanced diatomaceous earth lung disease. It turned out that the man had worked in Boston for over 30 years in a sugar refinery, shovelling, cleaning, and screening diatomaceous earth to be used as a filter. It is likely that fibrogenic material was present in the diatomaceous earth that this worker was handling. Such single cases are rarely identified and reported.

The therapy for diatomaceous earth pneumoconiosis is the same as that in use for silicosis. If chest x-ray changes are present, even though the patient has no clinical complaints, the worker should be removed from further exposure to diatomaceous earth because of the hazard of serious impairment of health from the pathologic changes due to the inhalation of the crystalline forms of silica.

References

Ahlmark A, Bruce T, Nyström A: *Silicosis and Other Pneumoconioses in Sweden,* Stockholm, Svenska Bokförlaget, 1960.

Cooper WC, Cralley LJ, Clark WH, et al: *Pneumoconiosis in Diatomite Mining and Processing.* Washington, DC, Public Health Service Bull No. 601, 1958.

Gross P: Pathology of diatomite dust pneumoconiosis, in Lanza AJ (ed): *The Pneumoconioses.* New York, Grune & Stratton, 1963, pp 59–61.

Legge RT, Rosencrantz E: Observations and studies on silicosis by diatomaceous silica. *Am J Publ Health* 1932;22:1055–1060.

Smith KW: Diatomaceous earth pneumoconiosis, in Lanza AJ (ed): *The Pneumoconioses.* New York, Grune & Stratton, 1963, pp 26–33.

Vigliani EC, Mottura G: Diatomaceous earth silicosis. *Br J Ind Med* 1948;5:148–160.

Vitums VC, Edwards MJ, Niles NR, et al: Pulmonary fibrosis from amorphous silica dust, a product of silica vapor. *Arch Environ Health* 1977;32:62–68.

Asbestos

Disease related to the inhalation of asbestos dust appears to have been the occupational illness of the 1960s and 1970s, very much like beryllium poisoning in the 1940s and 1950s. There is an enormous literature on asbestos-caused illness, of which only a small fraction can be referred to here.

The fire-resistant properties of asbestos were known to Herodotus in the fifth century B.C., who recorded its use in royal garments for cremation rites. Charlemagne is said to have owned a tablecloth made of asbestos, cleaned by passage through fire (Lee and Selikoff, 1979). But much earlier, in the Stone Age 4500 years ago, people in Finland strengthened earthenware pots and cooking utensils with anthophyllite asbestos fibers (Huuskonen, 1980).

The exact composition of the various mineral dusts referred to as asbestos in industrial use and inhaled by workers or city dwellers may be difficult to discover in individual instances. The terminology of geology is frequently different from that of industry. At the present time, the industrially used forms of asbestos are the amphiboles (actinolite, amosite, anthophyllite, crocidolite, and tremolite), all of which contain varying amounts of ferrous iron, and fibrous serpentine (mainly chrysotile). These chemically different magnesium silicates also contain varying amounts of calcium, chromium, nickel, silicon dioxide, and water. The industrial uses of various forms of asbestos are given in Table 12, taken in part from NIH (1978). In the United States in 1974 over 94% of asbestos fiber used was chrysotile, and almost all of the crocidolite was used for asbestos-cement pipe. In general, longer fibers are used for textiles while shorter fibers are employed for less demanding applications. Exposure to asbestos dust occurs during mining (largely a surface operation), milling and crushing, packaging, transport, manufacturing operations of asbestos-containing products, and in certain applications of these products.

Certain problems need to be kept in mind in evaluating reports of pulmonary asbestosis. Because asbestos occurs in the earth along with other minerals, the recorded disease may be due to a mixture of inhaled materials, although the specific hazard of asbestos dust has been pretty well established by now. More important, perhaps, is the difficulty in retrospectively establishing the precise character of the asbestos dust exposure in an individual worker-patient or for groups of workers. For example, New England shipyard workers studied by HLH in the 1960s were found to have handled three forms of industrial asbestos in the course of removing old insulation from ships' boilers and pipes. Another important problem is whether asbestos fibers acting as mechanical irritants deep in the lung are alone responsible for the disease (Smith et al., 1972). Finely divided dust generated by uncontrolled dry operations such as milling, bagging, or cutting asbestos insulation may, when inhaled, act as a chemical provoking fibrosis and/or neoplasia (Enterline and Henderson, 1973).

Table 12
Industrial Uses of Asbestos

Air filtration	Heat insulation
Asbestos-cement products (e.g., pipes)	Laboratory hoods for corrosives
Asbestos paper	Paint filler
Asbestos textiles, clothing	Pipe and furnace coverings
Asphalt filler	Pump packings and gaskets
Brake linings and clutch facings	Shingles, asbestos boards, sheets
Electric wire insulation	Vinyl asbestos tile
Filtration media	
Fireproof steel beams	

The first case of pulmonary fibrosis in an asbestos worker was reported in 1906 in England by Murray, and was based on a postmortem examination performed in 1899. A photomicrograph of tissue from this case was recently published by Lee and Selikoff (1979). Similar reports did not appear until the mid-1920s when Cooke (1927) used the term "asbestosis" for the first

time. He also described what later came to be called "asbestos bodies" in 1929. Subsequent reports of lung fibrosis came from the United States, and from Germany and Italy.

The first reports of lung carcinoma in asbestos workers came from Lynch and Smith (1935) in the United States and from Gloyne (1935) in Britain. Other reports followed rapidly and the truly impressive increase in lung malignancy was confirmed by Lynch and Cannon (1948) in the United States. Further publications from Britain in the 1950s established the carcinogenic behavior of asbestos (Gloyne, 1951; Doll, 1955). Isselbacher et al. (1953) suggested that, since the asbestos millworker whose case was presented was a heavy smoker, the malignancy was the result of two carcinogens — asbestos dust and tobacco.

Pleural plaques due to calcification were described in asbestotic lungs by Lynch and Smith (1935) and by Lanza (1938). The etiology of such plaques was complicated when Kiviluoto (1960) published the x-ray findings of pleural plaques, confirmed by Meurman (1966) in necropsies in Finnish populations, without associated illness. It was later established that the victims lived on soil rich in asbestiform material although the exposures were too small to induce pulmonary parenchymal fibrosis. Mesothelioma of the pleura and pericardium was first reported in an asbestos worker in 1947 by Mallory et al., and other reports followed in the 1950s from Germany. In 1960, Wagner et al. of South Africa published their now well-confirmed finding of malignant mesothelioma of the pleura in workers and their neighbors in asbestos mining communities.

Gilson of the United Kingdom made a significant interpretation of the accumulated experience with asbestos disease (1965). He pointed out that a decrease in the amount of asbestos in workroom air acts to control the occurrence of pulmonary fibrosis and reveals a significant increase in asbestos-related lung cancer. At still lower doses, malignant mesothelioma occurs. Many questions are still unanswered with respect to asbestos disease. For example, what are the pathogenetic factors in asbestos-produced disease that differ from those of other dusts? Does asbestos cause malignancy without a second potentially active carcinogen, such as cigarette smoking, chemicals such as nickel, or the hydrocarbons derived from the earth where asbestos is mined, as suggested by Harrington (1965)? The vast literature to date is still confusing, and it is difficult to present dependable and consistent clinical, radiologic, pathologic, and lung function findings in asbestos-produced disease. Part of the difficulty stems from the fact that recorded reports rarely supply information on the character and duration of the exposure to asbestos (Gibbs and Lachance, 1972).

Clinical syndromes Several major clinical syndromes have been described in connection with exposure to asbestos: diffuse interstitial pulmonary fibrosis (asbestosis), benign pleural effusion, carcinoma of the lung, pleural plaques, and mesothelioma. Other consequences, such as laryngeal and gastrointestinal carcinomas may also occur. Progressive pulmonary fibrosis is the most frequent occurrence, but its onset is usually gradual, and is characterized by the worker's awareness of dyspnea on exertion. Because of this slow course and since the fibrogenic effect of asbestos is progressive, there is an apparent delay in onset since last exposure that makes the diagnosis more difficult. The dyspnea increases in severity with time and is the chief cause of disability. Even in the absence of infection, a nonproductive cough may be troublesome. In some reported series, clubbing of the fingers is an early sign, appearing before shortness of breath. Pleuritic pain is common, hemoptysis rare. On auscultation, many cases of asbestosis are found to have persistent dry râles at both bases that are referred to as asbestotic râles. These fine basal crackles may appear before abnormalities are evident on chest radiography (Shirai et al., 1981). As the disease progresses, such râles or crepitations may be heard more widely, late in inspiration, but rarely above the tips of the scapulae (Parkes, 1973). These sounds are thought to be due to bronchiectasis caused by the local action of asbestos fibers that act as local irritants in fine bronchioles and favor continuing low-grade infection. It is not usual to hear a pleuritic rub. If, as is frequently the case, there is thickening of the pleura — or in late stages, emphysema — breath sounds are decreased. If pulmonary fibrosis exists alone, breath sounds are increased.

The patient may first visit the physician after the abrupt onset of severe dyspnea because of lung collapse due to an asbestos-induced tumor. The case reported by Isselbacher et al. (1953) was that of an asbestos worker who complained chiefly of chronic backache, a symptom not unusual but not easily recognized as being due to asbestos. The patient, an asbestos textile worker, had marked clubbing, cyanosis, cough, and dyspnea, all hardly noticed by the sick man because of their gradual onset and slow progression, and thought by him to be due to heavy cigarette smoking. Necropsy revealed advanced pulmonary fibrosis in all lobes with a striking number of asbestos bodies that reflected previous exposure, together with a bronchial malignancy metastatic to the spine.

The variation in clinical findings is dependent on the duration, intensity, and quality of the exposure to asbestos (Hardy, 1965; McDonald et al., 1972). As in all chronic illness, the patient's reaction to his complaints has much to do with the clinical picture when he first decides to seek medical help. In occupational disease, loss of job, retirement age, and compensation claims may influence the patient's action, and hence the signs and symptoms a physician has to deal with in making a correct diagnosis. As asbestosis progresses, all the signs of chronic lung illness appear, including anorexia, weight loss, secondary infection difficult to control, dyspnea severe enough to cause orthopnea, and right heart involvement. In cases of asbestosis with malignancy, chest pain usually becomes intractable.

A number of cases of asbestosis have been reported with tuberculosis as a complication. Such reports belong to the days when this infection was common. Secondary infection is so usual in asbestosis that it is likely that an occasional case will suffer tuberculous infection in areas where this disease is still common. Caplan's syndrome, an unusual response to dust in the lungs of those suffering from rheumatoid arthritis, was first reported in Welsh coal miners. This syndrome, considered to be a genetically determined pathologic response, has also been reported in cases of asbestosis (Morgan, 1964; Solomon et al., 1971) although one of the earliest cases, reported by Tellesson (1961), was found on necropsy 17 years later to have multiple chronic rheumatoid nodules but no interstitial fibrosis (Greaves, 1979).

Asbestos corns or warts are occasionally seen. These are increases in the horny layer of the skin stimulated by the local action of asbestos fibers introduced traumatically. These warts produce no pathologic change leading to impairment.

Reports in the literature do not agree as to whether or not the pulmonary fibrosis of asbestosis progresses once exposure has stopped. From her experience, HLH believes that if the amount of asbestos that reaches the lower respiratory tract is large enough to excite a pathologic response and great enough to cause measurable lung function abnormality, the asbestosis becomes progressive, a view supported by Murphy et al., (1972). It may be that infection, easily established in the asbestotic lung, explains the progression to increasing fibrosis and varying degrees of emphysema, which in turn leads to right heart strain. Before asbestos dust was controlled in industry, the chief cause of death was cor pulmonale. Wyers' 1949 report, the 1966 publications of Kleinfeld et al., and the review of Becklake (1976) are helpful clinical reviews of asbestosis and its complications.

Benign pleural effusion may occur with other asbestos-produced lung diseases or may appear as a primary manifestation. Such "idiopathic" effusions have been reported by Eisenstadt (1965, 1974) and by Gaensler and Kaplan (1971) and are characterized by recurrent, often bilateral, chest pain, dry râles, signs of effusion (which is sterile, and serous or blood-tinged), and clubbing. The condition may be self-limited or it may progress to chronic pleural thickening that is relieved by decortication.

Plaques of the parietal pleura are the most common form of non-malignant pleural disease related to asbestos (Hillerdal, 1981). Other lesions of the pleura are the benign exudative disease discussed above, progressive pleural fibrosis, and thickening of the visceral pleura. The latter is seldom seen but is thought to be demonstrable radiographically by the appearance of calcium in a localized area of interlobular thickening (Solomon et al., 1979). Pleural calcifications have been associated with household exposures to chrysotile in southeastern Turkey (Yazicioglu, 1976). Progressive pleural fibrosis usually follows heavy exposure (Hillerdal, 1981) and results in severe dyspnea (Wright et al., 1980).

Malignant mesotheliomas of pleura, peritoneum, and pericardium were called to world attention by the report of Wagner et al. (1960) of cases in a crocidolite mining area in North Western Cape Province, South Africa. Similar reports have now come from Britain, continental Europe, Australia, and the United States, and have been summarized by Becklake (1976). At the present time about 400 deaths occur annually in the United States as a result of pleural mesothelioma (Legha and Muggia, 1977). This disease is characterized clinically by chest pain and pleural effusion, and chest radiography reveals irregular pleural thickening or pleural densities. Severe pleuritic pain, breathlessness, cough, weight loss, and fatigue follow. Peritoneal mesotheliomas produce dull pain followed by swelling and weight loss. Progression is rapid with average survival time from onset of symptoms of about six months for pleural tumors and 13 to 14 months for peritoneal tumors (Becklake, 1976). Distant visceral metastases may be seen in half of the cases of pleural mesothelioma (Roberts, 1976). Hyponatremia is common among mesothelioma victims, and its treatment may improve the comfort of these patients (Perks et al., 1979). A disturbing feature of mesothelioma is its occasional occurrence in persons who deny exposure to asbestos and in whom microscopic examination of postmortem tissues has failed to demonstrate previous exposure to asbestos (Hasan et al., 1977). The risk of mesothelioma appears to be greater with amosite than with chrysotile, and is particularly great with crocidolite. This risk is probably related to fiber configuration and penetration (Kleinfeld, 1973).

That carcinoma of the lung is associated with asbestos exposure has been confirmed many times by epidemiologic studies (Becklake, 1976). Such tumors are frequently bronchogenic carcinomas but the preponderance is that of adenocarcinomas (Whitwell et al., 1974). When they occur, the patients are almost always tobacco smokers (Selikoff et al., 1967; Berry et al., 1972). Hammond et al. (1979) have recently published a 10-year study of 12,051 asbestos insulation workers each of whom had at least 20 years of work experience. Nonsmoking asbestos workers had a fivefold greater risk of dying of lung cancer than did nonsmoking workers in the control group. Asbestos workers who smoked had a fivefold greater risk of dying of lung cancer than did members of the control group who also smoked. Analysis of the data showed the combined effect of smoking and asbestos exposure to be multiplicative rather than additive, with a mortality ratio of 53.24 for those exposed to both hazards compared to 1.0 for non-smoking, non-asbestos control workers. Similar results were reported by Meurman et al. (1979) for anthophyllite miners and millers in Finland.

Malignant pleural mesothelioma causes pleural effusion leading to collapse of lung and, if peritoneal mesothelioma is present, severe ascites and cachexia can occur. In striking contrast are Finnish reports of plaques of parietal pleurae and diaphragm causing no symptoms or measurable disability (Meurman, 1966).

Other cancers have been associated with exposure to asbestos. Laryngeal carcinoma has been reported by a number of observers (Stell and McGill, 1973; Newhouse and Berry, 1973; Guidotti et al., 1975), and it has a long latent period (Libshitz et al., 1974). Here, too, there is a strong association between both asbestos exposure and smoking in the induction of this tumor (Shettigara and Morgan, 1975). Asbestos bodies have been detected in two of five larynges from patients who had occupational exposure to asbestos (Roggli et al., 1980). Increased risk of death from cancers of the esophagus, colon, and rectum was found by Selikoff et al. (1979) in their survey of 17,800 asbestos insulation workers in the United States and Canada for the period from 1943 to 1976. Ovarian cancers, once attributed to exposure to asbestos, are now believed to have been malignant mesotheliomas of the peritoneum (Becklake, 1976). An excess of lymphosarcoma and malignant lymphoma found by Robinson et al. (1979) among asbestos workers confirmed earlier suggestions that these diseases, too, might be associated with exposure to asbestos (Lieben, 1966; Gerber, 1970).

Chest radiography The many reports of roentgenographic findings resulting from excessive asbestos exposure underline the diversity of chest x-ray abnormalities (Lanza, 1938; Hurwitz, 1961; Rossiter et al., 1972; Soutar et al., 1974; Felton et al., 1980). Such variability is undoubtedly related to the character of the inhaled asbestos either alone or with another dust of fibrogenic potential, plus the changes produced by complicating infection, emphysema, and smoking in long-standing disease. Careful studies have also established the presence of considerable variation in interpretation among observers (Eyssen, 1980).

In individual cases there may be no x-ray evidence of asbestosis even though clubbing is present, lung function studies show measurable impairment, and an experienced physician detects fine dry râles at the bases. In some reported series, thickened pleura is seen without visible parenchymal involvement. This finding is usually bilateral in contrast to the unilateral change due to emphysema, hemothorax, and tuberculosis. The usually reported chest x-ray appearance of asbestosis alone is that of bilateral density involving the lower third of the lung initially, giving what is referred to as a "ground glass" effect. As the disease progresses, especially if exposure continues, more and more of the lungs are involved but the apices are spared. The right heart shadow increases in size as the disease puts a heavier load on that organ. Experienced observers consider that blurring of the heart is an early sign of disease in the lung parenchyma. Reports of x-ray findings include scattered nodular densities of varying sizes that are consistent with Caplan's syndrome, emphysema, pleural effusion, infection, or the development of malignancy. Except in groups of asbestos workers whose exposures are well documented, the x-ray findings can rarely be diagnostic for pulmonary asbestosis.

The finding of pleural effusion, with or without pulmonary infiltrates, associated with a history of asbestos exposure, may be a sign of benign disease or of malignant mesothelioma. Gaensler and Kaplan (1971) reported pleural effusion without malignancy as an early sign of asbestosis. Sluis-Cremer and Webster (1972) published nine case reports of pleurisy with effusion—some with and some without asbestosis. Such pleural reactions may occur without asbestosis or malignancy. Solomon et al. (1979) suggested that a high incidence of thickened interlobular fissures is a valuable sign of prior exposure to asbestos.

Lung function abnormalities Dependable studies of lung function of asbestos workers complaining of dyspnea date from 1960 when a defect in gas diffusing capacity was reported by Williams and Hugh-Jones (1960). Since then a number of studies have documented the pulmonary function changes due to the fibrosis of asbestosis. Lung volume is reduced. If the pleural response is marked, expansion of the lung is severely limited, a change easily documented by measurement of vital capacity (Soutar et al., 1974). Decrease in diffusing capacity and increase in alveolar-arterial oxygen difference have so often been discovered to be associated with disabling asbestos effect, even in the absence of x-ray changes, that they are considered to be an essential finding in the diagnosis. As the disease worsens, ventilation-perfusion abnormalities and decrease in pulmonary compliance are indices of the extent of the pathologic changes of asbestosis and readily explain the patients' complaints of dyspnea on the slightest effort (Kleinfeld et al., 1966; Gandevia, 1967; Becklake et al., 1972). Serial lung function tests, however, are thought by Britton et al. (1977) to have little value in assessing the prognosis of individual cases of asbestosis.

Pathologic changes Pathologic changes due to the inhalation of asbestos fibers and dust vary with the quantity and kind of material. Benign pleural plaques first described in Finland by Meurman (1966) in parietal pleura are located at the sites of greatest respiratory movement. These plaques consist of collagenous connective tissue with secondary calcification. Such plaques may occur in the absence of lung fibrosis even though asbestos bodies are found in the lung.

The pathologic changes of asbestosis are those of a nonspecific pulmonary fibrosis, the severity of which can be correlated with exposure. According to Lynch and Cannon (1948), the initial reaction to asbestos particles that are forced into respiratory bronchioles and alveoli is edema, followed by chronic changes due to the action of phagocytes attacking the mineral dust. Ultimately, interstitial fibrosis leads to disruption of the normal anatomy, with asbestos-containing macrophages in the walls of the involved alveoli. The fibrotic affected areas of the lung may contain emphysematous air sacs or greatly dilated bronchioles.

In all necropsy reports of chest disease due to asbestos, the parietal, and in severe cases the visceral, pleurae are thickened. Similar involvement of the diaphragm and the pericardium are reported. While it has not yet proved to be useful as a diagnostic tool, the finding of hyaluronic acid in asbestos-caused malignant mesotheliomas and in pleural fluid is of great interest (Wagner et al., 1960).

Asbestos bodies, also called ferruginous or "curious" bodies in the past, are of great importance in the diagnosis of asbestos disease. They appear in various shapes. Some of these are as long as 75 μm, and they are found in lung, sputum, and feces. Inhalation of talc results in bodies of similar appearance. Asbestos bodies are brownish or black in color, and are often dumbbell in shape. The protein gel coating is twice as thick at the ends of the asbestos fiber as it is along the shaft, a morphological feature accounting for the dumbbell shape. Eventually, the asbestos fiber disintegrates in the tissues. Asbestos bodies were first described by McDonald (1927), Simson (1928), and Lynch and Smith (1930). The activity of macrophages in trying to engulf the asbestos fiber results in an iron-containing protein coating that is readily stained by Prussian Blue or other stains with an affinity for iron, hence the appellation "ferruginous."

Discovery of asbestos bodies in the lungs of city dwellers, reported by Thomson (1965), led to the suggestion that the rise in rates of lung malignancy in this population might be related to asbestos from brake linings in street dirt. Other studies have shown that similar ferruginous bodies were present in lungs of persons who died before the days of heavy motor traffic. Nevertheless, the proportion of lungs containing asbestos bodies has increased during the period from 1940 to 1972 in the necropsies performed in a large Baltimore hospital (Bhavagan and Koss, 1976). The finding of asbestos bodies in sputum or lung biopsy proves exposure only.

Epidemiology Epidemiologic studies have confirmed the fact that bronchogenic carcinoma and malignant mesothelioma are significant risks in those persons exposed to unkown quantities of certain forms of asbestos (Wagner et al., 1971). In Canada, for example, where only chrysotile occurs, there was only a slight increase in bronchogenic carcinoma associated with heavy exposure and no cases of mesothelioma in early studies. Later reports of both mesotheliomas and bronchogenic cancers in this work population were the expression of prolonged latency of malignant response (Robinson et al., 1979). Other recent studies have confirmed the hazard of Canadian chrysotile with respect to these malignancies (McDonald et al., 1980; Nicholson et al., 1979). Enterline and Henderson (1973) showed that exposure to crocidolite and chrysotile asbestos in combination in the manufacture of asbestos-cement pipe entailed a greater risk of cancer than exposure to chrysotile alone. Crocidolite exposures have led to a high incidence of mesothelioma among women working in gas mask manufacture (McDonald and McDonald, 1978; Jones et al., 1979). Selikoff et al. (1972) published a report suggesting that amosite alone carries a significant hazard of malignancy, and this conclusion has been reinforced by the studies of Anderson (1979) and of Seidman et al. (1979). This finding is important since at one time in the mid-1970s industry contemplated a change to amosite because of the fear of the cancerogenic properties of crocidolite. There is no doubt that amosite causes asbestosis since its fibers remain longer in the lung and are fragile, and hence are readily fractured to respirable size.

In summary, with present knowledge it may be said that all of the major forms of asbestos present a hazard and that proper engineering controls are required to prevent serious long-term adverse effects.

Treatment There is no specific therapy for asbestosis. Control of respiratory infection may influence prognosis. Steroids have been tried without success. Because of the gas diffusion defect, the use of oxygen has been helpful in the control of symptoms. Decortication of pleural thickening may also be helpful.

While there are no entirely convincing studies to prove the point, a worker with recognized asbestosis should be urged to leave such exposure. This recommendation is based on the fact that clinical experience shows the pulmonary fibrosis of asbestosis to be a progressive disease. Because of reports of increased asbestos-related malignancy in smokers, it is especially important for an asbestos worker to stop smoking.

Control   The so-called safe limit for asbestos has been frequently revised downward. A limit of 5 fibers per ml for fibers of respirable size greater than 5 μm in length was suggested by the British Occupational Hygiene Society in 1968 (*Ann Occup Hyg* 1968;11:47). The United States adopted this value but reduced it to 2 fibers/ml in 1972. In 1975, the exposure limit in the United States was further reduced to 0.5 fibers/ml. NIOSH (1976) recommended a more stringent limit of 0.1 fibers/ml ($= 10^5$ fibers/m^3), a level supported by an *ad hoc* committee in 1980 (NIOSH/OSHA, 1980).

The problems of sampling methods and counting are complex and not standardized. Complete respiratory protection with an outside air supply is essential for dusty asbestos operations. Substitution of less harmful fiberglass or magnesia with low asbestos content should be employed wherever possible. Wet methods and local exhaust ventilation may be adequate for some less dusty operations, but care must be taken to avoid contamination of the neighborhood and the general environment.

References

Anderson H, Lilis R, Daum S, et al: Household exposure to asbestos and risk of subsequent disease, in Lemen R, Dement JM (eds): *Dusts and Disease*. Park Forest South, IL, Pathotox Publishers, 1979, pp 145-156.

Becklake MR: Asbestos-related diseases of the lung and other organs: Their epidemiology and implications for clinical practice. *Am Rev Resp Dis* 1976;114:187-227.

Becklake MR, Fournier-Massey G, Rossiter CE, et al: Lung function in chrysotile mine and mill workers of Quebec. *Arch Environ Health* 1972;24:401-409.

Berry G, Newhouse ML, Turok M: Combined effects of asbestos exposure and smoking on mortality from lung cancer in factory workers. *Lancet* 1972;2:476-479.

Bhavagan BS, Koss LG: Secular trends in prevalence and concentration of pulmonary asbestos bodies — 1940 to 1972. *Arch Pathol Lab Med* 1976;100:539-541.

Britton MG, Hughes DTD, Wever AMJ: Serial pulmonary function tests in patients with asbestosis. *Thorax* 1977;32:45-52.

Cooke WE: Pulmonary asbestosis. *Br Med J* 1927;2:1024-1025.

Cooke WE: Asbestos dust and the curious bodies found in pulmonary asbestosis. *Br Med J* 1929;2:578-580.

Doll R: Mortality from lung cancer in asbestos workers. *Br J Ind Med* 1955;12:81-86.

Eisenstadt HB: Benign asbestos pleurisy. *J Am Med Assoc* 1965;192:419-421.

Eisenstadt HB: Pleural effusions in asbestosis. *New Engl J Med* 1974;290:1025.

Enterline PE, Henderson V: Type of asbestos and respiratory cancer in the asbestos industry. *Arch Environ Health* 1973;27:312-317.

Eyssen G McK: Development of radiographic abnormality in chrysotile miners and millers. *Chest* 1980 78(suppl):411 — 414.

Felton JS, Sargent EN, Gordonson JS: Radiographic changes following asbestos exposure: Experience with 7,500 workers. *J Occup Med* 1980; 22:15-20.

Gaensler EA, Kaplan AI: Asbestos pleural effusion. *Ann Intern Med* 1971;74:178-191.

Gandevia B: Pulmonary function in asbestos workers: A three-year follow-up study. *Am Rev Resp Dis* 1967;96:420-427.

Gerber MA: Asbestosis and neoplastic disorders of the hematopoietic system. *Am J Clin Pathol* 1970;53:204-228.

Gibbs GW, Lachance M: Dust exposure in the chrysotile asbestos mines and mills of Quebec. *Arch Environ Health* 1972;24:189-197.

Gilson JC: Problems and perspectives: The changing hazards of exposure to asbestos. *Ann NY Acad Sci* 1965;132:696-705.

Gloyne SR: Two cases of squamous carcinoma of the lung occurring in asbestosis. *Tubercle* 1935; 17:5-10.

Gloyne SR: Penumoconiosis. A histological survey of necropsy material in 1205 cases. *Lancet* 1951;1:810-814.

Greaves IA: Rheumatoid "pneumoconiosis" (Caplan's syndrome) in an asbestos worker: a 17 years' follow-up. *Thorax* 1979;34:404–405.

Guidotti TL, Abraham JL, DeNee PB: Asbestos exposure and cancer of the larynx. *West J Med* 1975;122:75.

Hammond EC, Selikoff IJ, Seidman H: Asbestos exposure, cigarette smoking and death rates. *Ann NY Acad Sci* 1979;330:473–490.

Hardy HL: Asbestos related disease. *Am J Med Sci* 1965;250:381–389.

Harrington JS: Chemical studies of asbestos. *Ann NY Acad Sci* 1965;132:31–47.

Hasan FM, Nash G, Kazemi H: The significance of asbestos exposure in the diagnosis of mesothelioma: A 28-year experience from a major urban hospital. *Am Rev Resp Dis* 1977;115:761–768.

Hillerdal G: Non-malignant asbestos pleural disease. *Thorax* 1981;36:669–675.

Hurwitz M: Roentgenologic aspects of asbestosis. *Am J Roentgenol* 1961;85:256–262.

Huuskonen MS, Ahlman K, Mattsson T, et al: Asbestos disease in Finland. *J Occup Med* 1980;22:751–754.

Isselbacher K, Klous H, Hardy HL: Asbestosis and bronchogenic carcinoma: Report of one autopsied case and review of available literature. *Am J Med* 1953;15:721–732.

Jones JSP, Smith PG, Pooley FD, et al: The consequences of asbestos dust exposure in a wartime gas mask factory. *Symposium on Biological Effects of Mineral Fibers,* International Agency for Research on Cancer, IARC, Lyon, France, Sept 25–27, 1979.

Kiviluoto R: Pleural calcification as a roentgenologic sign of nonoccupational endemic anthophyllite asbestosis. *Acta Radiol* 1960;194 (suppl 1):1–67.

Kleinfeld M: Biological response to kind and amount of asbestos. *J Occup Med* 1973;15:296–300.

Kleinfeld M, Messite J, Kooyman JO, et al: Effect of asbestos dust inhalation on lung function. *Arch Environ Health* 1966;12:741–746.

Kleinfeld M, Messite J, Shapiro J: Clinical, radiological, and physiological findings in asbestosis. *Arch Intern Med* 1966;117:813–819.

Lanza AJ: *Silicosis and Asbestosis.* New York, Oxford University Press, 1938.

Lee DHK, Selikoff IJ: Historical background to the asbestos problem. *Environ Res* 1979;18:300–314.

Legha SS, Muggia FM: Pleural mesothelioma: clinical features and therapeutic implications. *Ann Intern Med* 1977;87:613–621.

Libshitz HI, Wershba MS, Atkinson GW, et al: Asbestos and carcinoma of the larynx. *J Am Med Assoc* 1974;228:1571–1572.

Lieben J: Malignancies in asbestos workers. *Arch Environ Health* 1966;13:619–621.

Lynch KM, Cannon WM: Asbestosis. VI. Analysis of forty necropsied cases. *Dis Chest* 1948;14:874–889.

Lynch KM, Smith WA: Asbestosis bodies in sputum and lung. *J Am Med Assoc* 1930;95:659–661.

Lynch KM, Smith WA: Pulmonary asbestosis. III. Carcinoma of lung in asbesto-silicosis. *Am J Cancer* 1935;24:56–64.

Mallory TB, Castleman B, Parris EE: Case study 33111. (Mesothelioma of pleura and pericardium). *New Engl J Med* 1947;236:407–412.

McDonald AD, McDonald JC: Mesothelioma after crocidolite exposure during gas mask manufacture. *Environ Res* 1978;17:340–346.

McDonald JC, Liddell FDK, Gibbs GW, et al: Dust exposure and mortality in chrysotile mining, 1910–1975. *Br J Ind Med* 1980;37:11–24.

McDonald JC, Becklake MR, Fournier-Massey G, et al: Respiratory symptoms in chrysotile asbestos mine and mill workers of Quebec. *Arch Environ Health* 1972;24:358–363.

McDonald S: Histology of pulmonary asbestosis. *Br Med J* 1927;2:1025–1026.

Meurman L: Asbestos bodies and pleural plaques in a Finnish series of autopsy cases. *Acta Pathol Microbiol Scand* 1966;suppl 181:1–107.

Meurman LO, Kiviluoto R, Hakama M: Combined effect of asbestos exposure and tobacco smoking on Finnish anthophyllite miners and millers. *Ann NY Acad Sci* 1979;330:491–495.

Morgan WKC: Rheumatoid pneumoconiosis in association with asbestosis. *Thorax* 1964;19:433–435.

Murphy RLH Jr, Gaensler EA, Redding RA, et al: Low exposure to asbestos. *Arch Environ Health* 1972;25:253–264.

Newhouse ML, Berry G: Asbestos and laryngeal carcinoma. *Lancet* 1973;2:615.

Nicholson WJ, Selikoff IJ, Seidman H, et al: Long-term mortality experience of chrysotile miners and millers in Thetford mines, Quebec. *Ann NY Acad Sci* 1979;330:11–21.

NIH: *Asbestos: An Information Resource.* Washington, DC, National Institutes of Health, NIH 78-1681 1978.

NIOSH: *Revised Recommended Asbestos*

358

Standard. Washington, DC, National Institute for Occupational Safety and Health (NIOSH 77-169) 1976.

NIOSH/OSHA: *Workplace Exposure to Asbestos. Review and Recommendations.* Washington, DC, National Institute for Occupational Safety and Health: Occupational Safety and Health Administration (NIOSH 81-103) 1980.

Parkes WR: Asbestos-related disorders. *Br J Dis Chest* 1973;67:261-300.

Perks WH, Stanhope R, Green M: Hyponatraemia and mesothelioma. *Br J Dis Chest* 1979; 73:89-91.

Roberts GH: Distant visceral metastases in pleural mesothelioma. *Br J Dis Chest* 1976;70: 246-250.

Robinson C, Lemen R, Wagoner JK: Mortality patterns, 1940-1975, among workers employed in an asbestos textile friction and packing products manufacturing facility, in Lemen R, Dement JM (eds): *Dusts and Disease.* Park Forest South, IL, Pathotox Publishers, 1979, pp 131-143.

Roggli VL, Greenberg SD, McLarty JL, et al: Asbestos body content of the larynx in asbestos workers. *Arch Otolaryngol* 1980;106:533-535.

Rossiter CE, Bristol LJ, Cartier PH, et al: Radiographic changes in chrysotile asbestos mine and mill workers in Quebec. *Arch Environ Health* 1972;24:388-400.

Seidman H, Selikoff IJ, Hammond EC: Short-term asbestos work exposure and long-term observation. *Ann NY Acad Sci* 1979;330:61-89.

Selikoff IJ, Bader RA, Bader ME, et al: Asbestos and neoplasia. *Am J Med* 1967;42: 487-496.

Selikoff IJ, Hammond EC, Churg J: Carcinogenicity of amosite asbestos. *Arch Environ Health* 1972;25:183-186.

Selikoff IJ, Hammond EC, Seidman H: Mortality experience of insulation workers in the United States and Canada, 1943-1976. *Ann NY Acad Sci* 1979;330:91-116.

Shettigara PT, Morgan RW: Asbestos, smoking, and laryngeal carcinoma. *Arch Environ Health* 1975;30:517-519.

Shirai F, Kudoh S, Shibuya A, et al: Crackles in asbestos workers: Auscultation and lung sound analysis. *Br J Dis Chest* 1981;75:386-396.

Simson FW: Pulmonary asbestosis in South Africa. *Br Med J* 1928;1:885-887.

Sluis-Cremer GK, Webster I: Acute pleurisy in asbestos exposed persons. *Environ Res* 1972;5: 390-392.

Smith WE, Hubert D, Badollet M: Biological differences in response to long and short asbestos fibers. (Abstract). *Am Ind Hyg Assoc J* 1972; 33:67.

Solomon A, Goldstein B, Webster I, et al: Massive fibrosis in asbestosis. *Environ Res* 1971;4:430-439.

Solomon A, Irwig LM, Sluis-Cremer GK, et al: Thickening of pulmonary interlobular fissures: Exposure-response relationship in crocidolite and amosite workers. *Br J Ind Med* 1979;36:195-198.

Solomon A, Sluis-Cremer GK, Goldstein B: Visceral pleural plaque formation in asbestosis. *Environ Res* 1979;19:258-264.

Soutar CA, Simon G, Turner-Warwick M: The radiology of asbestos-induced disease of the lungs. *Br J Dis Chest* 1974;68:235-252.

Stell PM, McGill T: Asbestos and laryngeal carcinoma. *Lancet* 1973;2:416-417.

Tellesson WG: Rheumatoid pneumoconiosis (Caplan's syndrome) in an asbestos worker. *Thorax* 1961;16:372-377.

Thomson JG: Asbestos and the urban dweller. *Ann NY Acad Sci* 1965;132:196-214.

Wagner JC, Sleggs CA, Marchand P: Diffuse pleural mesothelioma and asbestos exposure in the North Western Cape Province. *Br J Ind Med* 1960;17:260-271.

Wagner JC, Gilson JC, Berry G, et al: Epidemiology of asbestos cancers. *Br Med Bull* 1971;27:71-76.

Whitwell F, Newhouse ML, Bennett DR: A study of the histological cell types of lung cancer in workers suffering from asbestosis in the United Kingdom. *Br J Ind Med* 1974;31:298-303.

Williams R, Hugh-Jones P: The significance of lung function changes in asbestosis. *Thorax* 1960;15:109-119.

Wright PH, Hanson A, Kreel L, et al: Respiratory function changes after asbestos pleurisy. *Thorax* 1980;35:31-36.

Wyers H: Asbestosis. *Postgrad Med* 1949; 25:631-638.

Yazicioglu S: Pleural calcification associated with exposure to chrysotile asbestos in Southeast Turkey. *Chest* 1976;70:43-47.

Talc

Pure talc is very similar in composition to certain forms of asbestos: it and anthophyllite, chrysotile, and tremolite are all hydrated magnesium silicates. Talc occurs in mineral deposits in two forms: non-fibrous (platy, or nonasbestiform) and fibrous (tremolite). In its form in nature it is known as steatite or soapstone, in industrial use as talc or French chalk. As used in industry, talc may vary from the pure form to mixtures with asbestos, quartz, and other minerals (Blejer and Arlon, 1973; Dement and Zumwalde, 1979). However, the identification of mineral contaminants in talc can be a difficult task requiring precise and sophisticated analytical techniques (Hamer et al., 1976; Krause, 1977). In general, industrial talcs are mixed mineral dusts while cosmetic grade talc is free of detectable fibrous asbestos (Hildick-Smith, 1977).

Talc is used as a filler for paper, soaps, paints, roofing materials, cosmetic powders, and leather dressings. It is also used in ceramics, in the manufacture of electric switchboards, and, like asbestos, to insulate steam pipes. Large amounts of talc are used in the cable and rubber industry.

The greatest cause of pulmonary disease due to talc occurs in workers engaged in mining and milling so-called tremolite talc, a subject well documented by a series of papers by Kleinfeld and his colleagues (1955, 1963, 1964, 1965, 1967, 1974). In the United States, early reports of pulmonary fibrosis came chiefly from New York, Vermont, and Georgia (Dreessen, 1933). Other talc-producing areas in the United States are California, North Carolina, Montana, and Texas. About 30% of the world's talc comes from the United States with Manchuria, India, France, Italy, Austria, and Japan supplying the rest.

Not all forms of naturally occurring talc are equally fibrogenic for reasons that are not well understood (Schulz and Williams, 1942; Weiss and Boettner, 1967). Certain talcs used to powder surgeons' gloves, for cosmetic powders, and to stimulate adhesion formation in lung collapse therapy have been found to vary in fibrogenic properties. Talc is no longer used to dust surgical gloves because of well documented experience that some talcs cause granulomas and adhesions when accidentally spilled into surgical wounds.

Dyspnea on effort and cough are presenting symptoms in talc pneumoconiosis. As pathologic changes progress, cyanosis, clubbing, and increasing dyspnea are the usual complaints. Diminished breath sounds, diffuse râles, and limitation of chest expansion have also been noted (Kleinfeld et al., 1963). Tuberculosis, emphysema, and right heart disease are complications of pulmonary talcosis. The chest x-ray films show diffuse bilateral infiltration of the bases and mid-lung fields, with varying degrees of widespread nodula-

tion, usually with thickened pleurae (Kleinfeld et al., 1955, 1963). Secondary infection alters the x-ray picture which is at no time specific. Lung function abnormalities, reported by Kleinfeld et al., (1965), indicate that both ventilatory function and diffusing capacity are impaired. Talc bodies, very much like asbestos bodies, may be found in the sputum as evidence of exposure, and macrophages containing absorbed dust particles may be found in the diffusely fibrotic areas of the lung. The cases seen by HLH in Boston arose after many years of exposure to talc in cable and rubber manufacturing. They ran an indolent course, steadily progressing to terminal bouts of respiratory and/or cardiac failure.

Postmortem studies show that talc causes a nonspecific pulmonary fibrosis of the lung (Seeler, 1959). In addition, foreign body granulomas containing talc fibers are to be found in the lung, pleura, diaphragm, pericardium, and gastric wall. X-ray diffraction studies of affected lung have shown that less than 0.1% of free silica is present. This fact is mentioned because for some years the opinion was held that the presence of silica explained cases of so-called talc penumoconiosis. Asbestos and talc, which as already noted are very much alike mineralogically, also have some similar biological effects. However, there are few reports of significant risk of lung cancer in workers exposed to enough talc to cause pulmonary fibrosis. One exception is the group of talc miners and millers studied by Kleinfeld et al. (1967, 1974) where mortality from carcinoma of the lung and pleura was four times greater in the 60 to 79 year age group than in the control population. Recent studies of mortality patterns among upper New York State talc miners and millers have shown an excess incidence of bronchogenic cancer especially after 20 to 28 years of exposure (Brown et al., 1979). Rubino et al. (1976) maintained that pure talc does not cause cancer and suggested that the findings of Kleinfeld and his group resulted from the presence of fibrous asbestos. Norwegian and Swedish reports that exposure to soapstone over many years caused only mild fibrosis visible on x-ray films illustrate the variation in biological behavior of various talcs (Ahlmark et al., 1960).

The permissible exposure limits for talc depend upon whether it is nonfibrous (nonasbestiform) or fibrous. For the former the TLV is 20 mppcf (million particles per cubic foot), equivalent approximately to 700 million particles per m^3; for the latter, the asbestos limit of 5/ml of fibers greater than 5 μm in length has been recommended. However, in 1975 the exposure limit for these asbestos fibers was lowered to 0.5/ml, and NIOSH (1976) further recommended a limit of 0.1 fibers/ml, or 100,000/m³.

References

Ahlmark A, Bruce T, Nyström A: *Silicosis and Other Pneumoconioses in Sweden.* Stockholm, Svenska Bokförlaget, 1960.

Blejer HP, Arlon R: Talc: A possible occupational and environmental carcinogen. *J Occup Med* 1973;15:92-97.

Brown DP, Dement JM, Wagoner JK: Mortality patterns among miners and millers occupationally exposed to asbestiform talc, in Lemen R, Dement JM (eds): *Dusts and Disease.* Park Forest South, IL, Pathotox Publishers, 1979, pp 317-324.

Dement JM, Zumwalde RD: Occupational exposure to talcs containing asbestiform materials, in Lemen R, Dement JM (eds): *Dusts and Disease.* Park Forest South, IL, Pathotox Publishers, 1979, pp 287-305.

Dreessen WC: Effects of certain silicate dusts on lungs. *J Ind Hyg* 1933;15:66-78.

Hamer DH, Rolle FR, Schelz JP: Characterization of talc and associated minerals. *Am Ind Hyg Assoc J* 1976;37:296-304.

Hildick-Smith G: Talc—Recent epidemiological studies. *Inhaled Particles* 1977;IV Part 2: 655-665.

Kleinfeld M, Messite J, Tabershaw IR: Talc pneumoconiosis. *Arch Ind Health* 1955;12:66-76.

Kleinfeld M, Giel CP, Majeranowski JF, et al: Talc pneumoconiosis: Report of six patients with postmortem findings. *Arch Environ Health* 1963;7:101-115.

Kleinfeld M, Messite J, Shapiro J: Lung function in talc workers. *Arch Environ Health* 1964; 9:559-566.

Kleinfeld M, Messite J, Shapiro J: Effect of talc dust on lung function. *Arch Environ Health* 1965;10:431-437.

Kleinfeld M, Messite J, Kooyman O, et al: Mortality among talc miners and millers in New York State. *Arch Environ Health* 1967;14:663-667.

Kleinfeld M, Messite J, Zaki MH: Mortality experiences among talc workers: A follow-up study. *J Occup Med* 1974;16:345-349.

Krause JB: Mineralogical characterization of cosmetic talc products. *J Toxicol Environ Health* 1977;2:1223-1226.

NIOSH: *Revised Recommended Asbestos Standard.* Washington, DC, National Institute for Occupational Safety and Health (NIOSH 77-169) 1976.

Rubino GF, Scansetti G, Piolatto G, et al: Mortality study of talc miners and millers. *J Occup Med* 1976;18:186-193.

Schulz RZ, Williams CR: Commercial talc: Animal and mineralogical studies. *J Ind Hyg Toxicol* 1942;24:75-79.

Seeler AO, Gryboski JS, MacMahon HE: Talc pneumoconiosis. *Arch Ind Health* 1959;19: 392-402.

Weiss B, Boettner EA: Commercial talc and talcosis. *Arch Environ Health* 1967;14:304-308.

4 • *Mixed Dusts*

Introduction

Mineral pneumoconiosis is rarely caused by the inhalation of a single dust and should, therefore, be referred to as mixed dust pneumoconiosis. Much of the literature on the subject is confusing because of failure to measure and report the nature and quantity of dust of respirable size that the worker-patient has inhaled. A number of dusts have been judged to be inert biologically, and the action of associated harmful dusts is reported to explain pathologic change. Many students of dust disease have speculated on the additive, synergistic, or modifying effects of different dusts in combination. A variety of animal experiments have been undertaken to explore such possibilities without uniform agreement as to the meaning of the findings in explaining the development of pneumoconiosis in human lungs (Zaidi, 1969).

Mixed dust pneumoconioses are found in foundries where controls are inadequate and the workers are exposed to dust composed of iron, silicates, and silica (McLaughlin and Harding, 1956). Hamlin's (1953) report of a case of anthrasilicosis in a foundry worker is often cited as an illustration of pulmonary disease caused by two dusts inhaled simultaneously. Hematite miners and boiler scalers develop a chest disease that, because they are exposed to silica as well as to iron, is named siderosilicosis. Granite drillers suffer from mixed dust disease because of the high silica content of the rock. Barrie and Harding (1947) described the microscopic pathologic changes in cases of argyrosiderosis in the lungs of workers who polished silver with rouge (pure iron oxide). These cases showed deposits of iron in the lymphatic drainage and silver in the elastica of the arterial and alveolar walls. Emphysema but no fibrosis was encountered. Although these workers developed a cough productive of rust-colored sputum, no obvious physical impairment has been reported with argyrosiderosis. Other examples of mixed dust pneumoconioses discussed by Mark et al. (1979) usually have silica as one of the constituent minerals. In such cases, mixed dust fibrosis (MDF) occurs, a term originally proposed by McLaughlin (1950) for a condition encountered in foundry workers.

Chest x-ray abnormalities in such cases are a severe hindrance to a worker seeking employment, and in most medical centers in the United States excessive diagnostic procedures including lung biopsy are the usual fate of such a worker.

There are a number of reports of other pneumoconioses considered to be associated with exposure to a wide variety of mineral dusts of differing geologic and chemical character. Diagnostic titles usually refer to the incriminated dusts. Some, but not all, of these conditions are described in this chapter for reference and to help the physician correctly diagnose pulmonary disease in a patient or in a group of workers in the dusty trades.

References

Barrie HJ, Harding HE: Argyro-siderosis of the lungs in silver finishers. *Br J Ind Med* 1947; 4:225–229.

Hamlin LE: Anthracosilicosis occurring in a foundry employee. *Arch Ind Hyg Occup Med* 1953;7:339–351.

Mark GJ, Monroe CB, Kazemi H: Mixed pneumoconiosis: Silicosis, asbestosis, talcosis, and berylliosis. *Chest* 1979;75:726–728.

McLaughlin AIG: *Industrial Lung Diseases of Iron and Steel Foundry Workers*. London, H. M. Stationery Office, 1950.

362

McLaughlin AIG, Harding HE: Pneumoconiosis and other causes of death in iron and steel foundry workers. *Arch Ind Health* 1956;14: 350–378.

Zaidi SH: *Experimental Pneumoconiosis.* Baltimore, MD, Johns Hopkins, 1969.

Graphite

Graphite, one of the two forms of mineral carbon (the other being diamond), is also known as plumbago or black lead. It is one of the softest minerals known, and on rare occasions is found in hexagonal crystal form. It occurs in nature in granite and other metamorphosed rock, and when it is mined, free silica becomes airborne. It is also manufactured and synthetic graphite has a well developed crystalline structure. Graphite is used in foundries, in the electrical industry, in lead pencils, in the manufacture of carbon black and electrodes, in the rubber industry, and in heat exchangers, pumps, and valves. For certain nuclear reactor operations, the graphite must be pure, i.e., free of naturally occurring traces of other metals and silica.

That pneumoconiosis does occur among graphite workers appears to be established, although pure graphite, like carbon, is biologically inert. The amount of graphite inhaled and the quantity of free silica are the clinical and pathologic determinants. The case reports have varying interpretations as to precisely which dust is causative and hence what the disease course and prognosis may be. Pneumoconiosis has been reported from graphite dust exposure in mining, milling, and grinding; in carbon electrode manufacture; and from carbon and soot dust in pure carbon production. Case reports from Europe, the United Kingdom, Japan, Ceylon, and the United States make clear the fact that high-level exposure to graphite or other relatively pure forms of carbon dust produce chest x-ray and pathologic changes like those caused by coal with low silica content. Because varying amounts of fibrogenic silicon dioxide (silica) dust are inhaled with graphite in all but a few work exposures, the clinical picture may be more or less like silicosis. Iron dust may also be inhaled with graphite to produce a modified dust effect (Watson et al., 1959; Gaensler et al., 1966; Pendergrass et al., 1967; Ranasinha and Uragoda, 1972).

There are no unique chest radiographic features of graphite pneumoconiosis. The apices are often reported to be first and most heavily involved. Bilateral small x-ray opacities, without accompanying impairment of the worker, are very much like the so-called simple pneumoconiosis due to coal. Massive lesions seen on chest radiographs are thought to be due to large amounts of dust or to infection plus dust. In severe cases of graphite pneumoconiosis all indices of lung function may be abnormal and removal from exposure does not stop progression of the disease. Right heart failure or overwhelming infection are the usual causes of death.

In tissue sections, graphite can be identified by its birefringence and its resistance to conventional incineration (Johnson, 1980). The pathologic findings in the lung, like those of other mineral dust diseases, include thickened pleura, various forms of emphysema, and collections of dust with little or no inflammatory reaction. In severe cases, cavitation may occur in areas of aseptic necrosis caused by graphite encroaching on blood vessels (Dunner and Bagnall, 1946; MacMahon, 1952). If silica as well as graphite has been inhaled, a fibrotic reaction may be superimposed on the other pathologic findings, although fibrosis can occur in the absence of silica (Lister and Wimborne, 1972). Spencer (1977) made the point that giant cells containing crystalline particles may be found in the alveoli and blood vessels and in subpleural tissue, a finding that is absent in coal pneumoconiosis. Graphite bodies resembling talc or asbestos bodies can be found in the alveolar spaces, a nonspecific finding reflecting exposure not disease.

The best judgment is that pneumoconiosis caused by graphite or carbon dust is probably a mixed dust pneumoconiosis. Parmeggiani (1950) suggested that the mild disease that he found in graphite miners was due to the coating of silica by inert graphite dust. According to Hirsch et al. (1959), atypical mycobacteria may become pathogenic in a lung containing graphite, while Ranasinha and Uragoda (1972) felt that, at least in Ceylon, massive fibrosis was associated with tuberculous infection.

References

Dunner L, Bagnall DJT: Graphite pneumoconiosis complicated by cavitation due to necrosis. *Br J Radiol* 1946;19:165–168.

Gaensler EA, Cadigan JB, Sasahara AA: Graphite pneumoconiosis of electrotypers. *Am J Med* 1966;41:864–882.

Hirsch MJ, Kass I, Schaefer WB, et al: Infection with atypical tubercle bacilli in graphite pneumoconiosis. *Arch Intern Med* 1959;103: 814–817.

Johnson FB: Identification of graphite in tissue sections. *Arch Pathol Lab Med* 1980;104: 491–492.

Lister WB, Wimborne D: Carbon pneumoconiosis in a synthetic graphite worker. *Br J Ind Med* 1972;29:108–110.

MacMahon HE: The application of x-ray diffraction in pathology (with particular reference to pulmonary graphitosis). *Am J Pathol* 1952;28: 531–532.

Parmeggiani L: Graphite pneumoconiosis. *Br J Ind Med* 1950;7:42–45.

Pendergrass EP, Vorwald AJ, Mishkin MM, et al: Observations on workers in the graphite industry. *Med Radiog Photog* 1967;43:70–99.

Ranasinha KW, Uragoda CG: Graphite pneumoconiosis. *Br J Ind Med* 1972;29:178–183.

Spencer H: *Pathology of the Lung.* ed 3. Philadelphia, W. B. Saunders, 1977.

Watson AJ, Black J, Doig AT, et al: Pneumoconiosis in carbon electrode makers. *Br J Ind Med* 1959;16:274–285.

Coal

History and background   In 1661 the English diarist John Evelyn published an essay, *Fumifugium,* in which he protested the foul, smoky air of London and first used the now popular term "black lung." This term was used for the first time in describing a coal miner's lung in 1831 (Kerr, 1980). In the 19th century, attention to coal mining was focused on social problems such as child labor and long hours of work for women. Twentieth-century medical reports of lung damage appeared from all coal mining countries at about the same time, 1928–1936. After World War II, considerable effort was spent in the study of diseases of coal miners and their control, an activity continuing to the present time. Economic interests, strengthening of unions, health legislation, and the action of citizen groups, including miners and their families, have been factors playing a part in forcing control of coal-mining diseases. Efforts culminated in the United States with the passage of the Federal Coal Mine Health and Safety Act of 1969. The vast literature on the subject of coal dust disease can be approached by reference to the *Pneumoconiosis Abstracts* (1926–1950) and volumes such as Key et al. (1971).

Reports of medical problems among coal miners include a variety of injuries, nystagmus, vascular damage from the use of heavy vibrating tools, the effect of mine gases, and Weil's disease (Hunter, 1978). The latter is a spirochetal infection transmitted by rats living in the water in mines. Only chronic respiratory disease of workers exposed to coal dust will be dealt with here.

A number of occupational factors influence the symptoms and signs of chest disease in addition to the individual coal miner's personal or medical history or the health of the community where he lives. Since coal mining may be done near ground level in open pits, or at varying depths underground or far under the sea, a variety of risks may be encountered. Variations in methods of mining cause critical differences in the particle size distribution and the quantity of dust inhaled by the worker. In the United States at the present time, advances in mechanization have led to increased output of coal with accompanying clouds of dust. Much of this dust is small in size and is, therefore, respirable and difficult to control. Coal occurs in ore varying in content in the fibrogenic dust of quartz (silica). Silica in the form of sand may also be applied to underground tracks with compressed air to provide traction for heavily laden cars, a practice leading to a serious risk of silicosis, especially to motormen. Rock dust used to prevent explosions may create a dust hazard. Deep mines are hard to ventilate, and this problem may involve exposure not only to dust but also to irritating chemicals arising from blasting charges, and to dangerous levels of carbon monoxide and methane. Blasting may produce oxides of nitrogen, and in some mines irritating vapors and fumes arise from burning cable insulation. Wages in small mines are often paid on the amount of coal an individual delivers in a day, with the result that the miner does not wait for blasting fumes to clear and he so endures exposure to harmful chemicals in spite of cough, sternal pain, and dyspnea. There has been recent interest in the possibility that the metals that occur in nature with the coal being mined may play a part in the pathologic changes found in miners' lungs (Crable et al., 1967).

In Europe and in the United Kingdom, many coal miners stay at a single job in one mine for a working lifetime. In the United States, a coal miner may always maintain a single job but a number of men work intermittently or move from mine to mine in the search for better opportunities. Such variables in work patterns need to be taken into account in deciding, both in individual cases and in studies of groups of miners, what quantities of dust have been inhaled that may be harmful, either acting alone or in concert with certain chemicals. A medical history of an ill coal miner must include knowledge of smoking habits, chronic bacterial infections, and the presence of tuberculosis or allergies in the worker or his relatives, in addition to the work history for accurate assessment of the etiologic factors in his chest disease.

Terminology A commonly used term for chest disease caused by inhalation of coal dust is "coal worker's pneumoconiosis." The word "worker" rather than "miner" is used because, for example, men who load coal in ships suffer disease identical to that of men working in mines. A term used often is "anthracosilicosis," an accurate description that reflects the nature of the inhaled dust since all coals contain not only the carbon of fossil coal but also varying amounts of silica. Confusion in the literature arises from the concept that coal without silica is responsible for a unique lung disease. Nevertheless, Morgan and Lapp (1976) in their review of respiratory disease in coal miners distinguish between simple coal worker's pneumoconiosis (CWP) resulting from carbon particles alone and progressive massive fibrosis (PMF) in which silica is also incriminated.

Considerable knowledge of chronic respiratory disease of coal workers comes from South Wales where coal is said to contain only 2% silica or less in contrast to deposits elsewhere. Coal mined in the United States rarely contains as little as 2% silica. This fact accounts, in part, for the great variation in published reports of the prevalence of CWP in the United States and other parts of the world (Morgan et al., 1973). Other important reasons for regional differences in numbers of cases are mining methods, possibility of respiratory protection, and the failure of chest radiographs alone accurately to detect the presence and character of underlying chest disease (Naeye and Dellinger, 1972; Key et al., 1971).

A variety of terms such as conglomerate, pseudo-tumerale, complicated, and massive fibrosis refer to patterns of chest x-ray abnormalities produced by infection, or dusts, or to coalescence and/or cavitation of lesions (Kilpatrick et al., 1954; Key et al., 1971). All countries where coal or metal ores are mined have adopted some variant of these terms so that the literature on the subject is confusing (Andrews and Morgan, 1972; Reger et al., 1973). Stoeckle et al. (1962) introduced the term "disabling respiratory disease of coal miners" to convey the fact that chronic bronchitis and lung damage due to chemicals, as well as finely divided coal dust and infection, are etiologic factors in varying combinations that explain disease and disability. These authors argued that the terms "coal worker's pneumoconiosis," "black lung," and "anthrocosilicosis," referring as they do to damaging dust in the lung, ignore a number of etiologic factors, some of which are still poorly understood.

Clinical syndrome There is nothing distinctive about the clinical picture of chronic respiratory disease of coal workers. The onset is gradual, often forcing the patient to seek medical advice for the first time only after a bacterial infection or heavy exposure to fumes in a mine accident (Stoeckle et al., 1962; Key et al., 1971). Cough, wheezing, severe dyspnea, and complaint of sputum production varies with infection and smoking habits. The sputum is usually black, and in advanced disease large amounts of thick material referred to as melanosis are produced as a result of cavities caused by aseptic necrosis. Once the disease is symptomatic, the clinical course is that of chronic lung disease of any etiology. Tuberculosis and bacterial pneumonia, although more manageable with modern chemotherapy, are serious complications. Pulmonary arterial circulation involvement and right heart failure, secondary to emphysema and hypoxia, lead to increased impairment and to death. O'Brien (1972) reported pleural adhesions in coal miners.

The diagnosis of penumoconiosis in a single, individual coal miner (James and Thomas, 1956; Naeye and Dellinger, 1970) requires an accurate assessment of work exposures, and knowledge that has accumulated regarding chest x-ray abnormalities and lung function changes from studies of groups of coal workers. Data from many sources—earlier from abroad and more recently from the United States—describe the quality and quantity of inhaled dust and its correlation with disease, and makes possible accurate diagnosis.

Chest radiography Many schemes of classification of chest x-rays have been proposed as an aid to diagnosis and understanding the reaction of the lung to mineral dusts of underground mining. Jones and Dreessen (1936) suggested a classification of x-ray changes showing correlation with dose of coal dust inhaled. In the years since then, many changes in terminology and technique have been tried. Fletcher and Oldham (1949) introduced the important concept of "observer error" and modern practice has come to require that more than one radiologist read a film. Even so, considerable observer variation exists in evaluation of chest radiographs (Reger et al., 1973). The International Classification of Radiographs, developed by the International Labour Office in Geneva (ILO, 1959) has been widely distributed. An expansion of this system was developed in 1965 by the International Union Against Cancer (UICC) and was further refined by an international conference of experts in Cincinnati in 1967. This revised system is now known as the *UICC/ Cincinnati Classification of the Radiographic Appearances of Pneumoconioses* and was published as a special report (*Chest* 1970;58:57–67). This classification is based on a systematic and quantitative assessment of small opacities (rounded or irregular), large opacities, pleural thickening and uncalcified plaques, ill-defined diaphragm and/or cardiac outline, and pleural calcification. Chest x-rays of coal workers interpreted by use of this system have been a standard procedure in the United States since the passage of the 1969 Federal Coal Mine Health and Safety Act (Seaton et al., 1972). The x-ray findings and their position in the classification are used to decide what disability benefits are to be awarded. Hall et al. (1975) and Jagoe and Paton (1975) have independently proposed computer programs for measuring and classifying chest radiographs in series of simple pneumoconioses.

Hardy (1967) questioned the value of x-ray classifications, especially in the absence of accurate exposure histories. Because of the many causes of pulmonary fibrosis characterized by bilateral lung densities on x-rays, there appears to be little merit in insisting on any classification as an aid to diagnosis in an individual patient. For example, category zero, implying no disease, thus excludes cases of emphysema with too little dust to be radiopaque. However, there may be great value in the application of chest x-ray classification in the study of groups of workers. Cochrane (1960), studying well-defined South Wales mining populations and using chest x-ray classification, has contributed important knowledge of the epidemiology of coal dust disease and has provided a model for study of pneumoconiosis of any cause in groups exposed to an identifiable and measurable dust. Clinical judgment and aware-

ness that disease may be present despite a so-named normal radiograph will lead to a wiser method of settling coal miners' claims for compensation (Amandus et al., 1973). A study by Rossiter (1972) showing a dose response relation between dust inhaled and x-ray classification points to one method of improving the present system of awarding benefits or taking a miner from his job on the basis of x-ray changes alone.

Lung function changes   Lapp and Seaton (1971) have summarized the many studies first published by British and Belgian authors, except for the 1949 report of Gordon et al. Depending on the severity of the disease, all lung function indices may be abnormal, and, as is true of disability, the chest x-ray findings may not be correlated with lung function changes. In his study of West Virginia coal miners, Hyatt (1971) found the prevalence of individual symptoms (cough, phlegm, dyspnea, wheezing, aggravation by inclement weather, and increased frequency of episodes of illness) to be associated with decrease in pulmonary function as measured by lowered maximal midrespiratory flow.

It is important that there may be an increase in alveolar-arterial difference in simple pneumoconiosis as well as evidence of emphysema undetected by x-ray (Lavenne, 1960; Reid, 1967; Rasmussen 1971; Morgan et al., 1972). These findings mean that x-ray pneumoconiosis Categories 0 and 1 of the International Classification can be associated with disabling disease. Furthermore, the influence of inhaled lung toxicants that cause bronchitis, pneumonitis, and emphysema may be best measured by pulmonary function studies. These facts require the attention of United States physicians because the 1969 federal legislation awards benefits on the basis of chest x-ray abnormalities. There is a confusing and serious defect in the law inasmuch as disabling disease of coal workers can occur, as shown by lung function studies and pathologic findings, without demonstrable radiographic abnormalities.

Pathologic findings   Coal particles penetrate the lower respiratory tract and are taken up by the lung macrophages if they are below 5 μm in diameter. In contrast to silica, coal does not harm the macrophages that distribute the dust throughout the lung. During a bacterial infection, the coal-laden macrophage may "dump" the coal particles in the involved lung area, a process that may account for conglomerate lesions visible on x-ray. Inhaled coal containing less than 2% silica is held in a reticulin network without causing a fibrotic reaction; this is called simple pneumoconiosis (Gough, 1949). This stage, depending on the quantity of dust in the lung, appears on chest radiographs as bilateral, widely disseminated shadows described as linear or nodular opacities. Heppleston (1954) showed that, by accumulation of coal dust both inside and adjacent to the respiratory bronchioles, distortion of the normal anatomy occurs that leads to local emphysema, which he named focal. Leopold and Gough (1957) pointed out that infection plus dust further destroys the structures leading into the alveoli to produce what is now called centrilobular emphysema. Reid (1967) preferred to call it centriacinar emphysema. Depending upon the quantity inhaled, coal dust may be distributed throughout the lung, and the lesions of centrilobular emphysema can result in disabling disease. Distortions thus produced lead to shadows on x-ray variously described as confluent, complicated, or as characteristic of progressive massive fibrosis (PMF). Reid's study made the critical point that severe degrees of emphysema are not associated with accumulation of coal dust. This situation explains a patient's disability in spite of x-rays read as showing no disease or emphysema with no opacities due to dust.

James and Thomas (1956) described pulmonary vascular disease caused by excess coal deposition in and around blood vessels leading to their stenosis and eventual right heart hypertrophy. Cavities of considerable size may result from aseptic necrosis. Rasmussen (1971) stressed the concept that perivascular coal particles deposited in the lungs of coal miners in the southeastern United States accounted for early pulmonary hypertension, a finding not agreed to by all students of lung disease of coal miners.

Lungs containing large amounts of coal dust may be invaded by bacterial or mycobacterial infection, a process creating large amounts of nonfunctioning tissue. In addition, large amounts of dust and areas of focal and centrilobular emphysema result in pulmonary hypertension and cor pulmonale. Death usually results from overwhelming infection or right heart failure.

There have been suggestions that the pathologic response to coal dust deposited in the lung depends on an abnormal host response (Vigliani and Pernis, 1958). A striking example of such response is the Caplan syndrome. Caplan (1953) observed that coal miners with rheumatoid ar-

thritis present a unique chest x-ray appearance once the dust in the lung is of such quantity as to cause confluent lesions. Recent work by Heise and colleagues (1977, 1979) has examined the possible role of immunologic factors in coal workers' pneumoconiosis. The results of a study of histocompatability (HL-A) antigens in Pennsylvania and West Virginia coal miners suggested an association between W18 antigen and resistance to the development of progressive massive fibrosis. HL-A1 appeared to be associated with resistance to the development of both simple and complicated coal workers' pneumoconiosis. Such studies, while essentially preliminary, point to a more thorough understanding of the complex factors that govern individual susceptibility or resistance to coal dust exposure and the expression of consequent disease.

Necropsy studies have shown that coal miners have a lowered incidence of lung cancer, although the x-ray changes in dust disease make the diagnosis of lung malignancy difficult. Those miners with cancer who come to surgery survive longer than nonminers, perhaps as Goldman (1965) suggested because the coal dust slows the spread of the malignant cells. Reports are contradictory. Scarano et al., (1972) found an excess of lung cancer deaths in United States anthracite miners but Rooke et al. (1979) concluded from their study of Lancashire coal miners that there appeared to be no positive association of carcinoma of the lung and pneumoconiosis.

Prognosis   Because of the economic problems and the human misery involved, dust disease of coal workers has rightly received considerable attention. Surveys of large groups in Britain suggest that chest disease of miners has little influence on mortality. Morbidity, however, is very real and is unfavorably influenced by infection and tobacco smoking. It has been shown that dust disease, even that caused by coal alone, if it is visible on chest x-ray or sufficient to cause lung function abnormalities, may progress without further dust exposure. Years may elapse before a worker with mild simple pneumoconiosis by x-ray develops disabling symptoms and then only because of intercurrent infection.

The therapy of chest disease in coal workers is that of chronic lung disease of any cause. Prevention of progression of this dust disease in an individual patient rests on wise decision and the economic possibility of early removal from further exposure. In all coal mining countries, efforts are being made to assess the quality of the coal and its biological effects, to measure accurately the amount inhaled, and to develop techniques to reduce exposure.

References

Amandus HE, Reger RB, Pendergrass EP, et al: The Pneumoconioses: Methods of measuring progression. *Chest* 1973;63:736–743.

Andrews CE, Morgan WKC: Terminology of coal miner's pneumoconiosis. *J Am Med Assoc* 1972;221:88.

Caplan A: Certain unusual radiological appearances in the chest of coal miners suffering from rheumatoid arthritis. *Thorax* 1953;8:29–37.

Cochrane AL: Epidemiology of coalworkers' pneumoconiosis, in King EJ, Fletcher CM (eds): *Industrial Pulmonary Disease.* Boston, Little Brown, 1960, pp 221–231.

Crable JV, Keenan RG, Wolowicz FR, et al: The mineral content of bituminous coal miners' lungs. *Am Ind Hyg Assoc J* 1967;28:8–12.

Fletcher CM, Oldham PD: The problem of consistent radiological diagnosis in coalminers' pneumoconiosis. *Br J Ind Med* 1949;6:168–183.

Goldman KP: Mortality of coal-miners from carcinoma of the lung. *Br J Ind Med* 1965;22:72–77.

Gordon B, Motley HL, Theodos PA, et al: Anthrasilicosis and its symptomatic treatment. *W Va Med J* 1949;45:125–132.

Gough J: The pathology of pneumoconiosis. *Postgrad Med* 1949;25:611–618.

Hall EL, Crawford WO Jr, Roberts FE: Computer classification of pneumoconiosis from radiographs of coal workers. *IEEE Trans Biomed Eng* 1975;BME-22:518–527.

Hardy HL: Current concepts of occupational lung disease of interest to the radiologist. *Semin Radiol* 1967;2:225.

Heise ER, Major PC, Mentnech MS, et al: Predominance of histocompatibility antigens W18 and HL-A1 in miners resistant to complicated coalworkers' pneumoconiosis. *Inhaled Particles IV* 1977, pp 495–507.

Heise ER, Mentnech MS, Olenchock SA, et al: HLA-A1 and coalworkers' pneumoconiosis. *Am Rev Resp Dis* 1979;119:903–908.

Heppleston AG: The pathogenesis of simple pneumoconiosis in coal workers. *J Pathol Bact* 1954;67:51–63.

Hunter D: *The Diseases of Occupations,* ed 6. London, Hodder and Stoughton, 1978.

Hyatt RE: Pulmonary function in coal miners' pneumoconiosis. *J Occup Med* 1971;13:123–130.

ILO: Meeting of experts on the international classification of radiographs of the pneumoconioses, Geneva, Oct 27–Nov 7, 1958. *Occup Safety Health* 1959;9:63–70.

Jagoe JR, Paton KA: Reading chest radiographs for pneumoconiosis by computer. *Br J Ind Med* 1975;32:267–272.

James WRL, Thomas AJ: Cardiac hypertrophy in coalworkers' pneumoconiosis. *Br J Ind Med* 1956;13:24–29.

Jones RR, Dreessen WC: Medical Studies. *Anthracosilicosis Among Hard Coal Miners.* Washington, DC, Publ Health Bull No. 221, 1936.

Kerr LE: Black lung. *J Publ Health Policy* 1980;1:50–63.

Key MM, Kerr LE, Bundy M (eds): *Pulmonary Reactions to Coal Dust.* New York, Academic Press, 1971.

Kilpatrick GS, Heppleston AG, Fletcher CM: Cavitation in the massive fibrosis of coalworkers' pneumoconiosis. *Thorax* 1954;9:260–272.

Lapp NL, Seaton A: Pulmonary function, in Key MM, Kerr LE, Bundy M (eds): *Pulmonary Reactions to Coal Dust.* New York, Academic Press, 1971, pp 153–176.

Lavenne F: The heart in coal miners' pneumoconiosis — Cor pulmonale. *Proceedings of Pneumoconiosis Conference held at the University of Witwatersrand, Johannesburg, South Africa,* Feb 9–24, 1959. London, Churchill, 1960, pp 217–219.

Leopold JC, Gough J: The centrilobular form of hypertrophic emphysema and its relation to chronic bronchitis. *Thorax* 1957;12:219–235.

Morgan WKC, Burgess DB, Jacobsen G, et al: The prevalence of coal workers' pneumoconiosis in U.S. Coal miners. *Arch Environ Health* 1973;27:221–226.

Morgan WKC, Lapp NL: Respiratory disease in coal miners. *Amer Rev Resp Dis* 1976;113:531–559.

Morgan WKC, Lapp NL, Seaton A: Respiratory impairment in simple coal workers' pneumoconiosis. *J Occup Med* 1972;14:839–844.

Naeye RL, Dellinger WS: Lung disease in Appalachian soft-coal miners. *Am J Pathol* 1970;58:557–564.

Naeye RL, Dellinger WS: Coal workers' pneumoconiosis: Correlation of roentgenographic and postmortem findings. *J Am Med Assoc* 1972;220:223–227.

O'Brien RJ: Pleural calcification in coal miners. *J Occup Med* 1972;14:922–924.

Pneumoconiosis Abstracts. New York, Pitman, vol I, 1926–1938; vol II, 1939–1950.

Rasmussen DL: Impairment of oxygen transfer in dyspneic, nonsmoking soft coal miners. *J Occup Med* 1971;13:300–305.

Reger RB, Amandus HE, Morgan WKC: On the diagnosis of coalworker's pneumoconiosis. Anglo-American disharmony. *Am Rev Resp Dis* 1973;108:1186–1191.

Reid L. *The Pathology of Emphysema.* Chicago, Yearbook Publishers, 1967.

Rooke GB, Ward FG, Dempsey AN, et al: Carcinoma of the lung in Lancashire coalminers. *Thorax* 1979,34:229–233.

Rossiter CE: Evidence of dose-response relation in pneumoconiosis. *Trans Soc Occup Med* 1972;22:83–87.

Scarano D, Fadali AMA, Lemole GM: Carcinoma of the lung and anthracosilicosis. *Chest* 1972;62:251–253.

Seaton A, Lapp NL, Morgan WKC: Relationship of pulmonary impairment in simple coal workers' pneumoconiosis to type of radiographic opacity. *Br J Ind Med* 1972;29:50–55.

Stoeckle JD, Hardy HL, King WB Jr, et al: Respiratory disease in United States soft coal miners: Clinical and etiological considerations. A study of 30 cases. *J Chron Dis* 1962;15:887–905.

Vigliani EC, Pernis B: Immunological factors in the pathogenesis of the hyaline tissue of silicosis. *Br J Ind Med* 1958;15:8–14.

Clays

Clays are natural fine-grained materials found in the earth that have particle sizes that do not exceed 4 μm in diameter. They are formed by sedimentation, hydrothermal action, or by weathering. The clay mineral components of clay materials are crystalline hydrous aluminum silicates. A large variety of clays are found in nature, and many of them have specific applications in industry.

Brick clays are used for building, and fireclay is employed where resistance to high temperature is required. China clay, also called kaolin, is used for the manufacture of porcelain, as a textile dressing, as a filler in paper, and it is well-known as an ingredient in certain medications. Kaolin clay contains, before purification, some quartz and mica from the granitic rock in which it oc-

curs, and from which it is formed. Shales are related to clays since they are impure silicates of aluminum and are mined for the extraction of mineral oils.

Worker exposure to clays is considered to be harmless but there are a few reports of pneumoconiosis after long years of exposure. Because there may be free silica inhaled in some operations where clay is the chief dust and where there is little control of dust levels, cases of mixed dust pneumoconiosis may occur with the fibrogenic behavior of silica dominating the clinical and pathologic findings. Due to mechanization of some industries and especially the replacement of the older wet process for preparation of kaolin, overwhelming amounts of dust may reach the lung. The ensuing simple or complicated pneumoconiosis resembling that seen in coal workers may end fatally because of massive fibrosis, associated in some cases with pulmonary tuberculosis (Lynch and McIver, 1954; Hale et al., 1956; Edenfield, 1960).

References

Edenfield RW: A clinical and roentgenological study of kaolin workers. *Arch Environ Health* 1960;1:392–403.

Hale LW, Gough J, King EJ, et al: Pneumoconiosis of kaolin workers. *Br J Ind Med* 1956; 13:251–259.

Lynch KM, McIver FA: Pneumoconiosis from exposure to kaolin dust: kaolinosis. *Am J Pathol* 1954;30:1117–1127.

Fuller's Earth

Fuller's earth is a variable material that will decolorize mineral and vegetable oils. Its name is derived from an old process of cleaning raw wool by kneading it in water to which earths have been added to absorb dirt and oil, a practice known as fulling. Fuller's earth is frequently a clay composed of an aluminum silicate (usually montmorillonite) and traces of quartz. It is also used as a filter material, in soaps and pigments, in oil-drilling muds, as an insecticide carrier, and as a paper filler. There are published reports of bilateral chest x-ray changes in workers exposed over a period of years to fuller's earth. These are reported as fine punctate mottling with some coalescence. The response of workers to exposures is quite variable with some showing massive mid-lung shadows on chest x-ray (McNally and Trostler, 1941). A few postmortem reports describe a scattered pneumoconiosis without the pathological changes of silicosis (Campbell and Gloyne, 1942; Tonning, 1949).

References

Campbell AH, Gloyne SR: Case of pneumo-koniosis due to inhalation of fuller's earth. *J Pathol Bact* 1942;54:75–80.

McNally WD, Trostler IS: Severe pneumoconiosis caused by inhalation of fuller's earth. *J Ind Hyg Toxicol* 1941;23:118–126.

Tonning HO: Pneumoconiosis from fuller's earth. *J Ind Hyg Toxicol* 1949;31:41–45.

Sillimanite

This mineral is one of a group of aluminum silicates (Al_2SiO_5) that also includes kyanite and andalusite. It is used as a high-grade refractory in the manufacture of porcelain and fire-bricks for kilns and furnaces. There is a report of nondisabling changes on chest x-ray thought to be due to the dust of sillimanite (Middleton, 1936).

Reference

Middleton EL: Industrial pulmonary disease due to the inhalation of dust, with special reference to silicosis. *Lancet* 1936;2:1–9, 59–64.

Granite

Granite is an igneous rock composed primarily of quartz and feldspar, with an admixture of mica and granules of other minerals. Studies of quarry workers and granite cutters show that granite dust produces a lung disease very much like silicosis and with a predisposition to tuberculosis in the past. Studies of granite workers in Vermont over a long period illustrate the life history of a dust disease as influenced by control of dust exposure and tuberculous infection (Russell, 1941; Ashe and Bergstrom, 1964).

Some investigators consider the chest disease of granite workers to be silicosis (Ahlmark et al., 1965). Theriault et al. (1974) found that it is pos-sible to measure diminution in lung function as long as an average of 13.5 years before chest x-ray abnormalities appear in granite shed workers. Such studies have made it clear that after chronic silica exposures the severity of disease in granite quarry workers can be measured by both lung function studies and chest radiographs.

References

Ahlmark A, Bruce T, Nyström Å: Silicosis from quarrying and working of granite. *Br J Ind Med* 1965;22:285–290.

Ashe HB, Bergstrom DE: Twenty-six years' experience with dust control in the Vermont granite industry. *Ind Med Surg* 1964;33:73–78.

Russell AE: The health of workers in the dusty trades. VI. Restudy of a group of granite workers. *Publ Health Bull No. 269.* Washington, DC, 1941.

Theriault GP, Peters JM, Johnson WM: Pulmonary function and roentgenographic changes in granite dust exposure. *Arch Environ Health* 1974;28:23–27.

Mica

Mica occurs in nature in several forms (muscovite, phlogopite, and others) and is composed of potassium-aluminum silicate. This mineral, which occurs in flat sheets, is used for stove and lantern windows, paper and paint manufacture, and in insulators and dielectrics in the electric and electronic industries. There are reports of pneumoconiosis as a result of heavy exposure to mica over a period of five years or more. Complaints of dyspnea and cough have been described with changes in the lungs, especially the mid-zones, on chest x-ray.

Despite earlier reports that sericite, a variety of muscovite, caused pulmonary disease, later reports have suggested that sericite, as used in industry, does not cause disease (Dreessen et al., 1940; Heimann et al., 1953).

References

Dreessen WC, Dallavalle JM, Edwards TI, et al: Pneumoconiosis among mica and pegmatite workers. *Publ Health Bull No. 250*, Washington, DC, 1940.

370

Heimann H, Moskowitz S, Iyer CRH, et al:
Note on mica dust inhalation. *Arch Ind Hyg
Occup Med* 1953;8:531–532.

___

Slate

Slate is a term applied to a group of fine-grained rocks derived from sedimentary deposits and transformed by metamorphism. The flaky crystal structure is due in part to mica, and other constituents of slate include quartz and other minerals. There are a number of reports of pneumoconiosis in workers who handle slate as well as in those who mine and quarry it (Dreessen, 1933; Jones et al., 1967). The reports vary from descriptions of slight x-ray changes to severe dust disease. It is probable that inhalation of varying percentages of free silica explains this difference since the amount of such free silica is said to vary from 7% to as much as 35%.

References

Dreessen WC: Effects of certain silicate dusts on the lungs. *J Ind Hyg* 1933;15:66–78.
Jones JG, Owen TE, Corrado HA: Respiratory tuberculosis and pneumoconiosis in slate workers. *Br J Dis Chest* 1967;61:138–143.

___

Calcium Dusts

This category includes lime, limestone, gypsum, marble, and cement, which is a complex compound of lime. Many dusts of calcium are soluble in lung tissue and thus cannot be held responsible for a pneumoconiosis. Most series of cases reported for workers with heavy or long exposures to calcium dusts describe ill-defined or no chest x-ray changes. Workers disabled as a result of exposure to calcium dusts are considered to suffer damage because of the silica content of such dust (Doig, 1955; Davis and Nagelschmidt, 1956).

Because cement varies in composition, the literature on its effects on the lungs is confusing. Cement is described as 62% calcium oxide (CaO) and 22% silicon dioxide (SiO_2), but the amount of silica may be reduced to 6.5% in some processes and only 1% in finished cement. While there are scattered case reports of pneumoconiosis diagnosed by x-ray or at necropsy, surveys of cement workers suggest that cement is a relatively harmless dust. Two older reports described marked changes on x-ray along with disabling symptoms that probably reflected excessive dustiness or exposure to high quartz levels (Thompson et al., 1928; Russell, 1933). A number of later reports considered cement to be pathogenic but Sander (1958) stated that only exposure to "raw" or "mixed," but not to finished, cement caused pneumoconiosis. Animal studies have supported the view that cement dust is biologically harmless (Zaidi, 1969). Cement, however, is irritating and causes dermatitis, rhinitis, and pharyngitis without proper engineering controls and personal protection. Kalačić (1973) studied cement workers along with appropriate control groups. He found that smoking, age, and economic factors did not account for the higher prevalence of chronic nonspecific lung disease with obstructive ventilatory impairment that he noted among the cement workers.

References

Davis SB, Nagelschmidt G: A report on the absence of pneumoconiosis among workers in pure limestone. *Br J Ind Med* 1956;13:6–8.
Doig AT: Disabling pneumoconiosis from limestone dust. *Br J Ind Med* 1955;12:206–216.
Kalačić I: Chronic nonspecific lung disease in cement workers. *Arch Environ Health* 1973a;26:78–83.
Kalačić I: Ventilatory lung function in cement workers. *Arch Environ Health* 1973b;26:84–85.
Russell AE: The effect of cement dust upon workers. *Am J Med Sci* 1933;185:330–338.
Sander OA: Roentgen resurvey of cement workers. *Arch Ind Health* 1958;17:96–103.
Thompson LR, Brundag DK, Russell AE, et al: The health of workers in the dusty trades. 1. Health of workers in a Portland cement plant. *Publ Health Bull No. 176,* Washington, DC, 1928.
Zaidi AH: *Experimental Pneumoconiosis.* Baltimore, MD, Johns Hopkins, 1969.

___

Amorphous Silica

Physicians may be given a history of exposure to amorphous silica in workers with an abnormal chest x-ray and a complaint of dyspnea. The literature on the subject is confusing because of the variety of dusts referred to as amorphous silica.

Fused silica, kieselgur, flint, and quartz glass are sometimes referred to as amorphous silica, so-called because of the absence of crystalline structure, the established cause of fibrotic response in the lung. The crucial factor is probably the fact that the particle sizes of amorphous silica are at least two orders of magnitude smaller than the crystalline dusts that produce silicosis (Iler, 1979).

Silica flour, a finely milled crystalline silica, is sometimes incorrectly labelled as amorphous silica, but it has serious fibrogenic capabilities, as a recent report from Australia demonstrated. Acute silicosis developed in a young man who handled silica flour, with a rapidly fatal outcome (Zimmerman and Sinclair, 1977).

Comparisons of quartz, cristobalite, tridymite, and amorphous silica showed all of them to be fibrogenic when introduced as suspensions of the same particle size (1 to 4 µm) into rat lungs, although the effects of amorphous silica were least severe (King et al., 1953; Engelbrecht et al., 1958). It is possible, therefore, that clinically recognizable pneumoconiosis may occur in some workers exposed to amorphous silica if the quantity inhaled is great enough. Pulmonary fibrosis has been reported from workers exposed to amorphous silica (Vitums et al., 1977) but pulmonary function appears to be unaffected by such exposures (Wilson et al., 1979).

References

Iler RK: The Chemistry of Silica. New York, Wiley-Interscience, 1979.

Engelbrecht FM, Yoganathan M, King EJ, et al: Fibrosis and collagen in rats' lungs produced by etched and unetched free silica dusts. Arch Ind Health 1958;17:287–294.

King EJ, Mohanty GP, Harrison CV, et al: The action of different forms of pure silica on the lungs of rats. Br J Ind Med 1953;10:9–17.

Vitums VC, Edwards MJ, Niles NR, et al: Pulmonary fibrosis from amorphous silica dust, a product of silica vapor. Arch Environ Health 1977;32:62–68.

Wilson RK, Stevens PM, Lovejoy HB, et al: Effects of chronic amorphous silica exposure on sequential pulmonary function. J Occup Med 1979;21:399–402.

Zimmerman PV, Sinclair RA: Rapidly progressive fatal silicosis in a young man. Med J Aust 1977;2:704–706.

5 • Man-Made Materials

Man-Made Mineral Fibers

Man-made mineral fibers (MMMF) are usually amorphous silicates made from glass, rock, or fusible slag. They are known as rock wool or fibrous glass, and have various uses. Those that are continuous filaments with diameters of 9 to 25 μm are used in textiles and for reinforcing plastics. Fibers ranging from 1 to 6 μm in diameter are used for insulation against heat and sound, with the finer diameter "wools" having special applications in acoustic protection. Fibrous material less than 1 μm in diameter is used for special purposes such as scientific filter papers (Hill, 1977).

These artificial fibers are frequently coated with inert thermosetting resin binders of the phenol formaldehyde type. Dust is produced by sawing, grinding, cutting, and other forms of handling. It is of interest that these fibers break transversely but do not split longitudinally in the manner of asbestos to produce thinner fibers. Because the fibers are very hard, the dust that becomes airborne does not contain particles small enough to penetrate beyond the larger bronchi (Wright, 1968). While inhalation of fiber glass dust does not cause an identified pneumoconiosis, its sharp spicules can be very troublesome to those who are exposed (Gross et al., 1960, 1971). Wright (1980) has published correspondence from a British naval surgeon to his superiors in 1891 reporting the chest discomfort in workmen as a result of breathing the dust of "Cotton Silicate" fibers used for insulating boilers and steam pipes. The Fleet Surgeon, in turn, questioned the use of cough mixtures to relieve the distress because they might suppress expectoration of the irritating dust and recommended instead the use of protective face masks.

While occasional reports have appeared describing individual cases of chest illness at-tributable to the inhalation of fibrous glass particles (summarized by Hill, 1977), studies of groups of glass and rock wool workers have not revealed disease as a result of occupational exposure (Carpenter and Spolyar, 1945; Bjure et al., 1964; Wright, 1968; Utidjian and de Treville, 1970; Nasr et al., 1971). Investigation of workers who had left work with MMMF (Bayliss et al., 1976) or who have retired (Enterline and Henderson, 1975) also failed to reveal a significant health hazard.

Irritation of the skin can result from the mechanical irritant properties of MMMF dust, especially by fibers greater than 5 μm in diameter (Heisel and Hunt, 1968). Punctate erythema and itching may be produced by the release of histamine induced by the embedded fibers (Possick et al., 1970) but "hardening" of the skin develops with continued exposure and the discomfort subsides. Nevertheless, paronychia and warts due to implanted splinters of fiber glass, and irritation of the skin and conjunctivae are real problems (Longley and Jones, 1966). The direct trauma of inhaled fiber glass can cause cough, epistaxis, and sore throat (Nasr, 1967). HLH knows of two cases in which fiber glass ruptured small arteries in the upper respiratory tract with resultant bleeding severe enough to require surgical intervention. The use of lubricants and epoxy resins with fiber glass may complicate its irritant effect, especially to skin.

Some newer mineral fibers, based on aluminum oxide and zirconium oxide, have been developed for use as insulating materials at very high temperatures and for special applications as filters. *In vitro* tests with rat peritoneal macrophages in cell culture indicated a low order of toxicity for these fibers and a low probability of causing fibrosis. Introduction of these fibers into rat peritoneal cavities led to collagen deposition around alumina fibers, but no inhalation studies have been reported (Styles and Wilson, 1976).

References

Bayliss DL, Dement JM, Wagoner JK, et al: Mortality patterns among fibrous glass production workers. *Ann NY Acad Sci* 1976;271:324-335.

Bjure J, Soderholm B, Widimsky J: Cardiopulmonary function studies in workers dealing with asbestos and glasswool. *Thorax* 1964;19:22-27.

Carpenter JL, Spolyar LW: Negative chest findings in the mineral wool industry. *J Indiana Med Assoc* 1945;38:389-390.

Enterline PE, Henderson V: The health of retired fibrous glass workers. *Arch Environ Health* 1975;30:113-116.

Gross P, Westrick ML, McNerney JM: Glass dust: A study of its biologic effects. *Arch Ind Health* 1960;21:10-23.

Gross P, Tuma J, de Treville RTP: Lungs of workers exposed to fiber glass. A study of their pathologic changes and their dust content. *Arch Environ Health* 1971;23:67-76.

Heisel EB, Hunt FE: Further studies in cutaneous reactions to glass fibers. *Arch Environ Health* 1968;17:705-711.

Hill JW: Health aspects of man-made mineral fibres. A review. *Ann Occup Hyg* 1977;20:161-173.

Longley EO, Jones RC: Fiberglass conjunctivitis and keratitis. *Arch Environ Health* 1966; 13:790-793.

Nasr ANM: Pulmonary hazards from exposure to glass fibers. *J Occup Med* 1967;9:345-348.

Nasr ANM, Ditchek T, Scholtens PA: The prevalence of radiographic abnormalities in the chests of fiber glass workers. *J Occup Med* 1971; 13:371-376.

Possick PA, Gellin GA, Key MM: Fibrous glass dermatitis. *Am Ind Hyg Assoc J* 1970;31:12-15.

Styles JA, Wilson J: Comparison between *in vitro* toxicity of two novel fibrous mineral dusts and their tissue reactions *in vivo*. *Ann Occup Hyg* 1976;19:63-68.

Utidjian HMD, de Treville RTP: Fibrous glass manufacturing and health: report of an epidemiological study. Parts I and II. Proceedings of the 35th Annual Meeting of the Industrial Health Foundation, Pittsburgh, 1970.

Wright DS: Man-made mineral fibres: A historical note. *J Soc Occup Med* 1980;30:138-140.

Wright GW: Airborne fibrous glass particles. Chest roentgenograms of persons with prolonged exposure. *Arch Environ Health* 1968;16:175-181.

Silicon Carbide

Silicon carbide (carborundum) is produced by reduction of silica with excess carbon. It is extremely hard and has wide use in the manufacture of synthetic abrasives. It is also used as a refractory material in ceramics. Animal experiments have shown that silicon carbide does not produce fibrosis. However, there are two reports of nodular shadows in the chest x-rays of workers exposed to this material (Smith and Perina, 1948; Doig, 1949). Exact knowledge of the dust composition, the amount inhaled, and biopsy or necropsy study of the affected lungs are missing. Doig suggested that the harmful effect is caused by the liberation ‚of fibrogenic silica from the carbide by tissue fluids.

References

Doig AT: Other lung diseases due to dust. *Post Grad Med J* 1949;25:639-649.

Smith AR, Perina AE: Pneumoconiosis from synthetic abrasive materials. *Occup Med* 1948;5:396-402.

6 • Organic Dusts

Extrinsic allergic alveolitis and hypersensitivity pneumonitis are the British and United States terms that are in use at the present time to describe worker illness arising from exposure to a number of organic dusts. The diagnosis, to be accurate, requires the use of sophisticated tests, mainly immunologic, that may have a variable interpretation (McCombs, 1972). Workers reported as suffering from such diseases include farmers, grain handlers, maple-bark strippers, bird fanciers, duck and goose feather handlers, and mushroom workers. More unusual occupations that may also be involved are those of paprika splitters, cheese workers, and preparers of medicinal snuff made of porcine and bovine posterior pituitary powder. Although this list is incomplete, it serves to draw attention to the nonspecificity of the biological responses available to the respiratory tract and the variety of causes associated with occupational inhalation of organic dusts.

The organic dusts that have occupational significance can be divided into major groups such as plant dusts, animal dusts, mycotoxins, and proteolytic enzymes.

Plant Dusts

There are reports of respiratory disease due to various plant dusts, frequently termed vegetable dusts, as a result of occupational exposure. Unless such reports describe an epidemic occurrence associated with inhalation of a common etiologic agent producing similar clinical and pathologic findings, their attributions may not be correct. There are two disease patterns common to respiratory disease resulting from inhalation of vegetable dust. Most common is bronchospasm that, after long continued exposure, may cause bronchitis, bronchiectasis, emphysema, and right heart failure. The other pattern, more serious, is the development of an inflammatory reaction in the lower respiratory tract with formation of nonspecific granulomata that leads, with or without continuing exposure to the offending material, to pulmonary fibrosis of varying degrees of severity.

This section summarizes some of the knowledge of respiratory illness thought to be due to the inhalation of dusts of plant origin. A number of mechanisms of action of such dusts have been suggested, including direct irritant effect of finely divided dust particles, specific pharmacologically active agents in the dust, immunologic response of the sensitized worker to allergens in the dust, and contamination with molds, fungi, or bacteria that elaborate harmful products (Pernis et al., 1961; Fink, 1973). Thermophilic actinomycetes are frequently the antigenic agents responsible for the diseases caused by moldy hay (farmer's lung) and sugar cane (bagassosis), and even grow in heating and air-conditioning systems in offices and residences. Silica in the soil in which vegetation is grown is of such large particle size that action of this fibrogenic material is thought not to be an etiologic factor in this group of occupational respiratory diseases.

References

Fink JN: Organic dust-induced hypersensitivity pneumonitis. *J Occup Med* 1973;15:245–247.

McCombs R: Diseases due to immunologic reactions of the lungs. *N Engl J Med* 1972;286: 1245–1252.

Pernis B, Vigliani EC, Cavagna C, et al: The role of bacterial endotoxins in occupational diseases caused by inhaling vegetable dusts. *Br J Ind Med* 1961;18:120–129.

Grain dusts Respiratory symptoms occur in farmers, grain elevator workers, dockworkers, and others handling stored grain. The persons who are affected load and unload grain, or serve as threshers, millers, malsters, and elevator laborers. The chief complaints are cough and dyspnea that begin on exposure and, depending upon the length and level of exposure, may persist after the work has stopped. Grain fever, characterized by malaise, chills, and fever, occurs in some workers several hours after leaving work (Kleinfeld et al., 1968). It is thought to be a type III allergic reaction to the fungi in damp, moldy grain (Cotton and Dosman, 1978). There are a number of reports of an asthmatic syndrome that, after long continued exposure, causes chronic disabling pulmonary insufficiency (Skoulas et al., 1964). This asthmatic response may represent a type I immunologic response to allergens in the grain dust (Cotton and Dosman, 1978). Smoking habits have been shown to be a significant factor in the aggravation of grain-induced disease, but even in nonsmokers abnormalities of lung function are demonstrable. However, the findings are complicated and depend on whether the individual grain-handler has evidence of atopy (Gerrard et al., 1979; Patel et al., 1981). Tse et al. (1973) and Chan-Yeung et al. (1979) confirmed the role of smoking but they could find no significant correlation by skin prick and precipitin tests between positive results of such tests and clinical disease.

Abnormal lung function was also noted by doPico et al. (1977) who concluded that inhaled grain dust can cause acute inflammation of the respiratory tract mucosa and probably produces chronic airway disease. The respiratory disease of grain handlers appears to be a response to the dust itself but the role of fungal spores, which may number over $10^6/m^3$ (Farant and Moore, 1978), has not been clearly delineated.

A syndrome now called baker's asthma has been known since antiquity and was described by Ramazzini in 1700. Individual bakers develop cough and wheezing on exposure to flour dust. Spores of fungi have been found in bakers' sputum and in bakery air, but the immunologic reaction appears to be to defined antigens in wheat and rye flours mediated by IgE antibodies (Blands et al., 1976; Wilbur and Ward, 1976; Baldo and Wrigley, 1978). Continued employment can be accomplished by avoidance of undue exposure and by regular treatment with sodium cromoglycate (Hendrick et al., 1976).

References

Baldo BA, Wrigley CW: IgE antibodies to wheat flour components. *Clin Allergy* 1978;8: 109–124.

Blands J, Diamant B, Kallós P, et al: Flour allergy in bakers. I. Identification of allergenic fractions in flour and comparison of diagnostic methods. *Intern Arch Allergy Appl Immunol* 1976;52:392–406.

Chan-Yeung M, Wong R, MacLean L: Respiratory abnormalities among grain elevator workers. *Chest* 1979;75:461–467.

Cotton DJ, Dosman JA: Grain dust and health. I. Host factors. *Ann Intern Med* 1978;88:840–841.

Farant J-P, Moore CF: Dust exposures in the Canadian grain industry. *Am Ind Hyg Assoc J* 1978;39:177–194.

Gerrard JW, Mink J, Cheung SC, et al: Non-smoking grain handlers in Saskatchewan: Airways reactivity and allergic status. *J Occup Med* 1979;21:342–346.

Hendrick DJ, Davies RJ, Pepys J: Bakers' asthma. *Clin Allergy* 1976;6:241–250.

Kleinfeld M, Messite J, Swencicki RE, et al: A clinical and physiologic study of grain handlers. *Arch Environ Health* 1968;16:380–384.

Patel KR, Symington IS, Pollock R, et al: A pulmonary survey of grain handlers in the West of Scotland. *Clin Allergy* 1981;11:121–129.

doPico GA, Reddan W, Flaherty D, et al: Respiratory abnormalities among grain handlers. A clinical, physiologic, and immunologic study. *Am Rev Resp Dis* 1977;115:915–927.

Skoulas A, Williams N, Merriman JE: Exposure to grain dust. II. A clinical study of the effects. *J Occup Med* 1964;6:359–372.

Tse KS, Warren P, Janusz M, et al: Respiratory abnormalities in workers exposed to grain dust. *Arch Environ Health* 1973;27:74–77.

Wilbur RD, Ward GW Jr: Immunologic studies in a case of baker's asthma. *J Allergy Clin Immunol* 1976;58:366–372.

Farmer's lung The respiratory disease known as farmer's lung has been associated with exposure to moldy hay, oats, barley, and millet grain (Dickie and Rankin, 1958; Johnson, 1966; McCombs, 1972). This disease of humans, first documented by Campbell (1932), appears to be related to the disabling disease of horses known as "broken wind" or "heaves" and to the pulmonary

376

disease of cattle known as "fog fever," both due to the feeding of moldy fodder.

The onset of farmer's lung may occur insidiously or may take place several hours after exposure. Severe dyspnea, cough, cyanosis, and fever after exposure to the spore-laden dust of moldy hay are reported most often, and these symptoms occur after the worker has been sensitized by previous exposure to the causative agents present in the dust. Wheezing, expectoration, malaise, and occasionally hemoptysis, also occur. This acute phase may be accompanied by râles audible throughout the chest and by bilateral densities on the chest x-ray. Biopsy at this stage shows pulmonary edema as well as inflammatory changes in the alveolar walls, typical of a Type III, Arthus, reaction. Freedom from exposure will bring about relief of symptoms and reversal of the chest x-ray changes to normal.

The subsequent course depends on repeated exposures and the level of dustiness. Cases of chronic dyspnea after a single acute episode have been reported, but in most well-studied cases a subacute and later chronic phase are related to further exposure. Clinical and pathologic changes may reflect a chronic granulomatous interstitial pneumonitis, although granulomata may not be present in the acute phase (Emanuel et al., 1964). Lung function abnormalities, consisting of lowered vital capacity, total lung capacity, and CO diffusing capacity, were more often found in patients who had five or more symptomatic recurrences of disease, events that may be the most important factors in the development of progressive disease (Braun et al., 1979).

Farmer's lung in many cases becomes very much like the pulmonary fibrosis and emphysema of pulmonary sarcoidosis of long duration, both clinically and pathologically (Barbee et al., 1968). Knowledge of exposure to moldy grain or hay facilitates the differentiation of farmer's lung from miliary tuberculosis, beryllium disease, and Boeck's sarcoid. Farmer's lung is favorably influenced by steroid therapy, as are many other sarcoid-like diseases. It should be remembered that silo-filler's disease, which also occurs in farm workers, is a very different entity, a bronchiolitis of severe degree due to inhalation of oxides of nitrogen (see chapter on nitrogen compounds).

The cause of farmer's lung is thought to be an allergen present in the dust of moldy hay. Many fungal spores are found in such moldy vegetable dust and in the sputum of exposed farmers. That some cases of farmer's lung were said to improve

only after iodide therapy led to the earlier view that this was primarily a fungal disease (Törnell, 1946). Farmer's lung, however, does not behave clinically like one of the mycoses. The present view is that this disease is an extrinsic allergic alveolitis or hypersensitivity pneumonitis and that the antigenic material comes from the thermophilic actinomycetes, *Micropolyspora faeni* and *Thermoactinomyces vulgaris.* This view is supported by the finding of precipitins in the sera of patients with farmer's lung, thought to be mediated by IgG antibodies (Pepys and Jenkins, 1965). IgE antibodies, however, are absent in patients with farmer's lung or with pigeon-breeder's disease, a finding that separates these illnesses from allergic bronchopulmonary aspergillosis (Patterson et al., 1976). IgG antibodies to *M. faeni* have also been detected by enzyme-linked immunosorbent assay (ELISA) in patients with farmer's lung (Bamdad, 1980). Spores of thermophilic actinomycetes can be detected by electron microscopy in pulmonary alveolar macrophages obtained by simple lavage (Romet-Lemonne et al., 1980). Both the absolute numbers and the percentages of T lymphocytes are reduced in the peripheral blood of patients with farmer's lung or even of those exposed to moldy hay, while B lymphocytes are unaffected (Flaherty et al., 1976).

Whatever the exact etiology, available knowledge clearly shows that this agricultural lung disease is more common than had been thought and carries an unfavorable prognosis without prompt therapy and change of job (Wenzel et al., 1970). Respiratory protection with a suitable mask has not proved capable of preventing recurrence of symptoms in a sensitized worker on re-exposure to moldy vegetable dust. Robinson (1976) encountered two patients with allergic alveolitis from exposure to moldy hay who also had malabsorption due to coeliac disease, and he made the interesting suggestion that other patients needed to be screened to ascertain the extent of coexistence of these two conditions.

References

Bamdad S: Enzyme-linked immunosorbent assay (ELISA) for IgG antibodies in farmers' lung disease. *Clin Allergy* 1980;10:161–171.

Barbee RA, Callies Q, Dickie HA, et al: The long-term prognosis in farmer's lung. *Am Rev Resp Dis* 1968;97:223–231.

Braun SR, doPico GA, Tsiatis A, et al: Farmer's lung disease: long-term clinical and physiologic outcome. *Am Rev Resp Dis* 1979;119: 185–191.

Campbell JM: Acute symptoms following work with hay. *Br Med J* 1932;2:1143–1144.

Dickie HA, Rankin J: Farmer's lung: An acute granulomatous interstitial pneumonitis occurring in agricultural workers. *J Am Med Assoc* 1958; 167:1069–1076.

Emanuel DA, Wenzel FJ, Bowerman CI, et al: Farmer's lung. Clinical, pathologic, and immunologic study of twenty-four patients. *Am J Med* 1964;37:392–401.

Flaherty DK, Surfus JE, Chmelik F, et al: Lymphocyte subpopulations in the peripheral blood of patients with farmer's lung. *Am Rev Resp Dis* 1976;114:1093–1098.

Johnson JE: Farmer's lung in Maryland. Clinical, microbiological, and immunological studies. *Ann Intern Med* 1966;64:860–872.

McCombs R: Diseases due to immunologic reactions of the lungs. *N Engl J Med* 1972;286: 1245–1252.

Patterson R, Roberts M, Roberts RC, et al: Antibodies of different immunoglobulin classes against antigens causing farmer's lung. *Am Rev Resp Dis* 1976;114:315–324.

Pepys J, Jenkins PA: Precipitin (F.L.H.) test in farmer's lung. *Thorax* 1965;20:21–35.

Robinson TJ: Coeliac disease with farmers' lung. *Br Med J* 1976;1:745–746.

Romet-Lemonne JL, Lemarie E, Choutet P: Ultrastructural study of bronchopulmonary lavage liquid in farmer's lung disease. *Lancet* 1980;1:777.

Törnell E: Thresher's lung. Fungoid disease resembling tuberculosis or morbus Schaumann. *Acta Med Scand* 1946;125:191–219.

Wenzel FJ, Gray RL, Emanuel DA: Farmer's lung, its geographic distribution. *J Occup Med* 1970;12:493–496.

Bagasse dust Bagasse, from an Anglo-Saxon word meaning "worthless" by way of Provençal, is what remains of sugar-cane after the sugar has been extracted. This residual fiber is used in the manufacture of acoustic and thermal insulation, paper, refractory brick, and as bedding in stables and for fowl. Illness has resulted from exposure to its dust, and case reports have come from Louisiana and Puerto Rico in the United States, and from England, Italy, Peru, India, and the Philippines. The disease was first described by Jamison and Hopkins (1941) in a worker in a hard-board factory in New Orleans. They used the term "bagasscosis" but subsequent reports beginning with that of Castleden and Hamilton-Paterson (1942) have employed the term "bagassosis." Nicholson's (1968) suggestion that the diagnostic title be changed to "bagasse worker's lung" is helpful, and this name should probably be adopted. It is, however, a mistake to refer, as Nicholson does, to this and other occupational chest diseases caused by organic dusts as pneumoconioses (Hardy, 1967).

Bagassosis begins abruptly with chest pain, fever, severe dyspnea, and violent cough after exposure to dry bagasse dust, such as that produced by shredding machines, for periods averaging two months (Buechner, 1960; Buechner et al., 1964). Blood-tinged sputum may be produced, and moist râles may be heard, especially over the upper lung fields. Chest radiographs show bilateral irregular areas of infiltration that are easily confused with a number of diseases, such as tuberculosis, partly because of the severity of the clinical illness. Studies of lung function report abnormalities of all of the indices (Weill et al., 1966; Jenkins et al., 1971), particularly diminished ventilatory capacity (Hearn, 1968). The pathologic changes in bagassosis are said to be those of bronchiolitis, bronchopneumonia, bronchiectasis, and, in a few reports, the appearance of giant cells and inflammatory changes closely resembling those of farmer's lung. Some patients with bagasse worker's lung are said to recover completely while others, as in some cases of Boeck's sarcoid, develop disabling pulmonary fibrosis and emphysema (Nicholson, 1968). Pathologic material has been scarce for deaths have been few and most knowledge has been derived from lung biopsy specimens (Sodeman and Pullen, 1944; Bradford et al., 1961; Boonpucknavig et al., 1973). These have shown chronic interstitial infiltrates of lymphocytes and macrophages in the alveolar walls with eventual interstitial alveolar fibrosis.

A number of agents have been suggested as the cause for bagassosis. After finding as many as 20 different species of fungi in a single gram of bagasse, Jamison and Hopkins (1941) described bagassosis as a bronchopulmonary mycosis. Others considered the disease to be a result of mechanical irritation by bagasse dust plus bacterial infection. While there is a small amount of free silica in bagasse, the particles are over 20 to 30 μm in diameter and, as a result, few of them reach the lower respiratory tract (Hunter and

Perry, 1946). Bagasse worker's lung is now considered to be an extrinsic allergenic alveolitis or hypersensitivity pneumonitis, probably produced by *Thermoactinomyces vulgaris* but not also by *Micropolyspora faeni* (as is the case with farmer's lung). This conclusion is based on reactions to inhalation of extracts of these organisms (Hearn and Holford-Strevens, 1968) and the finding of precipitating antibodies to bagasse in the sera of patients with this illness (Salvaggio et al., 1966). Changes in methods of storage, with reduction of airborne organic dust and retardation of microbial decay, has resulted in a marked reduction in cases of bagasse illness in one Louisiana paper mill (Lehrer et al., 1978).

References

Boonpucknavig V, Bhamarapravati N, Kamtorn P, et al: Bagassosis: A histopathologic study of pulmonary biopsies from six cases. *Am J Clin Pathol* 1973;59:461–472.

Bradford JK, Blalock JB, Wascom CM: Bagasse disease of the lungs. Early histopathologic changes demonstrated by lung biopsy. *Am Rev Resp Dis* 1961;84:582–585.

Buechner HA: Bagassosis: Peculiarities of its geographic pattern and report of the first case from Peru and Puerto Rico. *J Am Med Assoc* 1960;174:1237–1241.

Buechner HA, Aucoin E, Vignes AJ, et al: The resurgence of bagassosis in Louisiana. *J Occup Med* 1964;6:437–442.

Castleden LIM, Hamilton-Paterson JL: Bagassosis; Industrial lung disease. *Br Med J* 1942;2: 478–480.

Hardy HL: Current concepts of occupational lung disease of interest to the radiologist. *Semin Radiol* 1967;2:225.

Hearn CED: Bagassosis: an epidemiological, environmental, and clinical survey. *Br J Ind Med* 1968;25:267–282.

Hearn CED, Holford-Strevens V: Immunological aspects of bagassosis. *Br J Ind Med* 1968;25:283–292.

Hunter D, Perry KMA: Bronchiolitis resulting from the handling of bagasse. *Br J Ind Med* 1946; 3:64–74.

Jamison SC, Hopkins J: Bagasscosis: a fungus disease of the lungs. *New Orleans Med Surg J* 1941;93:580–582.

Jenkins DE, Malik SK, Figueroa-Casas JC, et al: Sequential observations on pulmonary functional derangements in bagassosis. *Arch Intern Med* 1971;128:535–540.

Lehrer SB, Turer E, Weill H, et al: Elimination of bagassosis in Louisiana paper manufacturing plant workers. *Clin Allergy* 1978;8:15–20.

Nicholson, DP: Bagasse worker's lung. *Am Rev Resp Dis* 1968;97:546–560.

Salvaggio JE, Buechner HA, Seabury JH, et al: Bagassosis. I. Precipitins against extracts of crude bagasse in the serum of patients. *Ann Intern Med* 1966;64:748–758.

Sodeman WA, Pullen RL: Bagasse disease of the lungs. *Arch Intern Med* 1944;73:365–374.

Weill H, Buechner HA, Gonzalez E, et al: Bagassosis: A study of pulmonary function in 20 cases. *Ann Intern Med* 1966;64:737–747.

Bird-breeder's disease The description of pigeon-breeder's disease by Reed et al. (1965) was quickly followed by reports of similar illness in bird-fanciers (Hargreave et al., 1966) and in persons exposed to the droppings of domestic fowl (Korn et al., 1968). The illness has acquired a variety of similar names, such as bird-fancier's lung, budgerigar-fancier's lung (Hendrick et al., 1978), parakeet-fancier's lung (Sahn and Rickerson, 1972). This hypersensitivity pneumonitis is thought to be the most common variety of extrinsic allergic alveolitis in Great Britain, and is a reaction to proteins in bird droppings inhaled as dust. The illness is associated with high levels of serum-precipitating, complement-fixing antibodies against several antigens derived from either pigeon serum or pigeon droppings (Boren et al., 1977). Such precipitins have been detected, for example, in 40% of persons free from disease attending a national convention of pigeon breeders (Fink et al., 1972).

The acute form of the disease is characterized by chills, cough, and dyspnea developing suddenly after contact with birds or their droppings. Leucocytosis, eosinophilia, reduced vital capacity, and impaired alveolar diffusion are common. Chest x-ray abnormalities consist of diffuse, finely nodular shadows and reticular linear densities (Unger et al., 1968; Hargreave et al., 1972; Zylak et al., 1975). In the chronic illness, severe dyspnea, bronchitis, basal râles, and weight loss are prominent features, and the illness may occasionally be fatal (Edwards and Luntz, 1974).

A large literature has developed dealing with various immunologic aspects of the disease. Avian erythrocyte agglutination by sera from exposed persons can quickly detect avian-specific anti-bodies (Diment and Pepys, 1977). The agglutination reactions are mediated by antibodies directed against pigeon IgG and IgM. T lymphocyte reactivity to pigeon antigens has also been demonstrated (Moore et al., 1974; Schatz et al., 1976). Cessation of exposure to the provoking antigen results in recovery in some but not all patients (Allen et al., 1976).

Bird-fancier's lung should be distinguished from ornithosis and from histoplasmosis. *Ornithosis,* sometimes called psittacosis or parrot-fever from the bird with which it is most prominently associated, is an infectious disease caused by *Chlamydia psittaci.* This organism is an obligate intracellular parasite that enters the body through the respiratory tract as a result of inhalation of infected dried bird feces or, in poultry processing plants, of inhalation of an infected aerosol. The illness has a sudden onset with malaise, fever, anorexia, sore throat, headache, and pneumonitis. Attacks may occur frequently in poultry farm workers.

Histoplasmosis is a mild infection that results from the inhalation of dust contaminated with the spores of *Histoplasma capsulatum,* a fungus that grows abundantly where infected bird feces have been mixed with soil. Such contaminated soil is common in poultry farms and farmyards, and at roost sites of blackbirds (Chick et al., 1981), throughout central United States. With heavy exposure, pneumonitis and occasionally cavitation may occur, but most cases are asymptomatic or mild, and are detected on chest x-ray by calcific nodulation. Such chest x-ray changes have led to loss of work when the clinician has failed to make the proper diagnosis or has not known the benign prognosis.

References

Allen DH, Williams GV, Woolcock AJ: Bird breeder's hypersensitivity pneumonitis: Progress studies of lung function after cessation of exposure to the provoking antigen. *Am Rev Resp Dis* 1976;114:555-566.

Boren MN, Moore VL, Abramoff P, et al: Pigeon breeder's disease. Antibody response of man against a purified component of pigeon dropping extract. *Clin Immunol Immunopathol* 1977;8:108-115.

Chick EW, Compton SB, Pass T III, et al: Hitchcock's birds, or the increased rate of exposure to Histoplasma from blackbird roost sites. *Chest* 1981;80:434-438.

Diment JA, Pepys J: Avian erythrocyte agglutination tests with sera of bird fanciers. *J Clin Pathol* 1977;30:29-34.

Edwards C, Luntz G: Budgerigar-fancier's lung: Report of a fatal case. *Br J Dis Chest* 1974;68:57-64.

Fink JN, Schlueter DP, Sosman AJ, et al: Clinical survey of pigeon breeders. *Chest* 1972;62:277-281.

Hargreave FE, Hinson KF, Reid L, et al: The radiological appearances of allergic alveolitis due to bird sensitivity (bird fancier's lung). *Clin Radiol* 1972;23:1-10.

Hargreave FE, Pepys J, Longbottom JL, et al: Bird breeder's (fancier's) lung. *Lancet* 1966;1:445-449.

Hendrick DJ, Faux JA, Marshall R: Budgerigar-fancier's lung: The commonest variety of allergic alveolitis in Britain. *Br Med J* 1978;2:81-84.

Korn DS, Florman AL, Gribetz I: Recurrent pneumonitis with hypersensitivity to hen litter. *J Am Med Assoc* 1968;205:44-45.

Moore VL, Fink JN, Barboriak JJ, et al: Immunologic events in pigeon breeders' disease. *J Allergy Clin Immunol* 1974;53:319-328.

Reed CE, Sosman A, Barbee RA: Pigeon-breeders' lung. A newly observed interstitial pulmonary disease. *J Am Med Assoc* 1965;193:261-265.

Sahn SA, Rickerson HB: Extremes of clinical presentation in parakeet fanciers lung. *Arch Intern Med* 1972;130:913-917.

Schatz M, Patterson R, Fink J, et al: Pigeon breeder's disease. II. Pigeon antigen induced proliferation of lymphocytes from symptomatic and asymptomatic subjects. *Clin Allergy* 1976;6:7-17.

Unger JD, Fink JN, Unger GF: Pigeon breeder's disease: A review of the roentgenographic pulmonary findings. *Radiology* 1968;90:683-687.

Zylak CJ, Dyck DR, Warren P, et al: Hypersensitive lung disease due to avian antigens. *Radiology* 1975;114:45-49.

Wood dusts and wood products   Wood, sawdust, and occasionally other substances produced or extracted from wood can have adverse effects on persons occupationally exposed to these materials. Contact with many types of woods or their dusts has been known to result in irritant or sensitization dermatitis, while inhalation has produced

380

nasal mucosal irritation, asthma, and malignant tumors of the paranasal sinuses. A comprehensive review of wood toxicity has been prepared by Woods and Calnan (1976) who pointed out that irritant chemicals are often found in sap, latex, bark, and other outer parts of the tree and affect timber workers. Sensitizing substances, on the other hand, are more often found in the heartwood and therefore involve woodworkers who are exposed to fine dust. In one study of total suspended particles collected from wood machining operations, the highest measured dust levels were from hardwood sanding, with lower values for softwood (pine) sanding (Whitehead et al., 1981). Still lower levels were gathered from detailed wood working, such as finish-milling and furniture assembly.

The literature contains reports of reversible bronchial obstruction caused by exposure to the dust of boxwood, cottonwood, and evergreens used as Christmas trees. Sosman et al. (1969) reviewed these reports and, after study of four patients, considered that a hypersensitivity reaction plus a nonspecific irritant were responsible. Schlueter et al. (1972) described a hypersensitivity pneumonitis in men working with wood pulp and named it wood-pulp workers disease. Michaels (1967) studied necropsy material from woodworkers and suggested that there may exist a pneumoconiosis associated with furniture manufacture and the timber trade. Two cases of severe respiratory difficulty were recently described from a furniture factory as a result of exposure to imported abiruana wood (Booth et al., 1976).

Occupational asthma and rhinitis have been particularly noticeable among workers with Western (or Canadian) red cedar (*Thuja plicata*) in Canada, Australia, Japan, and elsewhere (Gandevia and Milne, 1970; Chan-Yeung et al., 1973; Ishizaki et al., 1973). Typically, workers processing this wood first develop nocturnal attacks of cough and asthma. Continued exposure leads to symptoms occurring earlier in the day. Many workers also have rhinitis. Improvement occurs during weekends and holidays, and recovery appears to be complete within six months after exposure ceases. Diagnosis can be confirmed by the inhalation provocation test. Plicatic acid appears to be the ingredient in red cedar extract that causes bronchoconstriction (Chan-Yeung, 1973). Asthma has also been reported in a patient who worked with redwood (*Sequoia sempervirens*) as a hobby (doPico, 1978), a finding reminiscent of the interstitial granulomatous

pneumonitis that followed prolonged inhalation of redwood sawdust that was described by Cohen (1967), who called the disease sequoiosis. Suberosis, reported from Portugal, is an example of a problem caused by inhalation of dust from cork oaks, the trees from which corks are made (Cancella, 1963). Australian corkwood (*Duboisia*) contains high concentrations of atropine-like alkaloids, especially hyoscine, for which the leaves are harvested and dried. Clinical poisoning has occurred from occupational and accidental field exposure, with symptoms of mydriasis, loss of visual accommodation, conjunctival hyperemia, dry throat, flushed face, and, when severe, delirium, irrationality, or depression, all of which subside on cessation of exposure (Pearn, 1981).

The association between woodworking and nasal adenocarcinomas was suggested by Macbeth (1965) for the furniture-making industry in Buckinghamshire. Acheson et al. (1968) confirmed this association between exposure to wood dust and the development of malignant tumors of the nose and paranasal sinuses. Further substantiation of this finding soon came from Denmark, France, and Belgium, and more recently from Australia (Ironside and Matthews, 1975), Sweden (Engzell et al., 1978), Italy (Cecchi et al., 1980), and the United States (Gamez-Araujo et al., 1975; Brinton et al., 1977). In the Houston series, males in the fifth decade of life were most frequently affected, and the mucinous adenocarcinomas were papillary or solid. Impairment of nasal mucociliary clearance has been demonstrated in woodworkers and is thought to be a factor in the etiology of malignant disease in cases of wood dust inhalation (Black et al., 1974; Andersen et al., 1976). Other respiratory cancers, but not gastrointestinal malignancies, have been reported to occur in excess in furniture woodworkers in Sweden (Esping and Axelson, 1980).

References

Acheson ED, Cowdell RH, Hadfield E, et al: Nasal cancer in woodworkers in the furniture industry. *Br Med J* 1968;2:587–596.

Andersen HC, Solgaard J, Andersen I: Nasal cancer and nasal mucus-transport rates in woodworkers. *Acta Otolaryngol* 1976;82:263–265.

Black A, Evans JC, Hadfield EH, et al: Impairment of nasal mucociliary clearance in woodworkers in the furniture industry. *Br J Ind Med* 1974;31:10–17.

Booth BH, LeFoldt RH, Moffitt EM: Wood dust hypersensitivity. *J Allergy Clin Immunol* 1976;57:352–357.

Brinton LA, Blot WJ, Stone BJ, et al: A death certificate analysis of nasal cancer among furniture workers in North Carolina. *Cancer Res* 1977;37:3473–3474.

Cancella L de C: Suberosis: A pneumoconiosis due to cork dust. *Ind Med Surg* 1963;32:435–445.

Cecchi F, Buiatti E, Kriebel D, et al: Adenocarcinoma of the nose and paranasal sinuses in shoemakers and woodworkers in the province of Florence, Italy (1963–1977). *Br J Ind Med* 1980; 37:222–225.

Chan-Yeung M: Maximal expiratory flow and airway resistance during induced bronchoconstriction in patients with asthma due to western red cedar (*Thuja plicata*). *Am Rev Resp Dis* 1973;108:1103–1110.

Chan-Yeung M, Barton GM, MacLean L, et al: Occupational asthma and rhinitis due to western red cedar (*Thuja plicata*). *Am Rev Resp Dis* 1973; 108:1094–1102.

Cohen HI, Merigan TC, Kosek JC, et al: Sequoiosis. A granulomatous pneumonitis associated with redwood sawdust inhalation. *Am J Med* 1967;43:785–794.

Engzell U, Englund A, Westerholm P: Nasal cancer associated with occupational exposure to organic dust. *Acta Otolaryngol* 1978;86:437–442.

Esping B, Axelson O: A pilot study on respiratory and digestive tract cancer among woodworkers. *Scand J Work Environ Health* 1980;6:201–205.

Gamez-Araujo JJ, Ayala AG, Guillamondegui O: Mucinous adenocarcinomas of nose and paranasal sinuses. *Cancer* 1975;36:1100–1105.

Gandevia B, Milne J: Occupational asthma and rhinitis due to western red cedar (*Thuja plicata*), with special reference to bronchial reactivity. *Br J Ind Med* 1970;27:235–244.

Ironside P, Matthews J: Adenocarcinoma of the nose and paranasal sinuses in woodworkers in the State of Victoria, Australia. *Cancer* 1975;36:1115–1121.

Ishizaki T, Shida T, Miyamoto T, et al: Occupational asthma from western red cedar dust (*Thuja plicata*) in furniture factory workers. *J Occup Med* 1973;15:580–585.

Macbeth R: Malignant disease of the paranasal sinuses. *J Laryngology* 1965;79:592–612.

Michaels L: Lung changes in woodworkers. *Can Med Assoc J* 1967;96:1150–1155.

Pearn J: Corked up. Clinical hyoscine poisoning with alkaloids of the native corkwood, *Duboisia*. *Med J Aust* 1981;2:422–423.

doPico GA: Asthma due to dust from redwood *(Sequoia sempervirens)*. *Chest* 1978;73:424–425.

Schlueter DP, Fink JN, Hensley GT: Woodpulp workers' disease: A hypersensitivity pneumonitis caused by *Alternaria*. *Ann Intern Med* 1972;77:907–914.

Sosman AJ, Schlueter DP, Fink JN, et al: Hypersensitivity to wood dust. *New Engl J Med* 1969;281:977–980.

Whitehead LW, Freund T, Hahn LL: Suspended dust concentrations and size distributions, and qualitative analysis of inorganic particles, from woodworking operations. *Am Ind Hyg Assoc J* 1981;42:461–467.

Woods B, Calnan CD: Toxic woods. *Br J Dermatol* 1976;95(suppl 13):1–97.

Turpentine   Turpentine, which has been the most familiar liquid vehicle for paints, has largely been displaced in recent years by less expensive thinners, especially petroleum distillates and chlorinated hydrocarbons. Oil of turpentine is produced by steam distillation of pine wood and of gum turpentine derived by tapping pine trees. It is still used under the name of gum spirits in artists' paints, and in high-grade work in ship and house painting, but turpentine has been nearly eliminated from formulas of ready-made interior oil-based paints. Turpentine is used in shoe polishes and as a chemical raw material for the manufacture of synthetic camphor and terpin hydrate.

Distilled or wood turpentine, produced by the destructive distillation of pine brush, stumps, and sawdust, also contains methyl alcohol, formaldehyde, phenols, and pyridine. Some of these compounds are irritating to the skin, and the use of this kind of turpentine has been followed by outbreaks of dermatitis in the United States, Britain, and Italy (McCord, 1926). One of the ingredients of sulfate turpentine, produced mainly in Sweden, Finland, and Russia, is Δ^3-carene, which is highly allergenic for the skin. However, since 1950 the declining use of oil of turpentine has been accompanied by such a decrease in incidence of sensitization that the International Contact Dermatitis Group has recomended that oil of turpentine be removed from standard patch test series (Cronin, 1979).

Chapman (1941) made a careful review of the

382

effect of paint on the kidneys with particular reference to the role of turpentine. His interest was aroused by two cases, both fatal, of extensive glomerulonephritis. One of the victims became ill after many years of work with turpentine paint, the other, after a brief exposure to turpentine vapor from freshly painted walls. Chapman cited instances from the earlier literature of what was apparently acute kidney damage, with lumbar pain, albuminuria, hematuria, scanty urine, and the appearance of casts and blood cells in the urine sediment. But in those cases that were followed, chronic glomerulonephritis did not appear. The changing use of turpentine in recent years may account for absence of current reports of kidney damage associated with its use.

References

Chapman EM: Observations on the effect of paint on the kidneys with particular reference to the role of turpentine. *J Ind Hyg Toxicol* 1941; 23:277–289.

Cronin E: Oil of turpentine – A disappearing allergen. *Contact Derm* 1979;5:308–311.

McCord CP: Occupational dermatitis from wood turpentine. *J Am Med Assoc* 1926;86:1979.

Textile dust Mill fever is an illness that has been known by many names according to the dust or operation that produces it – flax, combers, hackling, grain or malt fever, cotton cold, or dust fever (Hardy, 1967). This is an acute temporary illness, occurring at the onset of exposure and not returning except after long absence from the dust or with excessive exposure. The symptoms include chills, headache, malaise, fever, gastric upset, sneezing, and sore throat lasting 24 to 48 hours. No serious complications are described.

Weaver's cough is a disease that occasionally affects workers in epidemic numbers and is thought to be due to mildewed yarn or to low grade stained cotton that favors the growth of fungi. In one well-studied United States outbreak, the disease was thought to be caused by the endotoxin of *Bacillus aerobacter cloacae* (Caminita et al., 1947). Chest tightness, nonproductive cough, dyspnea, malaise, and headache are the usual complaints. The cough may become very disabling and may persist for weeks after exposure ceases. HLH studied an epidemic of this syndrome among workers in a weave room but where

workers performing the same tasks in an adjacent room had no symptoms. The sick workers were thought to be suffering from an "allergy" or from hysteria. More than half of those in the affected work room were ill, some so dyspneic that they had to be taken by ambulance to home or to a hospital. A heavy growth of *Penicillium notatum, Cladosporium,* and *Aspergillus fumigatus* was found in the workroom air, but there was no growth in the air of the adjacent unaffected weave room. Careful cleaning and a heavy coat of paint resulted in the disappearance of all symptoms.

Another instance of weaver's cough was reported by Murray et al. (1957) to be associated with the use of tamarind seed kernel powder as a sizing adhesive for viscose cloth. Within four months after the use of this material, weavers handling viscose yarn complained of cough and dyspnea in epidemic numbers. Discontinuation of this sizing material resulted in cessation of symptoms.

References

Caminita BH, Baum WF, Neal PA, et al: A review of the literature relating to affections of the respiratory tract in individuals exposed to cotton dust. *Publ Health Bull No. 297,* Washington, DC, 1947.

Hardy HL: Respiratory diseases among textile workers (Editorial). *N Engl J Med* 1967;277:209–210.

Murray R, Dingwall-Fordyce I, Lane RE: An outbreak of weaver's cough associated with tamarind seed powder. *Br J Ind Med* 1957;14:105–110.

Cotton dust The unusual and somewhat misnamed diagnostic title "byssinosis," derived from the Latin *byssinum*, linen garment, refers to a group of occupational respiratory diseases in workers exposed to the dusts of cotton, flax, and hemp. In the cotton mills of Lancashire, England, a disease termed "cotton spinner's phthisis" was described in 1831 by Kay and has been under study since the middle of the 19th century (Schilling, 1956). There are well-documented reports of the disease from Sweden, Spain, Holland, Italy, Egypt, and India (Bouhuys, 1966). More recent reports have also come from Australia (Gandevia and Milne, 1965), Sudan (Khogali, 1976), and Tanzania (Mustafa et al., 1979). McKerrow and Schilling (1961) and Bouhuys et al. (1967) showed that byssinosis also occurred in the United States cotton industry. Subsequent studies by Merchant et al. (1972) and by Harris et al. (1972) confirmed the fact that this disease was indeed a problem in the United States although the papers of Schrag and Gullet (1970) and Bouhuys et al. (1969) suggested that the disease in American cotton mills may differ in character from other outbreaks of byssinosis.

Exposure in certain industrial operations to some, but not all, kinds of dirty cotton, flax, and hemp over a period of years has been shown to be a chief cause of byssinosis. Such procedures include opening bales, removing dust and impurities, carding, cleaning, stripping, and grinding the teeth of machines in cotton mills and textile plants. HLH has maintained that it is a mistake to use the term byssinosis to apply to all respiratory complaints among all workers exposed to cotton, flax, and hemp. Further elucidation of the variation in the character of the exposures, of clinical syndromes, and of the mechanism of disease production may be hampered by such a specific title. Recent use of the term "brown lung" to push legislation for worker benefits hinders the scientific investigation of disabling occupational lung disease in the textile industry because of its inappropriate analogy with the term "black lung" that is applied popularly to coal worker's pneumoconiosis (Kilburn, 1981).

The worker's clinical story of the onset of byssinosis is unique. After a few hours of work in certain operations, symptoms begin with a sense of tightness in the chest. Cough, asthmatic wheezing, various degrees of dyspnea, and increase in sputum follow. Because these complaints occur on the first day of the work week, or after a vacation, the syndrome is also known as "Monday morning dyspnea" or "Monday morning asthma." Students of byssinosis, such as Schilling, have classified the disease into four categories. Grade ½ is characterized by occasional chest tightness on the first day of the work week while Grade 1 requires such tightness every first day of the work week. Grade 2 includes workers with this symptom every work day. Grade 3 byssinotics suffer Grade 2 symptoms that are constant and are accompanied by signs of permanent incapacity such as diminished effort tolerance and/or reduced ventilatory capacity. Patients in Grades 2 and 3 give a history of at least ten years' exposure and usually more than 20 years. Workers with Grade 3 byssinosis are severely disabled by dyspnea with exacerbation at the time of any respiratory infec-

tion. Death is usually due to right heart failure. As might be expected, cigarette smokers have a higher prevalence and greater severity of symptoms.

As the disease becomes established, its clinical course is that of chronic bronchitis and emphysema. Edwards et al. (1975) described centrilobular or paracinar emphysema in 23% and 14%, respectively, of 43 byssinotic patients, while the others were free of this complication. In this series, no excessive fibrosis, granuloma formation, or other lesion was present to suggest an extrinsic alveolitis. Hypertrophy and hyperplasia of the smooth muscles in the larger, but not in the segmental, bronchi appeared to reflect an irritant action on these structures rather than an allergic alveolitis or asthma. Byssinosis bodies up to 50 μm $\times$ 200 μm and consisting of hyalinized fibrous nodules containing a dark staining core presumably of cellulose have been described in some lung specimens of workers exposed to cotton dust (Spencer, 1977).

There is no specific chest x-ray picture, and numerous lung function studies have reflected decreasing ventilatory capacity (Bouhuys, 1971; Merchant et al., 1974). Edwards et al. (1970) and Bouhuys (1971) concluded from their studies with normal subjects that inhaled cotton dust causes narrowing of the airways throughout the bronchial tree without changes in the "static elastic properties or transer factor of the lung." This bronchoconstriction caused by exposure to textile dusts is inhibited by antihistamine drugs and by ascorbic acid while prior administration of disodium cromoglycate protects many workers against challenges with hemp dust or its extract (Zuskin and Bouhuys, 1975). Indeed, the release of histamine by pig platelets can be produced by incubation of these elements with cotton mill dust extracts (Ainsworth et al., 1979). Whether the active factor is a component of the cotton plant such as bract, which is the most abundant constituent of respirable raw cotton dust (Morey, 1979), or comes from gram-negative bacterial contaminants (Rylander et al., 1979) is not yet clear. Atopy in individual workers is also involved in the identification of susceptible workers (Jones et al., 1980). Since the production of prostaglandin $F_2\alpha$, a potent bronchoconstrictor, is stimulated by extracts of bract from glanded cotton cultivars acting on rabbit alveolar macrophages, this prostaglandin may be involved in the etiologic chain of events that lead to byssinosis (Ziprin et al., 1981).

Prevention of respiratory disease of cotton

384

workers depends on control of dust, especially the fine, easily inhaled material. Lung function tests should be done at time of pre-employment and can be used for routine medical monitoring to screen for early harmful effects of exposure to cotton dust. Improvement in ventilatory capacity as a result of reduced dust levels may be accomplished by steaming of the cotton (Imbus and Suh, 1974), which may also remove, at least temporarily, some of the bronchoconstricting properties of the dust.

In the United States, a new cotton dust standard became effective in 1980. The limits for lint-free respirable cotton dust averaged over an 8-hour period are 200 $\mu g/m^3$ for yarn manufacture, 750 $\mu g/m^3$ for slashing and weaving operations, and 500 $\mu g/m^3$ for nontextile industries.

References

Ainsworth SK, Neuman RE, Harley RA: Histamine release from platelets for assay of byssinogenic substances in cotton mill dust and related materials. *Br J Ind Med* 1979;36:35–42.

Bouhuys A: Byssinosis in textile workers. *Trans NY Acad Sci* 1966;28:480–490.

Bouhuys A: Byssinosis. *Arch Environ Health* 1971;23:405–407.

Bouhuys A, Heaphy LJ, Schilling RSF, et al: Byssinosis in the United States. *New Engl J Med* 1969;277:170–175.

Bouhuys A, Wolfson RL, Horner DW, et al: Byssinosis in cotton textile workers: Respiratory survey of a mill with rapid labor turnover. *Ann Intern Med* 1969;71:257–269.

Edwards C, Macartney J, Rooke G, et al: The pathology of the lung in byssinotics. *Thorax* 1975;30:612–623.

Edwards J, McCarthy P, McDermott M, et al: The acute physiological, pharmacological and immunological effects of inhaled cotton dust in normal subjects. *J Physiology* 1970;208:63P–64P.

Gandevia B, Milne J: Ventilatory capacity changes on exposure to cotton dust and their relevance to byssinosis in Australia. *Br J Ind Med* 1965;22:295–304.

Harris TR, Merchant JA, Kilburn KH, et al: Byssinosis and respiratory diseases of cotton mill workers. *J Occup Med* 1972;14:199–206.

Imbus HR, Suh MW: Steaming of cotton to prevent byssinosis—A plant study. *Br J Ind Med* 1974;31:209–219.

Jones RN, Butcher BT, Hammad YY, et al: Interaction of atopy and exposure to cotton dust in the bronchoconstrictor response. *Br J Ind Med* 1980;37:141–146.

Kay JP: Observations and experiments concerning molecular irritation of the lungs as one source of tubercular consumption, and on spinners' phthisis. *North of England Med Surg J* 1831; 1:348–363.

Khogali M: Byssinosis: A follow-up study of cotton ginnery workers in the Sudan. *Br J Ind Med* 1976;33:166–174.

Kilburn KH: Byssinosis 1981. *Am J Ind Med* 1981;2:81–88.

McKerrow CB, Schilling RSF: A pilot enquiry into byssinosis in two cotton mills in the United States. *J Am Med Assoc* 1961;177:850–853.

Merchant JA, Halprin GM, Hudson AR, et al: Responses to cotton dust. *Arch Environ Health* 1975;30:222–229.

Merchant JA, Kilburn KH, O'Fallon W, et al: Byssinosis and chronic bronchitis among cotton textile workers. *Ann Intern Med* 1972;76:423–433.

Merchant JA, Lumsden JC, Kilburn KH, et al: Intervention studies of cotton steaming to reduce biological effects of cotton dust. *Br J Ind Med* 1974;31:261–274.

Morey PR: Botanically what is raw cotton dust? *Am Ind Hyg Assoc J* 1979;40:702–708.

Mustafa KY, Bos W, Lakha AS: Byssinosis in Tanzanian textile workers. *Lung* 1979;157:39–44.

Rylander R, Imbus HR, Suh MW: Bacterial contamination of cotton as an indicator of respiratory effects among card room workers. *Br J Ind Med* 1979;36:299–304.

Schilling RSF: Byssinosis in cotton and other textile workers. *Lancet* 1956;2:261–265,319–325.

Schrag PE, Gullet AD: Byssinosis in cotton textile mills. *Am Rev Resp Dis* 1970;101:497–503.

Spencer H: *Pathology of the Lung, ed 3.* Philadelphia, WB Saunders, 1977.

Ziprin R, Folwer SR, Greenblatt GA, et al: The etiology of byssinosis—comparison of prostaglandin F_2 synthesis by alveolar macrophages stimulated with extracts from glanded and glandless cotton cultivars. *Am Ind Hyg Assoc J* 1981;42:876–879.

Zuskin E, Bouhuys A: Byssinosis: Airway responses in textile dust exposure. *J Occup Med* 1975;17:357–359.

Sisal, hemp, jute, and flax   Sisal, hemp, jute, and flax are fibers that have considerable industrial use around the world. *Sisal* is derived from *Agava sisilana,* a plant of the amaryllis family native to Central America and Mexico but now also grown in the West Indies, East Indies, Hawaii, and Africa. The fibers are used for binder twine, rope, brush bristles, and upholstering. *Hemp* fiber come from *Cannabis sativa,* which is also a source of marijuana and cannot be freely grown legally in the United States. The fiber is used for making rope, twine, yarns, and in some special papers. *Jute* is a fiber derived from *Corchorus* species, annual shrub-like plants grown mostly in India. It is used for coarse fibers, burlap and gunny sacks, twine, carpets, cushions, and curtains. *Flax* is a fiber derived from the flax plant, *Linum usitatissimum,* which is also the source of linseed oil. Flax culture is an old industry, dating back to ancient Egypt, largely for the production of linen fabrics, thread, twine, and canvas.

After long and heavy exposures to dusts of these fibers, workers may develop respiratory syndromes that closely resemble the various clinical stages of byssinosis from cotton dust or such nonspecific diseases as acute and chronic bronchitis, emphysema, and bronchiectasis. Sisal and jute dusts are less likely to produce symptoms of either byssinosis or chronic respiratory disease than are cotton, hemp, or flax (Valić and Žuškin, 1972). Sisal ropemaking also involves the use of a lubricant to soften the fiber and this mixture may be responsible for the respiratory effects sometimes seen in this industry (Baker et al, 1979). Histamine release from lung tissue and consequent bronchoconstriction have been demonstrated for extracts of sisal but not for the oil additive (Nicholls et al., 1973), so that a mechanism similar to that of byssinosis may be involved with sisal as well as cotton.

Workers with soft-hemp have chronic respiratory symptoms and lung function alterations typical of obstructive lung disease after 20 years' exposure to hemp dust (Bouhuys and Žuškin, 1976). Since disodium cromoglycate given to healthy volunteers protects against the bronchoconstriction induced by challenge aerosols of hemp dust extract (Žuškin and Bouhuys, 1976), this pharmacologic agent may have prophylactic application in industry in place of antihistamines.

Flax dust produces typical byssinosis, although not all exposed workers are affected. Susceptibility may be related to genetic factors such as HLA antigens, for HLA-B27 is significantly more common in flax byssinotics, although it is not necessary for occurrence of the disease (Middleton et al., 1979). The basis for industrial hygiene standards for flax dust was set forth by the British Occupational Hygiene Society (BOHS) in 1980.

References

Baker MD, Irwig LM, Johnston JR, et al: Lung function in sisal ropemakers. *Br J Ind Med* 1979; 36:216–219.

BOHS: British Occupational Hygiene Society: A basis for hygiene standards for flax dust. *Ann Occup Hyg* 1980;23:1–26.

Bouhuys A, Žuškin E: Chronic respiratory disease in hemp workers. A follow-up study, 1967–1974. *Ann Intern Med* 1976;84:398–405.

Middleton D, Logan JS, Magennis BP, et al: HLA antigen frequencies in flax byssinosis patients. *Br J Ind Med* 1979;36:123–126.

Nicholls PJ, Evans E, Valić F, et al: Histamine-releasing activity and bronchoconstricting effects of sisal. *Br J Ind Med* 1973;30:142–145.

Valić F, Žuškin E: Effects of different vegetable dust exposures. *Br J Ind Med* 1972;29: 293–297.

Žuškin E, Bouhuys A: Protective effect of disodium cromoglycate against airway constriction induced by hemp dust extract. *J Allergy Clin Immunol* 1976;57:473–479.

Castor beans Among the many plants that may cause dermatitis, the castor bean has, in addition, the ability to produce asthma, rhinitis, conjunctivitis, and urticaria. Anaphylaxis was reported in one woman who wore a necklace made of dried castor beans (Lockey and Dunkelberger, 1968). After castor oil extraction, pomace, the crushed residue, contains a potent allergen. Persons living near or working in extraction plants, farmers using pomace as a fertilizer, and dockworkers may all react to the castor bean dust. Severe reactions have occurred in these persons as well as in men handling burlap bags that once contained castor bean pomace (Ordman, 1955; Panzani, 1957). IgE antibodies to castor beans have been detected in Sudanese dockworkers sensitive to this plant seed (Kemeny et al., 1981). The persistence of the allergenic principle is illustrated by an outbreak of coughing, sneezing, sore eyes, and chest tightness at night in a group of furniture factory upholsterers who handled felt made from

386

sacks that earlier had been used to store castor beans. Radio-allergosorbent test (RAST) assays showed that the sera of the sensitized workers contained specific IgE antibodies against both the felt and castor bean extract (Topping et al., 1981).

References

Kemeny DM, Frankland AW, Fakhri ZI, et al: Allergy to the castor bean in Sudan: measurement of serum IgE and specific IgE antibodies. *Clin Allergy* 1981;11:463–471.

Lockey SD Jr, Dunkelberger L: Anaphylaxis from an Indian necklace. *J Am Med Assoc* 1968; 206:2900–2901.

Ordman D: An outbreak of bronchial asthma in South Africa affecting more than 200 persons, caused by castor bean dust from an oil processing factory. *Intern Arch Allergy Appl Immunol* 1955;7:10–24.

Panzani R: Respiratory castor bean dust allergy in the south of France with special reference to Marseilles. *Intern Arch Allergy Appl Immunol* 1957;11:224–236.

Topping MD, Tyrer FH, Lowing RK: Castor bean allergy in the upholstery department of a furniture factory. *Br J Ind Med* 1981;38:293–296.

Coffee and tea Coffee industry workers, especialy those handling green coffee beans, may develop occupational hypersensitivity asthma, rhinitis, or dermatitis as a result of exposure to dust in the manufacturing establishments (Bernton, 1973). Ventilatory function changes have been demonstrated, and the decreases in flow rates at low lung volumes have been interpreted to indicate that the bronchoconstrictor action of the dust mostly affects the smaller airways (Žuškin et al., 1979). These investigators have warned that continued exposure to dust in both green coffee handling and roasted coffee processing may lead to a persistent loss of pulmonary function.

Different sources have been proposed for the offending allergen: chlorogenic acid, which is also present in citrus fruits and castor beans (Freedman et al., 1964), or green coffee bean protein (Layton et al., 1965). Recent work involving the immunologic responses of mice indicates that the green coffee bean is the major source of the allergen in this disease (Lehrer et al., 1978), although the possible role of castor allergen has not been excluded (Lehrer et al., 1981). It should

also be recalled that inhaled soot from coffee roasting plants may have carcinogenic properties, at least for mice, rats, and guinea pigs (Hueper and Payne, 1960).

Tea manufacture is also characterized by occupational illnesses among some workers, and these conditions have been called tea taster's disease, tea factory cough, and tea maker's asthma. Tea taster's disease has been thought to result from the inhalation of micro-organisms while sniffing tea leaves. Both the cough and the asthma are consequences of inhaling the fine dust known as tea fluff (Uragoda, 1970). Systematic study of tea workers in Sri Lanka who were exposed to tea fluff during blending operations showed a prevalence of chronic bronchitis and asthma greater than that in the general population, where chronic bronchitis is uncommon (Uragoda, 1980). The inciting allergen has not yet been characterized or identified.

References

Bernton HS: On occupational sensitization – A hazard to the coffee industry. *J Am Med Assoc* 1973;233:1146–1147.

Freedman SO, Shulman R, Drupey J, et al: Antigenic properties of chlorogenic acid. *J Allergy* 1964;35:97–107.

Hueper WC, Payne WW: Carcinogenic studies on soot of coffee-roasting plants. *Arch Pathol* 1960;69:716–727.

Layton LL, Panzani R, Greene FC, et al: Atopic hypersensitivity to a portion of the green coffee bean and absence of allergic reactions to chlorogenic acid, low molecular weight components of green coffee, or to roasted coffee. *Intern Arch Allergy Appl Immunol* 1965;28:116–127.

Lehrer SB, Karr RM, Salvaggio JE: Extraction and analysis of coffee bean allergens. *Clin Allergy* 1978;8:217–226.

Lehrer SB, Karr RM, Salvaggio JE: Analysis of green coffee bean and castor bean allergens using RAST inhibition. *Clin Allergy* 1981;11:357–366.

Uragoda CG: Tea maker's asthma. *Br J Ind Med* 1970;27:181–182.

Uragoda CG: Respiratory disease in tea workers in Sri Lanka. *Thorax* 1980;35:114–117.

Žuškin E, Valić F, Skurić Z: Respiratory function in coffee workers. *Br J Ind Med* 1979;36: 117–122.

Tobacco   Apart from the harmful effects produced by smoking, workers in the tobacco industry have other problems associated with their occupation. Cigarette cutter's asthma is much less prevalent since the introduction of modern mechanization. However, harmful amounts of respirable free silica particles of a size that could reach the lower respiratory tract were found in one study of industrial drying and stemming of tobacco (McCormick et al., 1948). On the other hand, an investigation of the respiratory response to tobacco dust exposure by nonsmoking workers in three cigarette factories showed comparatively low prevalences of chronic respiratory symptoms (Valić et al., 1976). Only chest tightness and wheezing were more common in the exposed group, while no chronic deficits in ventilatory capacity were found except for acute effects during the work shift.

Green-tobacco illness is experienced by tobacco harvesters who handle uncured damp leaves in the fields. It is a self-limited illness characterized by headache, nausea, severe vomiting, pallor, and prostration, with recovery within 24 hours (Gehlbach et al., 1974). Most interesting is the finding that cigarette smokers rarely become ill. The cause of the disease appears to be dermal absorption of nicotine from the wet tobacco leaves since a tenfold increase in urinary cotinine (the major metabolite of nicotine) was found in affected workers (Gehlbach et al., 1975; Ghosh et al., 1980). Use of rubberized nylon rainsuits effectively protects workers against nicotine absorption from wet tobacco (Gehlbach et al., 1979).

Occupational tobacco dermatitis also occurs and appears to be unrelated to nicotine absorption (Rycroft, 1980). It may be an allergic reaction but the antigen is not known and does not appear to be in tobacco smoke (Gleich et al., 1980).

References

Gehlbach SH, Williams WA, Perry LD, et al: Green-tobacco sickness. An illness of tobacco harvesters. *J Am Med Assoc* 1974;229:1880–1883.

Gehlbach SH, Williams WA, Perry LD, et al: Nicotine absorption by workers harvesting green tobacco. *Lancet* 1975;1:478–480.

Gehlbach SH, Williams WA, Freeman JI: Protective clothing as a means of reducing nicotine absorption in tobacco harvesters. *Arch Environ Health* 1979;34:111–114.

Ghosh SK, Parikh JR, Gokani VN, et al: Studies on occupational health problems in agricultural tobacco workers. *J Soc Occup Med* 1980;29:113–117.

Gleich GJ, Welsh PW, Yunginger JW, et al: Allergy to tobacco: An occupational hazard. *New Engl J Med* 1980;302:617–619.

McCormick WE, Smith M, Marsh SP: A study of the health hazards of the tobacco stemming and redrying industry. *J Ind Hyg Toxicol* 1948;30:43–52.

Rycroft RJG: Tobacco dermatitis. *Br J Dermatol* 1980;103:225–229.

Valić F, Beritić D, Butković D: Respiratory response to tobacco dust exposure. *Am Rev Resp Dis* 1976;113:751–755.

Proteolytic enzymes   Experience with occupational illnesses attributable to proteolytic enzymes has been with two groups of substances: proteases derived from papaya and pineapple, and enzyme detergents used in the manufacture of household laundry detergents.

Laundry detergents   A proteolytic enzyme prepared from *Bacillus subtilis,* a nonpathogenic organism, has been added to detergent soaps for the removal of certain stains from clothing. Workers in this industry developed signs and symptoms of harmful effects of fine dust of this material, and these findings were reported by Flindt (1969) and Newhouse et al. (1970) in England and by McMurrain (1970) in the United States. Numerous papers from these and other countries followed and an international conference was held in 1976 that summarized the work of the intervening years (Gilson et al., 1976).

Symptoms associated with heavy exposure were striking and were progressively more severe with continued exposure. Lacrimation, rhinorrhea, cough with minimal sputum, and wheezing were the usual symptoms. The patient became increasingly breathless and had to sit upright at night in order to breathe. Occasionally, a worker reported mild hemoptysis and episodes of mild fever. Before proper controls were installed, re-exposure after an interval, such as a vacation or holiday, resulted in return of symptoms. If, by accident or job change, a worker with tolerated mild symptoms received a heavy dose in a short period, he suffered a violent reaction with dyspnea, choking, and cyanosis severe enough to require oxygen inhalation. At the time of such an episode, the chest x-ray is said to have shown transient infiltrates.

388

Dermatitis due to sensitization was not seen in detergent factories although palmar eczema did occur in workers producing the concentrated enzyme (Zachariae et al., 1973).

Shore et al (1971) reported lung function abnormalities that persisted in eight of 17 workers after removal from exposure for periods up to nine months. The workers interviewed complained that exposure to house dust or tobacco smoke caused symptoms, and that accustomed exercise was no longer possible. The men in this study were young, with a mean age of 36 years. By 1973 the lung function values in this group returned to normal in all of the cases where there was no further exposure (Kazemi, personal communication to HLH, 1973). Franz et al. (1971) reported a similar clinical syndrome followed by recovery. Weill et al. (1973) found reductions in lung volumes and in expiratory flow rates to be associated with past exposures, but they also noted a reversal in the downward trend in pulmonary function, presumably because of improved working conditions. In contrast to these reported improvements, Musk and Gandevia (1976) found a significant loss of pulmonary elastic recoil in workers formerly exposed to detergent proteolytic enzymes, with only partial recovery in some cases.

Pepys et al. (1969,1973) considered the illness to be an allergic reaction on the basis of the results of skin testing and finding precipitins in sera. Atopic patients were more likely than non-atopics to become skin prick-test positive, and a good correlation was found between skin-prick tests and the presence of enzyme-specific IgE in sera (Juniper et al., 1977). The findings of Shore et al. (1971) suggest that at high doses and/or with continued exposure, the proteolytic enzyme may act to produce lower respiratory tract damage as suggested by Falk and Briscoe (1970) in their discussion of alpha-antitrypsin deficiency. It is possible that spores of *B. subtilis* remaining in the material supplied to the detergent industry may in part be responsible for the asthmatic component of the syndrome. Mitchell and Gandevia (1971) described an acute bronchiolitis as a result of provocative inhalation of the industrially used enzyme, a finding confirming the specificity of this material. Zetterström's (1977) studies showed that even sensitized patients were free from symptoms during and after the normal laundry use of enzyme-containing detergents that was followed by adequate rinsing.

Bronchodilators give temporary relief, as do steroids. Adequate engineering controls and newer methods of coating the small harmful products with inert material may reduce the severity of this occupational hazard.

References

Falk GA, Briscoe WA: Alpha₁-antitrypsin deficiency in chronic obstructive pulmonary disease. *Ann Intern Med* 1970;72:427–429.

Flindt MLH: Pulmonary disease due to inhalation of derivatives of Bacillus subtilis containing proteolytic enzyme. *Lancet* 1969;1:1177–1184.

Franz T, McMurrain KD, Brooks S, et al: Clinical, immunologic, and physiologic observations in factory workers exposed to *B. subtilis* enzyme dust. *J Allergy* 1971;47:170–180.

Gilson JC, Juniper CP, Martin RB, et al: Biological effects of proteolytic enzyme detergents. *Thorax* 1976;31:621–634.

Juniper CP, How MJ, Goodwin BFJ, et al: *Bacillus subtilis* enzymes: A 7-year clinical, epidemiological, and immunological study of an industrial allergen. *J Soc Occup Med* 1977;27:3–12.

McMurrain KD Jr: Dermatologic and pulmonary responses in the manufacturing of detergent enzyme products. *J Occup Med* 1970;12:416–420.

Mitchell CA, Gandevia B: Acute bronchiolitis following provocative inhalation of "Alcalase"—A proteolytic enzyme used in the detergent industry. *Med J Aust* 1971;1:1363–1367.

Musk AW, Gandevia B: Loss of pulmonary elastic recoil in workers formerly exposed to proteolytic enzyme (alcalase) in the detergent industry. *Br J Ind Med* 1976;33:158–165.

Newhouse ML, Tagg B, Pocock SJ, et al: An epidemiological study of workers producing enzyme washing powders. *Lancet* 1970;1:689–693.

Pepys J, Hargreave FE, Longbottom JL, et al: Allergic reactions of the lungs to enzymes of *Bacillus subtilis*. *Lancet* 1969;1:1181–1184.

Pepys J, Wells ID, D'Souza MF, et al: Clinical and immunological responses to enzymes of *Bacillus subtilis* in factory workers and consumers. *Clin Allergy* 1973;3:143–160.

Shore NS, Greene R, Kazemi H: Lung dysfunction in workers exposed to *Bacillus subtilis* enzyme. *Environ Res* 1971;4.512–519.

Weill H, Waggenspack C, DeRouen T, et al: Respiratory reactions to B. subtilis enzymes in detergents. *J Occup Med* 1973;15:267–271.

Zachariae H, Thomsen K, Rasmussen OG: Occupational enzyme dermatitis. Results of patch testing with alcalase. *Acta Derm-Venerol* 1973; 53:145–148.

Zetterström O: Challenge and exposure test reactions to enzyme detergents in subjects sensitized to subtilisin. *Clin Allergy* 1977;7:355–363.

———

Papain and bromelain Respiratory disease and other allergic reactions have occurred in persons occupationally exposed to dusts of papain and bromelain, proteolytic enzymes derived from specific fruits. Papain is a sulfhydryl-linked protease derived from the unripe fruit of the papaya tree, *Carica papaya.* It is used for tenderizing meat, clearing beer, cleaning cloudy contact lenses, lysing wound adhesions, and treating Hymenoptera and jellyfish stings (Novey et al., 1979). Although papain produces emphysematous changes in laboratory animals when instilled or inhaled, such changes have not been reported for man in whom the effects are largely allergic.

Occupational asthma, coughing, and dyspnea have been reported as a result of exposure to papain dust in meat tenderizer factories (Flindt, 1978; Novey et al., 1979), by a blood bank technician and by pharmaceutical plant employees (Tarlo et al., 1978; Baur and Fruhmann, 1979), and by food research biochemists (Milne and Brand, 1975). Employees who developed rhinitis and asthma also showed positive skin and radioallergosorbent (RAST) tests with papain (Baur and Fruhmann, 1979). The presence of IgE and IgG antibodies have been demonstrated in numerous studies, including those already cited. The potential seriousness of the situation in sensitized workers was demonstrated by the case of asthma and anaphylactic death within 30 minutes reported by Flindt (1978). Theophylline, beta adrenergic bronchodilators, and steroids are helpful but may not control symptoms unless the patient is removed from exposure.

Similar though less common problems exist with bromelain (also called bromelin), a purified protease derived from pineapple, *Ananas comosus.* Asthma and rhinitis have been reported in sensitized pharmaceutical laboratory employees exposed to bromelain dust, sometimes in massive amounts (Galleguillos and Rodriguez, 1978; Baur and Fruhmann, 1979). RAST and skin-prick tests by the latter investigators have demonstrated that bromelain can induce IgE mediated respiratory and gastrointestinal reactions, and there is evidence for immunologic cross-reactions between bromelain and papain in human subjects.

References

Baur X, Fruhmann G: Allergic reactions, including asthma, to the pineapple protease bromelain following occupational exposure. *Clin Allergy* 1979;9:443–450.

Flindt MLH: Respiratory hazards from papain. *Lancet* 1978;1:430–432.

Galleguillos F, Rodriguez JC: Asthma caused by bromelin inhalation. *Clin Allergy* 1978;8:21–24.

Milne J, Brand S: Occupational asthma after inhalation of dust of the proteolytic enzyme, papain. *Br J Ind Med* 1975;32:302–307.

Novey HS, Marchioli LE, Sokol WN, et al: Papain-induced asthma—Physiological and immunological features. *J Allergy Clin Immunol* 1979;63:98–103.

Tarlo SM, Shaikh W, Bell B, et al: Papain-induced allergic reactions. *Clin Allergy* 1978;8:207–215.

———

Miscellaneous plant dusts Occupational exposures to an array of vegetable dusts or to toxic or allergenic substances or organisms present in plant materials have resulted in a variety of illnesses. Although most of the major diseases from offending plant agents have already been discussed, a rapid survey of some of the other occupational conditions may be instructive.

Mushroom grower's (or mushroom picker's) lung has occurred among persons handling reputedly pasteurized compost used for growing these edible fungi (Bringhurst et al., 1959; Sakula, 1967). The illness consists of fever, cough, and tightness of the chest. Earlier attribution of this disease to hypersensitivity to *Micropolyspora phaeni* has been questioned by Møller et al. (1976) since they found precipitating antibodies against this organism in sera of workers who never experienced the respiratory symptoms of the disease.

A case of asthma, progressive dyspnea, malaise, fever, and intermittent arthralgia occurred in a teacher who had an acute recurrence of symptoms on return to his home after hospitalization. The wood in his apartment was extensively infected with the fungus of dry rot, *Merulius lacrymans,* to which the patient had developed an extrinsic allergic alveolitis (O'Brien et al., 1978).

Maple-bark stripper's lung was described by Towey et al. (1932) among a group of men working in a railroad sleeper plant where they stripped bark from stored maple logs. More recent reports of the same disease have come from observers of sawmill employees in Wisconsin (Wenzel and Emanuel, 1967). The acute respiratory illness in these workers has been ascribed to a hypersensitivity state induced by spores of *Cryptostroma (Coniosporum) corticale* that occur in maple wood and English sycamore logs. Spores of this organism have been detected histologically in subpleural granulomatous nodules, from which they have also been cultured. Wood-cutter's disease, a recurrent eczema, has been reported to be the result of contact sensitization to lichens growing on ash bark (Champion, 1965).

Allergic alveolitis has been described in maltworkers who became hypersensitive to inhaled spores of *Aspergillus clavatus* that heavily contaminated the germinating barley on the malt floors in a Scottish whiskey distillery (Channell et al., 1969). This fungus was also recovered from the sputum of most of the employees, including those who developed overt pulmonary hypersensitivity.

Occupational exposure to psyllium (ispagula) powder used in bulk laxatives has led to rhinitis, conjunctivitis, or asthma in many employees of pharmaceutical firms processing or packaging this finely ground product, which is derived from the seeds of *Plantago ovata,* a member of the plantain-weed family (Busse and Schoenwetter, 1975; Göransson and Michaelson, 1979). Bronchial challenges with psyllium extract and intracutaneous tests have been positive in the sensitized employees. That soybean dust on occasion can also produce both immediate and delayed onset asthma in previously nonallergic persons when they are exposed to such dust at work has been reported several times, most recently by Bush and Cohen (1977).

Among other interesting conditions occurring as a result of occupational contact with plants are the phototoxic bullae seen in celery harvesters, perhaps due to the pink-rot fungus, *Sclerotinia sclerotiorum* (Birmingham et al., 1961); the allergic contact dermatitis from leatherleaf fern used by florists as a filler and background plant in bouquets and table decorations (Hausen and Schulz, 1978); the contact dermatitis from lettuce (*Lactuca sativa*) occasionally seen in gardeners and lettuce-packers, who also have a cross-sensitivity to endive (*Cichorium endivia*) (Krook,

1977); and the contact allergic sensitivity and photosensitivity seen in florists handling chrysanthemums, where the responsible allergen is thought to be a sesquiterpene lactone found in the leaves and flowers (Bleumink et al., 1976; Frain-Bell et al., 1979). Pyrethrum, a widely used insecticide made from the flowers of several chrysanthemum species, has been known to cause allergic rhinitis and asthma. Recently, a case of hypersensitivity pneumonitis, with pleuritic chest pain, nonproductive cough, and shortness of breath, was reported in a young woman who, for neurotic reasons, was repeatedly exposed to a pyrethrum-based insecticide (Carlson and Villaveces, 1977).

References

Birmingham DJ, Key MM, Tubich GE, et al: Phototoxic bullae among celery harvesters. *Arch Dermatol* 1961;83:73–87.

Bleumink E, Mitchell JC, Geissman TA, et al: Contact hypersensitivity to sesquiterpene lactones in chrysanthemum dermatitis. *Contact Derm* 1976;2:81–88.

Bringhurst LS, Byrne RN, Gershon-Cohen J: Respiratory disease of mushroom workers. *J Am Med Assoc* 1959;171:15–18.

Bush RK, Cohen M: Immediate and late onset asthma from occupational exposure to soybean dust. *Clin Allergy* 1977;7:369–373.

Busse WW, Schoenwetter WF: Asthma from psyllium in laxative manufacture. *Ann Intern Med* 1975;83:361–362.

Carlson JE, Villaveces JW: Hypersensitivity pneumonitis due to pyrethrum. Report of a case. *J Am Med Assoc* 1977;237:1718–1719.

Champion RH: Wood-cutter's disease: Contact sensitivity to lichen. *Br J Dermatol* 1965;77:285.

Channell S, Blyth W, Lloyd M, et al: Allergic alveolitis in maltworkers: A clinical, mycological, and immunological study. *Q J Med* 1969;38:351–376.

Frain-Bell W, Hetherington A, Johnson BE: Contact allergic sensitivity to chrysanthemum and the photosensitivity dermatitis and actinic reticuloid syndrome. *Br J Dermatol* 1979;101:491–501.

Göransson K, Michaelson NG: Ispagula powder: An allergen in the work environment. *Scand J Work Environ Health* 1979;5:257–261.

Hausen BM, Schulz KH: Occupational allergic contact dermatitis due to leatherleaf fern *Arachniodes adiantiformis* (Forst) Tindale. *Br J Dermatol* 1978;98:325–329.

Krook G: Occupational dermatitis from *Lactuca sativa* (lettuce) and *Cichorium* (endive). *Contact Derm* 1977;3:27–36.

Møller BM, Halberg P, Gravesen S, et al: Precipitating antibodies against *Micropolyspora phaeni* in sera from mushroom workers. *Acta Allergol* 1976;31:61–71.

O'Brien IM, Bull J, Creamer B, et al: Asthma and extrinsic allergic alveolitis due to *Merulius lacrymans*. *Clin Allergy* 1978;8:535–542.

Sakula A: Mushroom worker's lung. *Br Med J* 1967;3:708–710.

Towey JW, Sweany HC, Huron WH: Severe bronchial asthma apparently due to fungus spores found in maple bark. *J Am Med Assoc* 1932;99:453–459.

Wenzel FJ, Emanuel DA: The epidemiology of maple bark disease. *Arch Environ Health* 1967;14:385–389.

Animal Dusts and Animal Products

Reports occasionally appear that associate animal dusts and other animal products with disease. Anthrax is an infectious disease caused by penetration into the skin of spores of *Bacillus anthracis* in dust from wool, hides, crushed bones, and other products from infected animals. Occupational hypersensitivity diseases include feather picker's disease and duck fever among workers cleaning and sorting poultry feathers. Cough, dyspnea, chills, fever, nausea, and headache occur on first exposure. Some tolerance is developed within a week but substantial immunity and freedom from such symptoms requires several years of exposure.

Laboratory animal dander allergy has become a serious problem in research institutions (Lutsky and Neuman, 1975). Lincoln et al. (1974) quote estimates of 40 million mammals, of which 39 million are rodents, under study each year in the United States. Hypersensitivity reactions to animal dander and sera have become a problem among persons working with experimental animals. Such persons include animal caretakers, research technicians, veterinarians, as well as investigator scientists. Typical cases are those of young adults, with a family history of atopy, who develop hypersensitivity within three years of close contact with laboratory animals. Allergic rhinitis and asthma are the most common symptoms along with urticarial skin reactions and conjunctivitis. Angioedema may also occur but is less frequent.

Slaughterhouse workers may develop immediate-type hypersensitivity as a result of contact with fresh animal products, especially blood (Hjorth, 1978; Göransson, 1981), manifested as red, scaly eczema that heals spontaneously on cessation of exposure. Poultry processing has other hazards to the skin unrelated to dust, mainly lacerations, puncture wounds, and paronychial infections (Cohen, 1974).

Invertebrates may also be the cause of occupational hypersensitivity disease. Tussockosis, in persons exposed to fragments and dust of the fir tussock moth in the Pacific Northwest of the United States, involves the skin, eyes, and respiratory tract. Urticaria, itching, vesiculation, and eruptions affect the skin, while the eyes become swollen and pruritic. Rhinitis, chest discomfort and tightness, cough, dyspnea, and even epistaxis, are the chief airway symptoms (Perlman et al., 1976; Press et al., 1977). Skin tests with tussock moth materials gave positive results in most of the exposed workers.

Occupational asthma has been reported from a locust-breeding research center (Burge et al., 1980), while pulmonary hypersensitivity from inhaling grain weevil dust has been reported from another laboratory (Lunn and Hughes, 1967). Occupational dermatitis occurred from contact with grain itch mites in a manager of a store in Texas handling imported dried leaves and flowers for decorative purposes (Baggett et al., 1981). Bronchial asthma has been recorded in cultured oyster workers (Nakashima, 1969) and in workers exposed to prawn aerosols in a processing plant where compressed air was used to blow the edible meat out of the tails (Gaddie et al., 1980).

Occupational dermatitis from contact with animal proteins can occur in restaurant kitchens and food processing plants. The major sources of allergens of this type in Denmark appear to be fish and shellfish; here, the skin is mainly involved and inhalant allergies are rare (Hjorth and Roed-Petersen, 1976). Cheesemakers and cheese-washers may suffer from primary irritant hand dermatitis and from asthma induced by rennet (Niinimäki and Saari, 1978) or by the spores of *Penicillium casei*.

Pituitary snuff, prepared from porcine and cattle pituitaries, may give rise to a chronic interstitial pneumonitis in workers preparing this medicinal product (Mahon et al., 1967). Bronchospasm and eosinophilia may occur, and the pathologic changes in the lung resemble those seen in bird-breeder's lung.

References

Baggett DA, Davis BL, Elliot LB, et al: Occupational dermatitis associated with grain itch mites — Texas. *Morb Mort Weekly Rep* 1981;30:590–592.

Burge PS, Edge G, O'Brien IM, et al: Occupational asthma in a research centre breeding locusts. *Clin Allergy* 1980;10:355–363.

Cohen SR: Dermatologic hazards in the poultry industry. *J Occup Med* 1974;16:94–97.

Gaddie J, Legge JS, Friend JAR, et al: Pulmonary hypersensitivity in prawn workers. *Lancet* 1980;2:1350–1352.

Göransson K: Occupational contact urticaria to fresh cow and pig blood in slaughtermen. *Contact Derm* 1981;7:281–282.

Hjorth N: Gut eczema in slaughterhouse workers. *Contact Derm* 1978;4:49–52.

Hjorth N, Roed-Petersen J: Occupational protein contact dermatitis in food handlers. *Contact Derm* 1976;2:28–42.

Lincoln TA, Bolton NE, Garrett AS Jr: Occupational allergy to animal dander and sera. *J Occup Med* 1974;16:465–469.

Lunn JA, Hughes DTD: Pulmonary hypersensitivity to the grain weevil. *Br J Ind Med* 1967;24:158–161.

Lutsky IL, Neuman I: Laboratory animal dander allergy: I. An occupational disease. *Ann Allergy* 1975;35:201–205.

Mahon WE, Scott DJ, Ansell G, et al: Hypersensitivity to pituitary snuff with miliary shadowing in the lungs. *Thorax* 1967;22:13–20.

Nakashima T: Studies of bronchial asthma observed in cultured oyster workers. *Hiroshima J Med Sci* 1969;18:141–184.

Niinimäki A, Saari S: Dermatological and allergic hazards of cheesemakers. *Scand J Work Environ Health* 1978;4:262–263.

Perlman F, Press E, Googins JA, et al: Tussockosis: Reactions to Douglas fir tussock moth. *Ann Allergy* 1976;36:302–307.

Press E, Googins JA, Poareo H, et al: Health hazards to timber and forestry workers from the Douglas fir tussock moth. *Arch Environ Health* 1977;32:206–210.

APPENDIX

No attempt has been made in connection with the preparation of this edition to provide a comprehensive introduction or guide to the general literature on occupational medicine, industrial toxicology, or industrial hygiene. Reference is made in this Appendix to several series of monographs that may prove useful to readers who wish to pursue in greater detail the literature on selected specific topics. Monographs and other reviews are referred to in the individual reference lists that follow each topic in this revised edition.

NATIONAL INSTITUTE FOR OCCUPATIONAL SAFETY AND HEALTH (NIOSH)

Criteria Documents

The NIOSH "Criteria Documents" are so named because each of them has the common element in its title that reads: "Criteria for a Recommended Standard .... Occupational Exposure to ...". They are in a consistent format that includes biological effects of exposure to man and animals, environmental data, work practices, research needs, development of and recommendations for a standard, along with copious references and technical appendices. They are variously available from NIOSH, the Government Printing Office (GPO), or the National Technical Information Service (NTIS). For information on availabilities, see *NIOSH Publications Catalog,* 4th edition, 1980 (NIOSH 80-126), or a later edition, obtainable from NIOSH, Division of Technical Services, Cincinnati, OH 45226.

An alphabetic listing of "Criteria Documents" along with identifying NIOSH Publication Nos. follows:

Acetylene 76-195
Acrylamide 77-112
Acrylonitrile 78-116
Alkanes 77-151
Allyl Chloride 76-204
Ammonia 74-136

Antimony 78-216
Asbestos 72-10267
Asbestos (Revised) 77-169
Asphalt Fumes 78-106
Benzene 74-137
Benzoyl Peroxide 77-166
Benzyl Chloride 78-182
Beryllium 72-10268
Boron Trifluoride 77-122
Cadmium 76-192
Carbaryl 77-107
Carbon Black 78-204
Carbon Dioxide 76-194
Carbon Disulfide 77-156
Carbon Monoxide 73-11000
Carbon Tetrachloride 76-133
Chlorine 76-170
Chloroform 75-114
Chloroprene 77-210
Chromic Acid 73-11021
Chromium VI 76-129
Coal Gasification Plants 78-191
Coal Tar Products 78-107
Coke Oven Emissions 73-11016
Cotton Dust 75-118
Cresol 78-133
Crystalline Silica 75-120
Decomposition Products of Fluoro-
carbon Polymers 77-193
Dibromochloropropane (DBCP) 78-115
Diisocyanates 78-215
Dinitro-Ortho-Cresol 78-131
Dioxane 77-226
Epichlorohydrin 76-206
Ethylene Dibromide 77-221
Ethylene Dichloride 76-139
Ethylene Dichloride (1,2-Dichloroeth-
ane) (Revised) 78-211
Fibrous Glass 77-152
Formaldehyde 77-126
Furfuryl Alcohol 79-133
Glycidyl Ethers 78-166
Hot Environments 72-10269
Hydrazines 78-172
Hydrogen Cyanide and Cyanide Salts
77-108

NATIONAL COUNCIL ON RADIATION PROTECTION AND MEASUREMENTS (NCRP)

Reports

Many of the Reports of the NCRP are relevant to the field of occupational medicine and hygiene. They are authoritative statements and each is supported by an extensive bibliographic list. They are available from the National Council on Radiation Protection and Measurements, Suite 1016, 7910 Woodmont Avenue, Bethesda, Maryland 20814, at current prices.

A selected list follows. Reports marked with an asterisk (*) may be of particular interest to occupational physicians and industrial hygienists.

8* Control and Removal of Radioactive Contamination in Laboratories (1951)
9 Recommendations for Waste Disposal of Phosphorus-32 and Iodine for Medical Users (1951)
12 Recommendations for the Disposal of Carbon-14 Wastes (1953)
16 Radioactive Waste Disposal in the Ocean (1954)
22* Maximum Permissible Body Burdens and Maximum Permissible Concentrations of Radionuclides in Air and in Water for Occupational Exposure (1959)
30* Safe Handling of Radioactive Materials (1964)
32* Radiation Protection in Educational Institutions (1966)
35 Dental X-Ray Protection (1970)
36 Radiation Protection in Veterinary Medicine (1970)
37 Precaution in the Management of Patients Who Have Received Therapeutic Amounts of Radionuclides (1970)
38 Protection Against Neutron Radiation (1971)
39* Basic Radiation Protection Criteria (1971)
42 Radiological Factors Affecting Decision-Making in a Nuclear Attack (1974)

43* Review of the Current State of Radiation Protection Philosophy (1975)
44 Krypton-85 in the Atmosphere—Accumulation, Biological Significance, and Control Technology (1975)
45* Natural Background Radiation in the United States (1975)
46 Alpha-Emitting Particles in Lungs (1975)
47 Tritium Measurement Techniques (1976)
48* Radiation Protection for Medical and Allied Health Personnel (1976)
50* Environmental Radiation Measurements (1976)
52 Cesium-137 from the Environment to Man: Metabolism and Dose (1977)
53* Review of NCRP Radiation Dose Limit for Embryo and Fetus in Occupationally Exposed Women (1977)
54 Medical Radiation Exposure of Pregnant and Potentially Pregnant Women (1977)
55* Protection of the Thyroid Gland in the Event of Releases of Radioiodine (1977)
56 Radiation Exposure from Consumer Products and Miscellaneous Sources (1977)
57* Instrumentation and Monitoring Methods for Radiation Protection (1978)
58* A Handbook of Radioactivity Measurement Procedures (1978)
59* Operational Radiation Safety Program (1978)
60 Physical, Chemical, and Biological Properties of Radiocerium Relevant to Radiation Protection Guidelines (1978)
61* Radiation Safety Training Criteria for Industrial Radiography (1978)
62 Tritium in the Environment (1979)
63 Tritium and Other Radionuclide Labeled Organic Compounds Incorporated in Genetic Material (1979)
64 Influence of Dose and Its Distribution in Time on Dose-Response Relationships for Low-LET Radiations (1980)
65* Management of Persons Accidentally Contaminated with Radionuclides (1980)
66 Mammography (1980)
67 Radiofrequency Electromagnetic Fields—Properties, Quantities and Units, Biophysical Interaction, and Measurements (1981)

WORLD HEALTH ORGANIZATION (WHO)

Environmental Health Criteria

Monographs in this series are published by the World Health Organization with joint sponsorship by the United Nations Environment Programme. These reports, which contain information relating to occupational exposure, are available throughout the world from booksellers or at authorized WHO publications outlets.

1. Mercury (1976).
2. Polychlorinated Biphenyls and Terphenyls (1976).
3. Lead (1977).
4. Oxides of Nitrogen (1977).
5. Nitrates, Nitrites, and N-Nitroso Compounds (1977).
7. Photochemical Oxidants (1979).
8. Sulfur Oxides and Suspended Particulate Matter (1979).
9. DDT and its Derivatives (1979).
10. Carbon Disulfide (1979).
11. Mycotoxins (1979)
12. Noise (1979)
13. Carbon Monoxide (1979).
14. Ultraviolet Radiation (1979).
15. Tin and Organotin Compounds (1980).

GLOSSARY

This glossary, taken in large part from the previous edition of this book where the glossary was adapted from Johnstone and Miller (1960)*, has been included to help the reader understand the terms used by worker-patients. It makes no pretension to completeness and it may, in some cases, contain American terms that have not acquired world-wide use.

Abrasive blasting A process for cleaning surfaces by means of materials such as sand, aluminum, or steel grit in a stream of high pressure air.

Accelerator A substance that hastens or increases the speed of a chemical reaction, such as in vulcanizing rubber.

Acid pickling A bath treatment to remove scale and other impurities from metal surfaces prior to plating or other surface treatment. Sulfuric acid is commonly used.

Adiabatic Occurring without loss or gain of heat.

Alkylation The introduction of one or more alkyl radicals by addition or substitution into an organic compound.

Alloy A mixture of metals, such as in brass, and in some instances a metal and nonmetal.

Amalgamation The process of alloying metals with mercury. Used in extracting gold and silver from their ores.

Amazeine Machine process of beveling edges of leather strips preparatory to cementing them together in shoe manufacture.

Anneal To treat by heat with subsequent cooling for drawing the temper of metals and glass, i.e., to soften and render less brittle.

Anodize To coat a metal electrolytically with a protective film.

Antioxidant A chemical compound used in rubber and other formulations to prevent oxidation by exerting a "negative catalytic" action.

Arc welding One form of electric welding by use of uncoated or coated rods.

Artificial abrasives Materials, such as carborundum or emery, that are substituted for natural abrasives, such as sandstone.

Atomic hydrogen welding A shielded gas-electric welding process that uses hydrogen as the reducing atmosphere.

Azeotrope A liquid mixture that has a constant boiling point different from that of its constituents and that distills without change of composition.

Babbitt metal An alloy of tin that contains antimony and copper or an alloy of lead that contains tin and antimony; used to line bearings.

Back In hardrock mining, the roof or top surface of the excavation.

Bag house The housing containing bag filters for recovery of the fumes of arsenic, lead, and sulfur, from smelter flues.

Bakelite The trade name of a synthetic resin formed by the polymerization of formaldehyde and phenol.

Banbury mixer A mixing machine that permits control over the temperature of the batches commonly used in the rubber and plastic industries.

Beam house In a tannery, the area where hair, flesh, and grease are removed from hides or skins before tanning.

Beat elbow Bursitis of the elbow joint that results from the use of heavy vibrating tools.

Beat knee Bursitis of the knee joint due to friction or vibration; common in miners.

Beehive kiln A kiln shaped like a large beehive, usually used for calcining ceramics.

Beryl A silicate of beryllium and aluminum.

Billet A piece of semifinished iron or steel, nearly square in section, made by rolling and cutting an ingot.

Biscuit Unglazed earthenware or ceramic after the first firing.

Bisque ware Clay ware that has been fired in a bisque kiln but has not yet been glazed.

Blackdamp Chokedamp. Essentially carbon dioxide.

Blackhead itch Chloracne resulting from expo-

---

*Johnstone RT, Miller SE: *Occupational Diseases and Industrial Medicine,* Philadelphia, Saunders, 1960.

sure to chlorinated naphthalenes; also called "cable rash" by workmen.

Black liquor A liquor composed of alkaline and organic matter resulting from digestion of wood pulp and cooking acid during the manufacture of paper.

Blanching machine A device that automatically washes fruit or vegetables in hot water for canning.

Blast furnace A furnace in which combustion is forced by air under pressure.

Blooming mill A rolling mill for shaping heated metal ingots into rectangular blocks.

Blowhole A defect in a casting caused by the imprisonment of gas bubbles during solidification of the molten metal.

Boarding The process of softening leather and developing the grain by rubbing the surfaces together.

Boiling off Removing size and impurities from cloth preparatory to dyeing by circulating boiling caustic solution through cloth in a kier, or by running cloth through a boil-off machine.

Bone black Animal charcoal made by burning bone in a limited amount of air; bone char.

Bony coal High ash content slatey coal or carbonaceous shale found in coal seams.

Booster An explosive substance that transmits the impulse from the detonator to the main explosive.

Brake shoe A block, usually of cast iron or molded asbestos, shaped with a concave surface to contact a wheel or brake drum.

Brass An alloy of copper and zinc; may contain small proportions of lead or tin.

Brattice A plank and cloth partition constructed in underground passageways to control ventilation in mines.

Braze To solder with any alloy that is relatively infusible.

Briquette Coal or ore dust pressed into oval or brick-shaped blocks.

Broach A cutting tool for making nonround holes.

Broke Paper discarded from paper-making machines.

Bull ladle A refractory lined ladle designed to pour about 150 pounds (68 kg) of molten metal.

Burnishing iron A rotary wheel used to eliminate surface irregularities from shoe leather; also used in other trades.

Burr A thin rough edge on a machined piece of metal.

Bus bar Metal conductor forming a common junction between two or more electrical circuits.

Butt weld A butt joint made by welding.

Calcination The heat treatment of solid material to bring about decomposition, usually to a powder, but not by melting.

Calender An assembly of rollers for producing a smooth or glossy finish on cloth, paper, rubber, artificial leather, or plastic.

Carbon black A pure carbon, best known as common soot, produced commercially by incomplete combustion of hydrocarbons. Also called channel black, furnace black, acetylene black, or thermal black.

Carbonizing The immersion in sulfuric acid of semi-processed felt to remove any vegetable matter present.

Carborundum A trade name for silicon carbide widely used as an abrasive.

Carding The process of combing or untangling fibers such as wool or cotton.

Carrot A substance used for promoting felting of fur fibers.

Case-hardening A process of surface-hardening metals by increasing the carbon content of the outer surface.

Case mold A mold made of plaster of paris (partially dehydrated calcium sulfate) used as a pattern for making block molds.

Castellated A term applied to a nut that is radially grooved to form a seat for a cotter pin.

Casting The pouring of molten material into a mold and permitting it to solidify to the desired shape.

Catwalk A narrow suspended foot-way usually used for inspection or maintenance purposes.

Cellulose A complex polymeric carbohydrate that forms the cell walls of plants.

Cement, portland Portland cement commonly consists of hydraulic calcium silicates to which certain materials are added in limited amounts. Ordinarily, the mixture consists of calcareous materials such as limestone, chalk, shells, marl and clay, shale, and blast furnace slag. The mixture is calcined to incipient fusion at temperatures usually up to 1,500°C.

Ceramic A term applied to pottery, brick, and

tile products molded from clay and subsequently hardened by firing at high temperatures.

Chamfering The operation of rounding or beveling sharp edges and corners of a work piece.

Chaplet A specially shaped metal piece used to support a core of a foundry piece to hold it in place while the mold is being poured.

Chase A rectangular iron or steel frame to hold type in place during printing or plating.

Chelation The formation of a chemical ring structure containing a metal ion that is attached by coordinate links to two or more nonmetal atoms in the same molecule.

Chemical cartridge A type of absorption unit used with a respirator for removal of low concentrations of solvent vapors and certain gases.

Chicle The milky sap from a tropical tree, *Achras zapota,* a member of the sapodilla family, used for making chewing gum.

Chokedamp Same as blackdamp.

Christmas tree An elaborate assembly of pipes and valves that constitutes the above-ground control apparatus of an oil well.

Chuck An adjustable set of jaws that holds either a work piece or a cutting tool in a machine tool.

Clinker The rock-like product resulting from calcined or vitrified pulverized stone or other impurities formed in a furnace or kiln.

Coated welding rods Although the coatings of welding rods vary, most of them are fluoride coated. For the welding of iron and most steel, rods contain manganese, titanium, and a silicate.

Cofferdam A temporary watertight enclosure, built in water and pumped dry, to permit excavation in the floor of a waterway.

Coking High temperature carbonization of bituminous coal, coal tar, pitch, or petroleum residues to produce coke, a hard residue that is mainly carbon.

Colloid mill A machine that grinds materials into a very fine state of subdivision, and often simultaneously placing it in suspension in a liquid.

Coolants Transfer agents used in a flow system to convey heat from its source. Low temperature coolants include salt water, alcohols, glycols, and certain of the refrigerants such as ammonia, sulfur dioxide, methyl chloride, and fluorinated hydrocarbons ("Freons").

High temperature coolants include oil, mercury, tetraryl silicates, sodium-potassium alloy (NaK), and "Dowtherm."

Cope Top half of a flask used for preparing molds in a foundry.

Core A shaped hard-baked cake of sand and additives that is placed within a mold to form a cavity in the casting when it solidifies.

Core blower A mechanical device operated by compressed air that is used in a foundry for forming sand cores.

Cottrell precipitator A device for electrostatic precipitation of dust.

Cracker stillman In the petroleum industry, the operator of a cracking process who is usually located in a special control room that is some distance from the cracking units.

Cracking A term used almost exclusively in the petroleum industry, cracking is the thermal or catalytic decomposition of heavy hydrocarbons to form lighter products such as gasoline.

Crawfish A bucket-type conveyor system used to unload grain from boxcars.

Crib A room or enclosure from which tools, spare parts, and materials are dispensed.

Cribbing A framework of timber used to support heavy objects temporarily.

Crutcher A steam-jacketed mixing machine that incorporates fillers and perfumes into liquid soap.

Cullet Scrap glass.

Culls Rejected low-grade materials that have been sorted from kindred objects.

Culm Anthracite coal waste or inferior anthracite coal.

Cupola A vertical melting furnace consisting of a steel cylinder lined with refractory brick, open at the top and closed at the bottom with double doors. Commonly used in gray iron foundries.

Currying The finishing treatment of heavy leather products with oils and greases to increase strength, water repellancy, and pliability.

Cutting fluids and oils Cutting fluids are usually oils or oil-water emulsions used to cool and lubricate cutting tools. Cutting oils are usually light or heavy petroleum fractions; oil-water emulsions are most apt to use mineral oil.

Cyanide egg Sodium cyanide in shape of an egg.

Cyclone separator A centrifugal dust-collecting device for separating fine dust.

400

Dado cutter A cutter designed to cut grooves in wood.

Damp A harmful gas or mixture of gases in coal mines.

Den room A room where superphosphate is temporarily stored during fertilizer manufacture.

Deseaming Removal from steel ingots of superficial defects (cracks, cold drops, inclusions, and oxides and other impurities) by burning with oxygen-gas mixtures.

Die A hard metal or plastic form or device used to shape material to a particular contour or section.

Die casting To make a casting by forcing molten metal into a metal mold or die.

Digestor A large steel boilerlike still used to extract and vaporize turpentine oils from wood pulp or to prepare cellulose pulp.

Drag The under portion of a flask; the opposite of a cope.

Drop forge To forge between dies by a drop hammer or drop press.

Drop hammer A heavy hammer free to rise and fall between vertical guides.

Dross The scum that forms on the surface of molten metals, largely oxides and impurities.

Drumming The tumbling of hides or leather in a drum, either in dye or in solution, to soften the material or impregnate it with oil or dyes.

Ductile Capable of being drawn out into wire or thread.

Electrolysis The process of effecting chemical change by passing an electric current through a chemical solution.

Emery Corundum, aluminum oxide, a natural and synthetic abrasive.

Enamel A lead-free, oily paint that produces a glossy finish on a surface to which it is applied; often contains various synthetic resins. In contrast, ceramic enamel, i.e., porcelain enamel, contains lead.

Extrusion The forcing of raw material through a die or form in either a hot or cold state or in a partial solution. Long used with metals and clays, it is now extensively used in the plastics industry.

Facing In foundry work, the final touch-up of the mold surface to come in contact with the metal is called the facing operation, and the fine powdered material that is used is called the facing.

Ferrite Yellowish, reddish, or brownish discoloration in rock due to iron.

Fettle Any final trimming, cleaning, or smoothing operation, such as in pottery work. Fettling is common to many industries but the operation may vary greatly.

Fire brick A special clay brick that is capable of resisting high temperatures without melting or crumbling.

Firedamp In mining, the accumulation of explosive gas, chiefly methane. Miners refer to all dangerous underground gases as "damps."

Flameproofing material Substances resistant to the action of flames; includes chemicals that catalytically control the decomposition of cellulose material at flaming temperatures. Substances used as fire retardants include borax-boric acid, borax-boric acid-diammonium phosphate, ammonium bromide, stannic acid, antimony oxide, and combinations containing formaldehyde.

Flask In foundry work, the assembly of the cope and drag constitutes the flask. It is the wood or iron frame containing sand into which molded metal is poured. Some flasks may have three or four parts.

Flocculator A device for aggregating and coalescing fine particles.

Flotation A method of ore concentration in which the mineral is caused to float by chemical agents while the impurities sink.

Flume A trough in which water runs; used to transport materials, sometimes applied to a stream of water.

Flux Usually refers to a substance used to clean surfaces and promote fusion in soldering. Fluxes of various chemical natures are used in the smelting of ores, in the ceramic industry, in assaying silver and gold ores, and in other processes. The most common fluxes are silica, various silicates, lime, sodium and potassium carbonates, and litharge and red lead.

Forge A small open furnace used to heat metal so that it may be shaped, or the shaping process itself.

Forge welding The joining of metal parts by heating them to a high temperature and pressing or pounding them together.

Fractionation Separation of a mixture into different portions or fractions, usually by distillation.

Frit Partially fused minerals ground up for use in such operations as graniteware, pottery, and glass making.

Fuller's earth A clay-like material composed of colloidal hydrous aluminum silicate; used as a catalyst and as a filter medium in refining oils and fats.

Fume Gas-like emanation containing minute solid particles arising from the heating of a solid body, such as lead, in distinction to a gas or vapor.

Galvanizing An old method that is still used to provide a protective coating for metals by dipping them into a bath of molten zinc.

Gangue In mining or quarrying, useless chipped rock.

Gang welding A welding machine for conducting several welding operations simultaneously.

Garnet A complex silicate often found as crystals in gneiss and mica schist. Regarded as a semi-precious gem and used as an abrasive.

Gas welding Fusion welding with heat from a gas flame such as oxygen-acetylene.

Gauger In the petroleum industry, one who walks around the top of storage tanks, opens the "gauging hole" to measure the temperature and content level. Exposure is primarily to hydrogen sulfide.

Getter A chemically active substance placed inside a vacuum tube for removal of final traces of oxygen after the evacuation and sealing of the tube.

Glaze A compound of mineral, often containing lead, that is applied to pottery ware and then fired for a transparent glass-like finish.

Glazier A worker with finished glass but not a glass-maker.

Glory hole A peep-hole into a glass-making or steel furnace.

Gob Waste mineral material, such as from coal mines, but containing sufficient coal that gob pile fires may arise from spontaneous combustion.

Graphite A dark gray natural form of mineral carbon frequently referred to as plumbago; rarely found in pure form.

Gray iron Pig or cast iron containing graphitic carbon.

Grease monkey In many industries, the worker responsible for the oiling and greasing of machinery.

Grease stick In polishing and buffing, a stick containing an abrasive or polishing agent held against the revolving part.

Green ware Unfired pottery.

Grid A network of catwalks suspended from a ceiling. Also, part of a storage battery.

Grinder's asthma An obsolete term for silicosis.

Gyratory crusher A device for crushing rock by means of a heavy steel pestle, rotating in a steel cone, with the rock being fed in at the top and passing out of the bottom.

Halowax The trade name for chlorinated naphthalene waxes.

Heading In mining, a horizontal tunnel (drift); also, the end of a drift or gallery. In tanning, a layer of powdered bark over the tanning liquor.

Heat treatment Any of several processes of metal modification such as annealing or cyanide treatment.

Homogenizer A machine that forces liquids under high pressure through a perforated shield against a hard surface to blend or emulsify the mixture.

Hose mask A mask supplied with unmodified air through a hose or piping in contradistinction to a filter mask.

Hydration The process of converting raw material into pulp by prolonged beating in water. Also, to combine with water or with elements of water.

Hydro-blast Device used for removal of casting cores by means of an exceedingly high-pressure water stream.

Hydrogenation Reaction of molecular hydrogen with numerous organic compounds, e.g., the hydrogenation of olefins to paraffins or of the aromatics to naphthenes or the reduction of aldehydes and ketones to alcohols.

Inert gas welding An electric welding operation utilizing an inert gas such as helium to prevent oxidation of the metal being welded.

Ingot A block of iron or steel cast in a mold for ease in handling prior to processing.

Investment casting There are numerous types of investment casting, including the lost wax process. Materials used include fire-clay, silicon dioxide, silica flour, sillimanite, cristobalite, aluminum oxide, and zirconium oxide. The process that utilizes mercury that is frozen and later recovered at room temperatures may provide unrecognized harmful exposure to mercury vapor.

Jigger An apparatus for forming plastic clay that consists of a rotating head to mold the top and a shaping tool to shape the bottom. Also, a person operating a jig or device that shakes down grain during bagging. Other meanings also exist.

Jitterbug sander Electrically operated device for finishing aluminum, magnesium, and other materials.

Jolly A potter's apparatus similar to a jigger by which plastic clay is formed into flat ware and hollow ware.

Kaolin Aluminum silicate clays of mixed constituency; in some deposits, free silica may be present as an impurity.

Kapok A mass of silky fibers from pods of the ceiba tree used as a stuffing for mattresses, cushions, life preservers, and sleeping bags; also woven into fabric.

Kier A cylindrical iron tank lined with cement in which fabrics, yarns, and fibers are cleaned, bleached, or dyed.

Lacquer A colloidal dispersion or solution of nitrocellulose or similar resin-free film-forming compounds, or plasticizers in solvents or diluents, used to form a protective coating for various surfaces.

Lagging The removal of thermal insulation (also known as lagging) applied to pipes and other cylindrical objects.

Laminar flow Streamlined or layered flow in air or viscous fluid.

Lapping The operation of polishing or scraping surfaces such as metal or glass to a precise dimension.

Latex The milky sap exuded by many plants, chiefly applied to sap from rubber trees when the bark is cut. Also applied to materials produced synthetically for use in paints and other coatings, and in adhesives.

Lead burning The fusion of pieces of lead; used in the manufacture of lead plates for storage batteries.

Light end The portion of a mixture of liquids usually from a petroleum or by-product coke-oven source that distills at a lower boiling point range.

Liming The treatment of hides to loosen hair and to swell the fibers in order to obtain better impregnation of tanning solutions.

Linters Short cotton fibers that adhere to cotton seeds after ginning.

Litharge Lead monoxide obtained as a yellow flake or powder at temperatures above the melting point of the oxide.

Lithopone A white pigment and paint filler used in paints, printing inks, and linoleum in place of white lead; consists of zinc sulfide and barium sulfate.

Lode In mining, any vein of metal.

Macerator A power-driven machine that softens and mixes ingredients.

Make-up air Air introduced into a room to replace that removed by exhaust ventilation.

Mandrel A shaft used to support a work piece that is being processed.

Mask A stencil used in paint spraying to keep unwanted paint from an area.

Massicot Lead monoxide obtained as a yellow powder at temperatures below the melting point of the oxide.

Matcher A machine that planes and shapes boards; e.g., for tongueing and grooving.

Matte A crude mixture of metallic sulfides derived from sulfide ores.

Megger A high range ohmmeter used to measure resistance of electrical insulating materials.

Melt In the glass industry, the total batch of ingredients that may be introduced into pots or a furnace.

Mercerize To treat cotton cloth or yarn to obtain a shiny finish and to strengthen it by treatment with caustic soda under tension.

Metal In the glass industry, molten glass is "metal".

Metallizing The spraying of melted atomized metal onto a surface to be coated.

Micronizing A process for pulverizing certain minerals to an ultrafine particle size.

Millwright A mechanic engaged in the erection and maintenance of machinery.

Mineral pitch Tar from petroleum or coal in distinction to wood tar; asphalt.

Minium Red lead oxide (Pb_3O_4), usually prepared synthetically.

Mordant In dyeing, a chemical that fixes a dye

stuff by forming an insoluble compound.

Mortise A hole or slot into which is fitted a corresponding projection of another part to form a rigid joint.

Mosquitoes In the chemical industry, crystals floating in the air that are irritating to the eye.

Muffle furnace A closed furnace designed so that material placed in it does not come into direct contact with a flame or air.

Mule spinner In textile work, a machine that simultaneously draws and twists cotton or wool fibers into yarn; also called a mule jenny.

Muller (mull) Many different meanings in industry but generally a device for pounding, grinding, or mixing. In metal work, any of a number of rotating bearings in a cylinder for grinding.

Napper A machine that scratches the surface of yarn to produce a soft, fluffy texture.

Napper flock Waste from napping process.

Naumkeaging Smoothing the surface of a shoe sole and heel with a rubber buffing disc.

Ocher (or ochre) An earthy and often impure iron ore, usually red or yellow, extensively used as a pigment.

Opal Hydrated amorphous silica of many varieties and colors; some are gems but others are used as industrial abrasives.

Orange mineral A pigment lighter in color than red lead, and usually obtained by roasting white lead.

Paster In storage battery manufacture, the workman who spreads lead oxide of putty consistency into the battery grid; in leather work, the worker who stretches leather for drying by pasting it smoothly on surface materials.

Pearlite A mixture of ferrite and cementite found in slowly cooled iron-carbon alloys that is a common constituent of steel and cast iron. Not to be confused with *perlite,* a heat-expanded volcanic glass.

Pebble mill A rotating cylinder that contains hard, round pebbles to grind ceramic materials to a fine state.

Peel A long handled implement used to place products into an oven.

Peening To draw, bend, or flatten metal or leather by hammering or blasting with steel shot.

Perching A hand method of softening leather; also inspection of cloth in textile works.

Permanent mold A mold constructed of metal that can be used repeatedly in contrast to a sand mold, which is used only once.

Petrochemical A term applied to chemical substances produced from petroleum and natural gas.

Phosphors Naturally occurring or synthetic materials capable of absorbing radiant energy from suitable sources, such as x-rays, cathode rays, ultraviolet rays, and then emitting a portion of the energy in the ultraviolet, visible, or infrared region of the electromagnetic spectrum.

Pig In metal refining, a crude casting of small ingots from blast furnace metal.

Placer mining A method of mining in which mineral-bearing surface sands or gravels are washed or dredged with water to recover the mineral.

Plasticator A machine that kneads raw rubber by means of a worm screw enclosed in a heated housing.

Plasticizer A substance added to materials to produce or maintain elasticity, flexibility, and workability; widely used in plastics, resins, and rubbers.

Plastics Any of a large group of natural and synthetic organic materials of high molecular weight that may be molded into various shapes.

Plumbago A form of native mineralized carbon; graphite.

Polymerization A chemical reaction that produces very large molecules by a process of repetitive addition of smaller molecules.

Powderman In mining, quarrying, and road-building, the worker responsible for issuing explosives; at times, the powderman may be in charge of all blasting work. Also, a worker who blends and heats powders for molding plastics.

Producer gas The gas made in a producer furnace consisting chiefly of carbon monoxide, hydrogen, and nitrogen.

Proof room A room with controlled temperature and humidity in which bread dough is raised.

Puddler One who converts pig iron into wrought iron by remelting it in the presence of oxidizing substances to remove carbon and other impurities.

Pug mill A type of mill for grinding and mixing clay or for washing gold-bearing earth.

Pumice A natural silicate formed from volcanic ash or lava; used as an abrasive and for polishing.

Pyrites The sulfides of iron, copper, or tin, of which iron pyrites are the most common.

Quenching A hardening operation in which ferrous alloys raised to the desired temperature are quickly cooled by immersion in an oil bath.

Rad A unit of absorbed ionizing radiation equal to the absorption of 100 ergs of radiation energy per gram of absorbing material or 0.01 joules per kilogram of absorbing material.

Raw glaze A mixture of minerals in water to form a thick liquid that imparts a glass-like finish to ware when applied and fired in a kiln.

Reflux The portion of a condensed vapor that is returned to a still in contrast to the amount driven from the distilling apparatus.

Refractories A refractory material is one of a number of non-metallic ceramic substances that are especially resistant to the action of heat and hence used for the lining of furnaces; e.g., fire clay.

Rem The dose of any ionizing radiation that produces the same biological effect on human tissue as one roentgen of x-rays or gamma-rays.

Retting Treatment of vegetable fibers, such as flax or hemp, to promote bacterial decomposition with liberation of the wanted fibers.

Reverberatory A furnace or kiln in which the flame is reflected from the roof onto the material treated. Frequently used in the reclaiming of metals, such as lead from storage batteries.

Riddle A circular wire screen used for sifting impurities from sand.

Riser In metal casting, a channel in a mold to permit the escape of gases.

Roasting An ore refining operation in which high temperature is used, sometimes with catalytic agents, to drive off certain impurities, such as sulfur, or to promote oxidation.

Roentgen (R) A unit of radiation exposure; one R equals 2.58×10^{-4} coulomb per kilogram of air.

Rotary kiln A rotating cylindrical kiln, usually horizontal, used for the manufacture of portland cement and gypsum plaster.

Rotoclone The trade name of a type of dust collector that also serves as an air mover.

Rouge A finely powdered form of red ferric oxide used as a polishing agent.

Roving Cotton or other fiber prior to its passing through a spinning frame to become yarn.

Sagger In pottery, the ceramic container in which small pieces of pottery are fired; in metallurgy, a box in which cast-iron items are packed for placement in an oven.

Salamander A small furnace, usually cylindrical in shape, without grates or chimney, that is used for temporary heating purposes; a source of carbon monoxide.

Sand blasting A process for cleaning metal castings and other surfaces by a high-pressure air stream of sand.

Sand cutter A machine used in foundries for breaking up used molding sand and adding water to it for reuse; usually a portable unit.

Sand hog A worker doing tunneling operations under increased atmospheric pressure.

Sand slinger A power-driven machine that throws sand forcibly into flasks to produce evenly compacted molds.

Scoria The refuse from the melting of metals or reduction of ores; dross, slag.

Shakeout In foundries, the separation of a metal casting, still not cold, from its molding sand.

Shakes Workmen's name for metal fume fever.

Shale oil A tarry oil produces by distillation of bituminous shale.

Shoddy Reclaimed wool obtained by pulling apart soft rags or knitted or loosely woven woolens.

Shot blasting A process for cleaning metal castings and other surfaces by small steel shot in a high-pressure air stream; a substitute for sand blasting to avoid silicosis.

Silicone One of a group of organic silicon products, especially the polymerized organic siloxanes.

Sillimanite A natural aluminum silicate that usually appears as long, thin needle-like crystals and that is useful as a refractory material.

Silundum A mixture of silicon and carborundum; a hard, refractory substance produced in an electric furnace and widely used in the manufacture of resistors.

Sintering The process of making a coherent mass from earthy powders by heating but without melting.

Size A filler substance used to stiffen and strengthen a fabric or to retard penetration of liquids in paper.

Skelp Strips of metal used for making hollow cylinders such as pipe.

Skin Many different meanings in industry. In tanning, the outer coating of a small animal such as a lamb in distinction from a *hide* from a larger animal such as a horse. Also, the outer covering of an airplane or a door.

Slag The dross of flux and impurities, mostly silicates, that rise to the surface of molten metal during melting and refining.

Slate A dense fine-grain rock produced by compression of clays, shale, and other rocks; marked by a characteristic cleavage.

Slip A watery suspension of fine clay used in the manufacture of pottery; also, a watery suspension of pottery glaze.

Sludge In general, any muddy or slushy mass. Specifically, mud from a drill hole in boring; muddy sediment in a steam boiler; precipitated solid matter produced by sewage treatment.

Slurry A thick, creamy liquid resulting from the mixing and grinding of limestone, clay, and other raw materials with water.

Sly Mineral waste from the smelting of ores, such as the sly from blast furnace operations.

Smelting The melting or fusing of ore to separate the metal.

Smudging In horticulture, to protect an orchard or vineyard against frost or insect pests by heavy smoke.

Snag A ridge or jagged piece of metal projecting from the edge of a rough casting.

Snagging wheel A small-diameter, portable grinding wheel used for the removal of metal from rough castings.

Soaking pit A furnace in which steel ingots with still molten interiors stand in a heated upright chamber until solidification is complete.

Soapstone Complex silicate of varied composition similar to some talcs; with wide industrial application, such as in rubber manufacture.

Solder A metal or metallic alloy used for joining metal surfaces together by filling a joint or covering a junction. The most commonly used solder is one containing lead and tin. Silver solder may contain cadmium. Zinc chloride and fluorides are commonly used as fluxes to clean the surfaces.

Spelter Zinc castings in slab shape.

Spelter shakes Zinc chills.

Spinneret A small disc with very small holes through which viscose or other spinning solution are forced to emerge as thin filaments into a coagulating bath.

Spot welding One form of electrical resistance welding in which the current and pressure are restricted to the spots of metal surfaces directly in contact.

Sprue In a foundry, the hole in the flask through which metal is poured into the mold; in drop forging, the waste portion after the desired shape is hammered.

Stamping The crushing of ores by pulverizing with a stamp.

Steeping The process of soaking corn or other grains to swell and soften the kernels; also, the soaking of cellulose pulp in dilute sodium hydroxide to produce alkali cellulose.

Stink damp In mining, hydrogen sulfide.

Stoddard solvent A variable mixture of volatile inflammable petroleum distillates consisting of straight and branched paraffins, naphthenes, and alkyl aromatic hydrocarbons.

Stope A steplike underground excavation for the removal of ore.

Strip mine A mine in which coal or ore is extracted from the earth's surface after removal of overlayers of soil, clay, and rock.

Stripping The removal of previous paint coatings of faulty character to be followed by repainting.

Sublimation A process in which a metal, such as magnesium, passes directly from a solid into a gaseous state and condenses to form a solid again without liquefying.

Suint The dried perspiration of sheep deposited in the wool.

Surfacing machine A device used for trimming the surface of stone by repeated percussion of a square cut steel chipper against the surface.

Sweating The process of uniting metal parts by heating solder so that it runs between the parts.

Sweetening The process by which petroleum products are improved in odor by chemically changing certain sulfur compounds of objectionable odor into compounds having little or no odor.

Swing grinder A large power-driven grinding wheel mounted on a counterbalanced swivel supported arm and guided by two handles.

Tailings In mining or metal recovery processes, the worthless rock residue from which all or most of the metal has been extracted; also, reused tanning liquors.

Tar A loose term embracing wood, coal, or petroleum distillates; also derived from peat and shale.

Tawing   The tanning of light leathers.

Temper   To relieve the internal stresses in metal or glass and to increase ductility by heating the material to a point below its critical temperature and cooling slowly. See Anneal.

Template   A pattern made of wood or other hard material used as a guide in cutting, shaping, drilling, forming, scribing, or other operations to insure accuracy and consistency of the product.

Tenter frame   A device that dries and stretches cloth to its original width and straightens its weave after a finishing process by action of two diverging endless chains, each with a series of clips that hold an edge of the cloth and convey it past a heat source.

Tet   A common abbreviation for carbon tetrachloride.

Thermoplastic   Capable of being repeatedly softened by heat and becoming hard by cooling.

Thermosetting   Capable of becoming hard and rigid when heated.

Thermostable   Resistant to changes by heat.

Threshold limit value (TLV)   A time-weighted concentration of an airborne substance believed to be safe for most workers for repeated or continuous exposure during an 8-hour workday, 40-hour workweek.

Tinning   Any work with tin; in particular, in soldering, the primary coating with tin solder of the two surfaces to be united.

Toggling   The operation of tying hides or skins together to facilitate moving them from vat to vat, or tying them to screens or frames for drying.

Toner   An organic pigment that contains no inorganic constituent; also, a workman who modifies color in photography or the chemical solution used in this transformation.

Topaz   A fluosilicate of aluminum that is used as a semi-precious gem.

Tri   A common abbreviation for trichloroethylene.

Tripoli   A friable and dustlike silica used as an abrasive substance rubbed on the surface of a buffing wheel to polish metal.

Tumbling   An industrial process, such as in founding, in which small castings are cleaned by friction in a tumbling mill or tumbling barrel, which is a revolving drum containing sand, sawdust, stones, or other abrasives.

Tungsten carbide   An exceedingly hard alloy of tungsten and carbon bonded with cobalt or nickel; used for high-speed metal-cutting tools (also called diamond-cutting tools).

Tunnel kiln   In refractories, a horizontal kiln usually of considerable length through which objects to be fired move at a slow rate and emerge after complete firing; continuous kiln.

Turrel lathe   A power-driven metal working machine in which the stock is held and rotated about a horizontal axis to be machined successively by a number of cutting tools held in a turret.

Venturi scrubber   A wet dust collector employing a constricted tube through which water under high pressure is directed; this device acts as an air mover as well as a dust collector.

Viscose   A term applied to viscous liquid composed of cellulose xanthate in sodium hydroxide.

Viscose rayon   Rayon fiber produced by the reaction of carbon disulfide with cellulose and the hardening of the resulting viscous solution by passing it through dilute sulfuric acid; this final operation results in the evolution of hydrogen sulfide gas. Also, the yarn or fabric made from such fibers.

Vulcanizer   A machine in which raw rubber that has been mixed with sulfur or sulfur compounds is cured by heat and pressure to render it less plastic and more durable.

Water curtain or waterfall booth   Many different meanings in industry. In spray painting, the water running down a wall into which excess paint is drawn or blown by fans and by which the paint is carried downward to a collecting point; in mining, a sheet of water forming a screen to prevent the spread of fire.

Water gas tar   The tar that arises in the formation of water gas, and that resembles coal tar.

Water glass   A common name for sodium silicate in solution; often called "soluble glass".

Waterproofing agents   Usually these are formulations of three distinct materials: (1) a coating material, (2) a solvent, and (3) a plasticizer. Among the materials used in waterproofing are cellulose esters and ethers, polyvinyl chloride resins or acetates, and variations of vinyl chloride and vinylidine chloride polymers.

Welding   The several types of welding include electric arc welding, oxy-acetylene welding, spot welding, and inert or shielded gas welding that utilizes helium or argon. The hazards stem from (1) the fumes from the weld metal, such as lead or cadmium, or (2) the gases created by the process, or (3) the fumes or gases arising from the flux, or (4) exposure, especially of the eyes, to intense ultraviolet light.

Welding rod A rod or heavy wire that is melted and fused into metals in arc welding.

White damp In mining, carbon monoxide.

White souring An operation in the bleaching of cloth in which the fabric is immersed in a dilute sulfuric acid or hydrochloric acid solution to neutralize the action of chlorinated lime.

White spirit A petroleum distillation fraction that resembles naphtha.

Whiting A powdered calcium carbonate preparation used in the manufacture of putty and rubber, and in paper coatings.

Willemite A native zinc orthosilicate.

Work hardening The property of a metal to become harder and more brittle on being "worked" while cold, that is bent repeatedly or drawn in a press.

Working face The surface of ore, stone, or coal exposed by mining or quarrying operations.

Wort The liquid that is separated from the solid part of grain mash before fermentation and that after fermentation becomes ale or beer.

Xanthation A process in the viscose rayon industry in which sodium cellulose is reacted with carbon disulfide to form cellulose xanthate.

X-ray diffraction A method that utilizes the characteristic patterns of diffraction of x-rays by crystals; of value in determining the presence or absence of crystalline silica in industrial dust.

Yellow crumbs A term used in the viscose rayon industry to describe the cellulose xanthate as it is removed from the churn where it is produced by the reaction of sodium cellulose with carbon disulfide.

Zeolite Any of several hydrosilicates used in water softening processes.

Zoogler In lumbering, the workman who rides floating logs in ponds; also, the loader of logs onto trucks, cars, or sleds; a frogger or trailer.

INDEX

Accelerators, 282–283
Acetaldehyde, 209
Acetal resins, 272
Acetates, 284
Acetic acid, 203
Acetone, 210–211
Acetylcholine (AcCh)
  carbamate insecticides and, 294–295
  organophosphorus compounds and, 288, 289, 290, 291
Acetylcysteine, 242
Acetylene, 201
Acetylene dichloride, 234
Acetylene gas, 117
Acetylene tetrabromide, 243
Acetylene tetracholoride, 233
N-acetyl-D-penicillamine
  lead and, 77, 78–79
  mercury and, 100, 101–102
  thallium and, 132
Acidosis, metabolic, and methanol, 203–204
Acroanesthesia, 11
Acrolein, 161, 206
Acronitrile, 273
Acro-osteolysis, 275–276
Acrylamide, 278
Acrylics, 272, 284
Acrylonitrile, 273, 281
Actinium series, 315
Additives
  elastomer, 282–283
  polymer, 278–280
Adenocarcinomas, and wood dusts, 380
Adrenocorticotropic hormone (ACTH), 32
Aerosols, sodium hydroxide, 152–153
Air pollution, 4
  carbon monoxide and, 158, 162
  chemical compounds and, 149
  lead and, 80–82
Air systems, 6
Alcohols, 203–206
  allyl, 206
  amyl, 206
  n-butyl, 205–206
  calcium cyanamide and, 171
  carbon tetrachloride and, 230
  2-chloroethyl, 206
  ethyl, 205, 214
  grain, 205
  isopropyl, 205
  lead poisoning and, 67, 69, 70, 71
  metal fume fever and, 147

methyl, 203, 381
nitrate esters and, 222
pentyl, 206
propyl, 205
trichloroethylene and, 235
wood, 203
Aldehydes, 209–210, 269
Aldicarb, 295
Aliphatic esters, 219
Aliphatic hydrocarbons, 197–201
  exposure limits for, 201
  saturated, 197–200
  unsaturated, 201
Aliphatic nitro compounds, 223
Alkalies, 150–153
Alkyds, 270
Alkylbenzenes, 251–252
Alkyl nitrites, 223
Allergens, 4
Allyl alcohol, 206
Allyl chloride, 237–238
Allyl glycidyl ether, 217
Alpha particles, 314
Alpha rays, 314
Aluminosis, 10, 11
Aluminum, 9–12, 107, 136, 275
  animal studies of, 11, 12
  control measures for, 11–12
  fluorides and, 181
  grain fumigants with, 117
  industrial toxicity of, 9–11
  interpretation of reports on, 11–12
  selenium poisoning with, 124
  silicosis and, 347
  uses of, 9
Aluminum oxide, 10, 11, 372
Aluminum silicates, 369
Alveolitis, 390
Alzheimer's disease, 11
American Conference of Governmental Industrial Hygienists (ACGIH), 2
Amino compounds, 256–260
Aminophylline, 289
Amino resins, 268
Aminotriazole, 303
Amitrol, 303
Ammonia, 150–151, 269
  acute poisoning with, 150–151
  chronic poisoning with, 151
  control measures for, 151
  reactions at various concentrations of, 151
  uses of, 150

409

416

428